CLINICAL APPLICATION
OF
MECHANICAL VENTILATION

David W. Chang

CLINICAL APPLICATION
OF
MECHANICAL VENTILATION

THIRD EDITION

David W. Chang, Ed.D., RRT–NPS
Director of Clinical Education
Respiratory Therapy
Athens Technical College
Athens, Georgia

THOMSON

DELMAR LEARNING

Australia Canada Mexico Singapore Spain United Kingdom United States

THOMSON
DELMAR LEARNING

Clinical Application of Mechanical Ventilation, Third Edition
by David W. Chang

Vice President, Health Care Business Unit:
William Brottmiller

Editorial Director:
Matthew Kane

Acquisitions Editor:
Rhonda Dearborn

Developmental Editor:
Sarah Duncan

Editorial Assistant:
Debra S. Gorgos

Marketing Director:
Jennifer McAvey

Marketing Coordinator:
Christopher Manion

Production Director:
Carolyn Miller

Senior Production Editor:
James Zayicek

Library of Congress Cataloging-in-Publication Data

Chang, David W.
  Clinical application of mechanical ventilation/
David W. Chang.— 3rd ed.
    p. ; cm.
  Includes bibliographical references and index.
  ISBN-13: 978-1-4018-8485-7
  ISBN-10: 1-4018-8485-7
  1. Respiratory therapy. 2. Artificial respiration.
  [DNLM: 1. Respiration, Artificial. 2. Respiratory Therapy.
3. Ventilators, Mechanical. WF 145 C456c 2006] I. Title.
  RC735.I5C466 2006
  615.8'362—dc22

                                                    2005015179

Dedicated to

my wife, Bonnie

and our children, Michelle, Jennifer, and Michael

with love

CONTENTS

FOREWORD

In most large hospitals, the number of ventilator-hours per year may be dropping due to a change in patient demographics and the great success of therapist-driven ventilator management protocols. On the other hand, many centers report that patients who *do* require ventilator support are, in general, more sick than they have been in years past. These latter patients have higher acuity scores and include ultra-small low birth weight neonates on one end of the age spectrum and patients with dense ARDS or who have status-post lung transplantation problems on the other. This patient mix challenges the treating respiratory care practitioner as never before. The practitioner must understand the operative physiology and apply his or her management skills to the patient-ventilator interface in new and innovative ways if good outcomes are to be achieved.

In preparation of these few introductory remarks, I thought I would plunge right in and review the heart of the manuscript and bring myself up to speed on this ever-changing, ever-enlarging discipline, core to upper-end respiratory therapy knowledge and skill sets. I split the 3-inch manuscript in two and chose Chapter 11, Ventilation Waveform Analysis, to read in detail. Bad choice!

Just a few pages into that chapter, I realized how technically complex the field of mechanical ventilation has become, how greatly the technology has changed, and how badly out of date my knowledge (and competence) has become! I then went back to Chapter 1, Principles of Mechanical Ventilation, and took a more leisurely review of the material and ended up deciding that, yes, I could be instructed again in this field and that the organization and layout of this third edition would help me do it!

Over the years, authors have tried to compress knowledge and skills of ventilator management into two or, at best, three chapters of general respiratory care textbooks. This volume shows how naïve that approach really is, given the ever-enlarging theory, skill sets, and practice competencies required of today's respiratory care practitioner.

Most respiratory care training programs now devote a whole semester's classroom and laboratory experience to the art and science of ventilator management and the 18 chapters of this textbook should serve as an excellent source to the students and their instructors who navigate these treacherous shoals.

I particularly like the organization of Chapters 8–12 in this volume. One can imagine a patient progressing through initiation of ventilator support (Chapter 8), appropriate monitoring (Chapters 9–10), "tinkering" (Chapter 11), day-to-day ventilator management (Chapter 12), and eventual successful weaning (Chapter 15) in "bite-size pieces" of knowledge and skills. One of the strengths of this volume is its organization, and readers (at least first-time ones) would do well to let the authors pull and push them along as shallow a learning curve as the (admittedly complex) manuscript allows.

I particularly recommend the chapter Introductions (to see what is coming), Summaries (to review what has been presented), Self-Assessment Presentations (to see what has been learned and reviewed), and Case Studies (to bring it all together as might be done in the NBRC Registry Clinical Simulation Examinations).

My best wishes to all readers of this excellent volume! Take my advice: like Alice in Wonderland—start at the beginning, and when you come to the end, stop.

George G. Burton, M.D.
Associate Dean for Medical Affairs
Kettering College of Medical Arts
Kettering, Ohio

June 2005

PREFACE

For over half a century now, mechanical ventilation has been a fixture and an invaluable component of intensive care medicine. Technological innovations and techniques of ventilation have been developed to make mechanical ventilation more efficient and safer for patients. Numerous modes of ventilation are also available in traditional and noninvasive ventilators. The choices in equipment and methods of ventilation seem to be limitless. For this reason, in particular, respiratory therapists and other health care professionals are facing the challenge to keep up with the innovations and to become knowledgeable in the ever-changing techniques and clinical application of mechanical ventilation.

ORGANIZATION OF TEXT

Chapters 1 and 2 provide a review of the physiologic basis, rationale, and effects of positive pressure ventilation. Chapter 3 covers the common terminology in ventilator mechanics and the system used to classify mechanical ventilators. Chapter 4 describes the up-to-date operating modes of mechanical ventilation available in many newer ventilators. Chapter 5 provides the information on special airways that precedes the establishment of an artificial airway for positive pressure ventilation. Chapter 6 covers the rationale, techniques, management, and complications of artificial airways. Chapter 7 presents the clinical application of noninvasive positive pressure ventilation. Chapter 8 offers a step-by-step approach in the initiation of mechanical ventilation. The indications, contraindications, initial ventilator settings, and alarm settings relating to mechanical ventilation are also included. Chapter 9 outlines the essential methods of patient monitoring to include vital signs, chest auscultation, pulse oximetry, capnography, and transcutaneous blood gases. Chapter 10 covers the basics of hemodynamic monitoring. Normal and abnormal hemodynamic values are included along with noninvasive impedance cardiography. Chapter 11 gives a detailed discussion on ventilator waveform analysis and its applications. Chapter 12 presents the common and basic strategies to improve ventilation and oxygenation. It describes the basic strategies to correct common ventilator alarms and to recognize problems associated with fluid imbalance, electrolyte abnormalities, and nutritional concerns that may occur during mechanical ventilation. Chapter 13 includes special procedures associated with mechanical ventilation—chest tube and drainage system, fiberoptic bronchoscopy, and transport of mechanically ventilated patients. Chapter 14 summarizes the use of pharmacotherapy during mechanical ventilation. The drugs discussed in this chapter include bronchodilators, neuromuscular blocking agents, sedatives, narcotic analgesics, and barbiturates. Chapter 15 provides the weaning protocols. Weaning criteria, weaning indices, weaning failure, and terminal weaning are also included. Chapter 16 covers neonatal mechanical ventilation. An expanded coverage of high-frequency oscillatory ventilation is also included in this chapter. In a nontraditional setting, home mechanical ventilation is discussed in Chapter 17. Chapter 18 has 15 case studies including those essential cases that are commonly encountered by respiratory care practitioners in a critical care setting. As in the second edition, the key terms are boldfaced within the text and the definitions are placed in the margin for quick reference. Essential information is also highlighted in the margin and can be identified with a special icon (☑) .

CHANGES TO THE THIRD EDITION

This third edition provides updated information in many chapters—in particular, chapters 4, 10, 13 (new chapter), and 16. Chapter 4 includes many new modes (single and bi-mode) of ventilation that are commonly available in ventilators today. Chapter 10 provides information on impedance cardiography, a method for noninvasive hemodynamic monitoring. Chapter 13 is a new chapter and it includes three special procedures that are commonly associated with patients receiving mechanical ventilation. A detailed discussion is provided for each of these three special procedures—chest tube and drainage system, fiberoptic bronchoscopy, and transport of mechanically ventilated patients. Chapter 16 provides an extensive coverage of high frequency oscillatory ventilation and the information should be useful for the practitioners caring for premature infants. As in the past two editions, the goal of this edition of *Clinical Application of Mechanical Ventilation* is to provide the students a textbook they will enjoy reading and using at school and at home. It is also my goal to make this textbook a quick reference source for respiratory care practitioners and other health care professionals. I hope they will find this textbook a useful source of information for their clinical practice.

David W. Chang

ACKNOWLEDGMENTS

I am thankful to my colleagues, Terrell Ashe, Dr. George Burton, Frank Dennison, Tim Douds, Dr. Ian Gilmour, Brian J. Parker, Dr. Albert Santora, and Dr. W. John Russell, for making invaluable contributions to the third edition of *Clinical Application of Mechanical Ventilation*. Their insights and experience in different aspects of mechanical ventilation have helped make this book complete. Again, other individuals who contributed to the first and second editions of this book deserve my continued recognition. Their names, credentials, and professional affiliations are listed under the contributors' section.

I would also like to recognize my colleagues who reviewed the contents of this book for completeness and accuracy through all the stages of its development—from proposal to draft and manuscript. They provided accurate corrections, useful suggestions, and pertinent comments. Their input makes the third edition of *Clinical Application of Mechanical Ventilation* a valuable textbook for students and a helpful reference source for practitioners. The reviewers are:

Randall W. Anderson, RRT, RCP
Department Head, Respiratory Care
Spartanburg Technical College
Spartanburg, South Carolina

Dee Arkell, BS, RRT, CPFT
Director of Clinical Education, Respiratory
  Care
Spokane Community College
Spokane, Washington

Brian J. Parker, MPH, RRT-NPS, CPFT
Chair, Respiratory Care
Baptist College of Health Sciences
Memphis, Tennessee

Theresa P. Piurkowsky, MEd, RRT-NPS,
  CPFT
Department Head, Patient Care Services
Director of Clinical Education, Respiratory
  Care Program
Trident Technical College
Charleston, South Carolina

Ruben D. Restrepo, MD, RRT
Assistant Professor, Cardiopulmonary Care
  Sciences

Georgia State University
Atlanta, Georgia

Christopher Rowse, MS, RRT-NPS, RPFT,
Program Director, Respiratory Care
Northern Essex Community College
Lawrence, Massachusetts

Cynthia A. Smathers, MEd, RRT
Program Director
PIMA Medical Institute
Mesa, Arizona

Rita F. Waller, MSN, RRT, RN
Program Director, Respiratory Care
  Technology
Augusta Technical College
Augusta, Georgia

Jonathan B. Waugh, PhD, RRT, RPFT
Associate Professor and Director of
  Clinical Education
University of Alabama at Birmingham
Critical Care Dept, Respiratory Therapy
  Program
Birmingham, Alabama

To all manufacturers and organizations that granted permission to use their pictures and illustrations, I express my appreciation. Their willingness to share the original work enhances the clarity and delivery of the information in the book.

Publishing a textbook and its accompanying workbook and instructor's manual is definitely a coordinated team effort. The following individuals make my work on this textbook and the accompanying workbook and instructor manual smooth and fulfilling. I express my deepest gratitude to my publishing, editing, production, and marketing team members; to the editors and staff at Delmar Thomson Learning: Rhonda Dearborn, Sarah Duncan, Debra Gorgos, Christopher Manion, and James Zayicek; and the staff at ITC: Ben Kolstad and Mona Tiwary.

CONTRIBUTORS

Valerie Thomas Aston, RRT
Weber State University
Ogden, Utah

Walter C. Chop, MS., RRT
Southern Maine Technical College
South Portland, Maine

Frank Dennison, MEd, RRT, RPFT
Medical College of Georgia
Augusta, Georgia

Timothy Douds, BS, RRT-NPS
Gwinnett Medical Center
Lawrenceville, Georgia

Paul G. Eberle, MEd, RRT
Weber State University
Ogden, Utah

Sandra Gaviola, RRT
Greater Johnstown Career and
    Technology Center
Johnstown, Pennsylvania

Luis S. Gonzalez III, Pharm. D, BCPS
Conemaugh Memorial Hospital
Duquesne University
University of Pittsburg
Johnstown, Pennsylvania

Gary Hamelin, MS, RRT
Southern Maine Technical College
South Portland, Maine

James H. Hiers, MEd, RRT
Columbus State University
Columbus, Georgia

Wayne Lawson, MS, RRT
University of Texas
Health Science Center at San Antonio
San Antonio, Texas

Terry S. LeGrand, PhD, RRT
University of Texas
Health Science Center at San Antonio
San Antonio, Texas

Michell Oki, RRT, RPFT
Weber State University
Ogden, Utah

Angie Roberts, RRT
Columbus State University
Columbus, Georgia

Randon K. Parker, BS, RRT
Weber State University
Ogden, Utah

Kent B. Whitaker, MEd, RRT
formerly of Weber State University
Ogden, Utah

Gary C. White, MEd, RRT, CPFT
Spokane Community College
Spokane, Washington

CHAPTER ONE

PRINCIPLES OF MECHANICAL VENTILATION

David W. Chang

KEY TERMS

- airway resistance
- alveolar deadspace
- alveolar volume
- anatomic deadspace
- deadspace ventilation
- diffusion defect
- hypoventilation
- hypoxic hypoxia
- intrapulmonary shunting

- lung compliance
- oxygenation failure
- peak inspiratory pressure
- physiologic deadspace
- plateau pressure
- refractory hypoxemia
- ventilatory failure
- V/Q mismatch

INTRODUCTION

Mechanical ventilation is a useful modality for patients who are unable to sustain the level of ventilation necessary to maintain the gas exchange functions (oxygenation and carbon dioxide elimination). Indications for mechanical ventilation vary greatly among patients. Mechanical ventilation may be indicated in conditions due to physiologic changes (e.g., deterioration of lung parenchyma), disease states (e.g., chest trauma), medical/surgical procedures (e.g., postoperative recovery), as well as many other conditions leading to ventilatory failure or oxygenation failure.

Use of mechanical ventilation also varies greatly from short term to long term and from acute care in the hospital to extended care at home. One of the most frequent uses of mechanical ventilation is for the management of postoperative patients recovering from anesthesia and medications. In one study, postoperative procedures accounted for 35% of all patients who were placed on mechanical ventilation for more than 24 hours. Other major uses of mechanical ventilation include respiratory failure with multisystem failure, pre-existing lung disease, trauma, uncomplicated acute lung injuries, and other severe medical problems (Gillespie et al., 1986).

Regardless of the diagnosis or disease state, patients who require mechanical ventilation generally have developed ventilatory failure, oxygenation failure, or both. Specifically, when a patient fails to ventilate or oxygenate adequately, the problem may be caused by one of six pathophysiological factors: (1) increased airway resistance, (2) changes in lung compliance, (3) hypoventilation, (4) V/Q mismatch, (5) intrapulmonary shunting, and (6) diffusion defect.

AIRWAY RESISTANCE

airway resistance:
The degree of air flow obstruction in the airways.

Airway resistance is defined as air flow obstruction in the airways. In mechanical ventilation, the degree of airway resistance is primarily affected by the length, size, and patency of the airway, endotracheal tube, and ventilator circuit.

FACTORS AFFECTING AIRWAY RESISTANCE

Airway resistance causes obstruction of air flow in the airways. It is increased when the patency or diameter of the airways is reduced. Obstruction of air flow may be caused by changes: (1) inside the airway (e.g., retained secretions), (2) in the wall of the airway (e.g., neoplasm of the bronchial muscle structure), or (3) outside the airway (e.g., tumors surrounding and compressing the airway) (West, 2004a). When one of these conditions occurs, the radius of the airway decreases and airway resistance increases. According to the simplified form of Poiseuille's Law, the driving pressure (ΔP) to maintain the same air flow ($\dot{V}$) must increase by a factor of 16-fold when the radius (r) of the airway is reduced by only half of its original size.

$$\text{Simplified form of Poiseuille's Law: } \Delta P = \frac{\dot{V}}{r^4}$$

☑ Based on Poiseuille's Law, the work of breathing increases by a factor of 16-fold when the radius (r) of the airway is reduced by half its original size.

One of the most common causes of increased airway resistance is chronic obstructive pulmonary disease (COPD). This type of lung disease includes emphysema, chronic bronchitis, chronic asthma, and bronchiectasis. Mechanical conditions that may increase airway resistance include postintubation obstruction and foreign body aspiration. Infectious processes include laryngotracheobronchitis (croup), epiglottitis, and bronchiolitis (Cherniack et al., 1983). Table 1-1 lists three categories of clinical conditions that increase airway resistance.

☑ Airway resistance varies directly with the length and inversely with the diameter of the ET tube.

Normal airway resistance is between 0.6 and 2.4 cm H_2O/L/sec at a flow rate of 30 L/min (0.5 L/sec) (Burton et al., 1997). It is higher in intubated patients, depending on the size of the endotracheal (ET) tube. Airway resistance varies directly with the length and inversely with the diameter of the ET tube. In the clinical setting, the

TABLE 1-1   Clinical Conditions That Increase Airway Resistance

TYPE	CLINICAL CONDITIONS
COPD	Emphysema Chronic bronchitis Asthma Bronchiectasis
Mechanical obstruction	Postintubation obstruction Foreign body aspiration Endotracheal tube Condensation in ventilator circuit
Infection	Laryngotracheobronchitis (croup) Epiglottitis Bronchiolitis

ET tube is sometimes cut shorter for ease of airway management, reduction of mechanical deadspace, and reduction of airway resistance. However, the major contributor to increased airway resistance is the internal diameter of the ET tube. Therefore, during intubation, the largest appropriate size ET tube must be used so that the airway resistance contributed by the ET tube may be minimized. Once the ET tube is in place, its patency must be maintained as secretions retained on the inside wall of the ET tube greatly increase airway resistance.

Besides the ET tube, the ventilator circuit may also impose mechanical resistance to air flow and contribute to total airway resistance. This is particularly important when there is a significant amount of water in the ventilator circuit due to condensation.

AIRWAY RESISTANCE AND THE WORK OF BREATHING (ΔP)

Airway resistance is calculated by $\dfrac{\text{Pressure Change}}{\text{Flow}}$

$$\text{Raw} = \frac{\Delta P}{\dot{V}}$$

Raw = airway resistance
$\triangle P$ = pressure change (Peak Inspiratory Pressure − Plateau Pressure)
$\dot{V}$ = Flow

The pressure change ($\triangle P$) in the equation can be treated as the amount of work of breathing imposed on the patient. Since airway resistance is directly related to pressure change (the work of breathing), an increase in airway resistance means an increase in the work of breathing. In a clinical setting, airway obstruction is one of the most frequent causes of increased work of breathing (Beachey et al., 1990).

If pressure change (work of breathing) in the equation above is held constant, an increase in airway resistance will cause a decrease in flow and subsequently a decrease in minute ventilation. This is because airway resistance and flow in the equation are inversely related. In a clinical setting, **hypoventilation** may result if the patient is unable to overcome the airway resistance by increasing the work of breathing.

As a result of chronic air trapping, patients with chronic airway obstruction may develop highly compliant lung parenchyma and use a breathing pattern that is deeper but slower. Patients with restrictive lung disease breathe more shallowly but faster, since air flow resistance is not the primary disturbance in these patients.

EFFECTS ON VENTILATION AND OXYGENATION

The work of breathing imposed on a patient is increased when airway resistance is high. This creates a detrimental effect on the patient's ventilatory and oxygenation status. If an abnormally high airway resistance is sustained over a long time, fatigue of the respiratory muscles may occur, leading to ventilatory and oxygenation failure (Rochester, 1993). **Ventilatory failure** occurs when the patient's

☑ ↑ Airway resistance = ↑ Work of breathing.

hypoventilation: Inadequate alveolar ventilation leading to CO_2 retention, and increase in $PaCO_2$.

ventilatory failure: Failure of the lungs to eliminate carbon dioxide. Without supplemental oxygen, it leads to hypoxemia.

Figure 1-1 Increased bowing (from dotted to solid lines) of the pressure-volume loop suggests an increase in airflow resistance. Bowing of inspiratory limb (from A_1 to A_2) may be caused by excessive inspiratory flow. Bowing of the expiratory limb (from B_1 to B_2) may be caused by an increase in expiratory flow resistance such as bronchospasm.

oxygenation failure:
Failure of the heart and lungs to provide adequate oxygen for metabolic needs.

☑ An increased bowing of the P-V loop suggests an overall increase in airflow resistance.

☑ Excessive inspiratory flow → bowing of inspiratory limb. (A_1 to A_2)

☑ Increased expiratory flow resistance → bowing of expiratory limb. (B_1 to B_2)

lung compliance:
The degree of lung expansion per unit pressure change.

minute ventilation cannot keep up with CO_2 production. **Oxygenation failure** usually follows when the pulmonary system cannot provide adequate oxygen needed for metabolism.

AIRFLOW RESISTANCE

The airflow resistance of a patient-ventilator system may be monitored using the pressure-volume (P-V) loop display on a graphic-enabled ventilator (Tyco Healthcare, 2003). An increased bowing of the P-V loop suggests an overall increase in airflow resistance (Figure 1-1). The increase in airflow resistance may be caused by excessive inspiratory flow or increased expiratory flow resistance.

When the inspiratory flow exceeds a patient's tidal volume and inspiratory time requirement, bowing of the inspiratory limb may result (solid line A_2). In situations where the expiratory airflow resistance is increased (e.g., bronchospasm), bowing of the expiratory limb (solid line B_2) may occur.

LUNG COMPLIANCE

Lung compliance is volume change (lung expansion) per unit pressure change (work of breathing) and it is calculated by $C = \triangle V / \triangle P$ where C = compliance, $\triangle V$ = volume change, and $\triangle P$ = pressure change. A method to measure compliance is outlined in Table 1-2.

TABLE 1-2   Method to Measure Static and Dynamic Compliance

(1)   Obtain corrected expired tidal volume.

(2)   Obtain **plateau pressure** by applying inspiratory hold or occluding the exhalation port at end-inspiration.

(3)   Obtain **peak inspiratory pressure.**

(4)   Obtain **positive end-expiratory pressure** (PEEP) level, if any.

$$\text{Static Compliance} = \frac{\text{Corrected Tidal Volume}}{(\text{Plateau Pressure} - \text{PEEP})}$$

$$\text{Dynamic Compliance} = \frac{\text{Corrected Tidal Volume}}{(\text{Peak Inspiratory Pressure} - \text{PEEP})}$$

plateau pressure:
The pressure needed to maintain lung inflation in the absence of air flow.

peak inspiratory pressure: *The pressure used to deliver the tidal volume by overcoming non-elastic (airways) and elastic (lung parenchyma) resistance.*

✓ ↓ Lung compliance = ↑ Work of breathing

refractory hypoxemia: Low oxygen tension in blood that responds very poorly to oxygen therapy.

✓ In extreme high compliance situations, exhalation is often incomplete due to lack of elastic recoil by the lungs.

COMPLIANCE MEASUREMENT

Abnormally low or high lung compliance impairs the patient's ability to maintain efficient gas exchange. Low compliance typically makes lung expansion difficult and high compliance induces incomplete exhalation and CO_2 elimination. These abnormalities are often contributing factors to the need for mechanical ventilation.

Low Compliance.   Low compliance (high elastance) means that the volume change is small per unit pressure change. Under this condition, the lungs are *stiff* or *noncompliant*. The work of breathing is high when compliance is low. In many clinical situations (e.g., atelectasis), low lung compliance is responsible for **refractory hypoxemia.**

Low compliance measurements are usually related to conditions that reduce the patient's functional residual capacity. Patients with noncompliant lungs often have a restrictive lung defect, low lung volumes, and low minute ventilation. This condition may be compensated for by an increased respiratory rate. Table 1-3 shows some examples that lead to a decreased compliance measurement.

High Compliance.   High compliance means that the volume change is large per unit pressure change. In extreme high compliance situations, exhalation is often incomplete due to lack of elastic recoil by the lungs. Emphysema is an example of high compliance where the gas exchange process is impaired. This condition is due to chronic air trapping, destruction of lung tissues, and enlargement of terminal and respiratory bronchioles.

High compliance measurements are usually related to conditions that increase the patient's functional residual capacity. Patients with extremely compliant lungs often have an obstructive lung defect, air flow obstruction, incomplete exhalation, and poor gas exchange.

TABLE 1-3   Clinical Conditions That Decrease the Compliance

TYPE OF COMPLIANCE	CLINICAL CONDITIONS
Static compliance	Atelectasis ARDS Tension pneumothorax Obesity Retained secretions
Dynamic compliance	Bronchospasm Kinking of ET tube Airway obstruction

STATIC AND DYNAMIC COMPLIANCE

Assessment of compliance can be divided into static compliance and dynamic compliance measurements. The relationship and clinical significance of these measurements are discussed in the following sections.

Static Compliance.   Static compliance is measured when there is no air flow (using the plateau pressure – PEEP). When air flow is absent, airway resistance is not a determining factor. Thus, static compliance reflects the elastic resistance of the lung and chest wall.

Dynamic Compliance.   Dynamic compliance is measured when air flow is present (using the peak airway pressure–PEEP). Since air flow is present, airway resistance becomes a critical factor in the measurement of compliance. Dynamic compliance therefore reflects the condition of airway resistance (nonelastic resistance) as well as the elastic properties of the lung and chest wall (elastic resistance).

Plateau and Peak Inspiratory Pressure.   In general, conditions causing changes in plateau pressure and static compliance invoke similar changes in peak inspiratory pressure and dynamic compliance. For example, atelectasis causes an increase of plateau and peak inspiratory pressures (Figure 1-2, A to B). Since the plateau and peak inspiratory pressures are increased, the calculated static and dynamic compliance measurements are decreased. When atelectasis is resolved, the plateau and peak inspiratory pressures return to normal (Figure 1-2, B to A).

In conditions where the airflow resistance is increased (e.g., bronchospasm), the peak inspiratory pressure is increased while the plateau pressure stays unchanged (Figure 1-3, A to B). Since the peak inspiratory pressure is increased, the dynamic compliance is

✓ Static compliance reflects the elastic properties (elastic resistance) of the lung and chest wall.

✓ Dynamic compliance reflects the airway resistance (nonelastic resistance) and the elastic properties of the lung and chest wall (elastic resistance).

✓ Conditions causing changes in plateau pressure and static compliance invoke similar changes in peak inspiratory pressure and dynamic compliance.

Figure 1-2 In conditions where the lung compliance is decreased (e.g., atelectasis), the plateau pressure (P_{PLAT}) and peak inspiratory pressure (PIP) are both increased (from A to B).

☑ When the airflow resistance is increased (e.g., bronchospasm), the peak inspiratory pressure is increased while the plateau pressure stays unchanged.

decreased. The static compliance stays the same because there is no change in the plateau pressure. When bronchospasm is resolved, the peak inspiratory pressure and dynamic compliance measurements return to their previous states (Figure 1-3, B to A).

Pressure-Volume Loop. Since compliance is determined by $\Delta V/\Delta P$, the P-V loop provides useful information on the characteristics of a patient's compliance. Figure 1-4 shows a P-V loop during a mandatory breath. A slope is drawn from the beginning point dividing the inspiratory limb and the expiratory limb. A shift of the slope toward the pressure axis indicates a decrease in compliance. A shift of the slope toward the volume axis indicates an increase in compliance (Tyco Healthcare, 2003).

☑ A shift of the slope toward the pressure axis indicates a decrease in compliance.

In another P-V loop (Figure 1-5), a shift of the slope and P-V loop toward the pressure axis shows an increase in pressure ($\uparrow\Delta P$) required to deliver the same volume (ΔV). This condition shows a decrease in compliance ($\downarrow C$) (Tyco Healthcare, 2003).

Figure 1-3 In conditions where the airflow resistance is increased (e.g., bronchospasm), the peak inspiratory pressure (PIP) is increased while the plateau pressure (P_{PLAT}) stays unchanged (from A to B).

Figure 1-4 Shifting of the P-V slope toward the pressure axis (A) indicates a decrease in compliance. Shifting of the P-V slope toward the volume axis (B) indicates an increase in compliance.

☑ A shift of the slope toward the volume axis indicates an increase in compliance.

☑ $\triangle V/\uparrow\triangle P = \downarrow C$

Compliance measurements should be made so that a trend can be established. Interpretation is of little value with a single compliance measurement. It is also essential not to compare static compliance with dynamic compliance measurements as this can cause erroneous interpretations.

Figure 1-5 Shifting of the P-V slope and loop toward the pressure axis shows a higher pressure is required to deliver the same volume (decrease in compliance).

Clinical Ranges. For critically-ill patients, the dynamic compliance is between 30 and 40 mL/cm H_2O and static compliance is between 40 and 60 mL/cm H_2O. (Barnes, 1994) It is lower in intubated patients, depending on the internal diameter of the ET tube. See Table 1-2 for the method to measure compliance. The equations for static compliance (C_{ST}) and dynamic compliance (C_{DYN}) are:

☑ See Appendix 1 for example.

$$C_{ST} = \frac{\text{Corrected Tidal Volume}}{(\text{Plateau Pressure} - \text{PEEP})}$$

☑ See Appendix 1 for example.

$$C_{DYN} = \frac{\text{Corrected Tidal Volume}}{(\text{Peak Inspiratory Pressure} - \text{PEEP})}$$

COMPLIANCE AND THE WORK OF BREATHING

Since compliance is inversely related to pressure change (work of breathing), a decrease in compliance means an increase in the work of breathing. In a clinical setting, atelectasis is one of the frequent causes of increased work of breathing.

If the plateau pressure and peak inspiratory pressure (work of breathing) in the previous equations are held unchanged, a decrease in compliance will cause a decrease in volume. This is because compliance and volume change in the equation are directly related. In a clinical setting, hypoventilation usually results when a patient is unable to compensate for the decrease in compliance by increasing and maintaining a higher level of work of breathing. In low compliance situations such as ARDS, fibrosis, and kyphoscoliosis, the decrease in minute ventilation is characterized by small tidal volumes and fast respiratory rates—a sign of volume restriction (Cherniack et al., 1983).

EFFECTS ON VENTILATION AND OXYGENATION

Abnormal compliance impairs the gas exchange mechanism. When an abnormally low or high compliance is uncorrected and prolonged, muscle fatigue may occur and lead to the development of ventilatory and oxygenation failure (Rochester, 1993). Ventilatory failure develops when the patient's minute ventilation cannot keep up with the CO_2 production. Oxygenation failure usually follows when the pulmonary system cannot supply the oxygen needed for metabolism.

DEADSPACE VENTILATION

deadspace ventilation: Ventilation in excess of perfusion; wasted ventilation.

Deadspace ventilation is defined as wasted ventilation or a condition in which ventilation is in excess of perfusion. There are three types of deadspace: anatomic, alveolar, and physiologic.

ANATOMIC DEADSPACE

anatomic deadspace:
The volume occupy-
ing the conducting
airways that does
not take part in gas
exchange (estimated
to be about 1 mL/lb
ideal body weight).

Normally, the conducting airways contribute to about 30% of deadspace ventilation. For a tidal volume of 500 mL, about 150 mL of this volume is wasted since it does not take part in gas exchange. This volume in the conducting airways is called **anatomic deadspace** and it can be estimated to be about 1 mL/lb of ideal body weight (Shapiro et al., 1991).

Decrease in tidal volume causes a higher anatomic deadspace to tidal volume percent. Using the above example, the deadspace to tidal volume percent would increase from 30% (150/500) to 50% (150/300) if the tidal volume was decreased from 500 to 300 mL. See equations below for comparison:

☑ Decrease in tidal
volume causes
a higher anatomic
deadspace to tidal
volume percent.

$$\frac{150}{500} = 0.3 \text{ or } 30\%$$

$$\frac{150}{300} = 0.5 \text{ or } 50\%$$

ALVEOLAR DEADSPACE

alveolar deadspace:
The normal lung
volume that has
become unable to
take part in gas
exchange because of
reduction or lack of
pulmonary perfusion
(e.g., pulmonary
embolism).

In addition to anatomic deadspace, **alveolar deadspace** may occur in some clinical conditions. Alveolar deadspace contributes to wasted ventilation, and it occurs when the ventilated alveoli are not adequately perfused by pulmonary circulation. Pulmonary perfusion may be absent or low because of decreased cardiac output (e.g., congestive heart failure, blood loss), or due to obstruction of the pulmonary blood vessels (e.g., pulmonary vasoconstriction, pulmonary embolism) (Shapiro et al., 1991). Figure 1-6 shows the relationship between ventilation and perfusion during alveolar deadspace ventilation.

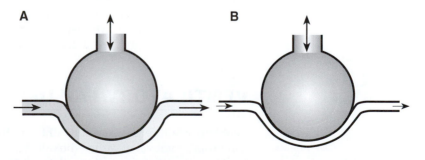

Figure 1-6   (A) Normal ventilation/perfusion relationship; (B) Alveolar deadspace ventilation occurs when the ventilated alveoli are not adequately perfused by pulmonary circulation (i.e., ventilation in excess of perfusion). Examples of deadspace ventilation include decrease in cardiac output and obstruction of pulmonary blood vessels.

TABLE 1-4   Clinical Conditions That Increase Physiologic Deadspace

TYPE OF CHANGE	CLINICAL CONDITIONS
↓ Tidal volume	Relative increase in V_D/V_T (drug overdose, neuromuscular disease)
↑ Alveolar deadspace	Decreased cardiac output (congestive heart failure, blood loss) Obstruction of pulmonary blood vessels (pulmonary vasoconstriction, pulmonary embolism)

PHYSIOLOGIC DEADSPACE

physiologic dead-space: Sum of ana-tomic and alveolar deadspace. Under normal conditions, it is about the same as anatomic deadspace.

Physiologic deadspace is the sum of anatomic and alveolar deadspace volumes. Under normal conditions, the physiologic deadspace approximates the anatomic deadspace. In diseased conditions where anatomic or alveolar deadspace ventilation is increased, physiologic deadspace is always higher than anatomic deadspace. Table 1-4 shows some clinical conditions that increase physiologic (anatomic and alveolar) deadspace.

Physiologic deadspace to tidal volume ratio (V_D/V_T) can be calculated as follows:

$$\frac{V_D}{V_T} = \frac{(PaCO_2 - P\bar{E}CO_2)}{PaCO_2}$$

✔ See Appendix 1 for example.

$PaCO_2$ is arterial CO_2 and $P\bar{E}CO_2$ is PCO_2 of a mixed expired gas sample. They are collected simultaneously. In patients on mechanical ventilation, V_D/V_T of less than 60% predicts normal ventilatory function upon weaning from mechanical ventilation (Shapiro et al., 1991).

Severe and prolonged deadspace ventilation causes inefficient ventilation, muscle fatigue, ventilatory and oxygenation failure.

VENTILATORY FAILURE

Ventilatory failure is the inability of the pulmonary system to maintain proper removal of carbon dioxide. Hypercapnia (increase in $PaCO_2$) is the key feature of ventilatory failure. When carbon dioxide production exceeds its removal, respiratory acidosis results. Hypoxemia can be the secondary complication of ventilatory failure but this type of hypoxemia usually responds well to oxygen therapy. Without supplemental oxygen, the degree of hypoxemia corresponds to the severity of ventilatory failure.

TABLE 1-5 Development of Ventilatory Failure

MECHANISM	CLINICAL FINDING
Hypoventilation	$PaCO_2$ greater than 45 mm Hg (>50 mm Hg for COPD patients)
Persistent V/Q mismatch	Hypoxemia that responds well to oxygen therapy
Persistent intrapulmonary shunt	Q_{SP}/Q_T greater than 20% (>30% in critical shunt)
Persistent diffusion defect	Gas diffusion rate less than 75% of predicted normal
Persistent reduction of P_IO_2	Low barometric pressure as in high altitude

V/Q mismatch: An abnormal distribution of ventilation and pulmonary blood flow. High V/Q is related to deadspace ventilation, whereas low V/Q is associated with intrapulmonary shunting.

intrapulmonary shunting: Pulmonary blood flow in excess of ventilation; wasted perfusion (e.g., atelectasis).

diffusion defect: Pathologic condition leading to impaired gas exchange through the alveolar-capillary membrane (e.g., interstitial or pulmonary edema).

alveolar volume: The portion of tidal volume that takes part in gas exchange.

☑ $\dot{V}_A = (V_T - V_D) \times RR$ (See Appendix 1 for example).

Table 1-5 lists five mechanisms leading to the development of ventilatory failure. They are (1) hypoventilation, (2) persistent ventilation-perfusion **(V/Q) mismatch,** (3) persistent **intrapulmonary shunting,** (4) persistent **diffusion defect,** and (5) persistent reduction of inspired oxygen tension (P_IO_2) (Greene et al., 1994).

HYPOVENTILATION

Hypoventilation can be caused by depression of the central nervous system, neuromuscular diseases, airway obstruction, and other conditions. In a clinical setting, hypoventilation is characterized by a reduction of alveolar ventilation (V_A) and an increase of arterial carbon dioxide tension ($PaCO_2$).

Alveolar Volume.   Alveolar volume (V_A) is the difference between tidal volume (V_T) and deadspace volume (V_D), as shown below:

$$V_A = V_T - V_D$$

The equation shows that alveolar volume can be increased by raising the tidal volume or by reducing the deadspace volume. In mechanical ventilation, a decrease in alveolar volume occurs when the tidal volume delivered to the patient is decreased or the deadspace volume is increased.

Hypoventilation caused by a reduction in tidal volume can be corrected by increasing the tidal volume on the ventilator. Unlike tidal volume, deadspace volume is difficult to change because anatomic deadspace stays rather constant and physiologic deadspace is caused by a lack of perfusion, thus requiring improvement of the pulmonary blood flow.

Minute Alveolar Ventilation ($\dot{V}_A$).   When the measurements are made over 1 min, minute alveolar ventilation ($\dot{V}_A$) becomes a function of the respiratory rate. Hypoventilation can result when the respiratory rate is too slow or absent (apnea). Hypoventilation due to a reduction in respiratory rate can be corrected by increasing the respiratory rate on the ventilator.

A patient's ventilatory status can best be monitored by the $PaCO_2$ measurement. The equation below shows the inverse relationship between $\dot{V}_A$ and $PaCO_2$. When the minute alveolar ventilation is low (hypoventilation), an elevated $PaCO_2$ is the typical finding in blood gas analysis.

☑ **Hypoventilation is characterized by an increase of $PaCO_2$.**

$$\dot{V}_A = \frac{\dot{V}CO_2}{PaCO_2}$$

VENTILATION/PERFUSION (V/Q) MISMATCH

The **ventilation/perfusion (V/Q)** ratio reflects the amount of ventilation in relation to the amount of pulmonary blood flow (perfusion). Since blood flow is gravity dependent, the V/Q ratio ranges from about 0.4 in the lower lung zone to 3.0 in the upper lung zone (West, 2004b).

Pulmonary embolism is an example that decreases pulmonary perfusion and leads to a high V/Q. Airway obstruction and interstitial lung disease are two examples that can cause a decrease in ventilation and lead to a low V/Q.

V/Q mismatch is responsible for the development of hypoxemia. With sufficient pulmonary reserve, a patient can usually compensate for the hypoxemic condition by hyperventilation. Hypoxemia caused by uncomplicated V/Q mismatch is readily reversible by oxygen therapy.

In mechanical ventilation, hypoxemia caused by V/Q mismatch can be compensated by increasing the rate, tidal volume, or F_IO_2 on the ventilator (Shapiro et al., 1991).

INTRAPULMONARY SHUNTING

☑ **Shunted pulmonary blood flow is not useful in gas exchange.**

In contrast with deadspace ventilation (ventilation in excess of perfusion), shunting refers to perfusion in excess of ventilation ("wasted" perfusion) (Figure 1-7). Shunted pulmonary blood flow is not useful

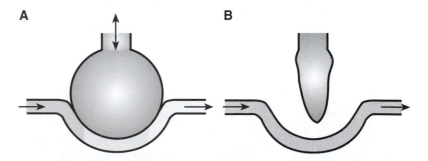

A

B

Figure 1-7 (A) Normal ventilation/perfusion relationship; (B) Intrapulmonary shunting occurs when the perfused alveoli are not adequately ventilated (i.e., perfusion in excess of ventilation). Atelectasis is an example that leads to intrapulmonary shunting.

TABLE 1-6 Interpretation of Shunt Percent

PHYSIOLOGIC SHUNT	INTERPRETATION
<10%	Normal
10% to 20%	Mild shunt
20% to 30%	Significant shunt
>30%	Critical and severe shunt

☑ Intrapulmonary
shunting
causes refractory
hypoxemia.

in gas exchange because it does not come in contact with ventilated and oxygenated alveoli. Intrapulmonary shunting causes refractory hypoxemia—low oxygen levels in the blood that respond very poorly to oxygen therapy alone.

In healthy individuals, the physiologic shunt approximates the anatomic shunt and it is less than 5%. For noncritically ill patients, the normal physiologic shunt is less than 10%. In other disease states, the physiologic shunt may be greater than 30% (Shapiro et al., 1994). See Table 1-6 for interpretation of shunt percent in hospitalized patients.

The shunt percent can be calculated or estimated by many methods, ranging from simple (less accurate) to complex (more accurate). The clinical use of two common calculations are discussed here: an estimated shunt equation and a classic shunt equation.

☑ The estimated
physiologic
shunt equation
requires only an arte-
rial blood sample.

Estimated Physiologic Shunt Equation. The estimated physiologic shunt equation requires only an arterial blood sample. It does not require a mixed venous blood sample from the pulmonary artery and therefore it is noninvasive and rather simple to compute. This estimated method is more meaningful when serial measurements are used to establish a trend. Two forms of this equation are possible: one for noncritical patients (e.g., spontaneously breathing, moderate level of F_1O_2, moderate level of continuous positive airway pressure) and one for critically ill patients (e.g., mechanical ventilation, high F_1O_2, high level of positive end-expiratory pressure).

☑ See Appendix 1
for example.

For noncritical patient:

$$\text{Estimated } \frac{Q_{SP}}{Q_T} = \frac{(CcO_2 - CaO_2)}{[5 + (CcO_2 - CaO_2)]}$$

For critical patient:

$$\text{Estimated } \frac{Q_{SP}}{Q_T} = \frac{(CcO_2 - CaO_2)}{[3.5 + (CcO_2 - CaO_2)]}$$

☑ The classic
physiologic
shunt equation
requires arterial
and mixed venous
blood samples.

Classic Physiologic Shunt Equation. The classic physiologic shunt equation requires an arterial blood sample and a mixed venous blood sample from the pulmonary artery. It is the most accurate among all shunt equations.

☑ See Appendix 1
for example.

$$\text{Classic } \frac{Q_{SP}}{Q_T} = \frac{(CcO_2 - CaO_2)}{(CcO_2 - C\dot{v}O_2)}$$

When the shunt percent is too high, oxygenation becomes an extremely difficult task for the cardiopulmonary system to support. Over time, the respiratory muscles will fatigue resulting in ventilatory failure. This is usually followed by oxygenation failure if ventilatory interventions are unsuccessful (Rochester, 1993).

DIFFUSION DEFECT

Diffusion of oxygen and carbon dioxide across the alveolar-capillary (A-C) membrane is due to the gas pressure gradients. Oxygen diffuses from the lungs ($P_AO_2 = 109$ mm Hg) to the pulmonary arteries ($P\dot{v}O_2 = 40$ mm Hg) with a pressure gradient of 69 mm Hg. Carbon dioxide diffuses from the pulmonary arteries ($P\dot{v}CO_2 = 46$ mm Hg) to the lungs ($P_ACO_2 = 40$ mm Hg) with a net pressure gradient of only 6 mm Hg. This is possible because the gas diffusion coefficient for carbon dioxide is 19 times greater than that for oxygen.

Diffusion of oxygen is greatly impaired when the inspired oxygen tension (P_IO_2) is reduced. The inspired oxygen tension is directly related to the barometric pressure. At high altitude where the barometric pressure is low, the inspired oxygen tension is also low. This leads to a condition known as **hypoxic hypoxia.**

hypoxic hypoxia:
Lack of oxygen
in the organs and
tissues due to a
reduction in inspired
oxygen tension.

The P_IO_2 is also reduced in a burning enclosure as combustion consumes oxygen in the air. Patients who suffer from smoke inhalation are at risk for developing hypoxic hypoxia. In addition to the reduced oxygen concentration and tension, the lung functions are impaired by the presence of carbon monoxide, toxic gases, and inert particles found in a fire (Wilkins et al., 1998).

In addition to the pressure gradient and diffusion coefficient, the gas diffusion rate is also affected by the thickness of the A-C membrane, the surface area of the A-C membrane, and the time available for diffusion to take place. Factors that can decrease the diffusion rate are shown in Table 1-7.

TABLE 1-7   Causes of Decreased Diffusion Rate

TYPE OF DIFFUSION PROBLEM	CLINICAL CONDITIONS
Decrease in $P(A-a)O_2$ gradient	High altitude Fire combustion
Thickening of A-C membrane	Pulmonary edema Retained secretions
Decreased surface area of A-C membrane	Emphysema Pulmonary fibrosis
Insufficient time for diffusion	Tachycardia

Conditions in Table 1-7 induce poor or inappropriate gas diffusion and can severely hinder the oxygenation process. Hypoxemia and hypoxia are usually the end results. Severe hypoxemia and hypoxia may lead to hypoxic pulmonary vasoconstriction, pulmonary hypertension, and cor pulmonale.

OXYGENATION FAILURE

Oxygenation failure is defined as severe hypoxemia ($PaO_2 < 40$ mm Hg) that does not respond to moderate to high levels (50% to 100%) of supplemental oxygen. It may be caused by hypoventilation, ventilation/perfusion mismatch, or intrapulmonary shunting. Regardless of the etiology of oxygenation failure, mechanical ventilation may be needed to minimize the work of breathing and provide oxygenation support.

HYPOXEMIA AND HYPOXIA

Hypoxemia is present when the oxygen level (e.g., PO_2, SaO_2) is decreased in arterial blood. The presence of hypoxia ($\downarrow PO_2$ in organs and tissues) may not be always apparent. Hypoxemia reflects the likelihood of hypoxia, but it is important to remember that hypoxia can occur in the absence of hypoxemia. For example, anemic hypoxia (e.g., $\downarrow$ hemoglobin, carbon monoxide poisoning), histotoxic hypoxia (e.g., cyanide poisoning), and circulatory hypoxia (e.g., $\downarrow$ cardiac output) may show normal PaO_2 measurements (Shapiro et al., 1991).

Hypoxemia. Hypoxemia is reduced oxygen in the blood. The PaO_2 is most often used to evaluate a patient's oxygenation status. Since PaO_2 reflects only the oxygen that is dissolved in the plasma, it does not represent all oxygen carried by the blood (hemoglobin and plasma). For precise assessment, oxygen content should be used as it includes the oxygen combined with hemoglobin as well as oxygen dissolved in the plasma.

When PaO_2 is used for oxygenation assessment, Table 1-8 may be used for interpretation of an adult's oxygenation status.

TABLE 1-8   Interpretation of Oxygenation Status Using PaO$_2$

HYPOXEMIA STATUS	PaO$_2$ (P$_B$ = 760 mm Hg)	PaO$_2$ (P$_B$ = 630 mm Hg)
Normal	80 to 100 mm Hg	60 to 79 mm Hg
Mild	60 to 79 mm Hg	50 to 59 mm Hg
Moderate	40 to 59 mm Hg	40 to 49 mm Hg
Severe	Less than 40 mm Hg	Less than 40 mm Hg

☑ Hypoxia can occur with a normal PaO$_2$.

☑ CaO$_2$ = (Hb × 1.34 × SaO$_2$) + (PaO$_2$ × 0.003)

☑ Oxygenation failure may develop when severe hypoxemia (PaO$_2$ <40 mm Hg) does not respond to a moderate to high level (50% to 100%) of supplemental oxygen.

☑ The important clinical signs of oxygenation failure and hypoxia include hypoxemia, dyspnea, tachypnea, tachycardia, and cyanosis.

☑ Mechanical ventilation is often used to support ventilatory or oxygenation failure.

Hypoxia. Hypoxia is reduced oxygen in the body organs and tissues. While hypoxemia and hypoxia are two terms sometimes used interchangeably, it is important to understand that hypoxia can occur with a normal PaO$_2$. For example, cyanide poisoning causes histotoxic hypoxia in which the tissues cannot carry out aerobic metabolism. In anemic hypoxia, the low hemoglobin level causes a low oxygen content while the PaO$_2$ may be normal. Since PaO$_2$ measures the oxygen tension of the plasma only, it cannot be used for assessment of anemic or histotoxic hypoxia. Arterial oxygen content (CaO$_2$) should be measured and used to assess the oxygenation status of a patient. In addition to the PaO$_2$ and CaO$_2$ measurements, hypoxia produces some clinical signs that may be used as a secondary assessment tool.

Signs of Hypoxia. In most clinical situations, hypoxemia is readily corrected by a moderate amount of supplemental oxygen. Oxygenation failure may develop when severe hypoxemia (PaO$_2$ <40 mm Hg) does not respond to moderate to high levels (50% to 100%) of supplemental oxygen.

The important clinical signs of oxygenation failure and hypoxia include hypoxemia, dyspnea, tachypnea, tachycardia, and cyanosis (Rochester, 1993). In addition, patients often appear to have shortness of breath and may become disoriented. These signs are usually readily available in the medical records or at the bedside. They should be used in conjunction with laboratory results during "routine" ventilator rounds to assess the patient so that appropriate action may be taken.

CLINICAL CONDITIONS LEADING TO MECHANCIAL VENTILATION

Mechanical ventilation is often used to support ventilatory or oxygenation failure. Failure to ventilate or oxygenate adequately may be caused by pulmonary or nonpulmonary conditions. For example, adult respiratory distress syndrome is a pulmonary condition commonly associated with mechanical ventilation and mortality. Many nonpulmonary conditions (e.g., hypovolemic shock, head trauma) also contribute to the need for mechanical ventilation (Gillespie et al., 1986; Kelly et al., 1993).

These pulmonary and nonpulmonary conditions often lead to a combination of deadspace ventilation, V/Q mismatch, shunt, diffusion defect, ventilatory failure, and oxygenation failure. For logical discussion and ease of patient management, they are separated into three distinct groups: (1) depressed respiratory drive (e.g., drug overdose), (2) excessive ventilatory workload (e.g., air flow obstruction), and (3) failure of ventilatory pump (e.g., chest trauma).

☑ Depressed or insufficient respiratory drive may lead to ventilatory and oxygenation failure.

DEPRESSED RESPIRATORY DRIVE

Depressed or insufficient respiratory drive may lead to a decrease in tidal volume, respiratory rate, or both. These patients may have normal pulmonary function but the respiratory muscles do not have adequate neuromuscular impulses to function properly. Mechanical ventilation is used to support these patients until the cause of insufficient respiratory drive has been reversed.

Table 1-9 lists the clinical conditions that may lead to a depressed respiratory drive. They are drug overdose (Parsons, 1994), acute spinal cord injury (Bach, 1991), head trauma (Hemmer, 1985), neurologic

TABLE 1-9   Causes of Depressed Respiratory Drive

TYPE OF RESPIRATORY DRIVE DEPRESSION	CLINICAL CONDITIONS
Drug overdose	Central hypoventilation (narcotics, alcohol, sedatives) Acute respiratory insufficiency (cocaine, heroin, methadone, propoxyphene, phenothiazines, alcohol, barbiturates) Severe pulmonary complications (poisons and toxins such as paraquat, petroleum distillates, organophosphates, mushrooms of *Amanita* genus, hemlock, botulism)
Acute spinal cord injury	Respiratory paralysis (tetraplegic with injury at C1-C3 level)
Head trauma	Abnormal respiratory patterns (apnea, tachypnea, Cheyne-Stokes respiration, apneustic breathing, ataxic breathing) Neurogenic pulmonary edema (increase in intracranial pressure) Delayed pulmonary dysfunction (intrapulmonary shunt, increased pulmonary vascular resistance, V/Q mismatch)
Neurologic dysfunction	Coma Cerebral vascular accident (stroke) Altered mental status (hypoxic brain)
Sleep disorders	Sleep apnea (central, obstructive, mixed) Sleep deprivation
Metabolic alkalosis	Hypoventilation to compensate for elevated pH in metabolic alkalosis

TABLE 1-10   Causes of Excessive Ventilatory Workload

TYPE	CLINICAL CONDITIONS
Acute airflow obstruction	Status asthmaticus Epiglotittis COPD
Deadspace ventilation	Pulmonary embolism Decrease in cardiac output Emphysema
Acute lung injury	ARDS IRDS
Congenital heart disease	Hypoplastic left heart syndrome Tetralogy of Fallot Persistent pulmonary hypertension
Cardiovascular decompensation	Decreased cardiac output V/Q mismatch Deadspace ventilation
Shock	Blood loss Peripheral vasodilation Congestive heart failure
Increased metabolic rate	Fever Increased work of breathing
Drugs	Acute pulmonary edema (narcotics, salicylates, nonsteroidal anti-inflammatory agents, naloxone, thiazide diuretics, contrast media, insulin) Bronchospasm (salicylates, nonsteroidal anti-inflammatory agents, hydrocortisone, beta-blockers, neuromuscular blocking agents, contrast media)
Decreased compliance	Atelectasis Tension pneumothorax Post-thoracic surgery Obesity Diaphragmatic hernia

TABLE 1-11   Causes of Ventilatory Pump Failure

TYPE	CLINICAL CONDITIONS
Chest trauma	Flail chest Tension pneumothorax
Premature birth	Idiopathic respiratory distress syndrome
Electrolyte imbalance	Hyperkalemia
Geriatric patients	Fatigue of respiratory muscles

dysfunction (Kelly et al., 1993), sleep disorders, and compensation for metabolic alkalosis (Greene et al., 1994).

EXCESSIVE VENTILATORY WORKLOAD

☑ Excessive ventilatory workload may lead to muscle fatigue, ventilatory and oxygenation failure.

Ventilatory workload is influenced by many clinical conditions (Table 1-10). When it exceeds the patient's ability to carry out the workload, ventilatory and oxygenation failure ensues and mechanical ventilation becomes necessary. The ventilatory workload is increased in the presence of acute air flow obstruction (Beachey et al., 1990), increased deadspace ventilation (Greene et al., 1994), acute lung injury (Kraus et al., 1993), congenital heart disease (DiCarlo et al., 1994), cardiovascular decompensation, shock (Hinson et al., 1992), increased metabolic rate, and decreased lung and chest wall compliance (Greene et al., 1994).

FAILURE OF VENTILATORY PUMP

☑ Failure of the ventilatory pump may lead to an increased work of breathing, eventual ventilatory and oxygenation failure.

Failure of the ventilatory pump is the structural dysfunction of the respiratory system to include the lung parenchyma, respiratory muscles, and thoracic skeletal structures. If uncorrected, this condition may lead to increased work of breathing and eventual ventilatory and oxygenation failure.

Table 1-11 lists some clinical examples of conditions that may lead to ventilatory pump failure. They include chest trauma, prematurity (Watchko et al., 1994), electrolyte imbalance (Freeman et al., 1993), and problems in geriatric patients (Krieger, 1994).

SUMMARY

Mechanical ventilation is used for many different clinical conditions. Essentially all uses of mechanical ventilation are targeted toward patients who fail to ventilate or oxygenate adequately. Ventilatory and oxygenation failure may be due to the adverse changes in a patient's physiologic functions (i.e., depressed respiratory drive, excessive ventilatory workload, and failure of ventilatory pump). These abnormal physiologic functions should be identified early on so that the indications for mechanical ventilation are clearly delineated.

While mechanical ventilation does not treat any ventilation or oxygenation abnormalities per se, it is a useful adjunct to support the gas exchange function until effective spontaneous breathing is restored.

Self-Assessment Questions

1. Airway resistance may be increased in all of the following clinical conditions *except:*

   A. airway obstruction.
   B. endotracheal tube with small internal diameter.
   C. condensation in ventilator circuit.
   D. tachycardia.

2. A mechanically ventilated patient has an increased airflow resistance due to unknown reasons. In assessing the patient-ventilator system, you would expect to see _____ on the pressure-volume (P-V) display.

   A. widening (bowing) of the P-V loop
   B. narrowing of the P-V loop
   C. shifting of the P-V slope toward the volume axis
   D. shifting of the P-V slope toward the pressure axis

3. Static compliance is primarily affected by a patient's _____ whereas the dynamic compliance is primarily affected by a patient's _____.

   A. elastic property of the lungs, airflow resistance
   B. elastic property of the lungs, minute ventilation
   C. airflow resistance, elastic property of the lungs
   D. airflow resistance, minute ventilation

4. The slope of a pressure-volume (P-V) loop is shifted toward the pressure axis. This condition is consistent with a(n):

   A. increase in compliance.
   B. increase in airflow resistance.
   C. decrease in compliance.
   D. decrease in airflow resistance.

5. The most recent blood gas report shows that a patient is hypoventilating ($PaCO_2$ = 65 mm Hg). The physician asks you to improve the patient's alveolar ventilation by making changes to the ventilator. You would proceed to:

   A. decrease the tidal volume.
   B. increase the mechanical deadspace on the ventilator circuit.
   C. increase the rate.
   D. decrease the tidal volume and rate.

6. Hypoventilation is characterized by a(n):

   A. increased PaO_2.
   B. increased pH.

   C. increased $PaCO_2$.
   D. decreased pH and $PaCO_2$.

7. Ventilation/perfusion (V/Q) mismatch is common in lung diseases. For example, a low V/Q may be seen in _____ and a high ratio in _____.

   A. atelectasis, pulmonary embolism.
   B. pulmonary embolism, atelectasis.

   C. atelectasis, airway obstruction.
   D. airway obstruction, atelectasis.

8. Which of the following causes of hypoxemia is *least* likely to be treated successfully by oxygen therapy alone?

   A. hypoventilation
   B. V/Q mismatch

   C. intrapulmonary shunting
   D. low P_1O_2

9. In managing a critically ill patient who has been on the ventilator for six days, the physician asks you to calculate the estimated shunt percent using only one arterial blood gas sample. You would use:

   A. Estimated $Q_{SP}/Q_T = (CcO_2 - CaO_2) / [5 + (CcO_2 - CaO_2)]$.
   B. Estimated $Q_{SP}/Q_T = (CcO_2 - CaO_2) / [3.5 + (CcO_2 - CaO_2)]$.

   C. Classic $Q_{SP}/Q_T = (CcO_2 - CaO_2) / (CcO_2 - C\dot{v}O_2)$.
   D. B or C only.

10 to 13. Match the types of gas diffusion problem with the clinical conditions affecting the diffusion rate.

TYPES OF DIFFUSION PROBLEM	CLINICAL CONDITIONS
10. Decreased pressure gradient	A. Emphysema
11. Thickening of A-C membrane	B. High altitude
12. Decreased surface area of A-C membrane	C. Tachycardia
13. Insufficient time for diffusion	D. Pulmonary edema

14. The ABG report for an abdominal postoperative patient shows respiratory acidosis with severe hypoxemia. In order to determine whether *hypoxia* is present, you would evaluate all of the following *except:*

   A. $PaCO_2$.
   B. heart rate.

   C. color of skin.
   D. spontaneous respiratory rate.

15 to 20. Ventilatory and oxygenation failure may occur when the respiratory drive is diminished. Match the types of respiratory depression with the respective clinical conditions.

TYPES OF DEPRESSION	CLINICAL CONDITIONS
15. Drug overdose	A. Altered mental status (hypoxic brain)
16. Acute spinal cord injury	B. Neurogenic pulmonary edema (increase of intracranial pressure)
17. Head trauma	C. Sleep apnea (central, obstructive, mixed)
18. Neurologic dysfunction	D. Hypoventilation to compensate for elevated pH
19. Sleep disorders	E. Respiratory paralysis (tetraplegic with injury at C1-C3 level)
20. Metabolic alkalosis	F. Narcotic and sedative use

21. Excessive and prolonged increase in the patient's respiratory workload may lead to fatigue of the _____ muscles. If uncorrected, _____ failure is the likely end result.

A. heart, ventilatory and oxygenation

B. heart, congestive heart

C. respiratory, ventilatory and oxygenation

D. respiratory, congestive heart

Answers to Self-Assessment Questions

1. D. tachycardia.

2. A. widening (bowing) of the P-V loop

3. A. elastic property of the lungs, airflow resistance

4. C. decreased in compliance.

5. C. increase the rate.

6. C. increased $PaCO_2$.

7. A. atelectasis, pulmonary embolism.

8. C. intrapulmonary shunting

9. B. Estimated $Q_{SP}/Q_T = (CcO_2 - CaO_2) / [3.5 + (CcO_2 - CaO_2)]$.

10. B. High altitude

11. D. Pulmonary edema

12. A. Emphysema

13. C. Tachycardia

14. A. $PaCO_2$

15. F. Narcotic and sedative use

16. E. Respiratory Paralysis (tetraplegic with injury at C1-C3 level)

17. B. Neurogenic pulmonary edema (increase of intracranial pressure)

18. A. Altered Mental Status (hypoxic brain)

19. C. Sleep apnea (central, obstructive, mixed)

20. D. Hypoventilation to compensate for elevated pH

21. C. respiratory, ventilatory and oxygenation

References

Bach, J. R. (1991). Alternative methods of ventilatory support for the patient with ventilatory failure due to spinal cord injury. *J Am Paraplegia Soc, 14*(4), 158–174.

Barnes, T. A., et al. (1994). Core textbook of respiratory case practice (2nd ed.). St. Louis, MO: Mosby.

Beachey, W. D., et al. (1990). Quantifying ventilatory reserve to predict respiratory failure in exacerbations of COPD. *Chest, 97*, 1086–1091.

Burton, G. G., et al. (1997). *Respiratory care: A guide to clinical practice* (4th ed.). Baltimore: Lippincott Williams & Wilkins.

Cherniack, R. M., et al. (1983). *Respiration in health and disease* (3rd ed.). Philadelphia: W.B. Saunders.

DiCarlo, J. V., et al. (1994). Respiratory failure in congenital heart disease. *Pediatr Clin North Am, 41*(3), 525–542.

Freeman, S. J., et al. (1993). Muscular paralysis and ventilatory failure caused by hyperkalemia. *Br J Anaesth, 70,* 226–227.

Gillespie, D. J., et al. (1986). Clinical outcome of respiratory failure in patients requiring prolonged (>24 hours) mechanical ventilation. *Chest, 90*(3), 364–369.

Greene, K. E., et al. (1994). Pathophysiology of acute respiratory failure. *Clin Chest Med, 15*(1), 1–12.

Hemmer, M. (1985). Ventilatory support for pulmonary failure of the head trauma patient. *Bull Eur Physiopathol Respir, 21,* 287–293.

Hinson, J. R., et al. (1992). Principles of mechanical ventilator use in respiratory failure. *Annu Rev Med, 43,* 341–361.

Kelly, B. J., et al. (1993). Prevalence and severity of neurologic dysfunction in critically ill patients—Influence on need for continued mechanical ventilation. *Chest, 104,* 1818–1824.

Kraus, P. A., et al. (1993). Acute lung injury at Baragwanath ICU, an eight-month audit and call for consensus for other organ failure in the adult respiratory distress syndrome. *Chest, 103,* 1832–1836.

Krieger, B. P. (1994). Respiratory failure in the elderly. *Clin Geriat Med, 10*(1), 103–119.

Parsons, P. E. (1994). Respiratory failure as a result of drugs, overdoses, and poisonings. *Clin Chest Med, 15*(1), 93–102.

Rochester, D. F. (1993). Respiratory muscles and ventilatory failure. *Am J Med Sci, 305*(6), 394–402.

Schuster, D. P. (1990). A physiologic approach to initiating, maintaining, and withdrawing mechanical ventilatory support during acute respiratory failure. *Am J Med, 88,* 268–278.

Shapiro, B. A., et al. (1991). *Clinical application of respiratory care* (4th ed.). St. Louis, MO: Mosby.

Shapiro, B. A., et al. (1994). *Clinical application of blood gases* (5th ed.). St. Louis, MO: Mosby.

Tyco Healthcare. (2003). *Ventilator waveforms—graphical presentation of ventilatory data.* Pleasanton, CA.

Watchko, J. F., et al. (1994). Ventilatory pump failure in premature newborns. *Pediatr Pulmonol, 17,* 231–233.

West, J. B. (2004a). *Pulmonary pathophysiology—The essentials* (6th ed.). Baltimore: Lippincott Williams & Wilkins.

West, J. B. (2004b). *Respiratory physiology—the essentials* (7th ed.). Philadelphia: Lippincott Williams & Wilkins.

Wilkins, R. L., et al. (1998). *Respiratory disease—Principles of patient care* (2nd ed.). Philadelphia, PA: F.A. Davis.

Suggested Reading

Chang, D. W. (1999). *Respiratory care calculations* (2nd ed.). Clifton Park, New York: Thomson Learning. Delmar.
Misasi, R. S., et al. (1994). The pathophysiology of hypoxia. *Crit Care Nurse, 14*(4), 55–64.

CHAPTER TWO

EFFECTS OF POSITIVE PRESSURE VENTILATION

David W. Chang
Terry S. LeGrand

——— OUTLINE ———

Introduction

Pulmonary Considerations
Spontaneous Breathing
Positive Pressure Ventilation
Airway Pressures
Compliance

Cardiovascular Considerations
Mean Airway Pressure and Cardiac
 Output
Decrease in Cardiac Output and O_2
 Delivery
Blood Pressure Changes
Pulmonary Blood Flow and Thoracic
 Pump Mechanism

Hemodynamic Considerations
Positive Pressure Ventilation
Positive End-Expiratory Pressure

Renal Considerations
Renal Perfusion
Indicators of Renal Failure
Effects of Renal Failure on Drug
 Clearance

Hepatic Considerations
PEEP and Hepatic Perfusion
Indicators of Liver Dysfunction
Effects of Decreased Hepatic
 Perfusion on Drug Clearance

Abdominal Considerations
Effects of PEEP and Increased
 Intra-abdominal Pressure

Gastrointestinal Considerations

Nutritional Considerations
Muscle Fatigue
Nutritional Support
Nutrition and the Work of Breathing

Neurologic Considerations
Hyperventilation
Ventilatory and Oxygenation Failure
Indicators of Neurologic Impairment

Summary

Self-Assessment Questions

Answers to Self-Assessment Questions

References

—————————————————— **KEY TERMS** ——————————————————

- **central venous pressure (CVP)**
- **continuous positive airway pressure (CPAP)**
- **gastrointestinal (GI)**
- **hepatic perfusion**
- **intra-abdominal pressure (IAP)**
- **mean airway pressure (mPaw or MAWP)**
- **oxygen delivery**
- **peak inspiratory pressure (PIP)**
- **positive end-expiratory pressure (PEEP)**

- **positive pressure ventilation**
- **pressure-limited**
- **pulmonary artery pressure**
- **pulmonary capillary wedge pressure**
- **renal perfusion**
- **stroke volume**
- **thoracic pump mechanism**
- **total parenteral nutrition (TPN)**
- **volume-limited**

—————————————————— **INTRODUCTION** ——————————————————

Positive pressure ventilation is an essential life support measure in the intensive care and extended care environments. The physiologic effects of positive pressure ventilation have complex interactions with the lungs and other organ systems. Some of these physiologic effects are beneficial while others may cause complications. This chapter discusses the side effects of positive pressure ventilation on the major organ systems of the body.

PULMONARY CONSIDERATIONS

This section compares the physiologic differences between spontaneous breathing and positive pressure ventilation. Two of the major effects are the changes in airway pressure and compliance.

SPONTANEOUS BREATHING

☑ During negative pressure ventilation, pressures in the airways, alveoli, and pleura are *decreased* during inspiration.

During spontaneous ventilation, the diaphragm and other respiratory muscles create gas flow by lowering the pleural, alveolar, and airway pressures. When alveolar and airway pressures drop below atmospheric pressure, air flows into the lungs (Pinsky, 1990). Negative pressure ventilation uses this principle by creating a negative pressure on the chest wall. When negative pressure is used for ventilation, the pressures in the airways, alveoli, and pleura are *decreased* during inspiration. Table 2-1 shows the relationship of barometric pressure (P_B) and alveolar pressure (P_{ALV}) during spontaneous breathing.

Pressures shown in Table 2-1 are for illustration purposes only. The barometric pressure is assigned 0 cm H_2O for easy comparison of pressure changes during spontaneous breathing. (Wilkins, 2003).

TABLE 2-1 Relationship of Barometric Pressure (P$_B$) and Alveolar Pressure (P$_{ALV}$) During Spontaneous Breathing

SPONTANEOUS BREATHING	P$_B$ (cm H$_2$O)	P$_{ALV}$ (cm H$_2$O)	ΔP	FLOW
Inspiration	0	−5	−5	Into lungs
End-inspiration	0	0	0	None
Expiration	0	+5	+5	Out of lungs
End-expiration	0	0	0	None

positive pressure ventilation:
Mechancial ventilation in which the volume is delivered by a positive pressure gradient (i.e., airway pressure higher than alveolar pressure).

pressure-limited:
Termination of the inspiratory cycle when the preset pressure is reached.

volume-limited:
Termination of the inspiratory cycle when the preset volume is reached.

POSITIVE PRESSURE VENTILATION

During **positive pressure ventilation,** gas flow is delivered to the lungs under a positive pressure gradient (i.e., airway pressure is greater than alveolar pressure). Therefore, the tidal volume delivered to the lungs is directly related to the positive pressure when a **pressure-limited** ventilator is used. In **volume-limited** ventilators, the level of positive pressure is dependent on the mechanical tidal volume, as well as the patient's compliance and airway resistance.

When positive pressure is used for ventilation, the pressures in the airways, alveoli, and pleura are *increased* during inspiration (Pinsky, 1990). Table 2-2 shows the relationship of inspiratory pressure (P$_I$) and alveolar pressure (P$_{ALV}$) during positive pressure ventilation. Pressures in Table 2-2 are for illustration purposes only. The barometric pressure is assigned 0 cm H$_2$O for easy comparison of pressure changes during positive pressure ventilation.

Since the pressure gradient and tidal volume are directly related, a higher peak inspiratory pressure observed during mechanical ventilation is usually related to a larger volume delivered. However, there are some exceptions to this relationship and some examples are presented in Table 2-3.

TABLE 2-2 Relationship of Inspiratory Pressure (P$_I$) and Alveolar Pressure (P$_{ALV}$) During Positive Pressure Ventilation

POSITIVE PRESSURE VENTILATION	P$_I$ (cm H$_2$O)	P$_{ALV}$ (cm H$_2$O)	ΔP	FLOW
Inspiration	20	0	+20	Into lungs
End-inspiration	20	20	0	No flow
Expiration	0	20	−20	Out of lungs
End-expiration	0	0	0	No flow

TABLE 2-3   Conditions That Limit the Volume Delivered by Positive Pressure Ventilation

CONDITIONS	EXAMPLES
Peak inspiratory pressure reached too soon	Airway obstruction
	Kinking of ET tube
	Bronchospasm
	Low lung compliance
	Pressure limit set too low
Unable to reach peak inspiratory pressure	ET tube cuff leak
	Ventilator circuit leak

AIRWAY PRESSURES

peak inspiratory pressure (PIP): *Maximum pressure measured during one respiratory cycle, usually at the end of inspiration.*

With a pressure-limited ventilator, the **peak inspiratory pressure (PIP)** is preset according to the estimated tidal volume requirement of a patient. The inspiratory phase terminates once the preset pressure is reached. For this reason, the patient may receive a smaller volume when the preset pressure is reached prematurely as would happen under conditions of low compliance or high airway resistance.

With a volume-limited ventilator, the volume is preset and the pressure used by the ventilator to deliver this preset volume is variable. The PIP observed at the end of the inspiratory phase is higher under conditions of low compliance or high airway resistance. On the other hand, the PIP is lower under conditions of high compliance or low airway resistance.

mean airway pressure (mPaw): *Average pressure within the airway during one complete respiratory cycle. It is directly related to the inspiratory time, respiratory rate, peak inspiratory pressure, and positive end-expiratory pressure (PEEP).*

When using a volume ventilator, all airway pressures (including PIP and **mean airway pressure [mPaw]**) are directly related to tidal volume, airway resistance, and peak inspiratory flow rate and inversely related to compliance.

These airway pressures (and lung volumes) have a direct impact on the intrathoracic pressure, blood flow, and blood pressure. Indirectly, they can affect the functions of different organ systems.

COMPLIANCE

In lungs with normal compliance, about 50% of the airway pressure is transmitted to the thoracic cavity. In noncompliant or stiff lungs (atelectasis, ARDS), the pressure transmitted to the thoracic cavity is much less due to the dampening effect of the nonelastic lung tissues. For this reason, high levels of PIP or positive end-expiratory pressure (**PEEP**) may be required to ventilate and oxygenate patients with low compliance. The decrease in cardiac output due to excessive PIP or PEEP is less severe, however, than if the same pressures are applied to lungs with normal or high compliance (Perkins et al., 1989).

CARDIOVASCULAR CONSIDERATIONS

Mechanical ventilation creates air flow by generating a pressure gradient. In turn, the pressures in the airways, thoracic cage, and pulmonary blood vessels are altered. In a clinical setting, the cardiovascular functions should be evaluated and monitored to prevent the adverse effects of mechanical ventilation on the heart and its vessels.

MEAN AIRWAY PRESSURE AND CARDIAC OUTPUT

Positive pressure ventilation increases mPaw and decreases cardiac output. Regardless of the mode of ventilation selected on the ventilator, a higher mPaw usually results in a lower cardiac output (Perkins et al., 1989). Since mPaw is a function of inspiratory time, respiratory rate, peak inspiratory pressure, and **positive end-expiratory pressure PEEP,** these four parameters should be kept to a minimum in order to maintain the mPaw at the lowest level possible.

In comparing **continuous positive airway pressure (CPAP)** and PEEP, PEEP reduces the cardiac output more severely as it causes a higher mPaw. This is because PEEP is used in addition to positive pressure ventilation, whereas CPAP is used in spontaneously breathing patients (Figure 2-1).

positive end-expiratory pressure (PEEP): *PEEP is an airway pressure strategy in ventilation that increases the end-expiratory or baseline airway pressure to a value greater than atmospheric pressure. It is used to treat refractory hypoxemia caused by intrapulmonary shunting.*

continuous positive airway pressure (CPAP): *The end-expiratory pressure applied to the airway of a spontaneously breathing patient.*

Figure 2-1 Comparison of mean airway pressure between (A) CPAP and (B) PEEP. The mean airway pressure is higher in (B) because PEEP (10 cm H_2O) is used in addition to positive pressure ventilation.

DECREASE IN CARDIAC OUTPUT AND O_2 DELIVERY

stroke volume:
Blood volume
output delivered
by one ventricular
contraction.

Use of positive pressure ventilation can reduce the amount of oxygen available to the body. An increase in positive airway pressure generally causes a higher intrathoracic pressure. In turn, this pressure is transmitted to the airways and alveoli, as well as to the mediastinum, great vessels that return blood to the heart (Marini, 2004). This change in pressure may lead to a reduction in **stroke volume** and cardiac output.

oxygen delivery:
Total amount of
oxygen carried by
blood. It is the prod-
uct of O_2 content and
cardiac output.

Since O_2 delivery is the product of O_2 content and cardiac output, reduction in stroke volume and cardiac output results in a decrease in **oxygen delivery.** As shown in the equation below and Figure 2-2, decreased cardiac output reduces O_2 delivery.

$$O_2 \text{ Content} \times \downarrow \text{Cardiac Output} = \downarrow O_2 \text{ Delivery}$$

Figure 2-2   Positive pressure ventilation leads to a decrease in O_2 delivery.

☑ For patients with cardiopulmonary disease or compromised cardiovascular reserve, positive pressure ventilation may cause blood pressure measurements to decrease.

BLOOD PRESSURE CHANGES

During spontaneous inspiration, there is a transient decrease of arterial blood pressure readings. In certain disease states, such as acute asthma exacerbation, this physiologic decrease becomes exaggerated and is referred to as *pulsus paradoxus* (Wright et al., 1996). During positive pressure ventilation, reverse pulsus paradoxus is observed in which the arterial blood pressure is slightly higher than that measured during spontaneous breathing. During positive pressure ventilation, pressures measured in the aorta, left atrium, pulmonary artery, and right atrium are also slightly higher than those measured during spontaneous ventilation. Because left ventricular end systolic volume has been shown to be reduced during a positive pressure inspiration while there is no change in left ventricular end diastolic volume, the mechanism of reverse pulsus paradoxus appears to be a reduction in left ventricular afterload (Abel, 1987). For patients with cardiopulmonary disease or compromised cardiovascular reserve, however, positive pressure ventilation may cause these pressure measurements to decrease. These measurements may also decrease when PIP or PEEP is at a level that compromises the cardiovascular function.

PULMONARY BLOOD FLOW AND THORACIC PUMP MECHANISM

During positive pressure ventilation, intrathoracic pressure changes according to the pressure transmitted across the lung parenchyma. In turn, changes in intrathoracic pressure can affect the pulmonary blood flow entering and leaving the ventricles.

Left ventricle. In the left ventricle, the effect of an increase in lung volume on pulmonary venous blood flow is dependent on the relative state of filling of the pulmonary circulation. In patients who are hypotensive, an increase in tidal volume causes a decrease in pulmonary venous return to the left ventricle (Figure 2-3) (Pinsky, 1990).

A   B

RT→   LT→   RT→   LT→

Figure 2-3 In hypotensive conditions, positive pressure ventilation decreases the blood flow to left heart. (A) Spontaneous breathing; (B) Positive pressure ventilation causes compression of the pulmonary blood vessels in hypotensive conditions.

Figure 2-4 In hypertensive conditions, positive pressure ventilation increases the blood flow to left heart in part due to the thoracic pump mechanism (see text). (A) Spontaneous breathing; (B) Positive pressure ventilation does not cause significant compression of the pulmonary blood vessels in hypertensive conditions.

thoracic pump mechanism:
Alternations in pulmonary blood flow caused by changes in intrathoracic pressure during positive pressure ventilation. In hypotensive conditions, positive pressure ventilation decreases the blood flow to the left heart. In hypertensive conditions, this mechanism enhances the outflow of blood from the right ventricle and into the left heart.

In hypertensive patients, use of large tidal volumes increases venous return to the left ventricle (Figure 2-4) (Pinsky, 1990). This is because compression of pulmonary blood vessels is minimal in hypertensive conditions. It is also due in part to the **thoracic pump mechanism** where the blood flow from right to left ventricle is enhanced during the expiratory phase of positive pressure ventilation (DiCarlo et al., 1994).

Right ventricle. In the right ventricle, high airway pressures and large tidal volumes used in positive pressure ventilation stretch and compress the pulmonary blood vessels and limit their capacity to hold blood volume. During expiration the pulmonary vessels, no longer under high pressure and large tidal volumes, are free to fill to their holding capacity with the blood leaving the right ventricle. This thoracic pump mechanism facilitates the outflow of blood from the right ventricle (Figure 2-5) (DiCarlo et al., 1994).

Figure 2-5 Thoracic pump mechanism. (A) During the inspiratory phase of positive pressure ventilation, the pulmonary blood vessels are compressed and the blood flow from right to left ventricle is decreased. (B) During the expiratory phase, the pulmonary blood vessels are no longer under alveolar compression and the blood flow from right to left ventricle is increased.

central venous pressure (CVP): *Pressure measured in the vena cava or right atrium. It reflects the status of blood volume in the systemic circulation. Right ventricular preload.*

pulmonary artery pressure (PAP): *Pressure measured in the pulmonary artery. It reflects the volume status of the pulmonary artery and the functions of the ventricles. Right ventricular afterload.*

pulmonary capillary wedge pressure (PCWP): *Pressure measured in the pulmonary artery with a balloon inflated to stop pulmonary blood flow. It reflects the volume status and functions of the left heart. Left ventricular preload.*

☑ PEEP increases peak inspiratory and mean airway pressures.

☑ PEEP increases CVP and PAP but decreases aortic pressure and cardiac output.

In children with right ventricular dysfunction, high positive pressure (up to 40 cm H_2O) and large tidal volumes (20 to 30 mL/kg) may reduce the workload of the right heart by the action of the thoracic pump mechanism (DiCarlo et al., 1994).

HEMODYNAMIC CONSIDERATIONS

One of the major adverse effects of mechanical ventilation is the changes in a patient's hemodynamic status. The major hemodynamic measurements affected by positive pressure ventilation include **central venous pressure (CVP)** and **pulmonary artery pressure.** The **pulmonary capillary wedge pressure** is not affected to a great extent because of the capability of the systemic venous circulation to compensate for changes in blood pressure and volume.

POSITIVE PRESSURE VENTILATION

Positive pressure ventilation causes an increase in intrathoracic pressure and compression of the pulmonary blood vessels. Partial recovery is observed during the expiratory phase. It is estimated that 15% to 20% of pulmonary blood volume is shifted to the systemic circulation at a tidal volume of 1L. An increase in intrathoracic pressure and compression of the pulmonary blood vessels causes an overall decrease in ventricular output, stroke volume, and pressure readings (Versprille, 1990).

Table 2-4 shows the general effects of positive pressure ventilation on hemodynamic measurements. It is essential to remember that the severity of these hemodynamic changes is dependent on the level of airway pressures, lung volume, and compliance characteristics of the patient.

POSITIVE END-EXPIRATORY PRESSURE

Positive end-expiratory pressure (PEEP) is a modality used in conjunction with positive pressure ventilation and it significantly increases the PAP and mPaw. In one study, when PEEP was initiated and increased to 15 cm H_2O over 90 sec, the central venous pressure and pulmonary artery pressure showed a drastic increase while the aortic pressure and cardiac output showed a significant decrease (Versprille, 1990). PEEP must be used with extreme care in a clinical setting because PEEP, in addition to positive pressure ventilation, can potentiate the reduction in cardiac output.

Table 2-5 outlines the general effects of PEEP on hemodynamic measurements. It is important to remember that PEEP is used in conjunction with positive pressure ventilation. For this reason, the hemodynamic changes may be different from those caused by positive pressure ventilation alone. The severity of these hemodynamic changes is also dependent on the lung volume and compliance.

TABLE 2-4 Effects of Positive Pressure Ventilation on Hemodynamic Measurements

PRESSURE OR VOLUME CHANGES	NOTES
Increase in intrathoracic pressure	Positive pressure applied to the lungs causes compression of the lung parenchyma against the chest wall.
Decrease in pulmonary blood volume and *increase* in systemic blood volume	During the inspiratory phase of positive pressure ventilation, a fraction of the pulmonary blood volume is shifted to the systemic circulation. This does not increase the central venous pressure (CVP) because the systemic venous circulation can readily absorb this extra volume.
Decrease in venous return (CVP)	Higher intrathoracic pressure impedes systemic blood return to right ventricle.
Decrease in right ventricular stroke volume*	Decreased venous return to right ventricle leads to lower right ventricular output.
Decrease in pulmonary arterial pressure (PAP)	Decreased right ventricular stroke volume leads to lower blood volume (pressure) in the pulmonary arteries.
Decrease in filling pressures	Lower blood volume entering and leaving the ventricles.
Decrease in left ventricular stroke volume*	Decreased right ventricular stroke volume and pulmonary artery pressure lead to lower left ventricular input and output.

NOTE: In the absence of compensation by increasing the heart rate, decrease in right and left ventricular stroke volumes generally leads to a decreased cardiac output.

TABLE 2-5 Effects of Positive End-Expiratory Pressure on Hemodynamic Measurements

PRESSURE OR CARDIAC OUTPUT CHANGE	NOTES
Increase in pulmonary artery pressure (PAP)	PEEP and positive pressure applied to the lungs cause significant compression of pulmonary blood vessels.
Increase in central venous pressure (CVP)	Incease in PAP causes a higher right ventricular pressure and hinders blood return from systemic circulation to right heart. This causes backup of blood flow and increase in pressure in the systemic venous circulation.
Decrease in aortic pressure	This is due to the significant increase in intrathoracic pressure and significant *decrease* in left and right ventricular stroke volumes.
Decrease in cardiac output	This is due to the significant increase in intrathoracic pressure and significant *decrease* in left and right ventricular stroke volumes.

The decrease in cardiac output due to positive pressure ventilation and PEEP can be managed by using appropriate intravascular volume expansion and positive inotropic support. A patient with adequate intravascular volume or one who receives a positive inotrope may have a smaller decline in cardiac output during positive pressure ventilation and PEEP (Perkins et al., 1989).

RENAL CONSIDERATIONS

Kidneys play an important role in eliminating wastes, clearance of certain drugs, and regulating fluid, electrolyte, and acid-base balance. The kidneys are highly vascular and at any one time receive about 25% of the body's circulating blood volume (Brundage, 1992). Because of these characteristics, they are highly vulnerable to decreases in blood flow as it would occur during positive pressure ventilation.

RENAL PERFUSION

renal perfusion: Blood flow to the kidneys. It is decreased when blood volume or cardiac output is low.

When **renal perfusion** or perfusion of the glomeruli of the kidneys is decreased, filtration becomes less effective (Baer et al., 1992). Subsequently, the urine output is decreased as the kidneys try to correct the hypovolemic condition by retaining fluid. If hypoperfusion of the kidneys persists or worsens, renal failure may result.

INDICATORS OF RENAL FAILURE

☑ Oliguria is defined as urine output <400 mL in 24 hours (or <160 mL in 8 hours).

For adequate removal of body wastes, urine output must be above 400 mL in a 24-hour period. Decreased urine output is an early sign of renal insufficiency or failure. This condition is called *oliguria* and is defined as urine output less than 400 mL in 24 hours (or less than 160 mL in 8 hours) (Kraus et al., 1993). Other early signs of renal failure include elevation of serum blood urea nitrogen (BUN) and creatinine, products of nitrogen metabolism (King, 1994). The kidney is responsible for eliminating these nitrogenous wastes to prevent toxic accumulation in the body; thus an increase in serum levels of BUN and creatinine indicates compromised renal function. See Table 2-6 for other major serum indicators of renal failure.

EFFECTS OF RENAL FAILURE ON DRUG CLEARANCE

Whenever the kidneys are not functioning properly, their performance is hindered. Renal dysfunction from any cause can affect all normal kidney functions, including fluid and electrolyte regulation and drug clearance.

Hypoperfusion.   Hypoperfusion of the kidneys may affect the rate of drug clearance. For example, the duration of neuromuscular blockade after short-term use of pancuronium or vecuronium may be

TABLE 2-6 Serum Indicators of Renal Failure

SERUM MEASUREMENTS	NORMAL	RENAL FAILURE
Blood urea nitrogen (BUN)	10 to 20 mg/dL	Increased
Creatinine	0.7 to 1.5 mg/dL	Increased
BUN to creatinine ratio	10:1	Normal or increased
Potassium	3 to 5 mEq/L	Usually increased
Sodium	138 to 142 mEq/L	Usually decreased

✓ Hypoperfusion of the kidneys may affect the rate of drug clearance and lead to a higher drug concentration in the circulation.

prolonged in renal failure. The duration of muscle paralysis may be as long as 7 days after receiving vecuronium for more than 2 days (Hansen-Flaschen et al., 1993). It is therefore essential to note the effects of renal failure and the possibility of prolonged neuromuscular blockade when measuring a patient's lung mechanics or attempting to wean a patient from mechanical ventilation.

Glomerular Filtration Rate (GFR). Decreased renal function caused by positive pressure ventilation may also affect other drugs whose clearance is mainly dependent on the GFR of the kidneys. Glomerular filtration results from high pressure within the glomerulus or renal capillary. This is caused by differences in the tone of the afferent and efferent arterioles, the vessels that lead into and out of the glomerulus. The afferent arteriole is maintained in a somewhat dilated state relative to the efferent arteriole, which is always somewhat constricted. When blood flow to the kidney is normal, a hydrostatic pressure head causes the high rate of renal perfusion seen in the normovolemic state. When coupled with back pressure from the partially constricted efferent arteriole, pressures within the glomerulus are maintained at an elevated state and are responsible for its ultrafiltration function. When renal perfusion drops, the pressure causing glomerular filtration decreases, leading to a decrease in filtration.

Examples of drugs that are eliminated by this mechanism include digoxin, vancomycin, beta-lactam antibiotics, and the aminoglycosides (e.g., gentamycin, tobramycin) (Perkins et al., 1989). A decrease in GFR causes a relatively higher concentration of these drugs in the circulation.

Tubular Secretion. Another group of drugs whose elimination could be reduced by a lower renal blood flow are drugs undergoing tubular secretion. Tubular secretion is the mechanism whereby substances are secreted from the blood via the peritubular capillaries into the renal tubule to become a part of the urine. Examples of drugs that are eliminated by this mechanism include digoxin, furosemide, procainamide, and some penicillins (Perkins et al., 1989). Decrease of renal tubular secretion causes a relatively higher concentration of these drugs in the circulation.

Reabsorption. The third group of drugs whose elimination could be decreased are those being reabsorbed at a higher rate. Reabsorption in the renal tubules is the mechanism whereby required substances that are filtered by the glomerulus are reclaimed by the cells lining the renal tubule and are ultimately reabsorbed into the blood. Some of these substances are reabsorbed down to an equal concentration gradient; thus an enhanced concentration gradient could lead to increased reabsorption.

As cardiac output is reduced by mechanical ventilation, renal blood flow and, thus, urine volume are also reduced. As the urine becomes more concentrated, the drugs in the glomerular filtrate also become more concentrated. This causes an increase in the reabsorption gradient of the drugs in the filtrate. Some of the drugs used in critically ill patients include aminoglycosides, theophylline, and phenobarbital (Perkins et al., 1989). Decreased renal perfusion causes a higher reabsorption rate of these drugs back into the circulation.

HEPATIC CONSIDERATIONS

hepatic perfusion:
Blood flow to the
liver. It is decreased
when the blood
volume or cardiac
output is low.

Hepatic perfusion accounts for about 15% of total cardiac output. Positive pressure ventilation alone does not alter the blood flow to the liver to any significant degree. But when PEEP is added to mechanical ventilation, the blood flow to the liver is noticeably reduced (Bonnet et al., 1982).

PEEP AND HEPATIC PERFUSION

The decrease in hepatic blood flow is inversely related to the level of PEEP. In one study, the hepatic blood flow decreased 3%, 12%, and 32% at PEEP of 10, 15, and 20 cm H_2O, respectively (Bonnet et al., 1982). The decrease in hepatic blood flow is solely caused by a reduction in cardiac output as a result of PEEP. This inference is made because the ratio of hepatic blood flow to cardiac output remains unchanged at 15% during mechanical ventilation without PEEP (Perkins et al., 1989).

INDICATORS OF LIVER DYSFUNCTION

☑ Impairment of liver function is likely when prothrombin time is >4 sec, bilirubin level is ≥50 mg/L, or albumin level is ≤20 g/L.

Liver dysfunction may be monitored by measuring the prothrombin time and bilirubin and albumin levels (Kraus et al., 1993). Impairment of liver function is likely when coagulation time is increased (prothrombin time >4 sec over control, bilirubin level is increased (≥50 mg/L), or albumin level is decreased (≤20 g/L).

EFFECTS OF DECREASED HEPATIC PERFUSION ON DRUG CLEARANCE

☑ Hypoperfusion of the liver may affect the rate of drug clearance and lead to a higher drug concentration in the circulation.

A decrease in hepatic blood flow may diminish the drug clearance mechanism of the liver. Drugs most likely to be affected by changes in hepatic blood flow are agents whose clearance relies on the liver and its perfusion. Examples of such drugs commonly used in the intensive care unit include lidocaine, meperidine, propranolol, and verapamil (Perkins et al., 1989). When hepatic perfusion is inadequate, use of these drugs may lead to a relatively higher serum concentration due to diminished drug clearance.

intra-abdominal pressure (IAP): *Pressure measured by a transducer via a transurethral bladder catheter.*

ABDOMINAL CONSIDERATIONS

Increases in **intra-abdominal pressure (IAP)** are related to clinical conditions such as bowel edema or obstruction and ascites. IAP may also be increased in procedures such as use of pneumatic antishock garments and surgical repair of abdominal wall hernias. When these patients are placed on mechanical ventilation, conditions that are conducive to an increase in IAP should be monitored to avert potential complications.

☑ Elevated intra-abdominal pressure transmits excessive pressure across the diaphragm to the heart and great vessels. In turn, this excess pressure leads to decreased cardiac output and decreased renal perfusion.

EFFECTS OF PEEP AND INCREASED INTRA-ABDOMINAL PRESSURE

An elevated IAP transmits excessive pressure across the diaphragm to the heart and great vessels. In turn, this excessive pressure leads to decreased cardiac output (Cullen et al., 1989) and decreased renal perfusion (Harman et al., 1982). Excessive IAP also compresses the lungs and reduces the functional residual capacity (Burchard et al., 1985).

TABLE 2-7   Effects of PEEP and Increased Intra-abdominal Pressure

SYSTEM	EFFECTS
Cardiovascular	Increased peripheral vascular resistance
	Decreased compliance of ventricles
	Decreased cardiac output
Renal	Decreased renal perfusion
	Decreased glomerular filtration rate
Pulmonary	Decreased functional residual capacity
	Increased atelectasis
	Impaired gas exchange
	Increased V/Q mismatch and venous admixture

It has been shown that use of PEEP on patients with elevated IAP may lead to cardiovascular, renal, and pulmonary dysfunction (Burchard et al., 1985; Cullen et al., 1989; Harman et al., 1982). These types of dysfunction are summarized in Table 2-7.

Use of high levels of PEEP (>15 cm H_2O) in the presence of high IAP (>20 mm Hg) requires caution because of potentiation of the pressures exerted on the heart and great vessels (Sussman et al., 1991). However, the pressures transmitted to the heart and great vessels are not as severe in patients with low pulmonary compliance due to the dampening effects of the noncompliant lungs and chest wall.

gastrointestinal (GI):
Organ system
including the stom-
ach and intestines.

GASTROINTESTINAL CONSIDERATIONS

☑ GI complications may be caused by a decrease in perfusion to the GI tract and medications that are commonly used in mechanically ventilated patients.

Positive pressure ventilation is associated with many organ-system complications and one of which involves the **gastrointestinal (GI)** tract. GI complications in patients who are being mechanically ventilated include erosive esophagitis, stress-related mucosal damage (SRMD), diarrhea, decreased bowel sounds, high gastric residuals, and constipation (Mutlu, 2000). These conditions are likely caused by a decrease in perfusion to the GI tract and medications that are commonly used in mechanically ventilated patients. Morphine sulfate is a medication commonly used for pain control. Some of the GI side effects of morphine include constipation and vomiting. Table 2-8 summarizes the factors that may adversely affect the normal GI functions (Mutlu, 2001).

TABLE 2-8 Major factors adversely affecting normal GI functions

FACTORS	NOTES
Mechanical ventilation (especially with high levels of PEEP)	Increase intrathoracic pressure Increase right atrial pressure Reduce pressure gradient between mean systemic venous and right atrial pressures Reduce cardiac output and GI perfusion
Splanchnic hypoperfusion	Due to decrease mean arterial pressure and/or increased resistance in the GI vascular bed May lead to stress-related mucosal damage (SRMD)
Medications (e.g., opiates, sedatives, vasopressors, antibiotics)	Decrease GI motility Impaired venous return via venodilation and/or diminution of response to vasopressors

NUTRITIONAL CONSIDERATIONS

Malnutrition in critically ill patients can create muscle fatigue, ventilatory insufficiency, and ventilatory failure. This sequence of events can lead to a need for mechanical ventilation. It can also make weaning from mechanical ventilation difficult or unsuccessful. Adequate nutritional support is therefore essential in the management of critically ill patients. However, excessive nutritional support is undesirable since it may cause excessive carbon dioxide production, as well as increased work of breathing in order to eliminate excessive CO_2 (van den Berg & Stam, 1988).

MUSCLE FATIGUE

☑ COPD patients have higher caloric needs because of the increased work of breathing associated with chronic air flow obstruction.

The work of breathing can be affected by mechanical aberrations such as changes in airway resistance and lung or chest wall compliance. In clinical conditions where there is a persistent increase in airway resistance (e.g., COPD) or reduction in compliance (e.g., atelectasis), the respiratory muscles must work strenuously to overcome the abnormal resistance and compliance. For instance, COPD patients use 430 to 720 kcal/day to carry out the work of breathing. This caloric cost of breathing for COPD patients is about 10 times that of normal individuals (normal = 38 to 72 kcal/day) (Brown et al., 1983) because of the increased work of breathing necessary to overcome the high airway resistance and V/Q abnormalities.

Over time, these abnormalities may cause fatigue of the respiratory muscles, and ventilatory failure with concurrent CO_2 retention and hypoxemia (Brown et al., 1994).

Other than the mechanical aberrations that can lead to increased work of breathing and eventual muscle fatigue, there are nonmechanical factors as well. Malnutrition is an example of a nonmechanical cause of muscle fatigue that may lead to ventilatory failure (Fiaccadori et al., 1991).

Table 2-9 shows the major mechanical and nonmechanical factors that may lead to reduced respiratory muscle efficiency and muscle fatigue.

NUTRITIONAL SUPPORT

Adequate nutrition is a therapeutic necessity in order to provide and preserve inspiratory muscle strength and prevent ventilatory failure. Patients who have respiratory disorders are likely to lose weight due to increased work of breathing, decreased nutritional intake, and infectious states causing increased metabolic rate (Mlynarek & Zarowitz, 1987).

Undernutrition in patients with or without COPD is found to deplete their stores of glycogen and protein in the diaphragm. In addition, COPD patients who suffer from decreased protein synthesis

TABLE 2-9   Factors Leading to Respiratory Muscle Fatigue

MECHANICAL FACTORS	NONMECHANICAL FACTORS
High airway resistance	Malnutrition
Low lung compliance	Endocrine diseases (high metabolic rate)
Low chest wall compliance	Electrolyte disorders
	Drugs
	Persistent hypoxemia

(Data from Fiaccadori et al., 1991; Grassino et al., 1984; Rochester, 1986.)

in the diaphragm may lose diaphragm muscle mass (Mlynarek & Zarowitz, 1987). Since the diaphragm is the major respiratory muscle, loss of muscle mass in the diaphragm may reduce the efficiency of ventilation.

It has been demonstrated that patients who receive 2,000 to 3,000 kcal per day exhibit better inspiratory strengths and endurance than those receiving only 400 kcal/day (Bassili et al., 1981). Energy requirements for critically ill patients are normally computed using the Harris-Benedict equation. This equation estimates the *resting energy expenditure* (REE) based on weight, height, age, and sex (Roza et al., 1984). In ventilator patients who are hypermetabolic or hypercatabolic (i.e., infection, trauma, burns), a correction factor is included to allow for additional metabolic needs. It ranges from 1.0 to 1.2 times the REE for maintenance of lean body mass and 1.4 to 1.6 times the REE for restoration of lean body mass (Mlynarek & Zarowitz, 1987).

total parenteral nutrition (TPN): *Complete nutritional support provided to the patient by any method (usually intravenous) other than the intestinal route.*

✔ Since fat emulsion provides 9.1 kcal/g, it provides maximum caloric intake with minimum CO_2 production.

NUTRITION AND THE WORK OF BREATHING

Total parenteral nutrition (TPN) or hyperalimentation is a complete nutritional program provided to patients by any method (usually intravenous) other than the intestinal route. It is often used to support and supplement a patient's nutritional needs with a hypertonic solution consisting of amino acids, glucose, vitamins, electrolytes, and fat emulsion. When TPN is used, it is essential to keep the amount of dextrose (a form of glucose) to a minimum as it can cause lipogenesis and increase O_2 consumption and CO_2 production. Contribution to the total caloric needs by glucose should be in the range of 40% to 60% (Brown et al., 1984).

Since hydrous dextrose generates 3.4 kcal/g and fat emulsion provides 9.1 kcal/g, fat is the ideal source of energy for patients who have restricted fluid intake. Fat also reduces CO_2 production, a by-product of glucose metabolism, thus reducing the work of breathing (Brown et al., 1983). A fat-based TPN should be considered for patients with significant or persistent CO_2 retention as fat emulsion may provide maximum caloric intake with minimum CO_2 production.

It is important to note that the work of breathing is significantly increased in patients receiving high caloric intake by means of TPN. The increase in work of breathing is primarily due to increases in oxygen consumption and carbon dioxide production during TPN (van den Berg & Stam, 1988). Mechanical ventilation and weaning strategies must take this fact into account in order to provide adequate support for a patient's ventilatory needs.

The increase in $\dot{V}CO_2$ causes a rise in $PaCO_2$, resulting in respiratory acidosis. Ventilatory failure can occur if the patient is unable to increase ventilation in proportion to the increase of CO_2 production. This is particularly important in patients with impaired ventilatory reserves such as those with obstructive or restrictive lung diseases.

NEUROLOGIC CONSIDERATIONS

Among many other monitoring systems that influence the respiratory drive, the central and peripheral chemoreceptors respond rapidly to the levels of CO_2, $H+$, and O_2 in the blood. For this reason, the degree of ventilation (CO_2, $H+$) and oxygenation (O_2) can affect the normal functions of the brain.

HYPERVENTILATION

☑ Sustained hyperventilation of less than 24 hours causes respiratory alkalosis and reduces cerebral blood flow and intracranial pressure.

Carbon dioxide acts as a vasodilator in cerebral blood vessels. During mechanical ventilation, intentional hyperventilation is sometimes used to constrict these blood vessels, and thus minimize intracranial pressure in patients with head injury. Sustained hyperventilation of less than 24 hours causes respiratory alkalosis, reducing cerebral blood flow and intracranial pressure. After 24 hours, the buffer systems of the body return the pH toward normal, negating the vasoconstrictor effect of controlled hyperventilation.

☑ 2,3-bisphospho-glycerate (2,3-BPG) is also known as 2,3-diphospho-glycerate P (2,3-DPG)

If hyperventilation is prolonged, cerebral tissue hypoxia may result due to the leftward shift of the oxyhemoglobin curve. A left shift causes higher oxygen affinity for hemoglobin but reduced oxygen release to tissues. Sustained hyperventilation also produces significant hypophosphatemia because of movement of phosphate into the cells. Hypophosphatemia interferes with cerebral tissue metabolism by reducing ATP stores and 2,3-BPG levels, which further increases the leftward shift of the oxyhemoglobin curve (Jozefowicz, 1989). Table 2-10 summarizes the neurologic changes in short-term (<24 hours) and sustained (>24 hours) hyperventilation.

VENTILATORY AND OXYGENATION FAILURE

Ventilatory and oxygenation failure has serious and detrimental effects on the central nervous system (CNS). Such failure may occur in patients on mechanical ventilation because of preexisting clinical conditions,

TABLE 2-10   Neurologic Changes in Hyperventilation

CONDITION	PATHOPHYSIOLOGIC CHANGES
Respiratory alkalosis (< 24 hours)	Decreased cerebral blood flow Reduced intracranial pressure
Respiratory alkalosis (Prolonged > 24 hours)	Leftward shift of oxyhemoglobin curve Increased O_2 affinity for hemoglobin Reduced O_2 release to tissues Cerebral tissue hypoxia Neurologic dysfunction Hypophosphatemia

making ventilation and oxygenation extremely difficult to accomplish in spite of high F_1O_2 and PEEP.

Abnormalities in ventilation and gas exchange can cause hypercapnia (increase in $PaCO_2$), respiratory acidosis (decrease in pH as a result of the increased $PaCO_2$), hypoxemia (decrease in PaO_2), secondary polycythemia (increase in red blood cell concentration and thus hemoglobin level), and electrolyte disturbances. These changes may lead to neurologic impairment.

☑ Headache, mental status changes, motor disturbances, and ocular abnormalities may be signs of neurologic impairment.

INDICATORS OF NEUROLOGIC IMPAIRMENT

When neurologic functions are impaired due to ventilatory and oxygenation failure, the patient may experience headache, mental status changes, motor disturbances, and ocular abnormalities (Jozefowicz, 1989).

The patient usually describes the headache as "pressure in the head" having a higher intensity during night and early morning hours. The headache is the result of cerebral vasodilation in response to hypoventilation and CO_2 retention during sleep.

Hypoxia, hypercapnia, and acidosis are responsible for the changes in a patient's mental status. Early mental disturbances include drowsiness, forgetfulness, and irritability. In severe or chronic cases of hypoxia and hypercapnia, stupor and coma may occur.

Hypercapnia may also cause muscle tremor and ocular abnormalities. Muscle tremor is the result of excessive stimulation of the sympathetic nervous system and catecholamine release from the adrenal medulla. Ocular abnormalities such as papilledema, swelling of the area where the optic nerve exits the back of the eye, is the result of cerebral vasodilation and elevated intracranial pressure. Table 2-11 illustrates some neurologic changes in hypercapnia and hypoxemia.

TABLE 2-11   Neurologic Changes in Hypercapnia and Hypoxemia

CONDITION	PHYSIOLOGIC CHANGES
Hypercapnia (with normal pH)	Increased cerebral blood flow Increased intracranial pressure
Hypercapnia (with low pH) Hypoxemia	Impaired cerebral metabolism Decreased mental and motor functions

SUMMARY

Positive pressure ventilation is beneficial to support a patient's ventilatory and oxygenation needs. However, it has many inherent physiologic side effects on other organ systems. When caring for critically ill patients with positive pressure ventilation, it is vital to observe and monitor the patients carefully for occurrence of side effects. If side effects and their causes are identified, appropriate strategies should be used to resolve them.

Self-Assessment Questions

1. During the inspiratory phase of positive pressure ventilation, gas flows into the lung because the pressure in the:

   A. airway is higher than the pressure in the lungs.
   B. airway is lower than the pressure in the lungs.
   C. lungs is higher than the barometric pressure.
   D. lungs and airway are the same.

2. A neonate is being ventilated by a pressure-limited ventilator. The physician asks you to adjust the ventilator to increase the patient's mechanical tidal volume. You would:

   A. increase the tidal volume setting.
   B. increase the pressure setting.
   C. decrease the flow rate.
   D. decrease the inspiratory time.

3. A postoperative patient is recovering in the intensive care unit on a volume-limited ventilator. For a volume-limited ventilator, the _____ is preset with a variable _____ depending on the compliance and airway resistance characteristics.

   A. peak inspiratory pressure, tidal volume
   B. peak inspiratory pressure, peak flow
   C. tidal volume, peak inspiratory pressure
   D. tidal volume, peak flow

4. Positive pressure ventilation decreases the oxygen delivery to a patient with normal hemodynamic status because it causes all of the following changes *except*:

   A. increase in intrathoracic pressure.   C. increase in pulmonary blood flow.
   B. reduction in stroke volume.   D. decrease in cardiac output.

5. In children with right ventricular dysfunction, the thoracic pump mechanism _____ the outflow of blood from the _____ ventricle.

   A. increases, left   C. increases, right
   B. decreases, left   D. decreases, right

6 to 11. For *positive pressure ventilation*, match the volume and pressure changes with the respective reasons.

PRESSURE OR VOLUME CHANGES	REASONS
6. *Increase* in intrathoracic pressure	A. Decreased venous return to right ventricle leads to lower right ventricular output.
7. *Decrease* in venous return or central venous pressure	B. Decreased right ventricular stroke volume and pulmonary artery pressure lead to lower left ventricular input and output.
8. *Decrease* in right ventricular stroke volume	C. Higher intrathoracic pressure impedes systemic blood return to right ventricle.
9. *Decrease* in pulmonary arterial pressure	D. Positive pressure applied to the lungs causes compression against the chest wall.
10. *Decrease* in ventricular filling pressures	E. Decreased right ventricular stroke volume leads to lower blood volume (pressure) in the pulmonary arteries.
11. *Decrease* in left ventricular stroke volume	F. Lower blood volume entering and leaving the ventricles.

12 to 15. For *positive end-expiratory pressure,* match the pressure and cardiac output changes with the respective reasons. You may use any answer *more than once.*

PRESSURE OR CARDIAC OUTPUT CHANGES	REASONS
12. *Increase* in pulmonary artery pressure	A. Increase in pulmonary artery pressure causes a higher right ventricular pressure and hinders the blood return from systemic circulation to right heart. This causes backup of blood flow and increase in pressure in the systemic venous circulation.
13. *Increase* in central venous pressure (CVP)	B. This is due to the significant increase in intrathoracic pressure and significant *decrease* in left and right ventricular stroke volumes.
14. *Decrease* in aortic pressure	C. PEEP and positive pressure applied to the lungs cause significant compression of pulmonary blood vessels.
15. *Decrease* in cardiac output	

16. A patient in the renal dialysis unit has recently been placed on a ventilator because of ventilatory and oxygenation failure. In caring for this patient, which of the following laboratory results would indicate that the patient's renal functions are failing?

   A. blood urea nitrogen of 30 mg/dL
   B. creatinine of 1.0 mg/dL

   C. potassium of 3 mEq/L
   D. sodium of 140 mEq/L

17. For patients with renal _____ or failure, the drug concentration in the circulation is usually _____ than normal when clearance of those drugs is dependent on proper renal perfusion.

   A. hyperperfusion, higher
   B. hyperperfusion, lower

   C. hypoperfusion, higher
   D. hypoperfusion, lower

18. Perfusion to the liver is usually affected by a high level of _____ and hepatic failure may be present when the _____.

   A. positive pressure ventilation; bilirubin level is less than 50 mg/L.

   B. positive pressure ventilation; albumin level is less than 20 mg/L.

   C. positive end-expiratory pressure; bilirubin level is greater than 50 mg/L.

   D. positive end-expiratory pressure; albumin level is greater than 20 mg/L.

19. Cardiovascular, renal, and pulmonary dysfunction may occur in patients with an intra-abdominal pressure _____ when positive end-expiratory pressure _____ is used during mechanical ventilation.

   A. greater than 15 mm Hg; greater than 15 cm H_2O
   B. greater than 20 mm Hg; greater than 15 cm H_2O
   C. less than 15 mm Hg; greater than 15 cm H_2O
   D. greater than 20 mm Hg; less than 15 cm H_2O

20. Gastrointestinal (GI) complications during mechanical ventilation may be caused by all of the following conditions *except*:

   A. increased intrathoracic pressure.
   B. increased cardiac output.
   C. hypoperfusion of the GI viscera.
   D. use of opiates and sedatives.

21. For patients with increased work of breathing and CO_2 retention, the caloric intake should be _____ than normal and the source of nutrition should be _____ based so as to provide maximum calorie intake and minimum CO_2 production.

   A. higher; fat
   B. higher; dextrose
   C. lower; fat
   D. lower; dextrose

22. Hyperventilation is sometimes provided for patients with increased intracranial pressure. This is done because respiratory _____ can reduce the intracranial pressure by _____ the cerebral blood vessels.

   A. acidosis; dilating
   B. acidosis; constricting
   C. alkalosis; dilating
   D. alkalosis; constricting

23. Headache, drowsiness, and irritability are some signs of altered _____ status resulting from hypoxemia and hypercapnia.

   A. renal
   B. hepatic
   C. nutritional
   D. neurologic

Answers to Self-Assessment Questions

1. A. airway is higher than the pressure in the lungs

2. B. increase the pressure setting.

3. C. tidal volume, peak inspiratory pressure

4. C. increase of pulmonary blood flow.

5. C. increases, right

6. D. Positive pressure applied to the lungs causes compression against the chest wall.

7. C. Higher intrathoracic pressure impedes systemic blood return to right ventricle.

8. A. Decreased venous return to right ventricle leads to lower right ventricular output.

9. E. Decreased right ventricular stroke volume leads to lower blood volume (pressure) in the pulmonary arteries.

10. F. Lower blood volume entering and leaving the ventricles.

11. B. Decreased right ventricular stroke volume and pulmonary artery pressure lead to lower left ventricular input and output.

12. C. PEEP and positive pressure applied to the lungs cause significant compression of pulmonary blood vessels.

13. A. Increase in pulmonary artery pressure causes a higher right ventricular pressure and hinders the blood return from systemic circulation to right heart. This causes backup of blood flow and increase of pressure in the systemic venous circulation.

14. B. This is due to the significant increase in intrathoracic pressure and significant *decrease* in left and right ventricular stroke volumes.

15. B. This is due to the significant increase in intrathoracic pressure and significant *decrease* in left and right ventricular stroke volumes.

16. A. Blood urea nitrogen of 30 mg/dL

17. C. hypoperfusion, higher

18. C. positive end-expiratory pressure, bilirubin level is greater than 50 mg/L.

19. B. greater than 20 mm Hg, greater than 15 cm H_2O

20. B. increased cardiac output.

21. A. higher, fat

22. D. alkalosis, constricting

23. D. neurologic

References

Abel, J. G., et al. (1987). Cardiovascular effects of positive pressure ventilation in humans. *Ann Thorac Surg, 43,* 198–206.

Baer, C. L., et al. (1992). Acute renal failure. *Crit Care Nurs Q, 14*(4), 1.

Bassili, H. R., et al. (1981). Effect of nutritional support on weaning patients off mechanical ventilators. *J Parenter Enter Nutr, 5,* 161–163.

Bonnet, F., et al. (1982). Changes in hepatic flow induced by continuous positive-pressure ventilation in critically ill patients. *Crit Care Med, 10,* 703–705.

Brown, B. R. (1994). Understanding mechanical ventilation: Indications for and initiation of therapy. *J Okla State Med Assoc, 87,* 353–357.

Brown, R. O., et al. (1984). Nutrition and respiratory disease. *Clin Pharm, 3,* 152–160.

Brown, S. E., et al. (1983). What is now known about protein-energy depletion: When COPD patients are malnourished. *J Respir Dis, 4*(5), 36–50.

Brundage, D. J. (1992). *Renal disorders.* St. Louis, MO: Mosby.

Burchard, K. W., et al. (1985). Positive end-expiratory pressure with increased intra-abdominal pressure. *Surg Gynecol Obstet, 161,* 313–318.

Cullen, D. J., et al. (1989). Cardiovascular, pulmonary and renal effect of massively increased intra-abdominal pressure in critically ill patients. *Crit Care Med, 17,* 118–121.

DiCarlo, J. V., et al. (1994). Respiratory failure in congenital heart disease. *Pediatr Clin North Am, 41*(3), 525–542.

Fiaccadori, E., et al. (1991). Pathophysiology of respiratory muscles in course of under-nutrition. *Ann Ital Med Int, 6,* 402–407.

Grassino, A., et al. (1984). Respiratory muscle fatigue and ventilatory failure. *Am Rev Respir Dis, 35,* 625–647.

Hansen-Flaschen, J., et al. (1993). Neuromuscular blockade in the intensive care unit—More than we bargained for. *Am Rev Respir Dis, 147,* 234–236.

Harman, P. K., et al. (1982). Elevated intra-abdominal pressure and renal function. *Ann Surg, 196,* 594–597.

Jozefowicz, R. F. (1989). Neurologic manifestations of pulmonary disease. *Neurol Clin, 7*(3), 605–616.

King, B. A. (1994, March). Detecting acute renal failure. *RN, 57*(3), 34–40.

Kraus, P. A., et al. (1993). Acute lung injury at Baragwanath ICU—An eight-month audit and call for consensus for other organ failure in the adult respiratory distress syndrome. *Chest, 103*(6),1832–1836.

Marini, J. J., (2004). *Critical care medicine: The essentials* (*3rd* ed.). Baltimore: Lippincott Williams & Wilkins.

Mlynarek, M., & Zarowitz, B. J. (1987). Individualizing nutrition in patients with acute respiratory failure requiring mechanical ventilation. *Drug Intell Clin Pharm (EBU), 21*(11), 865–870.

Mutlu, G. M., et al. (2000). Complications of mechanical ventilation, *Respir Care Clin North Am, 6*, 213–252.

Mutlu, G. M., et al. (2001). GI complications in patients receiving mechanical ventilation, *Chest, 119*(4), 1222–1241.

Perkins, M. W., et al. (1989). Physiologic implications of mechanical ventilation on pharmacokinetics. *DICP, Ann Pharmacother, 23,* 316–323.

Pinsky, M. R. (1990). The effects of mechanical ventilation on the cardiovascular system. *Crit Care Clin, 6*(3), 663–678.

Rochester, D. F. (1986). Respiratory effects of respiratory muscle weakness and atrophy. *Am Rev Respir Dis, 134,* 1083–1086.

Roza, A. M., et al. (1984). The Harris-Benedict equation reevaluated: Resting energy requirements and the body cell mass. *Am J Clin Nutr, 40,* 168–182.

Sussman, A. M., et al. (1991). Effect of positive end-expiratory pressure on intra-abdominal pressure. *Southern Med J, 84*(6), 697–700.

van den Berg, B., & Stam, H. (1988). Metabolic and respiratory effects of enteral nutrition in patients during mechanical ventilation. *Intensive Care Med, 14,* 206–211.

Versprille, A. (1990). The pulmonary circulation during mechanical ventilation. *Acta Anaesthesiol Scand, 34, Suppl. 94,* 51–62.

Wilkins, R. L., et al. (2003). *Egan's fundamentals of respiratory care* (8th ed.). St. Louis, MO: Mosby.

Wright, R. O., et al. (1996) Continuous, noninvasive measurement of pulsus paradoxus in patients with acute asthma. *Arch Pediatr Adoles Med, 150*(9), 914–918.

CHAPTER THREE

CLASSIFICATION OF MECHANICAL VENTILATORS

Gary C. White

OUTLINE

Introduction

Ventilator Classification

Ventilatory Work

Input Power

Drive Mechanism
Piston Drive Mechanism
Bellows Drive Mechanism
Reducing Valve Drive Mechanism
Microprocessor-Controlled
    Pneumatic Drive Mechanism

Control Circuit
Mechanical
Pneumatic
Fluidics
Electric
Electronic

Control Variables
Pressure Controller
Volume Controller
Flow Controller
Time Controller

Phase Variables
Trigger Variable
Limit Variable
Cycle Variable
Baseline Variable
Conditional Variable

Output Waveforms
Pressure Waveforms
Volume Waveforms
Flow Waveforms

Alarm Systems
Input Power Alarms
Control Circuit Alarms
Output Alarms

Summary

Self-Assessment Questions

Answers to Self-Assessment Questions

Suggested Reading

KEY TERMS

- compressor
- controller
- cycle
- flow triggered
- microprocessor
- pneumatic drive mechanism

- pressure triggered
- reducing valve
- servo
- sine wave
- solenoid valve
- time triggered

INTRODUCTION

The role of patient management in many situations is dependent on the respiratory care practitioner's understanding of mechanical ventilators and their characteristics. This applies to the acute care setting for all ages: adults, pediatrics, and neonatal patients. The same is also true in the transport and long-term care environments. Therefore, it is important for the respiratory care practitioner to understand classification of mechanical ventilators and the design characteristics employed by a ventilator to achieve the task of supporting a patient's ventilation.

In this chapter, you learn how ventilators are classified according to Chatburn's classification system and how the common ventilators employed in various patient care settings are classified.

VENTILATOR CLASSIFICATION

Ventilator technology has evolved since the introduction of Engström 100, the first volume-controlled mechanical ventilator in 1951. Since that time, a multitude of manufacturers have produced and marketed ventilators of all sizes, descriptions, and capabilities. Many manufacturers have coined new terms to describe their ventilators and to accentuate how their product is different from the others. Several different ventilator classification systems may be employed to describe mechanical ventilators. The majority of these systems focus on the differences between ventilators rather than the similarities.

Robert Chatburn (1992) has proposed a new way to classify mechanical ventilators based on related features, physics, and engineering. Chatburn's ventilator classification system has been featured in several articles and textbooks. It allows flexibility as ventilator technology evolves in contrast to other systems that employ more narrowly defined design principles or rely to a greater extent on manufacturer's terms.

With the evolution of ventilator technology over the next decade or more, the flexibility of Chatburn's classification system will be validated as it is increasingly adopted by practitioners. This author believes this system is important enough to include in this text and others that describe ventilator operational characteristics. Students and practitioners learning about this classification system should refer to the ("Suggested Reading" section) at the end of this chapter and read Chatburn's original contributions (Chatburn, 1991, 1992, 2001).

VENTILATORY WORK

Pulmonary physiologists have described the work ventilatory muscles perform during inspiration, and how muscles can actively assist during exhalation. During inspiration, the primary ventilatory muscles cause the size (volume) of the thoracic cage to increase, overcoming the elastic forces of the lungs and thorax and the resistance of the airways. As the volume of the thoracic cage increases, intrapleural pressure becomes more negative, resulting in lung expansion as the visceral pleura expands with the parietal pleura. Gas flows from the atmosphere into the lungs as a result of the transairway pressure gradient. During expiration, the muscles of inspiration relax. The elastic forces of the lung and thorax cause the chest to decrease in volume. Exhalation occurs as a result of the greater pressure at the alveolus when compared to atmospheric pressure. All of this muscle activity to overcome the elastic and resistance properties of the lungs and thorax requires energy and work.

The work that the muscles and/or the ventilator must perform is proportional to the pressure required for inspiration times the tidal volume. The pressure required to deliver the tidal volume is referred to as the *load* either the muscles or the ventilator must work against. There is an elastic load (proportional to volume and inversely proportional to compliance) and a resistance load (proportional to airway resistance and inspiratory flow). These variables are related by the equation of motion for the respiratory system:

$$\text{Muscle Pressure} + \text{Ventilator Pressure} = \frac{\text{Volume}}{\text{Compliance}} + (\text{Resistance} \times \text{Flow})$$

Compliance is defined as a change in volume divided by a change in pressure, which is a measure of the elastic forces of the lungs and thorax. Flow, as defined earlier, is a unit of volume divided by a unit of time. Resistance is the force that must be overcome to move gas through the conducting airways, which is best described by Poiseuille's Law.

A mechanical ventilator is simply a machine or device that can fully or partially substitute for the ventilatory work accomplished by the patient's muscles. If the patient's ventilatory muscles contribute no work (sedation, paralysis, etc.), the mechanical ventilator provides full ventilatory support. If the patient's muscles are able to sustain all of the patient's ventilatory requirements, no support is provided by the machine and ventilatory support is zero. Between the two extremes, partial support can be provided by the mechanical ventilator in assisting the ventilatory muscles.

INPUT POWER

Mechanical ventilators may be first classified as to the power source that is used to provide the energy required to support the patient's ventilation. As described earlier, ventilation requires work and therefore, energy.

Pneumatically powered ventilators use compressed gas as an energy source for their operation. Medical gases are anhydrous, and oil free at a pressure of 50 psi. Examples of ventilators that utilize pneumatic power include the Bennett PR-2, Bird Mark 7, Percussionaire IPV, Monaghan 225/SIMV, and the Percussionaire VDR.

Ventilators may also be electrically powered, utilizing 120 V 60 Hz alternating current (AC) or 12 V direct current (DC) for a power source. The electrical power can be used to run electric motors to drive pistons, **compressors,** or other mechanical devices that generate gas flow. Examples of electrically powered ventilators include the Emerson 3-MV, Puritan Bennett LP-10 and LP-20, and the Bear Medical Systems Bear 33.

Some ventilators are powered by a combination of both pneumatic and electric power sources. Many third-generation ventilators require both an electrical (for **microprocessor** control systems) and pneumatic power source. These ventilators include the BEAR 1000, Hamilton Veolar, Puritan-Bennett 840, and others.

DRIVE MECHANISM

The drive mechanism is the system used by the ventilator to transmit or convert the input power to useful ventilatory work. The type of drive mechanism determines the characteristic flow and pressure patterns each ventilator produces. The use of microprocessors and proportional **solenoid valves** allows these newer ventilators to produce a variety of user-selected inspiratory flow or pressure patterns. An understanding of the different drive mechanisms will allow you to apply a ventilator more effectively in the clinical environment. Drive mechanisms include pistons, bellows, **reducing valves,** and pneumatic circuits.

compressor: *A device capable of building up pressure by compressing the volume of air.*

microprocessor: *Minute computer that is designed to perform specific functions.*

solenoid valve: *A valve controlled by an electronic switching device that is used to regulate the specific functions of a ventilator.*

reducing valve: *A device that decreases the delivery pressure of a gas.*

Figure 3-1 A schematic diagram of a rotary-driven piston drive mechanism for a mechanical ventilator.

PISTON DRIVE MECHANISM

An electrically driven piston with an inspiratory one-way valve can be used to generate a pressure gradient to drive a ventilator (Figure 3-1). During the backstroke of the piston, gas enters the cylinder through the one-way valve. When the piston travels in the opposite direction, a second one-way valve opens, delivering the compressed gas to the patient.

Pistons are usually electrically powered. However, they may be rotary or linear driven. Figure 3-2 compares a linear-driven and

Figure 3-2 A comparison between (A) a rotary-driven piston and (B) a linear-driven piston drive mechanism for a mechanical ventilator.

Figure 3-3 A bellows drive mechanism for a mechanical ventilator.

rotary-driven piston. Output waveforms, which are discussed later in this chapter, vary depending on how the piston is driven.

BELLOWS DRIVE MECHANISM
Ventilators may also use a bellows to compress the gas for delivery to the patient (Figure 3-3). A bellows may be compressed by a spring, a weight, or by gas pressure if it is in a sealed chamber. A one-way valve admits gas to the bellows expanding the bellows. When it is compressed, the one-way valve closes, causing gas delivery to the patient.

REDUCING VALVE DRIVE MECHANISM
A reducing valve may be used to drive a ventilator and to provide enough of a pressure gradient to cause ventilation. The Bennett PR-2 is one example of a ventilator that uses a reducing valve.

MICROPROCESSOR-CONTROLLED PNEUMATIC DRIVE MECHANISM
Although technically both pistons and bellows are pneumatic systems, a separate classification is required for the newer ventilators that use proportional solenoid valves and microprocessor controls. Current

generation ventilators use programmed algorithms in the microprocessors to open and close the solenoid valves to mimic virtually any flow or pressure wave pattern.

This is called a microprocessor-controlled **pneumatic drive mechanism.** Furthermore, with advances in clinical medicine, the microprocessors can be reprogrammed to deliver new patterns that may not yet be described in the literature. Ventilator manufacturers, using microprocessors and the associated proportional solenoid valves, have greater flexibility in designing and updating ventilator technology.

pneumatic drive mechanism: Operation of a ventilator with pressurized gas as a power source.

CONTROL CIRCUIT

The control circuit is the system that governs or controls the ventilator drive mechanism or output control valve. The control circuit is the system that is responsible for the characteristic output waveforms that will be discussed later in this chapter. Control circuits may be classified as open or closed loop control circuits, mechanical, pneumatic, fluidic, electric, and electronic.

An open loop control circuit is one where the desired output is selected and the ventilator achieves the desired output without any further input from the clinician or the ventilator itself.

A closed loop control circuit is one where the desired output is selected and then the ventilator measures a specific parameter or variable (flow, pressure, or volume) continuously, and the input is constantly adjusted to match the desired output. This type of control circuit may also be referred to as **servo** controlled.

servo: A feedback system that typically consists of a sensing element, an amplifier, and a servomotor, used in the automatic control of the mechanical device of a ventilator.

MECHANICAL
Mechanical control circuits employ simple machines such as levers, pulleys, or cams to control the drive mechanism. Early mechanical ventilators used these systems to control their outputs. Being mechanical, some of these control systems were very durable but lacked flexibility by being an open loop type control system.

PNEUMATIC
Pneumatic devices can be used as control circuits. These devices include valves, nozzles, ducted ejectors, and diaphragms. The IPPB ventilators and the Percussionaire IPV and VDR ventilators all use pneumatic control circuits.

FLUIDICS
Fluidics is the application of gas flow and pressure to control the direction other gas flows and to perform logic functions. The logic functions of fluidics have their origin in digital electronics. Fluidic elements, just as do digital electronic gates, control their outputs according to the

Figure 3-4   A schematic illustrating the Coanda effect.

inputs received. By combining fluidic elements in specific ways, a flu-idic ventilator (e.g. Monaghan 225) can be designed to function in a sim-ilar way to other ventilators that are electronically controlled.

Fluidic elements operate using the Coanda effect. If a jet of gas exits at high velocity adjacent to a wall (Figure 3-4), the gas flow will attach to the adjacent wall. An area of reduced pressure forms a sepa-ration bubble, which attaches the flow to the adjacent surface. Fluidic elements use a flow splitter located beside adjacent walls to control the direction of flow and to perform logic functions (Figure 3-5).

ELECTRIC
Electric control circuits use simple switches to control the drive mech-anism. Some home care ventilators control tidal volume delivery using electric switches to control the travel limit of the piston that

Figure 3-5   A schematic illustrating a fluidic flow splitter.

drives the ventilator. The Emerson 3-MV ventilator uses two micro-switches to control the inspiratory and expiratory time.

ELECTRONIC

Electronic devices such as resistors, diodes, transistors, integrated circuits, and microprocessors can be used to provide sophisticated levels of control over the drive mechanisms of contemporary ventilators. Electronic control systems provide greater flexibility but often at the expense of complexity.

CONTROL VARIABLES

When providing ventilatory support, the mechanical ventilator can control four primary variables during inspiration. These four variables are pressure, volume, flow, and time. Figure 3-6 illustrates an algorithm that can be applied to determine which variable the ventilator is controlling.

PRESSURE CONTROLLER

controller: The mechanism that provides a mode of ventilation within a specific parameter (pressure, time, volume, or flow).

A ventilator is classified as a pressure **controller** if the ventilator controls the transrespiratory system pressure (airway pressure minus body surface pressure). Further classification of a ventilator as a positive or negative pressure ventilator depends on whether the airway pressure rises above baseline (positive) or body surface pressure is lowered below baseline (negative).

A positive pressure ventilator applies pressure inside the chest to expand it. This type of ventilator requires the use of a tight-fitting

Figure 3-6 Criteria for determining the control variable during a ventilator-assisted inspiration. (From R. L. Chatburn (1991). *Respir Care, 36*(10). Used with permission.)

Figure 3-7 A schematic illustrating positive pressure ventilation.

mask, or more commonly, an artificial airway. A pressure greater than atmospheric pressure is applied to the lungs, causing them to expand (Figure 3-7). Once positive pressure is no longer applied, the patient is allowed to exhale passively to ambient pressure. Exhalation occurs because of the pressure differential between the lungs and the atmosphere and through the elastic recoil of the lungs and thorax. This is the type of ventilator most commonly used today.

Negative pressure ventilators apply subatmospheric pressure outside of the chest to inflate the lungs. The negative pressure causes the chest wall to expand, and the pressure difference between the lungs and the atmosphere causes air to flow into the lungs (Figure 3-8). Once negative pressure is no longer applied, the patient is allowed to exhale passively to ambient pressure. Positive pressure may also be applied to further assist the patient during exhalation.

Regardless of whether a ventilator is classified as positive or negative pressure, the lungs expand as a result of the positive transrespiratory system pressures generated. It is the transrespiratory pressure gradient that largely determines the depth or volume of inspiration. A typical pressure controller is unaffected by changes in the patient's compliance or resistance. That is, the pressure level that is delivered to the patient will not vary in spite of changes in patient compliance or resistance.

Figure 3-8 A schematic illustrating negative pressure ventilation.

VOLUME CONTROLLER

To be classified as a volume controller, volume must be measured and used as a feedback signal to control the output (volume) delivered. A volume controller allows pressure to vary with changes in resistance and compliance while volume delivery remains constant.

Volume controllers can measure volume by the displacement of the piston or bellows that serves as the ventilator's drive mechanism. If the displacement of the bellows or piston is controlled, volume therefore is also controlled. Examples of this type of ventilator include the Bennett MA-1 and MA-2+2 and the Emerson 3-MV. The Bennett ventilators control bellows displacement whereas the Emerson 3-MV controls piston displacement. Another way to control volume is to measure flow and turn it into a volume signal electronically.

FLOW CONTROLLER

Flow controllers allow pressure to vary with changes in the patient's compliance and resistance while directly measuring and controlling flow. Flow may be measured by vortex sensors, heated wire grids, venturi pneumotachometers, strain gauge flow sensors, and other devices. What is important is that the ventilator directly measures flow and uses the flow signal as a feedback signal to control its output.

Many ventilators are incorrectly classified as *volume ventilators*. Even though a tidal volume is set or displayed, many ventilators measure flow and then derive volume from the flow measurement [Volume (L) = Flow (L/sec) $\times$ Inspiratory Time (sec)]. However, if a ventilator is operated in pressure support or pressure control mode, the ventilator then becomes a pressure controller, since pressure is the variable that is measured and controlled.

TIME CONTROLLER

Time controllers are ventilators that measure and control inspiratory and expiratory time. These ventilators allow pressure and volume to vary with changes in pulmonary compliance and resistance. Since neither pressure or volume is directly measured or used as a control signal, time (inspiratory, expiratory, or both) remains the only variable that may be controlled.

PHASE VARIABLES

A ventilator-supported breath may be divided into four distinct phases: (1) the change from expiration to inspiration, (2) inspiration, (3) the change from inspiration to expiration, and (4) expiration. More detail can be learned by studying what occurs to the four variables (pressure, volume, flow, and time) during these phases. When the variable is examined during a particular phase, it is termed a *phase variable*.

TRIGGER VARIABLE

The trigger variable is the variable that determines the start of inspiration. Pressure, volume, flow, or time may be measured by the ventilator and used as a variable to initiate inspiration. Many ventilators may use time or pressure as trigger variables.

time triggered: Initiation of a mechanical breath based on the set time interval for one complete respiratory cycle (inspiratory time and expiratory time).

Control: Time Triggered.   A **time-triggered** breath is initiated and delivered by the ventilator when a preset time interval has elapsed. The respiratory rate control on the ventilator is a time-triggering mechanism.

For example, if the ventilator respiratory rate is preset at 12 breaths per minute (60 sec), the time-triggering interval for each complete breath is 5 sec. At this time-trigger interval, the ventilator automatically delivers one mechanical breath every 5 sec without regard to the patient's breathing effort or requirement.

60 sec/12 breaths = 5 sec/breath

pressure triggered: Initiation of a mechanical breath based on the drop in airway pressure that occurs at the beginning of a spontaneous inspiratory effort.

✓ Comparing to a sensitivity setting of −3 cm H₂O, −5 cm H₂O requires *more* patient effort to trigger the ventilator to inspiration.

Pressure Triggered.   A **pressure-triggered** breath is initiated and delivered by the ventilator when it senses the patient's spontaneous (negative pressure) inspiratory effort. The patient may trigger the ventilator by generating a pressure gradient or a flow gradient.

Pressure triggering uses the drop in airway pressure that occurs at the beginning of a spontaneous inspiratory effort to signal the ventilator to begin inspiration (Figure 3-9). The amount of negative pressure, below the patient's baseline airway pressure (or end-expiratory pressure), a patient must generate to trigger the ventilator into inspiration is the sensitivity level. The range of acceptable sensitivity levels for pressure triggering varies from -1 to -5 cm H_2O below the patient's baseline pressure.

For example, if the sensitivity for pressure triggering is set at -3 cm H_2O, then the patient must generate a pressure of -3 cm H_2O at the airway opening to trigger the ventilator into inspiration. If the sensitivity for pressure triggering is changed from -3 to -5 cm H_2O, the ventilator becomes *less* sensitive to the patient's inspiratory effort as more effort is needed to trigger the ventilator into inspiration. Changing the sensitivity from -3 to -5 cm H_2O is *decreasing* the sensitivity setting on the ventilator.

In situations where auto-PEEP is present, the triggering pressure would become greater. In order for the ventilator to sense a successful triggering effort, the patient must overcome both the auto-PEEP level and the sensitivity setting. See Figure 12-2 (Chapter 12) for further discussion on auto-PEEP and the strategy to compensate for the effects of auto-PEEP.

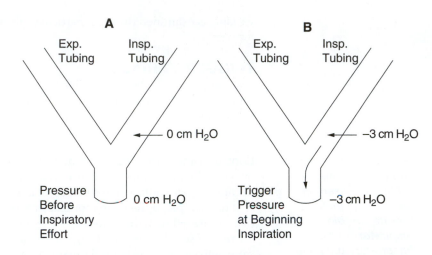

Figure 3-9 Pressure-trigger mechanism. (A) Before an inspiratory effort, the pressure in the airway and ventilator tubing equals 0 cm H_2O. A mechanical breath is not initiated because there is no pressure drop to trigger the ventilator sensitivity settings. (B) At beginning inspiration, the pressure in the airway and ventilator tubing is −3 cm H_2O. A mechanical breath is initiated because the pressure drop is sufficient to trigger the ventilator sensitivity setting (assuming it is set as −3 cm H_2O or less).

flow triggered:
Flow-triggering strategy uses a combination of continuous flow and demand flow. Before inspiration, the delivered flow equals the return flow. As the patient initiates a breath, the return flow to the ventilator is decreased and this flow differential triggers a mechanical breath.

Flow Triggered. Some ventilators are able to measure inspiratory and expiratory flows. When the patient's inspiratory flow reaches a specific value, a ventilator-supported breath is delivered. Flow triggering has been shown to be more sensitive and responsive to a patient's efforts than pressure triggering. A **flow-triggered** breath uses a strategy that combines the continuous flow and demand flow mechanisms, and it is used to reduce the inspiratory effort imposed on the patient during mechanical ventilation. It is considered to be more sensitive to the patient's inspiratory effort and therefore usually requires less inspiratory work than pressure triggering.

In flow triggering, a continuous flow passes through the ventilator circuit and returns to the ventilator (i.e., delivered flow = returned flow). As the patient initiates a breath, part of the delivered flow goes to the patient and the return flow to the ventilator is therefore reduced (i.e., delivered flow > return flow). The ventilator senses this flow differential and instantly supplies enough flow to satisfy the mechanical or spontaneous tidal volume. CMV, SIMV, and PSV can all be flow triggered (Figure 3-10).

One infant ventilator (Sechrist IV-200) uses inductive plethysmography to initiate a ventilator-supported breath. When the infant's chest expands, a small electrical signal is generated between two chest leads, which is commonly used to monitor the infant's respiratory rate. The ventilator is interfaced to the respiratory rate monitor, and inspiratory triggering occurs when the signal is detected by the ventilator. This type of triggering is much faster and responsive than

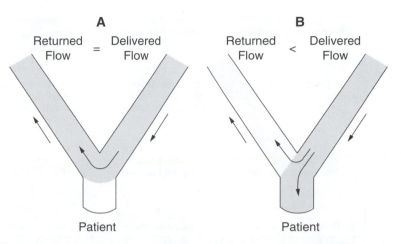

Figure 3-10 Flow-trigger mechanism. (A) Before an inspiratory effort, the delivered flow equals the returned flow. Flow trigger is not activated because there is no drop in returned flow. (B) At beginning inspiration, some of the delivered flow goes to the patient and this leads to a lower returned flow. Flow trigger is activated when the ventilator senses an inspiratory effort (the returned flow is lower than the delivered flow).

pressure or flow triggering, since it is directly measuring the infant's inspiratory efforts or exertions.

How hard the patient must work to initiate or trigger a breath is termed the ventilator sensitivity. If the ventilator is made more sensitive to the patient's efforts (pressure, flow, or volume), it is easier for the patient to trigger a breath. The converse is also true.

LIMIT VARIABLE

During a ventilator-supported breath, volume pressure and flow all rise above their respective baseline values. Inspiratory time is defined as the time interval between the start of inspiratory flow and the beginning of expiratory flow. If one or more variables (pressure, flow, or volume), is not allowed to rise above a preset value during the inspiratory time, it is termed a limit variable. Note that in this definition, inspiration does not end when the variable reaches its preset value. The breath delivery continues, but the variable is held at the fixed, preset value. Figure 3-11 provides a useful algorithm for determining the limit variable (pressure limited, volume limited, or flow limited) during the inspiratory phase.

CYCLE VARIABLE

cycle: The length of one complete breathing cycle.

Inspiration ends when a specific **cycle** variable (pressure cycled, volume cycled, flow cycled, or time cycled) is reached (Figure 3-11). This variable must be measured by the ventilator and used as a feedback signal to end inspiratory flow delivery, which then allows exhalation to begin.

Figure 3-11 Criteria for determining the phase variables during a ventilator-assisted breath. (From R. L. Chatburn (1991). *Respir Care, 36*(10). (Used with permission.)

Again it is easy to make false assumptions regarding many ventilators by classifying them as volume cycled. Most newer ventilators measure flow and are flow controllers. Since flow is measured and used as a feedback signal for gas delivery, volume becomes a function of flow and time [Volume (L) = Flow (L/sec) × Inspiratory Time (sec)]. Therefore, these ventilators are really time cycled, rather than "volume cycled." Inspiration ends because a preset time interval has passed, and volume has not been directly measured.

BASELINE VARIABLE

Expiratory time is defined as the interval between the start of expiratory flow and the beginning of inspiratory flow. This is also termed the expiratory phase. The variable that is controlled during the expiratory phase or expiratory time is termed the baseline variable. Most commonly, pressure is controlled during the expiratory phase.

Application of positive end-expiratory pressure (PEEP) and continuous positive airway pressure (CPAP) are used to increase the functional residual capacity (FRC), to improve gas distribution, and oxygenation. These pressures when applied above baseline (ambient pressure) during exhalation, maintain the lungs in a partially inflated state. This helps to prevent alveolar collapse, recruit previously collapsed alveoli, and distend those alveoli that are already patent. PEEP and CPAP pressures must be titrated carefully to monitor hemodynamic functions, blood gases or oximetry, and compliance to achieve the greatest benefit with the least amount of detrimental side effects.

CONDITIONAL VARIABLE

Conditional variables are defined as patterns of variables that are controlled by the ventilator during the ventilatory cycle. Early ventilators, such as the Puritan Bennett MA-1, used relatively simple conditional variables (volume cycled, pressure limited, pressure triggered, and PEEP). Newer third-generation microprocessor-controlled ventilators, such as the Puritan-Bennett 840, are capable of delivering complex ventilatory patterns. Figure 3-12 summarizes the ventilator classification system.

OUTPUT WAVEFORMS

Output waveforms are graphical representations of the control or phase variables in relation to time. Output waveforms are typically presented in the order of pressure, volume, and flow. The ventilator determines the shape of the control variable, whereas the other two depend on the patient's compliance and resistance. Convention dictates that flow values above the horizontal axis are inspiratory, whereas flow below the horizontal axis is expiratory. This corresponds to pressure and flow values rising above the horizontal axis for inspiration and falling back to the baseline during expiration. The ideal waveforms are represented in Figure 3-13.

Careful observation and assessment of waveforms during mechanical ventilation can provide useful information for the clinician. Waveforms can assist the clinician in the detection of inadvertent PEEP, the patient's ventilatory work, resistance and compliance changes as well as many other events or changes. Some ventilators are able to present pressure versus volume waveforms to assist in minimizing the patient's work of breathing. Still other ventilators can present flow versus volume waveforms, to aid in the assessment of bronchodilator therapy during mechanical ventilation and the assessment of airway obstruction. As waveforms become widely used, their usefulness will approach that of the ECG tracing in the assessment of the heart.

Mode	Mandatory Breath				Spontaneous Breath				Control Logic			
	Control	Trigger	Limit	Cycle	Control	Trigger	Limit	Cycle	Supported	Conditional Variable	Action
CMV	Pressure, volume, or flow	Time	Pressure, volume, or flow	Time, pressure, volume, or flow	—	—	—	—	—	—	—
A/C	Pressure, volume, or flow	Time, pressure, volume, or flow	Pressure, volume, or flow	Time, pressure, volume, or flow	—	—	—	—	—	Time or patient effort	Machine-to-patient triggered
AMV	Pressure, volume, or flow	Pressure, volume, or flow	Pressure, volume, or flow	Time, pressure, volume, or flow	—	—	—	—	—	—	—
IMV	Pressure, volume, or flow	Time	Pressure, volume, or flow	Time, pressure, volume, or flow	Pressure	Pressure, volume, or flow	Pressure	Pressure	No	—	—
SIMV	Pressure, volume, or flow	Time, pressure, volume, or flow	Pressure, volume, or flow	Time, pressure, volume, or flow	Pressure	Pressure, volume, or flow	Pressure	Pressure	No	Time or patient effort	Machine-to-patient triggered
CPAP	—	—	—	—	Pressure	Pressure, volume, or flow	Pressure	Pressure	No	—	—
PCV	Pressure	Time	Pressure	Time	—	—	—	—	—	—	—
PC-IMV	Pressure	Time	Pressure	Time	Pressure	Pressure, volume, or flow	Pressure	Pressure	No	—	—

Figure 3-12 Summary of the ventilator classification system as described by Robert L. Chatburn. (From R. L. Chatburn (1992). Technical description and classification of modes of ventilator operation. *Respir Care, 37*(9). Used with permission.)

(continued)

Mode	Mandatory Breath				Spontaneous Breath				Control Logic		
	Control	Trigger	Limit	Cycle	Control	Trigger	Limit	Cycle	Supported	Conditional Variable	Action
PC-SIMV	Pressure	Time, pressure, volume, or flow	Pressure	Time	Pressure	Pressure, volume, or flow	Pressure	Pressure	No	Time or patient effort	Machine-to-patient triggered
PCIRV	Pressure	Time	Pressure	Time	Pressure		Pressure				
APRV	Pressure	Time or pressure	Pressure	Time	Pressure	Pressure, volume, or flow	Pressure	Pressure	No	Time or patient effort	Machine-to-patient triggered
PSV	—	—	—	—	Pressure	Pressure, volume, or flow	Pressure	Volume	Yes		
MMV	Volume or flow	Time	Volume or flow	Time, volume, or flow	Pressure	Pressure, volume, or flow	Pressure	Pressure or volume	Yes	Minute ventilation, time	Sponta-neous to-mandatory breath
VAPS	Flow	Time or pressure	Flow	Time or volume	Pressure	Pressure or flow	Pressure	Flow	Yes	Tidal volume	Pressure-to-volume control
BiPAP	Pressure	Time	Pressure	Time	Pressure	Pressure	Pressure	Pressure	No	—	—

CMV = continuous mandatory ventilation; NA = not applicable; A/C = assist/control; AMV = assisted mechanical ventilation; IMV = intermittent mandatory ventilation; SIMV = synchronized mandatory ventilation; CPAP = continuous positive airway pressure; PCV = pressure-controlled ventilation; PC-IMV = pres-sure-controlled IMV; PCIRV = PC inverse-ratio ventilation; APRV = airway pressure release ventilation; PSV = pressure support ventilation; MMV = mandatory minute ventilation; VAPS = volume-assisted pressure support; BiPAP = bilevel positive airway pressure.

Figure 3-12 *(continued)*

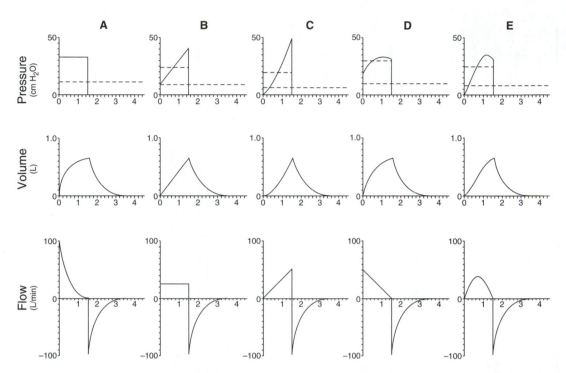

Figure 3-13 Theoretical output waveforms for (A) pressure-controlled inspiration with rectangular pressure waveform, identical to flow-controlled inspiration with an exponential-decay flow waveform; (B) flow-controlled inspiration with rectangular flow waveform, identical to volume-controlled inspiration with an ascending-ramp flow waveform; (C) flow-controlled inspiration with an ascending-ramp flow waveform; (D) flow-controlled inspiration with a descending-ramp flow waveform; and (E) flow-controlled inspiration with a sinusoidal flow waveform. The short dashed lines represent mean inspiration pressure, whereas the longer dashed lines denote mean airway pressure (assuming zero end-expiratory pressure). For the rectangular pressure waveform in A, the mean inspiratory pressure is the same as the peak inspiratory pressure. These output waveforms were created by (1) defining the control waveform (e.g., an ascending-ramp flow waveform is specified as flow = constant × time) and specifying that tidal volume equals 644 mL (about 9 mL/kg for a normal adult); (2) specifying the desired values for resistance and compliance (for these waveforms, compliance = 20 mL/cm H_2O and resistance = 20 cm H_2O/L/sec, according to ANSI recommendations); (3) substituting the above information into the equation of motion; and (4) using a computer to solve the equation for pressure, volume, and flow and plotting the results against time. (From R. L. Chatburn (1991). *Respir Care, 36* (10). Used with permission.)

PRESSURE WAVEFORMS

Pressure waveforms include rectangular, exponential, sinusoidal, and oscillating (Figure 3-14). Each of these waveforms would have these characteristic shapes, providing that pressure is the control variable. The descriptors used to describe each waveform are based on their respective shapes.

The rectangular waveform is characterized by a near instantaneous rise to a peak pressure value that is held to the start of exhalation. During expiration, the pressure rapidly drops to baseline.

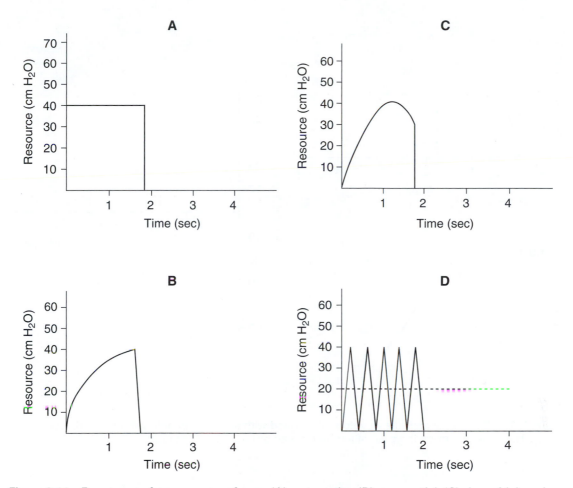

Figure 3-14 Four types of pressure waveforms: (A) rectangular; (B) exponential; (C) sinusoidal; and (D) oscillating.

sine wave: *A graphic presentation of flow and time that has a horizontal "S" appearance.*

The exponential waveform is depicted by a more gradual increase in pressure when compared with the rectangular waveform. This type of waveform is common in some infant ventilators and has become an option on some adult ventilators. Ventilator settings such as flow and inspiratory time regulate how steep the waveform rises toward peak inspiratory pressure.

The sinusoidal waveform resembles the positive half of a **sine wave.** Sinusoidal waveforms are characteristically produced by ventilators having a rotary-driven piston drive mechanism (Figure 3-15).

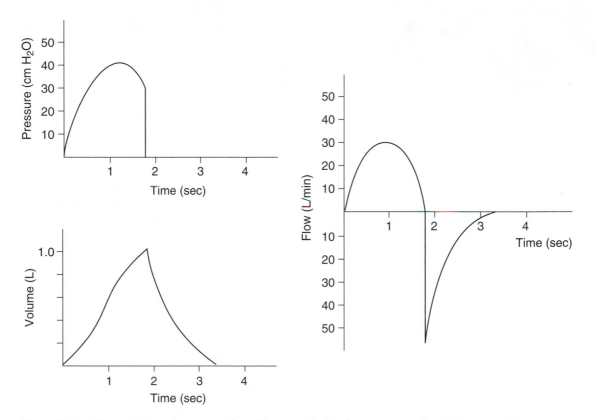

Figure 3-15 Sinusoidal pressure waveform illustrated with the corresponding volume and flow waveforms. This type of pattern is typical of a rotary-driven piston drive mechanism.

Ventilators using this drive mechanism include the Emerson 3-MV, Respironics PLV-100, BEAR 33, and Puritan-Bennett LP-10 and LP-20.

VOLUME WAVEFORMS

Volume waveforms can be classified into two types, ascending ramp and sinusoidal (Figure 3-16). The ascending ramp waveform is produced by a constant (i.e., rectangular) inspiratory flow pattern. The shape is characterized by a linear rise to the peak inspiratory pressure value. Sinusoidal volume waveforms are produced by ventilators that have a rotary-driven piston drive mechanism. Ventilators using this drive mechanism include the Emerson 3-MV, Respironics PLV-100, BEAR 33, and Puritan-Bennett LP-10 and LP-20.

FLOW WAVEFORMS

The four types of flow waveforms are shown in Figure 3-17. The waveforms include rectangular (constant), ascending ramp, descending ramp, and sinusoidal.

Figure 3-16 Two types of volume waveforms: (A) ascending ramp; and (B) sinusoidal.

The rectangular waveform is produced when volume is the control variable and the output is an ascending ramp. The flow waveform (a derivative of the volume waveform with respect to time), assumes the characteristic rectangular shape.

The ramp waveform can be ascending or descending. If flow rises as the breath is delivered, it is termed ascending. If flow falls during the ventilator-supported breath, it is called a descending ramp.

The sinusoidal waveform resembles the positive portion of a sine wave. It is generated by a rotary-driven piston drive mechanism.

ALARM SYSTEMS

Alarm systems are designed to alert the clinician to undesirable technical or patient events. Triggering of any alarm requires clinician awareness or action. As the complexity of mechanical ventilators has increased, so have the number and complexity of the alarm systems. Technical events are those events limited to the performance of the ventilator, while patient events are those relating to the patient's condition. Alarms can be visual, audible, or both depending on the seriousness of the event.

INPUT POWER ALARMS

Input power alarms can be further classified as to loss of electrical or pneumatic power.

Loss of electrical power usually results in the ventilator activating a backup alarm that is battery powered. Most battery backup alarms are powered by rechargeable nickel cadmium batteries, which are

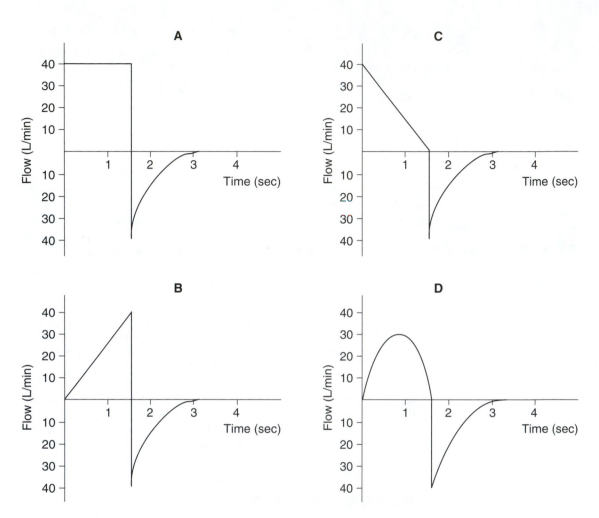

Figure 3-17   Four types of flow waveforms: (A) rectangular (constant); (B) ascending ramp; (C) descending ramp; and (D) sinusoidal.

recharged when AC power is available. When AC power is lost, the backup batteries activate audible and visual alarms.

Loss of either air or oxygen pneumatic sources will result in a technical event alarm. If either input pressure falls below a specified value from 50 psi, the alarm will result. Some alarms are electronic (BEAR 1000, BEAR I, II and III, Puritan-Bennett 840), whereas others are pneumatic reed alarms such as those employed in oxygen blenders.

CONTROL CIRCUIT ALARMS

Control circuit alarms alert the clinician to settings or parameters that are not within acceptable ranges or specifications, or they warn the clinician that the ventilator has failed some part of a self-diagnostic test. In the event of an incompatible setting or parameter, the clinician is allowed the opportunity to change the input to one that is compatible. Failure of the self-diagnostic test may render the ventilator inoperative, and the clinician is alerted by a message display that test failure has occurred.

OUTPUT ALARMS

Output alarms can be further subdivided into pressure, volume, flow, time, inspiratory, and expiratory gas.

Pressure alarms include high/low peak and mean and baseline airway pressures. High and low values may be set for each of these output parameters to alert the clinician of changes in the patient's respiratory status. Additionally, an alarm may be provided to detect failure of the airway pressure to return to the baseline valve. This could be caused by airway obstructions, circuit obstructions, or ventilator malfunctions.

Volume alarms include high/low exhaled tidal volumes for both ventilator-supported breaths and spontaneous breaths. Low volumes may result from sedation (spontaneous volumes), disconnection, or apnea (spontaneous volumes).

Flow alarms are limited to exhaled minute volume. High and low values may be set on some ventilators to alert the clinician to changes in the patient's minute ventilation.

Time alarms include high/low frequency or rate, excessive or inadequate inspiratory time, and excessive or inadequate expiratory time. High/low ventilatory rate alarms alert the clinician to changes in the patient's ventilatory rate. Inspiratory and expiratory time alarms may alert the practitioner to circuit obstructions or malfunctions, changes in gas distribution, or inappropriate ventilator settings.

Inspired gas alarms alert the clinician to changes in oxygen concentration or gas temperature. Some ventilators incorporate an oxygen analyzer to detect changes in F_IO_2. High/low alarms alert the clinician to these changes. Inspired gas temperature may be controlled by a servo-controlled humidifier or monitored by an independent ventilator temperature alarm. High/low temperature alarms can alert the clinician to changes in the inspiratory gas temperature.

Exhaled oxygen tension or end tidal carbon dioxide tension can be monitored, and high/low alarms can be sent to the exhaled gas monitoring system. These monitors can assist the clinician in determining the V_D/V_T, gas exchange, and the respiratory exchange ratio (R).

SUMMARY

As computer and medical technologies are getting more advanced, future mechanical ventilators are likely to have more new features than the current ventilators. No one knows for certain whether more new features will make the ventilators more complex and less user-friendly. But no matter what the future ventilators become, the practitioners who use mechanical ventilators must learn and maintain the theory, skills, and practice in the use of mechanical ventilation.

The ability to use mechanical ventilation will be enhanced if the practitioners are able to classify the ventilator properly and apply the unique characteristics of each ventilator in patient care situations.

Self-Assessment Questions

1. The primary forces that the ventilatory muscles must overcome include:

    I. Resistive forces
    II. Compliance forces
    III. Elastic forces
    IV. Inductive forces

    A. I and II.   C. II and III.
    B. I and III.   D. II and IV.

2. When the ventilator assumes all of the ventilatory work, this is termed:

    A. partial ventilatory support.   C. incomplete ventilatory support.
    B. full ventilatory support.   D. no ventilatory support.

3. A type of control circuit that relies on cams, pulleys, and levers is termed a/an:

    A. electronic control circuit.   C. electric control circuit.
    B. fluidic control circuit.   D. mechanical control circuit.

4. A ventilator that measures flow and uses that measurement to control the output of the ventilator is termed a:

    A. pressure controller.   C. volume controller.
    B. flow controller.   D. time controller.

5. If pressure rises to a preset level and is maintained at that level until inspiration ends, this is termed a:

    A. time limit.   C. pressure limit.
    B. volume limit.   D. flow limit.

6. An alarm that results from the loss of 50 psi gas pressure is termed a/an:

   A. input power alarm.   C. output alarm.
   B. control circuit alarm.   D. gas pressure alarm.

Answers to Self-Assessment Questions

1. B. I and III. (Resistive forces, Elastic forces)

2. B. full ventilatory support.

3. D. mechanical control circuit.

4. B. flow controller.

5. C. pressure limit.

6. A. input power alarm.

Suggested Reading

Barnes, T. A., et al. (1994). *Core textbook of respiratory care practice* (2nd ed.). St. Louis, MO: Mosby.

Branson, R. D. (1992). Intrahospital transport of critically ill, mechanically ventilated patients. *Respir Care, 37*(7), 775–795.

Branson, R. D., et al. (1992). Technical description and classification of modes of ventilator operation. *Respir Care, 37*(9), 1026–1044.

Chatburn, R. L. (1991). A new system for understanding mechanical ventilators. *Respir Care, 36*(10), 1123–1155.

Chatburn, R. L. (1992). Classification of mechanical ventilators. *Respir Care, 37*(9), 1009–1025.

Chatburn, R. L. (2001). A new system for understanding modes of mechanical ventilation. *Respir Care, 46*(6), 604–621.

Dupuis, Y. (1992). *Ventilators: Theory and clinical application* (2nd ed.). St. Louis, MO: Mosby.

Gietzen, J. W., et. al. (1991). Effect of PEEP-Valve placement on function of a home-care ventilator. *Respir Care, 36*(10), 1093–1098.

White, G. C. (2004). *Equipment theory for respiratory care* (4th ed.). Clifton Park, New York: Thomson Delmar Learning.

CHAPTER FOUR

OPERATING MODES OF MECHANICAL VENTILATION

David W. Chang
James H. Hiers

OUTLINE

Pressure Support Ventilation (PSV)
  Indications for the PSV Mode
Adaptive Support Ventilation (ASV)
Proportional Assist Ventilation (PAV)
Volume-Assured Pressure Support (VAPS)
Pressure-Regulated Volume Control (PRVC)
  Automode
Volume Ventilation Plus (VV+)
  Volume Control Plus (VC+)
  Volume Support (VS)
Pressure Control Ventilation (PCV)

Airway Pressure Release Ventilation (APRV)
  Indications for the APRV Mode
Inverse Ratio Ventilation (IRV)
  Physiology of IRV
  Adverse Effects of IRV
  Pressure Control-IRV (PC-IRV)
Automatic Tube Compensation (ATC)
Summary
Self-Assessment Questions
Answers to Self-Assessment Questions
References
Suggested Reading

KEY TERMS

- adaptive support ventilation (ASV)
- airway pressure release ventilation (APRV)
- assist/control (AC)
- automatic tube compensation (ATC)
- automode
- Bi-level positive airway pressure (BiPAP)
- continuous positive airway pressure (CPAP)
- control mode
- eucapnic ventilation
- intermittent mandatory ventilation (IMV)
- mandatory minute ventilation (MMV)
- positive end-expiratory pressure (PEEP)
- pressure control ventilation (PCV)
- pressure-regulated volume control (PRVC)
- proportional assist ventilation (PAV)
- synchronized intermittent mandatory ventilation (SIMV)
- volume-assured pressure support (VAPS)
- volume ventilation plus (VV+)

INTRODUCTION

This chapter provides an introduction to different operating modes available on most mechanical ventilators. Since the information associated with mechanical ventilation is immense, the reader should learn the operating modes and study them in the order presented in this chapter. The definition and unique characteristics of each operating mode are described here. The initiation and application of these operating controls may be found in subsequent chapters.

NEGATIVE AND POSITIVE PRESSURE VENTILATION

☑ Mechanical ventilators generate gas flow and volume by creating either a negative or positive pressure gradient.

Every ventilator must generate an inspiratory flow in order to deliver a tidal volume. Since gas flow requires a pressure gradient, a mechanical ventilator must produce a pressure gradient (i.e., pressure difference) between the airway opening and the alveoli in order to produce inspiratory flow and volume delivery. The pressure gradient that must be generated between the airway opening and the alveoli is known as the transairway pressure (Des Jardins, 2001).

> Transairway Pressure (P_{TA}) = Pressure at Airway Opening (P_{AO}) − Alveolar Pressure (P_{ALV})

At end-exhalation and prior to the beginning of inspiration, the pressures at the airway opening and the alveoli are both equal to atmospheric pressure. Since these two pressures are equal at this point, there is no pressure gradient and therefore no flow.

Since a pressure gradient is needed to generate gas flow and volume, mechanical ventilators achieve this condition by creating either a negative or positive pressure gradient.

NEGATIVE PRESSURE VENTILATION

Negative pressure ventilation creates a transairway pressure gradient by decreasing the alveolar pressures to a level below the airway opening pressure (i. e., below the atmospheric pressure). Unless airway obstruction is present, negative pressure ventilation does not require an artificial airway. Two classical devices that provide negative pressure ventilation are the "iron lung" and the chest cuirass or chest shell.

☑ The tidal volume delivered by a negative pressure ventilator is directly related to the negative pressure gradient.

Iron Lungs.   An "iron lung" ventilator encloses the patient's body except for the head and neck in a tank and the air in it is evacuated to produce a negative pressure around the chest cage. This negative pressure surrounding the chest and underlying alveoli results in chest wall and alveolar expansion. The tidal volume delivered to the patient is directly related to the negative pressure gradient. For example, a more negative pressure applied to the chest wall will yield a larger tidal volume. Since negative pressure ventilation does not require tracheal intubation, this noninvasive method of ventilation has been used extensively and successfully to support chronic ventilatory failure (Corrado et al., 1994; Frederick, 1994).

Disadvantages and complications associated with the iron lung type of negative pressure ventilator are (1) poor patient access and (2) potential for a decreased cardiac output known as "tank shock" (Frederick, 1994).

Since the iron lung encloses the patient, it restricts access to the patient for routine health care. Tank shock may result from a decreased venous blood return to the right atrium. Normally, the heart and vena cava are surrounded by negative pleural pressure while the remainder of the vascular system outside the thorax is subjected to atmospheric pressure. This creates a vascular pressure gradient between the vena cava and the venous drainage that enhances venous blood return to the right atrium. However, if a patient is placed in an iron lung, this vascular pressure gradient is lost because the peripheral vasculature is subjected to negative pressures that closely approximate the pleural pressure. This results in a potential decrease in venous return that could lead to a decreased cardiac output.

Chest Cuirass.   The chest cuirass or chest shell (see Figure 17-1, Chapter 17) is a form of negative pressure ventilation that was intended to alleviate the problems of patient access and tank shock associated with iron lungs. This shell device covers only the patient's chest and leaves the arms and lower body exposed. Although the chest shell improves patient access and decreases the potential for tank shock, ventilation with this device may be limited by the difficulties in maintaining an airtight seal between the shell and the patient's chest wall (Newman et al., 1988).

To overcome the problem of air leakage, individually designed cuirass "respirators" minimize air leaks, and they have been used successfully to ventilate patients with chest wall diseases such as scoliosis (Kinnear, Hockley et al., 1988; Kinnear, Petch et al., 1988). Because of the availability of positive pressure ventilators, chest cuirass ventilators are seldom used in an acute care facility. However, they are rather useful in selected home care settings because of the ease to maintain and the capability to ventilate without an artificial airway. All subsequent discussions on mechanical ventilation in this text refer to positive pressure ventilation unless negative pressure ventilation is specifically mentioned.

POSITIVE PRESSURE VENTILATION

The tidal volume delivered by a positive pressure ventilator is directly related to the positive pressure gradient.

Positive pressure ventilation is achieved by applying positive pressure (a pressure greater than atmospheric pressure) at the airway opening. Increasing the pressure at the airway opening produces a transairway pressure gradient that generates an inspiratory flow. This flow in turn results in the delivery of a tidal volume. Therefore, tidal volume is directly related to the transairway pressure gradient. All other factors being held constant, increasing the positive pressure being applied to the lungs will result in a larger tidal volume being delivered.

OPERATING MODES OF MECHANICAL VENTILATION

A ventilator mode can be defined as a set of operating characteristics that control how the ventilator functions. An operating mode can be described by the way a ventilator is triggered into inspiration and cycled into exhalation, what variables are limited during inspiration, and whether or not the mode allows only mandatory breaths, spontaneous breaths, or both.

Many different functions are commonly available on modern ventilators regardless of the mode. These functions include control of the F_IO_2, control of the inspiratory flow rate, and control of various alarms.

There are 19 essential ventilator modes available in different ventilators. Two or more of these modes are often used together to achieve certain desired effects. For example, spontaneous plus PEEP is the same as CPAP, and it is used to oxygenate a patient who has adequate ventilation. SIMV may be used with PSV to provide ventilation and reduce the work of breathing.

1. Spontaneous
2. Positive end-expiratory pressure (PEEP)
3. Continuous positive airway pressure (CPAP)
4. Bilevel positive airway pressure (BiPAP)
5. Controlled mandatory ventilation (CMV)
6. Assist control (AC)
7. Intermittent mandatory ventilation (IMV)
8. Synchronized intermittent mandatory ventilation (SIMV)
9. Mandatory minute ventilation (MMV)
10. Pressure support ventilation (PSV)
11. Adaptive support ventilation (ASV)
12. Proportional assist ventilation (PAV)
13. Volume-assured pressure support (VAPS)
14. Pressure-regulated volume control (PRVC)
15. Volume ventilation plus (VV+)
16. Pressure control ventilation (PCV)
17. Airway pressure release ventilation (APRV)
18. Inverse ratio ventilation (IRV)
19. Automatic tube compensation (ATC)

SPONTANEOUS

Spontaneous mode is not an actual mode on the ventilator since the rate and tidal volume during spontaneous breathing are determined by the patient. Even though the spontaneous mode is not a direct

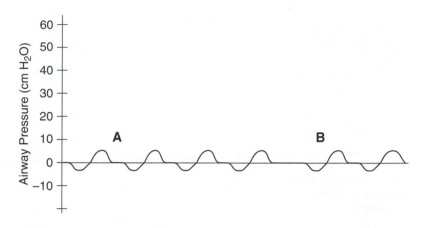

Figure 4-1 Spontaneous breathing pressure tracing. (A) The spontaneous rate is at a normal pattern. (B) The spontaneous breath is delayed by the patient.

ventilator function, the role of the ventilator during the spontaneous mode is to provide the (1) inspiratory flow to the patient in a timely manner, (2) flow adequate to fulfill a patient's inspiratory demand (i.e., tidal volume or inspiratory flow), and (3) provide adjunctive modes such as PEEP to complement a patient's spontaneous breathing effort. The graphical tracing of spontaneous breaths is shown in Figure 4-1.

APNEA VENTILATION

Apnea ventilation is a safety feature incorporated with the spontaneous breathing mode. In the event of apnea or an extremely slow respiratory rate, backup ventilation is invoked by the apnea ventilation feature and it delivers a predetermined tidal volume, respiratory rate, F_IO_2, and other essential ventilator functions to the patient.

positive end expiratory pressure (PEEP): PEEP is an airway pressure strategy in ventilation that increases the end-expiratory or baseline airway pressure to a value greater than atmospheric. It is used to treat refractory hypoxemia caused by intrapulmonary shunting.

POSITIVE END-EXPIRATORY PRESSURE (PEEP)

Positive end-expiratory pressure (PEEP) increases the end-expiratory or baseline airway pressure to a value greater than atmospheric (0 cm H_2O on the ventilator manometer). It is often used to improve the patient's oxygenation status, especially in hypoxemia that is refractory to high level of F_IO_2.

PEEP is not commonly regarded as a "stand-alone" mode, rather it is applied in conjunction with other ventilator modes. For example, when PEEP is applied to spontaneous breathing patients, the airway pressure *continuous positive airway pressure (CPAP):* CPAP is PEEP applied to the airway of a patient who is breathing spontaneously. It is used to treat refractory hypoxemia in patients who are able to maintain adequate spontaneous ventilation.

assist/control (AC): In the assist/control (AC) mode, the patient may increase the respiratory rate (assist) in addition to the preset mechanical respiratory rate (control). Each assist breath provides the preset mechanical tidal volume.

☑ PEEP is effective in refractory hypoxemia caused by intrapulmonary shunting.

☑ Refractory hypoxemia is present when the PaO_2 is ≤60 mm Hg at an F_IO_2 of ≥50%.

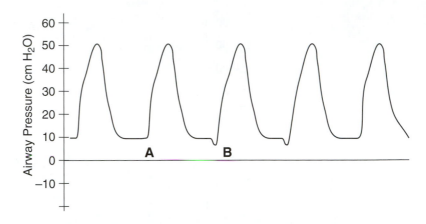

Figure 4-2 Positive end-expiratory pressure (PEEP). An assist/control pressure tracing with 10 cm H_2O of PEEP. (A) A controlled breath with PEEP. (B) An assisted breath with PEEP; note the negative deflection at the beginning of inspiration.

is called **continuous positive airway pressure (CPAP).** Figure 4-2 shows an **assist/control (AC)** pressure tracing with 10 cm H_2O of PEEP.

INDICATIONS FOR PEEP

Two major indications for PEEP are (1) intrapulmonary shunt and refractory hypoxemia and (2) decreased functional residual capacity (FRC) and lung compliance.

Intrapulmonary Shunt and Refractory Hypoxemia. The primary indication for PEEP is refractory hypoxemia induced by intrapulmonary shunting. This condition may be caused by a reduction of the FRC, atelectasis, or low V/Q mismatch (Tyler, 1983). Refractory hypoxemia is defined as hypoxemia that responds poorly to moderate to high levels of oxygen. A helpful clinical guideline for refractory hypoxemia is when the patient's PaO_2 is 60 mm Hg or less at an F_IO_2 of 50% or more.

Decreased FRC and Lung Compliance. A severely diminished FRC and reduced lung compliance greatly increase the alveolar opening pressure. If the patient is breathing spontaneously, a decreased lung compliance always increases the work of breathing and if severe enough can lead to fatigue of the respiratory muscles and ventilatory failure. Since PEEP increases the FRC, this pulmonary impairment may be prevented or improved by early application of PEEP therapy.

PHYSIOLOGY OF PEEP THERAPY

PEEP reinflates collapsed alveoli and maintains alveolar inflation during exhalation. Once "recruitment" of these alveoli has occurred, PEEP lowers the alveolar distending pressure and facilitates gas diffusion and oxygenation (Tyler, 1983).

Normally, the alveolar end-expiratory pressure equilibrates with atmospheric pressure (i.e., zero pressure) and the average pleural pressure is approximately –5 cm H_2O. Under these conditions, the alveolar distending pressure is 5 cm H_2O (alveolar-pleural). This distending pressure is sufficient to maintain a normal end-expiratory alveolar volume to overcome the elastic recoil of the alveolar wall. However, if the force of elastic recoil is increased due to a decrease in compliance, the alveolar volume will decrease. If the lung compliance continues to deteriorate, the elastic recoil forces can become great enough to completely overcome the normal alveolar distending pressure, thus resulting in alveolar collapse and the creation of intrapulmonary shunting. PEEP increases the alveolar end-expiratory pressure which increases the alveolar distending pressure, and therefore reexpands or recruits these collapsed alveoli.

PEEP
↓
Increases alveolar distending pressure
↓
Increases FRC by alveolar recruitment
↓
Improves ventilation
↓
(1) Increases V/Q
(2) Improves oxygenation
(3) Decreases work of breathing

COMPLICATIONS ASSOCIATED WITH PEEP

Complications and hazards associated with PEEP include (1) decreased venous return and cardiac output, (2) barotrauma, (3) increased intracranial pressure, and (4) alterations of renal functions and water metabolism.

Decreased Venous Return.   Assuming a normal intravascular volume, venous return to the right atrium is influenced by the difference in the central venous pressure and the negative pleural pressure that surrounds the heart. During PEEP, the pleural pressure becomes less negative and the pressure gradient between the central venous drainage and the right atrium will decrease resulting in a decreased venous return. This in turn results in a decreased cardiac output and hypotension (Qvist et al., 1975).

Experience has shown that significant increases in the mean airway pressure are more likely to increase pleural pressures sufficiently to decrease venous return. Since PEEP increases both peak inspiratory pressures and mean airway pressures, it has the potential to decrease venous return and cardiac output. It is vital to closely monitor the

☑ Since PEEP increases both peak inspiratory pressures and mean airway pressures, it has the potential to decrease venous return and cardiac output.

patient receiving PEEP therapy for any drop in blood pressure, especially when PEEP is either first applied or increased to high levels. If PEEP decreases the blood pressure, first be sure that the patient is not hypovolemic (Shapiro et al., 1991). If the blood volume is adequate, then the PEEP should be decreased until an adequate blood pressure is reestablished.

☑ **The detrimental effects of PEEP are dependent on the compliance characteristics of the patient.**

A given amount of PEEP does not impede venous return to the same degree in different patients. If a patient has an extremely low lung compliance, the airway pressure is less readily transmitted into the pleural space. In effect, the low lung compliance shields the pleural space from the full effects of the increased alveolar pressure. Patients with adult respiratory distress syndrome (ARDS) usually have a very low lung compliance and often require very high PEEP levels. However, despite high PEEP levels, hemodynamic instability is seldom a problem unless the patient has preexisting cardiovascular disease (Shapiro et al., 1991).

In contrast, if a patient has a normal or elevated lung compliance, the increased alveolar pressure due to the PEEP will more readily be transmitted into the pleural space. In other words, PEEP therapy in patients with normal or high lung compliance will more likely produce an elevated pleural pressure and therefore a decreased venous return (Shapiro et al., 1991).

Barotrauma.   Barotrauma is lung injury that results from the hyperinflation of alveoli past the rupture point. Although each patient is different, a PEEP greater than 10 cm H_2O (or mean airway pressure >30 cm H_2O, or a peak inspiratory pressure >50 cm H_2O) are associated with an increased incidence of alveolar rupture or barotrauma (Bezzant et al., 1994; Slutsky, 1994). Alveolar rupture can produce pneumothorax, tension pneumothorax, pneumomediastinum, pneumopericardium, and pneumoperitoneum. Subcutaneous emphysema or crepitus of unknown cause should always be interpreted as a sign that barotrauma has occurred.

☑ **PEEP greater than 10 cm H_2O (or mean airway pressure >30 cm H_2O, peak inspiratory pressure >50 cm H_2O) is associated with an increased incidence of barotrauma.**

Since PEEP increases alveolar pressures and alveolar volumes, it has the potential to produce barotrauma (Petersen et al., 1983), especially when combined with volume-cycled ventilation. Therefore plateau pressures should be closely monitored in these patients as well as being vigilant for any signs of barotrauma.

Increased Intracranial Pressure.   In patients with normal lung compliance, PEEP may increase the intracranial pressure (ICP) due to an impedance of venous return from the head. However, in patients with ARDS or noncompliant lungs, transmission of the excessive pressure generated by PEEP is minimal and it does not cause as much adverse effect on a patient's ICP.

☑ **In patients with normal lung compliance, PEEP may increase the intracranial pressure due to impedance of venous return from the head.**

☑ Positive pres-
sure ventilation
can reduce the blood
flow to the kidneys
and affect its normal
functions.

Alterations of Renal Functions and Water Metabolism. Kidneys play an important role in eliminating wastes, clearance of certain drugs, and regulating fluid, electrolyte, and acid-base balance. They are highly vascular and at any one time receive about 25% of the body's circulating blood volume (Brundage, 1992). Because of these characteristics, the kidneys are highly vulnerable to a decrease in blood flow as would occur during positive pressure ventilation.

When perfusion to the glomeruli of the kidneys is decreased, filtration becomes less effective (Baer et al., 1992). Subsequently, the urine output is decreased as the kidneys try to correct the hypovolemic condition by retaining fluid. If hypoperfusion of the kidneys persists or worsens, renal failure may result.

CONTINUOUS POSITIVE AIRWAY PRESSURE (CPAP)

eucapnic ventilation:
The amount of venti-
lation needed to
bring the patient's
PaCO₂ to normal.

Continuous positive airway pressure (CPAP) is PEEP applied to the airway of a patient who is breathing spontaneously (Figure 4-3). The indications for CPAP are essentially the same as for PEEP with the additional requirement that the patient must have adequate lung functions that can sustain **eucapnic ventilation** documented by the $PaCO_2$. In adults, CPAP may be given via a face mask, nasal mask, or endotracheal tube. In neonates, nasal CPAP is the method of choice.

Figure 4-3   Continuous positive airway pressure (CPAP) of 10 cm H_2O.

bilevel positive airway pressure (BiPAP): An airway pressure strategy that applies independent positive airway pressures (PAP) to both inspiration and expiration.

BILEVEL POSITIVE AIRWAY PRESSURE (BIPAP)

Bilevel positive airway pressure (BiPAP) allows the clinician to apply independent positive airway pressures to both inspiration and expiration. IPAP (inspiratory) and EPAP (expiratory) are used to define when the positive airway pressure is present. IPAP provides positive pressure breaths and it improves ventilation and hypoxemia due to hypoventilation. EPAP is in essence CPAP and it improves oxygenation by increasing the functional residual capacity and enhancing alveolar recruitment.

INDICATIONS FOR BIPAP

BiPAP appears to be of value in preventing intubation of the end-stage COPD patient (Ambrosino et al., 1992; Confalonieri et al., 1994; Renston et al., 1994) and in supporting patients with chronic ventilatory failure (Strumpf, 1990). Other indications of BiPAP include patients with restrictive chest wall disease (Hill, 1992), neuromuscular disease (Ellis et al., 1987), and nocturnal hypoventilation (Carroll et al., 1988; Waldhorn, 1992). See Chapter 7, "Noninvasive Positive Pressure Ventilation."

☑ BiPAP appears to be of value in preventing intubation of the end-stage COPD patient and in supporting patients with chronic ventilatory failure.

INITIAL SETTINGS

The BiPAP system may be used in one of three modes: spontaneous, spontaneous/timed, and timed. Mode selection depends on a patient's needs and ability to breath spontaneously. In general, if the patient is breathing spontaneously, the IPAP and EPAP may be set at 8 cm H_2O and 4 cm H_2O, respectively. The spontaneous/timed mode is used as a backup mechanism and the breaths per minute (BPM) is set two to five breaths below the patient's spontaneous rate. In the timed mode, set IPAP and EPAP as above and the BPM slightly higher than the patient's spontaneous rate. The %IPAP may be set at 33% or 50% for an I:E ratio of 1:2 or 1:1, respectively.

☑ The initial settings of IPAP and EPAP are 8 cm H_2O and 4 cm H_2O, respectively.

☑ A BiPAP device can be used as a CPAP device by setting the IPAP and EPAP at the same level.

ADJUSTMENTS OF IPAP AND EPAP

IPAP levels are generally determined by monitoring the patient's clinical and physiologic response to gradual changes of IPAP, rather than by directly measuring the volume delivered.

When the cardiopulmonary responses are positive, the IPAP may be increased in increments of 2 cm H_2O to enhance the "pressure boost" to improve alveolar ventilation, normalize $PaCO_2$, and reduce the work of breathing. Since IPAP does not provide volume-cycled ventilation, the volume delivered by IPAP is directly related to the IPAP and EPAP pressure difference and the compliance characteristics of the lung/thorax system. The volume delivered is inversely related to the air flow resistance. In other words, a larger delivered volume may be obtained

☑ IPAP may be increased in increments of 2 cm H_2O to enhance the "pressure boost" to improve alveolar ventilation, normalize $PaCO_2$, and reduce the work of breathing.

by (1) increasing the IPAP level, (2) decreasing the EPAP level, (3) increasing the compliance, and (4) reducing the air flow resistance.

✓ The EPAP should be increased by 2 cm H_2O increments to increase functional residual capacity and oxygenation in patients with intrapulmonary shunting.

The EPAP should be increased by 2 cm H_2O increments to increase functional residual capacity and oxygenation in patients with intrapulmonary shunting. When the EPAP is the same as the IPAP, CPAP results. It is not possible to increase the EPAP higher than the IPAP. Since IPAP and EPAP are methods to manipulate the airway pressures, all adverse effects of positive pressure ventilation and PEEP should be monitored. The patient should be advised to report any unusual chest discomfort, shortness of breath, or severe headache when using the BiPAP system.

CONTROLLED MANDATORY VENTILATION (CMV)

control mode: In control mode, the ventilator delivers the preset tidal volume at a set time interval (time-triggered respiratory rate).

With controlled mandatory ventilation (CMV) also known as continuous mandatory ventilation or **control mode,** the ventilator delivers the preset tidal volume at a time-triggered respiratory rate (Figure 4-4). Since the ventilator controls both the patient's tidal volume and respiratory rate, the ventilator "controls" the patient's minute volume. In the control mode, a patient cannot change the ventilator respiratory rate or breath spontaneously. For example, if the tidal volume and respiratory rate of a ventilator are set at 800 mL and 10 BPM, respectively, the minute volume will be 8,000 mL.

The control mode should only be used when the patient is properly medicated with a combination of sedatives, respiratory depressants,

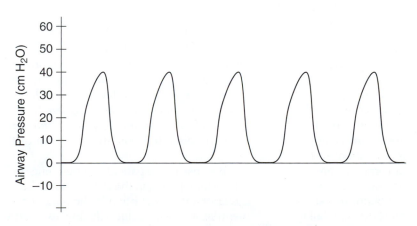

Figure 4-4 Control mode pressure tracing. The time intervals between mechanical breaths are equal when a control mode is used.

☑ The RCP must recognize any spontaneous breathing efforts during control mode ventilation.

and neuromuscular blockers. The control mode ventilation should not be instituted by decreasing the ventilator's triggering sensitivity to the point that no amount of patient effort can trigger the ventilator into inspiration. The problem with this approach should be obvious since any spontaneous inspiratory effort would be like attempting to inspire through a completely obstructed airway. Regardless of how vigorous the patient's inspiratory effort is, no gas flow would be delivered to the patient until the ventilator automatically becomes time triggered. If the control mode is improperly established in this way, it may not be physically harmful to the patient. However, it would most likely be psychologically devastating for the patient to realize that he or she has no control over his or her breathing requirements.

INDICATIONS FOR THE CONTROL MODE

The control mode is most often indicated if the patient "fights" the ventilator in the initial stages of mechanical ventilatory support. "Fighting" or "bucking" the ventilator often means that the patient is severely distressed and vigorously struggling to breathe. Their rapid spontaneous inspiratory efforts become asynchronous with the ventilator's ability to provide an adequate inspiratory flow. The typical result is that the patient will be attempting to actively exhale while the ventilator is delivering a breath. This results in high pressure limit cycling, which decreases the ventilator delivered tidal volume.

Other indications for control mode ventilation include (1) tetanus or other seizure activities that interrupt the delivery of mechanical ventilation (Linton et al., 1992), (2) complete rest for the patient typically for a period of 24 hours (Perel et al., 1992), and (3) patients with a crushed chest injury in which spontaneous inspiratory efforts produce significant paradoxical chest wall movement (Burton et al., 1997).

COMPLICATIONS ASSOCIATED WITH THE CONTROL MODE

☑ In a sedated or apneic patient, the primary hazard of the control mode is the potential for apnea and hypoxia if the patient should become disconnected from the ventilator or the ventilator should fail to operate.

Since the patient's spontaneous respiratory drive will have been blunted with sedation in the control mode, the patient is totally dependent on the ventilator for ventilation and oxygenation. As a result, the primary hazard associated with the control mode is the potential for apnea and hypoxia if the patient should become accidentally disconnected from the ventilator or the ventilator should fail to operate.

Because of the patient's dependence on the ventilator, the most important alarms in the control mode become those that alert the caregiver of any interruption in the patient's ventilation. The important ventilator alarms include the low exhaled volume alarm and the low inspiratory pressure alarm.

Table 4-1 summarizes the major characteristics of the control mode.

TABLE 4-1   Characteristics of the Control Mode

CHARACTERISTIC	DESCRIPTION
Type of breath	Each breath delivers a mechanical tidal volume.
Triggering mechanism	Every breath in the control mode is time triggered.
Cycling mechanism	Inspiration is terminated by the delivery of a preset tidal volume (volume cycled).

ASSIST CONTROL (AC)

With the assist/control (AC) mode, the patient may increase the ventilator respiratory rate (assist) in addition to the preset mechanical respiratory rate (control). Each control breath provides the patient with a preset, ventilator delivered tidal volume. Each assist breath also results in a preset, ventilator delivered tidal volume. The assist-control mode does not allow the patient to take spontaneous breaths (Figure 4-5).

ASSIST CONTROL TRIGGERING MECHANISM

The mandatory mechanical breaths may be either patient triggered by the patient's spontaneous inspiratory efforts (assist) or time triggered by a preset respiratory rate (control). If a breath is patient triggered, it is referred to as an assisted breath; if a breath is time triggered, the breath is referred to as a control breath.

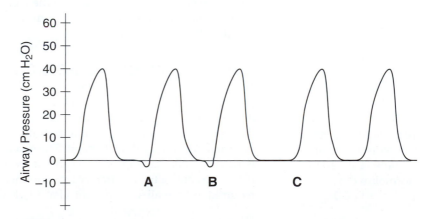

Figure 4-5   Assist/control mode pressure tracing. Each assisted or controlled breath triggers a mechanical tidal volume. (A) An assisted breath; note the negative deflection at the beginning of inspiration. (B) Another assisted breath that is initiated by the patient sooner than (A). (C) A controlled breath; note the absence of a negative deflection at the beginning of inspiration.

For example, if the patient has a stable assist rate of 12 BPM, then the patient is triggering breaths every 5 sec. If the control rate is preset at 10 BPM, the ventilator would deliver time-triggered breaths every 6 sec. However, since the interval between the assisted breaths is shorter than 6 sec, no time-triggered breaths will be delivered. If however, the patient's spontaneous breaths were to decrease less than the preset control rate, then the ventilator would begin delivering time-triggered breaths.

ASSIST CONTROL CYCLING MECHANISM

Inspiration in the AC mode is terminated by volume cycling. When the preset tidal volume is delivered, the ventilator is cycled to expiration.

INDICATIONS FOR THE AC MODE

The AC mode is most often used to provide full ventilatory support for patients when they are first placed on mechanical ventilation. Full ventilatory support is defined as any ventilator mode that provides all of the work of breathing.

The AC mode is typically used for patients who have a stable respiratory drive (a stable rate of spontaneous inspiratory efforts of at least 10 to 12 BPM) and can therefore trigger the ventilator into inspiration. Essentially, the time-triggering control rate is generally considered as a safety net to provide adequate ventilation in the event that the patient stops triggering the ventilator at an acceptable respiratory rate (Sassoon et al., 1990). The generally accepted minimum control respiratory rate in the AC mode is 2 to 4 BPM less than the patient's assist rate, or a minimum control rate of from 8 to 10 BPM.

ADVANTAGES OF THE AC MODE

There are two primary advantages with the AC mode. First, the patient's work of breathing requirement in the AC is very small when the triggering sensitivity (pressure or flow) is set appropriately and the ventilator supplies an inspiratory flow that meets or exceeds the patient's inspiratory flow demand. The second advantage of AC is that if the patient has an appropriate ventilatory drive, this mode allows the patient to control the respiratory rate and therefore the minute volume required to normalize the patient's $PaCO_2$ (Kirby, 1988).

COMPLICATIONS ASSOCIATED WITH THE AC MODE

The potential hazard associated with AC is alveolar hyperventilation (respiratory alkalosis). In two separate studies, the pH was found to be higher and the $PaCO_2$ was lower in the AC mode than the results

☑ The AC mode allows the patient to control the respiratory rate and therefore the minute volume required to normalize the patient's $PaCO_2$.

TABLE 4-2   Characteristics of the Assist Control Mode

CHARACTERISTIC	DESCRIPTION
Type of breath	Each breath, assist or control, delivers a preset mechanical tidal volume.
Triggering mechanism	Mechanical breaths may be either patient triggered (assist) or time triggered (control).
Cycling mechanism	Inspiration is terminated either by the delivery of a preset tidal volume (volume cycled) or by the high pressure limit (pressure cycled).

intermittent man-datory ventilation (IMV): IMV is a mode in which the ventilator delivers control (mandatory) breaths and allows the patient to breathe spontaneously to any tidal volume the patient is capable of between the mandatory breaths.

obtained in the **intermittent mandatory ventilation (IMV)** mode (Culpepper et al., 1985; Hopper et al., 1985). If the patient's respiratory center is either injured or diseased, the patient may have an inappropriately high respiratory drive leading to an excessive assist rate despite a low $PaCO_2$. If the patient is assisting at a high respiratory rate (i.e., >20 to 25 BPM) and the tidal volume is preset at 10 to 15 mL/kg, this will usually result in hypocapnia and respiratory alkalosis.

Mechanical deadspace may be used in this situation, but it is generally considered safer to switch the patient to another mode of ventilation (e.g., SIMV) that limits the patient's ability to generate excessive minute volumes.

Table 4-2 summarizes the major characteristics of the assist control mode.

INTERMITTENT MANDATORY VENTILATION (IMV)

✓ Since IMV breaths are delivered at a rate independent of the patient's spontaneous respiratory rate, breath stacking may occur.

Intermittent mandatory ventilation (IMV) is a mode in which the ventilator delivers control (mandatory) breaths and allows the patient to breathe spontaneously at any tidal volume the patient is capable of in between the mandatory breaths (Figure 4-6).

Historically, IMV was a separate circuit adapted to ventilators that were designed to provide either assist/control or control mode ventilation. As such, it was the first widely used mode that allowed partial ventilatory support (i.e., a mode that allowed the patient to breathe spontaneously in addition to receiving ventilator delivered breaths) (Heenan et al., 1980).

The primary complication associated with IMV was the random chance for breath stacking. This occurs when the patient is taking a spontaneous breath and the ventilator delivers a time-triggered mandatory breath at the same time. If this occurs, the patient's lung

Figure 4-6 Intermittent mandatory ventilation (IMV) pressure tracing with two mandatory breaths and five anticipated spontaneous breaths (only three active). IMV mode may cause breath stacking since the mandatory breaths are delivered at a set time interval with no regard to the patient's breathing frequency. Mandatory breath (A) begins before the patient is ready for the anticipated spontaneous breath #2. Mandatory breath (B) begins shortly after the initiation of the anticipated spontaneous breath #4. The anticipated spontaneous breaths #2 and #4 did not occur as they turned into mechanical breaths during the mandatory cycle.

volume and airway pressure could increase significantly. Setting appropriate high pressure limits will reduce the risk of barotrauma in the event of breath stacking. As long as the breath stacking only occurs occasionally, the IMV mode is an acceptable mode of ventilation with few complications.

The sophistication of ventilator technology has progressed to the point that no new adult ventilators offer the IMV mode. Rather, all ventilators currently available have been designed to provide synchronized IMV (SIMV) (Shapiro et al., 1976).

SYNCHRONIZED INTERMITTENT MANDATORY VENTILATION (SIMV)

Synchronized intermittent mandatory ventilation (SIMV) is a mode in which the ventilator delivers either assisted breaths to the patient at the beginning of a spontaneous breath or time-triggered mandatory breaths. The mandatory breaths are synchronized with the patient's spontaneous breathing efforts so as to avoid breath stacking (Figure 4-7).

synchronized inter-mittent mandatory ventilation (SIMV): SIMV is a mode in which the ventilator delivers control (mandatory) breaths to the patient at or near the time of a spontaneous breath. The mandatory breaths are synchro-nized with the patient's sponta-neous breathing efforts so as to avoid breath stacking.

Figure 4-7 Synchronized intermittent mandatory ventilation (SIMV) pressure tracing with two mandatory breaths and five anticipated spontaneous breaths (only three active). SIMV mode does not cause breath stacking since the mandatory breaths are delivered slightly sooner or later than the preset time interval but within a time window. Mandatory breaths (A) and (B) occur during a spontaneous inspiratory effort. The anticipated spontaneous breaths #2 and #4 did not occur as they turned into mechanical breaths during the mandatory cycle.

SIMV MANDATORY BREATH-TRIGGERING MECHANISM

The SIMV mandatory breaths may be either time triggered or patient triggered. The triggering mechanism is determined by whether or not the patient makes a spontaneous inspiratory effort just prior to the delivery of a time-triggered breath. For example, if the SIMV mandatory respiratory rate is set at 10 BPM, then the ventilator would time trigger a breath every 6 sec if the patient is not attempting to inspire spontaneously. However, if the patient is breathing spontaneously between the mandatory breaths, and if by random chance, the patient begins to inspire just prior to the point at which the ventilator would be expected to time trigger, then the ventilator senses this spontaneous effort and delivers the mandatory breath as an assisted patient-triggered breath. The mandatory breath whether time or patient triggered is controlled by all applicable mechanical tidal volume settings.

Synchronization Window. The time interval just prior to time triggering in which the ventilator is responsive to the patient's spontaneous inspiratory effort is commonly referred to as the *synchronization window* (Sassoon, 1991). Although the exact time interval of the synchronization window is slightly different from manufacturer to manufacturer, 0.5 sec is representative. For example, given an SIMV mandatory rate of 10 BPM, the ventilator would be expected to time trigger every 6 sec. If the synchronization window is 0.5 sec, then at 5.5 sec from the beginning of the previous mandatory breath, the ventilator automatically becomes sensitive to any spontaneous inspiratory effort, i.e., the synchronization window becomes active. If the patient makes a spontaneous inspiratory effort when the synchronization window is active, the ventilator is patient triggered to deliver an assisted mandatory breath. Patient triggering may be based either on pressure or flow. If, however, no spontaneous inspiratory effort exists while the synchronization window is active, the ventilator will time trigger when the full time triggering interval elapses.

SIMV SPONTANEOUS BREATH-TRIGGERING MECHANISM

☑ Spontaneous rate and tidal volume taken by the patient in the SIMV mode are totally dependent on the patient's breathing effort.

In between the mandatory breaths, SIMV permits the patient to breathe spontaneously to any tidal volume the patient desires. The gas source for spontaneous breathing in the SIMV mode is typically supplied by a demand valve. The demand valve is always patient triggered, either by pressure or flow depending on the ventilator.

It is important to understand that the spontaneous breaths taken by the patient in the SIMV mode are truly spontaneous. The ventilator provides the humidified gas at the selected F_1O_2, but the spontaneous rate and spontaneous tidal volume are totally dependent on the patient's breathing effort.

INDICATIONS FOR THE SIMV MODE

☑ The primary indication for SIMV is to provide partial ventilatory support to the patient.

The primary indication for SIMV is to provide partial ventilatory support, i.e., a desire to have the patient actively involved in providing part of the minute volume. In a practical sense, when a patient is first placed on ventilatory support, full ventilatory support is appropriate to provide a period of rest, typically for the first 24 hours. After this initial period of full ventilatory support, it is typical practice to place the patient on a trial run of partial ventilatory support with SIMV. It is customary to ease the patient from full support to partial support by gradually decreasing the mandatory rate as tolerated by the patient. This depends on, of course, reversal of the clinical conditions that committed the patient to the ventilator in the first place.

ADVANTAGES OF THE SIMV MODE

Since SIMV promotes spontaneous breathing and use of respiratory muscles, SIMV (1) maintains respiratory muscle strength/avoids muscle atrophy, (2) reduces ventilation to perfusion mismatch, (3) decreases mean airway pressure, and (4) facilitates weaning.

Maintains Respiratory Muscle Strength/Avoids Muscle Atrophy.
SIMV helps to maintain respiratory muscle activity and strength.

Patients maintained in full ventilatory support for extended periods tend to experience partial loss of ventilatory muscle strength. This can be minimized by using the respiratory muscles during spontaneous breathing (Zelt et al., 1972).

Reduces Ventilation to Perfusion Mismatch.   Deadspace ventilation (i.e., high ventilation to low perfusion) is typical in the upper zone of the lungs because pulmonary perfusion is gravity dependent and favors the lower lung zone. This problem is intensified during positive pressure ventilation as the lung units in the upper zone are hyperinflated. Spontaneous breathing during SIMV tends to distribute the spontaneous tidal volume more evenly thus reducing alveolar deadspace ventilation (Weisman et al., 1983).

Decreases Mean Airway Pressure.   The mean airway pressure is directly related to the peak inspiratory pressure and inspiratory time (Note: Two other factors are respiratory rate and positive end-expiratory pressure). Since spontaneous breaths during SIMV have a lower peak inspiratory pressure and inspiratory time, SIMV tends to have a lower mean airway pressure.

The mean airway pressure is an important consideration because the greater the mean airway pressure, the greater the potential for a reduced venous return, cardiac output, and arterial perfusion pressure. Reduction of the mean airway pressure during SIMV indirectly enhances the patient's cardiovascular functions (Wilkins et al., 2003).

Facilitates Weaning.   SIMV facilitates weaning due to its ability to decrease the mandatory rate in small increments. This may offer some advantage to those "hard-to-wean" patients who cannot tolerate an abrupt decrease of the mechanical respiratory rate (Downs et al., 1973).

COMPLICATIONS ASSOCIATED WITH THE SIMV MODE

The ideal approach of SIMV weaning is to provide a spontaneous breathing workload that gradually increases a patient's muscle strength and endurance. The primary disadvantage associated with SIMV is the desire to wean the patient too rapidly, leading first to a high work of spontaneous breathing and ultimately to muscle fatigue and weaning failure. The best way to avoid this is to decrease the SIMV mandatory respiratory rate slowly and monitor the patient closely for signs of fatigue (Wilkins et al., 2003).

Table 4-3 summarizes the major characteristics of the synchronized IMV mode.

Table 4-3   Characteristics of the Synchronized IMV Mode

CHARACTERISTIC	DESCRIPTION
Type of breath	The ventilator delivers mechanical tidal volume at a preset respiratory rate. The patient may breathe spontaneously between mandatory breaths.
Triggering mechanism	Mandatory breaths may be either time triggered or patient triggered. Spontaneous breaths are patient triggered (i.e., the demand flow valve opens in response to the patient's spontaneous inspiratory effort).
Cycling mechanism	The mandatory breaths are volume cycled. The patient controls spontaneous rate and volume.

MANDATORY MINUTE VENTILATION (MMV)

mandatory minute ventilation (MMV): MMV is a feature of some ventilators that causes an increase of the mandatory rate (Note: In Hamilton Veolar, the pressure support level), when the patient's spontaneous breathing level becomes inadequate. This compensation by the ventilator ensures a safe minimal minute ventilation.

Mandatory minute ventilation (MMV), also called minimum minute ventilation, is a feature of some ventilators that provides a predetermined minute ventilation when the patient's spontaneous breathing effort becomes inadequate. For example, an apnea episode (lack of spontaneous breathing) may cause the actual minute ventilation to drop below the preset level. When this occurs, the mandatory rate is increased automatically to compensate for the decrease in minute ventilation caused by the apnea. This compensation by the ventilator ensures a desired minute ventilation.

MMV is an additional function of the SIMV mode and is intended to prevent hypercapnia by "automatically" ensuring that the patient receives a minimum preset minute volume. It is especially useful in preventing hypoventilation and respiratory acidosis in the final stages of weaning with SIMV when the patient's spontaneous breathing is assuming a significant portion of the total minute volume.

For example, a patient may have been weaned down to a mandatory SIMV rate of 4/min with a mandatory tidal volume of 800 mL; the patient's ventilator delivered minute volume would then be 3.2 L/min ($\dot{V}_E = RR \times V_T$). If this patient's spontaneous minute volume is 6 L/min, then the total minute volume is the sum of the ventilator-delivered minute volume and the spontaneous breathing minute volume 9.2 L/min in this example. If the patient's spontaneous minute volume suddenly decreases by a significant amount or if the patient becomes apneic, then without MMV the reduced minute volume would cause hypercapnia and respiratory acidosis. However, on MMV-equipped ventilators, a decrease in the patient's spontaneous minute volume would trigger an automatic increase in the ventilator's mandatory respiratory rate.

The way that MMV functions on the majority of ventilators is that a desired minimum minute volume is preset on the ventilator; usually only slightly less than the minute volume required to "normalize" the $PaCO_2$. The ventilator then measures the total minute volume and compares it with the preset minimum minute volume. As long as the patient's total minute volume equals or exceeds the preset minimum minute volume, the MMV function is not activated. However, if the patient's spontaneous minute volume decreases to the point that the total minute volume becomes less than the preset mandatory minute volume, then the ventilator will automatically increase the SIMV mandatory respiratory rate until it reaches the preset mandatory minute volume.

In the MMV mode, it is important to monitor not only the patient's spontaneous minute volume, but also the patient's estimated spontaneous alveolar minute volume. The reason for this is that if the patient becomes distressed, the tendency is to increase the spontaneous respiratory rate at the expense of a decreased tidal volume (i.e., the patient will typically adopt the spontaneous breathing pattern that minimizes the work of breathing). A minute volume supported by a rapid respiratory rate and low tidal volume may avert the MMV function but at the same time provides a significant amount of deadspace ventilation. This results in a decreased alveolar minute volume.

☑ A minute volume supported by rapid respiratory rate and low tidal volume (e.g., distressed patient) may avert the MMV function but at the same time provides a significant amount of deadspace ventilation. This results in a decreased alveolar minute volume.

Perhaps the most efficient method of ensuring that this condition does not occur is to set the high respiratory rate alarm at approximately 10 BPM greater than the patient's "baseline" spontaneous respiratory rate.

Although MMV operates in the manner previously described on most ventilators, one exception is seen in the Hamilton Veolar ventilator. Selecting the MMV mode on this ventilator automatically places the patient in a "pure" pressure support mode (i.e., every breath is a spontaneous pressure-supported breath and no mandatory breaths are given). A minimum desired mandatory minute volume is selected and the ventilator automatically compares the patient's total minute volume with the preset minimum minute volume. On the Veolar, if the patient's total minute volume is less than the preset minimum minute volume, the ventilator automatically increases the pressure support level until the minimum minute volume is obtained (Wilkins et al., 2003).

Table 4-4 summarizes the major characteristics of the mandatory minute ventilation mode.

TABLE 4-4   Characteristics of the Mandatory Minute Ventilation Mode

CHARACTERISTIC	DESCRIPTION
Type of breath	The ventilator increases the mandatory respiratory rate (Note: Hamilton Veolar increases the pressure support level).
Triggering mechanism	Increase of the mandatory respiratory rate (or the pressure support level in the Hamilton Veolar) is triggered when the actual minute volume is less than the preset minimal minute volume.
Cycling mechanism	All mandatory breaths are volume cycled. Patients control their own spontaneous rates and volumes.

PRESSURE SUPPORT VENTILATION (PSV)

☑ PSV lowers the work of spontaneous breathing and augments the spontaneous tidal volume.

Pressure support ventilation (PSV) is used to lower the work of spontaneous breathing and augment a patient's spontaneous tidal volume. When PSV is used with SIMV, it significantly lowers the oxygen consumption requirement presumably due to the reduced work of breathing (Kanak et al., 1985).

PSV applies a preset pressure plateau to the patient's airway for the duration of a spontaneous breath (Figure 4-8). Pressure-supported breaths are considered spontaneous because (1) they are patient triggered, (2) the tidal volume varies with the patient's inspiratory flow demand, (3) inspiration lasts only for as long as the patient actively inspires, and (4) inspiration is terminated when the patient's inspiratory flow demand decreases to a preset minimal value. PSV can be used in conjunction with spontaneous breathing in any ventilator mode.

A pressure-supported breath is therefore patient triggered, pressure limited, and flow cycled. It is pressure limited because the maximum airway pressure cannot exceed the preset pressure support level. It is flow cycled because a pressure-supported breath cycles to expiration when the flow reaches a minimal level.

It is important to understand how the pressure plateau is created and maintained. Essentially, when the pressure-supported breath is patient triggered (either by pressure or flow), the ventilator demand valve generates a flow high enough to rapidly increase the airway

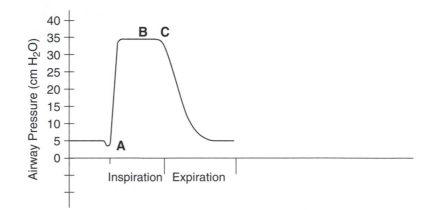

Figure 4-8 Pressure support ventilation (PSV) with PEEP of 5 cm H_2O. (A) Inspiratory effort; (B) Pressure support plateau of 30 cm H_2O (peak inspiratory pressure of 35 cm H_2O, PEEP of 5 cm H_2O); (C) Beginning expiratory phase when the inspiratory flow drops to 25% (or other predetermined %) of its peak flow.

pressure to the preset pressure limit and then maintain the pressure plateau (via servo control and demand valve) for the duration of the patient's spontaneous inspiratory effort. Typically, the flow pattern associated with pressure support is a steeply descending tapered flow pattern. As previously described, the demand valve flow terminates when it decreases to a preset lower flow limit. The point at which flow cycling occurs varies with different ventilators but 5L/min is representative.

INDICATIONS FOR THE PSV MODE

Pressure support is commonly applied in the SIMV mode when the patient takes spontaneous breaths. Pressure support is not active during the mandatory breaths. Pressure support has been advocated as a stand-alone mode by some clinicians; however, this requires close monitoring because as a stand-alone mode, every breath is patient triggered.

☑ Pressure support (1) ↑ spontaneous tidal volume, (2) ↓ spontaneous respiratory rate, and (3) ↓ work of breathing.

Pressure support is typically used in the SIMV mode to facilitate weaning in a difficult to wean patient. In this application, pressure support (1) increases the patient's spontaneous tidal volume, (2) decreases the patient's spontaneous respiratory rate, and (3) decreases the work of breathing.

☑ The level of pressure support is titrated until (1) spontaneous tidal volume = 10 to 15 mL/kg or (2) spontaneous respiratory rate < 25/min.

These three effects have been used to titrate the proper level of pressure support. For example, one physician may increase the pressure support level until a desired spontaneous tidal volume is achieved (e.g., 10 to 15 mL/kg). Another physician may increase the pressure support level until the patient's spontaneous respiratory rate decreases to a target value (usually 25 BPM or less) (MacIntyre, 1987).

The third endpoint for the pressure support level is to decrease the work of breathing (MacIntyre, 1986). This approach is probably less commonly used for the patient in immediate respiratory distress, but is more often used as a "routine" method to decrease the work of breathing. Since an endotracheal tube provides an increased airway resistance and increased the work of breathing, pressure support has been used successfully to overcome this gas flow resistance. The airway resistance on most modern ventilators may be obtained easily but in ventilators not equipped with this function, the following equation may be used to estimate the airway resistance:

☑ See Appendix 1 for example.

$$\text{Airway Resistance} = \frac{(\text{Peak Inspiratory Pressure} - \text{Plateau Pressure})}{\text{Mean Flow}}$$

Table 4-5 summarizes the major characteristics of the pressure support ventilation mode.

TABLE 4-5   Characteristics of the Pressure Support Ventilation Mode

CHARACTERISTIC	DESCRIPTION
Type of breath	Pressure-supported breaths are considered spontaneous. (Note: Pressure support may be applied in any mode that permits spontaneous breathing such as SIMV.)
Triggering mechanism	Pressure-supported breaths are patient triggered.
Cycling mechanism	Pressure-supported breaths are technically flow cycled by a minimum spontaneous inspiratory flow threshold. This minimum inspiratory flow is controlled entirely by the patient's spontaneous inspiratory flow demand.

NOTES: The tidal volume delivered by a pressure-supported breath is influenced both by the pressure support level (cm H_2O) and the patient's spontaneous inspiratory flow demand. The inspiratory time of the pressure-supported breath is also completely controlled by the patient's spontaneous inspiratory flow demand.

ADAPTIVE SUPPORT VENTILATION (ASV)

adaptive support ventilation (ASV): A mode of ventilation that changes the number of mandatory breaths and pressure support level according to the patient's breathing pattern.

☑ With increasing triggering efforts, the number of mandatory breaths decreases and the pressure support level increases until tidal volume = alveolar volume + 2.2 mL/kg of deadspace volume.

The **adaptive support ventilation (ASV)** mode is available in the Galileo ventilator. With this mode, the therapist inputs the patient's body weight and the percent minute volume. The body weight is used to estimate the deadspace volume. For an estimated minute ventilation requirement for a patient, the ventilator uses predetermined settings of 100 mL/min/kg for adults and 20 mL/min/kg for children. The therapist may select the percent minute volume ranging from 20% to 200% of the predetermined adult or child setting. For example, if 160% is selected for an adult, the minute ventilation delivered by the ventilator will be about 160 mL/min/kg.

In the ASV mode, the ventilator uses test breaths to measure the system compliance, airway resistance, and any intrinsic PEEP. Following determination of these variables, the ventilator selects and provides the frequency, inspiratory time, I:E ratio, and high pressure limit for mandatory and spontaneous breaths.

If there is no spontaneous triggering effort, the ventilator determines and provides the mandatory frequency, tidal volume, and high pressure limit needed to deliver the pre-selected tidal volume, inspiratory time, and I:E ratio. As the patient begins to trigger the ventilator, the number of mandatory breaths decreases and the pressure support level increases until a calculated tidal volume is able to provide adequate alveolar volume (i.e., tidal volume = alveolar volume + 2.2 mL/kg of deadspace volume).

PROPORTIONAL ASSIST VENTILATION (PAV)

proportional assist ventilation (PAV): A mode of ventilation that changes the pressure support level according to the volume, elastance, airflow resistance, and flow demand.

☑ The pressure support is in proportion to the patient's pulmonary characteristics (elastance and airflow resistance) and demand (volume or flow).

☑ PAV may be flow assist or volume assist and it is active in assist breaths only.

Proportional assist ventilation (PAV) (Evita 4, Dräger Medical) and proportional pressure support are similar modes of ventilation. With PAV, there is no target flow, volume, or pressure during mechanical ventilation. The pressure used to provide the pressure support is variable and is in proportion to the patient's pulmonary characteristics (elastance and airflow resistance) and demand (volume or flow) (Appendini et al., 1999). PAV is set to overcome 80% of the elastance and airflow resistance. For example, at 40 cm H_2O/L of elastance, 32 cm H_2O of pressure is generated to provide 1 L of volume.

PAV may be flow assist (FA) or volume assist (VA). In FA, the applied pressure is provided to meet the patient's inspiratory flow demand. FA reduces the inspiratory effort needed to overcome airflow resistance (Appendini et al., 1999). VA occurs when PAV provides the pressure to meet the patient's volume requirement. VA reduces the inspiratory effort needed to overcome systemic elastance such as restrictive lung defects (Navalesi et al., 1996).

PAV is achieved by a positive feedback control that amplifies airway pressure in proportion to instantaneous inspiratory flow and volume. Unlike the traditional modes of mechanical ventilation, PAV changes with the patient's breathing effort. The advantage of PAV is its ability to track changes in breathing effort over time. By varying the pressure to augment flow and volume, a more uniform breathing pattern becomes possible (Bigatello et al., 1997). PAV has been reported to provide mechanical ventilation while promoting patient-ventilator synchrony (Younes, 1992). However, in conditions where the elastance or airflow resistance shows sudden improvement, the pressure provided by PAV may be too high. This may lead to overdistension, increased air trapping, and barotrauma.

In terms of physiologic response, PAV improves ventilation and reduces the neuromuscular drive and work of breathing in ventilator-dependent patients with COPD. When PAV is used with CPAP, the reduction of inspiratory muscle work reaches values close to those found in normal subjects. Exercise tolerance may be improved with this strategy of combining PAV with CPAP (Appendini et al., 1999; Dolmage & Goldstein, 1997). Table 4-6 summarizes the major characteristics of the PAV mode.

TABLE 4-6 Characteristics of the Proportional Assist Ventilation Mode

CHARACTERISTIC	DESCRIPTION
Type of breath	PAV occurs during assisted breaths only
Triggering mechanism	Pressure or flow triggered
Cycling mechanism	PAV terminates once the patient's volume or flow demand is met

VOLUME-ASSURED PRESSURE SUPPORT (VAPS)

volume-assured pressure support (VAPS): A mode of ventilation that assures a stable tidal volume by incorporating inspiratory pressure support ventilation (PSV) with conventional volume-assisted cycles (VAV).

☑ VAPS incorporates pressure support ventilation with conventional volume-assisted cycles to provide stable tidal volume in patients with irregular breathing patterns.

☑ VAPS may prolong the inspiratory time. Patients with airflow obstruction should be monitored closely in order to prevent air trapping and other related side effects.

Pressure-regulated volume control (PRVC) provides volume support with the lowest pressure possible by changing the flow and inspiratory time.

Volume-assured pressure support (VAPS) is available in Bird 8400 STi and TBird ventilators. It is similar to pressure augmentation in Bear 1000 ventilator and is also known as volume-assisted pressure support.

VAPS incorporates inspiratory pressure support ventilation (PSV) with conventional volume-assisted cycles (VAV). This combination provides an optimal inspiratory flow during assisted/controlled cycles, reducing the patient's work of breathing commonly seen during VAV. Unlike typical PSV, VAPS assures stable tidal volume in patients with irregular breathing patterns.

In VAPS, the therapist must preset the desired minimum tidal volume and the pressure support level. During VAPS, the mechanical breaths may be patient or time triggered. Once a breath is triggered, the ventilator tries to reach the pressure support level as soon as possible. The delivered volume is then compared with the preset tidal volume for further action by the ventilator.

If the delivered volume equals the preset volume, the breath is considered a pressure support breath. Since pressure support breaths are dependent on the patient effort, the delivered volume may be larger than the preset volume. It is essential to set the pressure support level that provides a volume that is lower than the preset volume. On the other hand, if the delivered volume falls short of the preset volume, the ventilator switches from a pressure-limit breath to a volume-limited breath. This results in a longer inspiratory time (at a constant flow) until the preset volume is delivered.

Since VAPS may prolong the inspiratory time automatically, patients with airflow obstruction should be monitored closely in order to prevent air trapping and other undesirable cardiovascular effects associated with prolonged inspiratory time.

PRESSURE-REGULATED VOLUME CONTROL (PRVC)

Pressure-regulated volume control (PRVC) is available in Siemens 300 ventilator. It is also known as adaptive pressure ventilation in Hamilton Galileo ventilator, autoflow in Evita 4 ventilator, and variable pressure control in Venturi ventilator. In the Siemens 300 ventilator, PRVC is only active during CMV whereas in other ventilators, this type of dual control mode is also active in SIMV. Table 4-7 outlines the characteristics of the PRVC mode.

PRVC is used primarily to achieve volume support while keeping the peak inspiratory pressure (PIP) at a lowest level possible. This is

TABLE 4-7   Characteristics of the Pressure-Regulated Volume Control Mode

CHARACTERISTIC	DESCRIPTION
Type of breath	CMV in Siemens 300; SIMV in other ventilators
Triggering mechanism	Time triggered or patient triggered
Cycling mechanism	Volume cycled under normal operating conditions

✓ PRVC provides volume support while keeping the PIP at a lowest level possible by altering the peak flow and inspiratory time in response to changing airway or compliance characteristics.

achieved by altering the peak flow and inspiratory time in response to changing airway or compliance characteristics.

For example, Equation (1) below shows that at constant flow, the PIP is increased due to increasing airflow resistance. Note that the increasing airflow resistance may be due to increasing airway resistance (nonelastic resistance) or decreasing lung compliance (elastic resistance). Since PIP and flow have a direct mathematical relationship, PRVC lowers the flow (to reduce the driving pressure) so as to maintain the PIP at 5 cm H_2O below the pressure limit. See Equation (2). To compensate for a lower inspiratory flow, PRVC prolongs the inspiratory time to deliver the target volume.

(1) ↑ Airflow Resistance (nonelastic or elastic) = ↑ PIP / Flow

(2) ↑ Airflow Resistance (nonelastic or elastic) = PIP / ↓ Flow

AUTOMODE

automode: This mode provides time-triggered, PRVC breaths when prolonged apnea is detected (12, 8, and 5 sec in adult, pediatric, and neonatal modes respectively).

Automode is a feature of Siemens 300A ventilator and it combines PRVC and volume support. This mode alters between time-cycled and flow-cycled breaths depending on the degree of patient effort. If there is no spontaneous triggering effort for a time period (i.e., apnea for 12, 8, and 5 sec in adult, pediatric, and neonatal modes, respectively), the ventilator provides PRVC and the breaths are time triggered. The delivered volume is preset with a variable PIP up to the high pressure limit.

When the patient has two consecutive breaths that trigger the mechanical breaths, the automode switches to volume support in which all breaths become patient triggered, pressure limited, and flow cycled.

VOLUME VENTILATION PLUS (VV+)

volume ventilation plus: An option that combines volume control plus and volume support.

Volume ventilation plus (VV+) is available in the Puritan Bennett 840® ventilator (Tyco Healthcare). It is an option that combines two different dual mode volume-targeted breath types: volume control plus and volume support.

VOLUME CONTROL PLUS (VC+)

Volume control plus (VC+) is used to deliver mandatory breaths during AC and SIMV modes of ventilation. VC+ is intended to provide a higher level of synchrony than standard volume control ventilation.

☑ Following a test breath, the target pressures for subsequent breaths are adjusted accordingly to compensate for any tidal volume differences (Set V_T − Delivered V_T).

☑ In VC+, active spontaneous breaths are allowed during the inspiratory phase of a mandatory breath.

☑ In VS, the clinician sets the target tidal volume and the ventilator uses variable pressure support levels to provide the target tidal volume.

In VC+, the clinician sets the target tidal volume and inspiratory time. The ventilator delivers a single test breath using standard volume and decelerating flow and plateau to determine the relative compliance. The target pressures for subsequent breaths are adjusted accordingly to compensate for any tidal volume differences (Set V_T − Delivered V_T). Flow is adjusted automatically to reduce the likelihood of inadequate flow or aggressive flow demand.

Active spontaneous breaths are allowed during the inspiratory phase of a mandatory breath by way of a pressure control style of breath and the use of an active exhalation valve. Excessive pressure caused by breathing or coughing is vented, thus maintaining synchrony.

VOLUME SUPPORT (VS)

Volume support (VS) is intended to provide a control tidal volume and increased patient comfort. Weaning from anesthesia is a common application for VS.

In VS, the clinician sets the target tidal volume but not the inspiratory time or mandatory rate. The ventilator delivers a single spontaneous pressure support type of breath and uses variable pressure support levels to provide the target tidal volume. During weaning or awakening from anesthesia, the patient assumes a higher spontaneous tidal volume and the ventilator decreases the pressure support level accordingly. When the spontaneously tidal volume decreases, the ventilator increases the pressure support level automatically to maintain the target tidal volume.

During VS, the ventilator rate and minute ventilation are determined by the triggering effort of the patient. The inspiratory time is determined by the patient respiratory demand.

PRESSURE CONTROL VENTILATION (PCV)

pressure control ventilation (PCV): Once inspiration begins, a pressure plateau is created and maintained for a preset inspiratory time.

In **pressure control ventilation (PCV),** the pressure-controlled breaths are time triggered by a preset respiratory rate. Once inspiration begins, a pressure plateau is created and maintained for a preset inspiratory time. Pressure-controlled breaths are therefore time triggered, pressure limited, and time cycled.

Pressure control is a newer mode of controlled ventilation that has some functional similarities to pressure support ventilation, but they have very different indications. Pressure-controlled breaths are time triggered by a preset respiratory rate and as in the control mode, the patient should be sedated. Once a pressure-controlled breath has been time triggered, a pressure plateau is created and maintained by servo-controlled inspiratory flow in a manner similar to pressure support. Recall that the pressure plateau in pressure support is maintained for as long as the patient maintains a spontaneous inspiratory flow.

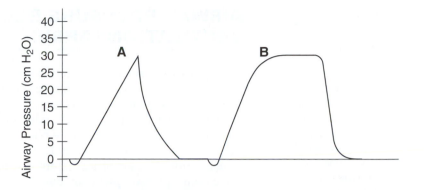

Figure 4-9 (A) Pressure tracing of a volume-controlled mechanical breath; (B) Pressure tracing of a pressure-controlled mechanical breath; note the prolonged inspiratory pressure plateau with pressure control ventilation.

✓ Pressure control can minimize the peak inspiratory pressure while still maintaining adequate oxygenation and ventilation.

In pressure control, however, the pressure plateau is maintained for a preset inspiratory time (Figure 4-9).

Pressure control is usually indicated for patients with severe ARDS who require extremely high peak inspiratory pressures during mechanical ventilation in a volume-cycled mode. As a result of these high airway pressures, they have a higher incidence of barotrauma (Gurevitch et al., 1986).

The advantage of switching these patients from conventional volume-cycled ventilation to pressure control is that by doing so, the peak inspiratory pressure can be reduced while still maintaining adequate oxygenation (PaO_2) and ventilation ($PaCO_2$) (Lain et al., 1989). Being able to decrease the PIP significantly reduces the risk of barotrauma for these patients.

Table 4-8 summarizes the major characteristics of the pressure control ventilation mode.

TABLE 4-8 Characteristics of the Pressure Control Ventilation Mode

CHARACTERISTIC	DESCRIPTION
Type of breath	Only mandatory breaths are available to the patient in the pressure control mode.
Triggering mechanism	The mandatory breaths in the pressure control mode are time triggered by a preset rate (may be patient triggered for additional breaths).
Cycling mechanism	The mandatory breaths are time cycled by a preset inspiratory time.

NOTES: The peak inspiratory pressure is controlled by the preset pressure limit. As with any pressure limited ventilator, the tidal volume will vary directly with lung compliance and inversely with airway resistance. It may be necessary to invert the I:E ratio beyond 1:2 to maintain oxygenation. I:E ratios as high as 4:1 have been reported with successful outcome.

AIRWAY PRESSURE RELEASE VENTILATION (APRV)

airway pressure release ventilation (APRV): A mode of ventilation in which the spontaneous breaths are at an elevated baseline (i.e., CPAP). This elevated baseline is periodically "released" to facilitate expiration.

Airway pressure release ventilation (APRV) is similar to CPAP in that the patient is allowed to breathe spontaneously without restriction. During spontaneous exhalation, the PEEP is dropped (released) to a lower level and this action simulates an effective exhalation maneuver. The length of pressure release time is usually between 1 and 2 sec. When the pressure release time is shorter than the spontaneous effort, it resembles pressure-controlled breath (from high to low baseline pressure) with an inverse inspiratory-expiratory (I:E) ratio.

To provide APRV, the ventilator must have a high flow CPAP circuit that has been modified with the addition of a release valve. When the release valve opens, the CPAP pressure is vented and the circuit pressure decreases to zero or a lower CPAP level. Figure 4-10 shows the airway pressure release during CPAP mode.

A mandatory inspiration begins with time-triggered closing of the release valve. The airway pressure rapidly increases to the baseline CPAP pressure and is maintained for the duration of

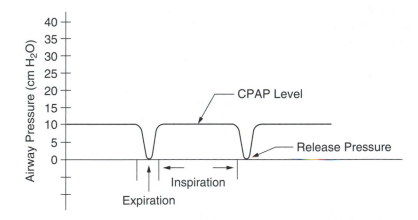

Figure 4-10   Airway pressure release ventilation (APRV) at a CPAP level of 10 cm H_2O and pressure release to 0 cm H_2O with a net release pressure gradient of 10 (10−0) cm H_2O. During APRV, the expiratory phase occurs when the airway pressure is released from 10 to 0 cm H_2O. On inspiration, the CPAP level is maintained at 10 cm H_2O. Since the pressure release time period is rather short, an inversed I:E ratio is usually observed when the mechanical rate is less than 20 breaths per minute (or more than 3 seconds per breath). The tidal volume during APRV is determined by the pressure gradient between CPAP and final pressure after pressure release.

✓ With APRV, the patient's tidal volume will vary directly with changes in lung compliance and inversely with changes in airway resistance.

✓ APRV can provide effective partial ventilatory support with lower peak airway pressure than that provided by the PSV and SIMV modes.

inspiration (for as long as the release valve remains closed). The mandatory inspiration ends with time-triggered opening of the release valve, which allows the circuit pressure to decrease as the patient exhales. What is unique about this mode is that the patient is allowed to inspire spontaneously at any point during a mandatory breath. Since APRV mandatory breaths are pressure limited, for a given pressure gradient (difference between the CPAP circuit pressure and the release pressure), the patient's tidal volume will vary directly with changes in lung compliance and inversely with changes in airway resistance. For this reason, the patient's exhaled tidal volume should be closely monitored.

When bilevel (two level-CPAP) mode on the Puritan Bennett 840 ventilator is in use, the spontaneous breaths have the option of PSV. This PSV feature helps to augment the spontaneous tidal volumes in condition of low compliance and high airflow resistance.

INDICATIONS FOR THE APRV MODE

This is a relatively new mode of ventilation that has yet to gain wide acceptance. At present, the primary indication for this mode is similar to that of pressure control, namely, as an alternative to conventional volume-cycled ventilation for patients with significantly decreased lung compliance such as patients with ARDS. Conventional volume-cycled ventilation in these patients is associated with excessive peak airway pressures and barotrauma. APRV can provide effective partial ventilatory support with lower peak airway pressure than that provided by the PSV and SIMV modes (Chiang et al., 1994). However, APRV may be less comfortable than the PSV and SIMV modes, and synchronization with mechanical breaths may also be a problem.

Table 4-9 summarizes the major characteristics of the airway pressure release ventilation mode.

TABLE 4-9   Characteristics of the Airway Pressure Release Ventilation Mode

CHARACTERISTIC	DESCRIPTION
Type of breath	Time-triggered mandatory breaths will continue in this mode and the patient is allowed to breathe spontaneously between mandatory breaths.
Triggering mechanism	The mandatory breaths are time triggered, and the patient assumes all spontaneous breaths.
Cycling mechanism	The mandatory breaths are time cycled by a preset inspiratory time.

INVERSE RATIO VENTILATION (IRV)

The ratio of inspiratory time (I time) to expiratory time (E time) is known as the I:E ratio. In conventional mechanical ventilation, the I time is traditionally lower than the E time so that the I:E ratio ranges from about 1:1.5 to 1:3. This resembles the normal I:E ratio during spontaneous breathing, and it is considered physiologically beneficial to normal cardiopulmonary function.

Since the mid-1980s, investigators have been extending the inspiratory time during mechanical ventilation to promote oxygenation in patients with ARDS (Gurevitch et al., 1986; Marcy et al., 1991). The inverse I:E ratio in use is between 2:1 and 4:1 and often it is used in conjunction with pressure control ventilation (Lain et al., 1989; Tharratt et al., 1988).

PHYSIOLOGY OF IRV

☑ Inverse ratio ventilation (IRV) improves oxygenation by (1) ↓ intrapulmonary shunting, (2) ↑ V/Q matching, and (3) ↓ deadspace ventilation.

Inverse ratio ventilation (IRV) improves oxygenation by (1) reduction of intrapulmonary shunting, (2) improvement of V/Q matching, and (3) decrease of deadspace ventilation. From the review of available literature, Shanholtz et al. (1994) concluded that these mechanisms were also achievable by use of conventional ventilation with PEEP. However, two notable changes are observed during IRV. They are (1) increase of mean airway pressure and (2) presence of auto-PEEP. These two changes are likely the reason for the improvement of shunting and hypoxemia in ARDS patients.

☑ The increase in mPaw during IRV helps to reduce shunting and improve oxygenation in ARDS patients.

Increase of Mean Airway Pressure.   To achieve the same degree of ventilation and oxygenation, IRV requires a lower peak airway pressure and PEEP, but a higher mean airway pressure (mPaw) than conventional mechanical ventilation. The increase in mPaw during IRV helps to reduce shunting and improve oxygenation in ARDS patients (Shanholtz et al., 1994).

☑ The presence of auto-PEEP during IRV may help to reduce shunting and improve oxygenation in ARDS patients.

Addition of Auto-PEEP.   Since IRV provides a longer I time and shorter E time, breath stacking with an increase of end-expiratory pressure is likely when there is not enough time for complete expiration (Duncan et al., 1987; Kacmarek et al., 1990). The presence of auto-PEEP during IRV may help to reduce shunting and improve oxygenation in ARDS patients (Shanholtz et al., 1994).

ADVERSE EFFECTS OF IRV

During IRV, the increase in mPaw and the presence of auto-PEEP both contribute to the increase of mean alveolar pressure and volume, the incidence of barotrauma may be as high as that obtained by conventional ventilation with high levels of PEEP (Tharratt et al., 1988).

TABLE 4-10 Observed Changes after Switching from PPV + PEEP to PC-IRV

INCREASE	DECREASE	NO CHANGE
Mean airway pressure	PEEP requirement	F_IO_2 requirement
Central venous pressure	Peak airway pressure	Intrinsic PEEP
Pulmonary artery pressure	Cardiac output	Blood pressure
PaO_2		$PaCO_2$

(Data from East et al., 1992; Lain et al., 1989, 1990.)

Another potential hazard of IRV is a higher rate of transvascular fluid flow or flooding induced by an increased alveolar pressure (Permutt et al., 1979). This condition may induce or worsen preexisting pulmonary edema.

Patients receiving IRV are often agitated. They may require sedation and neuromuscular blocking agents to facilitate ventilation. The associated complications with these drugs can be serious and they should be monitored carefully when used in conjunction with IRV (Hansen-Flaschen et al., 1993).

PRESSURE CONTROL-IRV (PC-IRV)

☑ When PC is used with IRV, the peak airway pressure may be kept at a safe level.

Since IRV may increase the mPaw, create auto-PEEP, and increase the incidence of barotrauma, it is sometimes used in conjunction with pressure control due to its pressure-limiting capability. By using pressure control, the peak airway pressure may be kept at a safe level. This strategy helps to minimize pressure-induced lung injuries. When an inverse I:E ratio is used with pressure control ventilation, it is called pressure control inverse ratio ventilation (PC-IRV).

Several studies compare the outcomes of ARDS patients before and after the implementation of PC-IRV. The changes that may occur when positive pressure ventilation with PEEP (PPV + PEEP) is switched over to the PC-IRV mode of ventilation are summarized in Table 4-10.

AUTOMATIC TUBE COMPENSATION (ATC)

automatic tube compensation (ATC): A mode of ventilation that offsets and compensates for the airflow resistance imposed by the artificial airway.

Automatic tube compensation (ATC) is available in the Evita 4 ventilator (Dräger Medical). PB840 ventilator has a similar feature which is called tubing compensation (TC). This tubing compensation can be applied in all ventilation modes. ATC offsets and compensates for the airflow resistance imposed by the artificial airway. It allows the patient to have a breathing pattern as if breathing spontaneously without an artificial airway. With ATC, the pressure delivered by the ventilator to compensate for the airflow resistance is active during inspiration and expiration. It is dependent on the airflow characteristics and the flow demand of the patient. For example, when the airway diameter decreases or flow demand increases, the pressure is raised to overcome a higher airflow resistance or increased flow demand.

SUMMARY

There are many different ventilator operating modes and the number is expected to increase in coming years. As each mode is designed to accomplish a set of specific functions, it is essential to understand its capabilities, as well as its limitations and complications. When two or more operating modes are used in tandem, care and caution must be used because the combined outcomes are often complex and difficult to predict or manipulate.

An excellent source of obtaining detailed technical information is to consult the operation manual or contact the technical professionals of each ventilator manufacturer. Quality patient care is possible when the appropriate operating modes are selected and applied. A willingness to participate in continuing education is highly desirable and sometimes mandatory in this ever-changing field of mechanical ventilation.

Self-Assessment Questions

1. Volume cycled ventilators deliver a predetermined _____ to the patient using variable _____ according to the changing compliance and resistance.

   A. tidal volume, peak inspiratory pressure
   B. tidal volume, PEEP

   C. peak airway pressure, tidal volume
   D. PEEP, pressure support

2. Positive end-expiratory pressure (PEEP) is most commonly used to correct:

   A. hypercapnia.
   B. mild hypoxemia.

   C. refractory hypoxemia.
   D. respiratory acidosis.

3. In the assist/control (AC) mode of a volume-limited ventilator, the tidal volume initiated by the assist breath should be _____ the tidal volume initiated by the control breath.

   A. greater than
   B. less than

   C. about 150 mL less than
   D. equal to

4. When PEEP is applied to the airway of a patient who is breathing spontaneously, it is called:

   A. airway pressure release ventilation.
   B. continuous positive airway pressure.

   C. pressure support ventilation.
   D. pressure control ventilation.

5. _____ is a mode in which the ventilator delivers control (mandatory) breaths and allows the patient to breathe spontaneously to any tidal volume the patient is capable of in between the mandatory breaths.

A. Intermittent mandatory ventilation
B. Continuous positive airway pressure
C. Mandatory minute ventilation
D. Airway pressure release ventilation

6. _____ delivers control (mandatory) breaths to the patient at or near the beginning of a spontaneous breath, thus avoiding breath stacking.

A. Continuous positive airway pressure
B. Airway pressure release ventilation
C. Intermittent mandatory ventilation
D. Synchronized intermittent mandatory ventilation

7. _____ best describes the mode of ventilation that changes the number of mandatory breaths and pressure support level according to the patient's breathing pattern.

A. Automatic tube compensation
B. Volume ventilation plus
C. Adaptive support ventilation
D. Volume-assured pressure support

8. _____ is primarily used to reduce the work of breathing imposed by the endotracheal tube and ventilator circuit.

A. Pressure support ventilation
B. Pressure control ventilation
C. Airway pressure release ventilation
D. Continuous positive airway pressure

9. _____ is a mode of ventilation that changes the pressure support level according to the changes in volume, elastance, airflow resistance, and flow demand.

A. Proportional assist ventilation (proportional pressure support)
B. Pressure support ventilation
C. Volume-assured pressure support
D. Automatic tube compensation

10. _____ is a mode of ventilation that assures a stable tidal volume by using pressure support ventilation and volume-assisted ventilation.

A. Automatic tube compensation
B. Pressure support ventilation
C. Proportional pressure support
D. Volume-assured pressure support

11. In pressure-regulated volume control, the peak inspiratory pressure is kept at a lowest level possible by altering the _____ in response to changing airway or compliance characteristics.

A. peak flow and tidal volume
B. peak flow and inspiratory time
C. plateau pressure and tidal volume
D. plateau pressure and inspiratory time

12. Volume ventilation plus (VV+) provides the following options:

   A. volume control plus, and pressure support.
   B. volume control plus and volume support.
   C. volume-assured pressure support and pressure support.
   D. volume-assured pressure support and volume support.

13. When the patient has no spontaneous breathing efforts, pressure control ventilation delivers _____ triggered breaths and a _____ is created and maintained for a preset inspiratory time.

   A. pressure, PEEP
   B. time, pressure plateau
   C. flow, pressure plateau
   D. patient, PEEP

14. One distinctive characteristic of airway pressure release ventilation is that during exhalation, the _____ level is lowered (released) to the baseline or a lower level.

   A. peak airway pressure
   B. plateau pressure
   C. continuous positive airway pressure
   D. positive end expiratory pressure

15. Inverse ratio ventilation has been used successfully to reduce intrapulmonary shunting and improve oxygenation. These effects are likely the result of _____ and _____.

   A. deadspace ventilation, increase of peak airway pressure.
   B. deadspace ventilation, auto-PEEP.
   C. increase of mean airway pressure, auto-PEEP.
   D. increase of peak airway pressure, auto-PEEP.

Answers to Self-Assessment Questions

1. A. tidal volume, peak inspiratory pressure

2. C. refractory hypoxemia.

3. D. equal to

4. B. continuous positive airway pressure.

5. A. Intermittent mandatory ventilation

6. D. Synchronized intermittent mandatory ventilation

7. C. Adaptive support ventilation

8. A. Pressure support ventilation

9. A. Proportional assist ventilation (proportional pressure support)

10. D. Volume-assured pressure support

11. B. peak flow and inspiratory time.

12. B. volume control plus and volume support

13. B. time, pressure plateau

14. C. continuous positive airway pressure

15. C. increase of mean airway pressure, auto-PEEP

References

Ambrosino, N., et al. (1992). Physiologic evaluation of pressure support ventilation by nasal mask in patients with stable COPD. *Chest, 101,* 385–391.

Appendini, L., Purro, A., & Gudjonsdottir, M., et al. (1999). Physiologic response of ventilator-dependent patients with chronic obstructive pulmonary disease to proportional assist ventilation and continuous positive airway pressure. *Am J Respir Crit Care Med, 159*(5 Pt 1), 1510–1517.

Baer, C. L., et al. (1992). Acute renal failure. *Crit Care Nurs Q, 14*(4), 1.

Bezzant, T. B., et al. (1994). Risk and hazards of mechanical ventilation: A collective review of published literature. *Dis Mon, 40*(11), 583–638.

Bigatello, I. M., Nishimura, M., Imanaka, H., et al. (1997). Unloading of the work of breathing by proportional assist ventilation in a lung model. *Crit Care Med, 25*(2), 267–272.

Brundage, D. J. (1992). *Renal disorders.* St. Louis, MO: Mosby.

Burton, G. B., et al. (1997). *Respiratory care: A guide to clinical practice* (4th ed.). Baltimore: Lippincott Williams & Wilkins.

Carroll, N., et al. (1988). Control of nocturnal hypoventilation by nasal intermittent positive pressure ventilation. *Thorax, 43,* 349–353.

Chiang, A. A., et al. (1994). Demand-flow airway pressure release ventilation as a partial ventilatory support mode: Comparison with synchronized intermittent mandatory ventilation and pressure support ventilation. *Crit Care Med, 22*(9), 1431–1437.

Confalonieri, M., et al. (1994). Severe exacerbations of chronic obstructive pulmonary disease treated with BiPAP by nasal mask. *Respiration, 61*(6), 310–316.

Corrado, A., et al. (1994). Iron lung treatment of acute or chronic respiratory failure: 16 years of experience. *Monaldi Arch Chest Dis, 49*(6), 552–555.

Culpepper, J. A., et al. (1985). Effect of mechanical ventilator mode on tendency towards respiratory alkalosis. *Am Rev Respir Dis, 132*(5), 1075–1077.

Des Jardins, T. R. (2001). *Cardiopulmonary anatomy and physiology: Essentials for respiratory care* (4th ed.). Clifton Park, NY: Thomson Delmar Learning.

Dolmage, T. E., & Goldstein, R. S. (1997). Proportional assist ventilation and exercise tolerance in subjects with COPD. *Chest, 111*(4), 948–954.

Downs, J. B., et al. (1973). Intermittent mandatory ventilation: A new approach to weaning patients from mechanical ventilators. *Chest, 64,* 331–335.

Duncan, S. R., et, al. (1987). Inverse ratio ventilation. PEEP in disguise? *Chest, 92,* 390–391.

East, T. D., et al. (1992). A successful computerized protocol for clinical management of pressure control inverse ratio ventilation in ARDS patients. *Chest, 101*(3), 697–710.

Ellis, E. R., et al. (1987). Treatment of respiratory failure during sleep in patients with neuro-muscular disease. *Am Rev Respir Dis, 135,* 148–152.

Frederick, C. (1994). Noninvasive mechanical ventilation with the iron lung. *Crit Care Nurs Clin North Am, 6*(4), 831–840.

Gurevitch M. J., et al. (1986). Improved oxygenation and lower peak airway pressure in severe adult respiratory distress syndrome: Treatment with inverse ratio ventilation. *Chest, 89,* 211–213.

Hansen-Flaschen, J., et al. (1993). Neuromuscular blockade in the intensive care unit: More than we bargain for. *Am Rev Respir Dis, 147,* 234–236.

Heenan, T. J., et al. (1980). Intermittent mandatory ventilation. *Chest, 77,* 598–602.

Hill, N. S. (1992). Efficacy of nocturnal nasal ventilation in patients with restrictive thoracic disease. *Am Rev Respir Dis, 145,* 365–371.

Hopper, R. G., et al. (1985). Acid-base changes and ventilator mode during maintenance ventilation. *Crit Care Med, 13*(1), 44–45.

Kacmarek, R. M., et al. (1990). Pressure-controlled inverse-ratio ventilation: Panacea or auto-PEEP? *Respir Care, 35,* 945–948.

Kanak, R., et al. (1985). Oxygen cost of breathing: Changes dependent upon mode of mechanical ventilation. *Chest, 87*(1), 126–127.

Kinnear, W., Hockley, S., Harvey, J., et al. (1988). The effects of one year of nocturnal cuirass-assisted ventilation in chest wall disease. *Eur Respir J, 1*(3), 204–208.

Kinnear, W., Petch, M., Taylor, G., et al. (1988). Assisted ventilation using cuirass respirators. *Eur Respir J, 1*(3), 198–203.

Kirby, R. R. (1988). Modes of mechanical ventilation. In R. M. Kacmarek et al. (Eds.), *Current respiratory care.* Philadelphia: B. C. Becker.

Lain, D. C., et al. (1989). Pressure control inverse ratio ventilation as a method to reduce peak inspiratory pressure and provide adequate ventilation and oxygenation. *Chest, 95*(5), 1081–1088.

Lain, D., et al. (1990). Reduction of peak inflation and positive end-expiratory pressures using pressure control with inverse-ratio ventilation: A case report. *Heart Lung, 19*(4), 358–361.

Linton, D. M., et al. (1992). Metabolic requirements in tetanus. *Crit Care Med, 20*(7), 950–952.

MacIntyre, N. R. (1986). Respiratory function during pressure support ventilation. *Chest, 89*(5), 677–683.

MacIntyre, N. R. (1987). Pressure support ventilation: Effects on ventilatory reflexes and ventilatory muscle workload. *Resp Care, 32,* 447–457.

Marcy, T. W., et al. (1991). Inverse ratio ventilation in ARDS: Rationale and implementation. *Chest, 100,* 494–504.

Navalesi, P., Hernandez, P., Wongsa, A., et al. (1996). Proportional assist ventilation in acute respiratory failure: Effects on breathing pattern and inspiratory effort. *Am J Respir Crit Care Med, 154*(5), 1330–1338.

Newman, J. H., et al. (1988). Fabrication of a customized cuirass for patients with severe thoracic asymmetry. *Am Rev Respir Dis, 137*(1), 202–203.

Perel, A., et al. (1992). *Handbook of mechanical ventilatory support.* Baltimore: Lippincott Williams & Wilkins.

Permutt, S., et al. (1979). Mechanical influences on water accumulation in the lungs. In A. E. Fishman (ed.), *Pulmonary edema* (pp. 175–193). Bethesda, MD: American Physiologic Society.

Petersen, G. W., et al. (1983). Incidence of pulmonary barotrauma in a medical ICU. *Crit Care Med, 11,* 67–69.

Qvist, J., et al. (1975). Hemodynamic responses to mechanical ventilation with PEEP. *Anesthesiology, 42,* 45–55.

Renston, J. P., et al. (1994). Respiratory muscle rest using nasal BiPAP ventilation in patients with stable severe COPD. *Chest, 105*(4), 1053–1060.

Sassoon, C. S. H., et al. (1990). Ventilator modes: Old and new. *Crit Care Clin, 6(*3), 605–634.

Sassoon, C. S. H. (1991). Positive pressure ventilation: Alternate modes. *Chest, 100,* 1421–1429.

Shanholtz, C., et al. (1994). Should inverse ratio ventilation be used in adult respiratory distress syndrome? *Am J Respir Crit Care Med, 149,* 1354–1358.

Shapiro, B. A., et al. (1976). Intermittent demand ventilation (IDV): A new technique for support ventilation in critically ill patients. *Respir Care, 21,* 521–525

Shapiro, B. A., et al. (1991). *Clinical application of respiratory care.* St. Louis, MO: Mosby.

Slutsky, A. S. (1994). Consensus conference on mechanical ventilation—January 28–30, 1993 at Northbrook, IL, USA, Part I. *Int Care Med, 20,* 64–79.

Strumpf, D. A. (1990). An evaluation of the Respironics BiPAP bi-level CPAP device for delivery of assisted ventilation. *Respir Care, 35,* 415–422.

Tharratt, R. S., et al. (1988). Pressure controlled inverse ratio ventilation in severe adult respiratory failure. *Chest, 94,* 755–762.

Tyler, D. C. (1983). Positive end expiratory pressure: A review. *Crit Care Med, 11*(4), 300–308.

Waldhorn, R. E. (1992). Nocturnal nasal intermittent positive pressure ventilation with bi-level positive airway pressure (BiPAP) in respiratory failure. *Chest, 101,* 516–521.

Weisman, L. M., et al. (1983). Intermittent mandatory ventilation. *Am Rev Respir Dis, 127,* 641–647.

Wilkins, R. L., et al. (2003). *Egan's fundamentals of respiratory care* (8th ed.) St. Louis , MO: Mosby.

Younes, M. (1992). Proportional assist ventilation, a new approach to ventilatory support: Theory. *Am Rev Respir Dis, 145,* 114–120.

Zelt, B. A., et al. (1972). Prolonged nasotracheal intubation and mechanical ventilation in the management of asphyxiating thoracic dystrophy: A case report. *Anesth Analg, 51,* 342–348.

Suggested Reading

Adaptive Support Ventilation
Petter A. H., et al. (2003). Automatic 'respirator/weaning' with adaptive support ventilation: The effect on duration of endotracheal intubation and patient management. *Anesth Analg,* 97(6), 1743–1750.

Airway Pressure Release Ventilation
Frawley P. M., et al. (2001). Airway pressure release ventilation: Theory and practice. *AACN Clin Issues,* 12(2), 234–246.

Mode of Ventilation
Chatburn, R. L., et al. (2001). A new system for understanding modes of mechanical ventilation. *Respir Care,* 46(6), 604–621.

PEEP/Pressure Support
MacIntyre, N. R., Cheng, K. C., & McConnell, R. (1997). Applied PEEP during pressure support reduces the inspiratory threshold load of intrinsic PEEP. *Chest, 111*(1), 188–193.

Proportional Assist Ventilation
Ambrosino, N., Vitacca, M., Polese, G., et al. (1997). Short-term effects of nasal *proportional* assist ventilation in patients with chronic hypercapnic respiratory insufficiency. *Eur Respir J, 10*(12), 2829–2834.

Bianchi, L., Foglio, K., Pagani, M., et al. (1998). Effects of *proportional* assist ventilation on exercise tolerance in COPD patients with chronic hypercapnia. *Eur Respir J, 11*(2), 422–427.

Marantz, S., Patrick, W., Webster, K., et al. (1996). Response of ventilator-dependent patients to different levels of proportional assist. *J Appl Physiol, 80*(2), 397–403.

Ranieri, V. M., Giuliani, R., Mascia, L., et al. (1996). Patient-ventilator interaction during acute hypercapnia: Pressure-support vs. proportional-assist ventilation. *J Appl Physiol, 81*(1), 426–436.

Ranieri, V. M., Grasso, S., Mascia, L., et al. (1997). Effects of proportional assist ventilation on inspiratory muscle effort in patients with chronic obstructive pulmonary disease and acute respiratory failure. *Anesthesiology, 86*(1), 79–91.

Tejeda, M., Boix, J. H., Alvarez, F., et al. (1997). Comparison of pressure support ventilation and assist-control ventilation in the treatment of respiratory failure. *Chest, 111*(5), 1322–1325.

Protective-Ventilation Strategy

Acute respiratory distress syndrome network. (2000). Ventilation with lower tidal volumes as compared with traditional tidal volumes for acute lung injury and acute respiratory distress syndrome. *NEJM,* 342, 1301–1308.

Amato, M., et al. (1998). Effects of a protective-ventilation strategy on mortality in the acute respiratory distress syndrome. *NEJM,* 338, 347–354.

Artigas, A., et al. (1998). The American-European consensus conference on ARDS, Part 2. *Am J Respir Crit Care Med,* 157, 1332–1347.

Volume-Controlled Ventilation

Kallet R., et al. (2000). The effects of pressure control versus volume control assisted ventilation on patient work of breathing in acute lung injury and acute respiratory distress syndrome. *Respir Care,* 45, 1085–1096.

CHAPTER FIVE

SPECIAL AIRWAYS FOR VENTILATION

David W. Chang

OUTLINE

KEY TERMS

- autoclave
- blind distal end
- blind intubation
- double-lumen endobronchial tube
- esophageal gastric tube airway (EGTA)

- esophageal obturator airway (EOA)
- laryngeal mask airway (LMA)
- oropharyngeal airway
- pharyngealtracheal lumen airway (PTLA)

INTRODUCTION

In situations involving respiratory arrest, bag and mask ventilation is typically used and may be followed by endotracheal intubation. Occasionally, endotracheal intubation may not be successful due to unusual anatomy or difficult intubation. In these cases, a special airway such as the esophageal obturator airway, the esophageal gastric tube airway, the laryngeal mask airway, and the pharyngealtracheal lumen airway may serve as a stopgap measure for providing ventilation when bag and mask ventilation is deemed inadequate. Double-lumen endobronchial tube is another special airway for conditions where independent lung ventilation is indicated.

OROPHARYNGEAL AIRWAY

oropharyngeal airway: A device to relieve upper airway obstruction.

☑ An oropharyngeal airway should be used in patients who are sedated or unconscious.

An **oropharyngeal airway** is used to relieve upper airway obstruction if airway maneuvers (e.g., head tilt-chin lift, jaw thrust) fail to open an unobstructed airway (White, 2004). During bag-mask ventilation, an oropharyngeal airway may facilitate effective ventilation. It may also be used as a bite block in intubated patients. An oropharyngeal airway should be used in patients who are sedated or unconscious. For conscious patients, insertion of this airway may cause gag reflex, vomiting, and aspiration of stomach contents into the lungs.

TYPES OF OROPHARYNGEAL AIRWAYS

There are two major types of oropharyngeal airways (Figure 5-1). The Berman airway has external side channels and ranges from size 43 mm for infants to size 110 mm for extra large adults. The common Guedel airway has one large internal channel and the Cath-Guide Guedel has three internal channels. Guedel airways have sizes ranging from 55 mm for infants to 120 mm for extra large adults. (Table 5-1)

Figure 5-1 A variety of oropharyngeal airways. Berman airways, a Guedel airway, and a Cath-Guide Guedel airway are shown.

SELECTION OF OROPHARYNGEAL AIRWAY

☑ The size of an oropharyngeal airway may be estimated by the distance from the center of the mouth to the angle of the jaw or from the corner of the mouth to the earlobe.

The appropriate size (from flange to distal tip) of an oropharyngeal airway may be estimated based on the length in millimeters from the center of the mouth to the angle of the jaw. Alternatively, the length in millimeters from the corner of the mouth to the earlobe may be used. The third method is to measure the distance from the central incisors to the angle of the jaw. To evaluate the size using this method, place the airway next to the patient's face. (http://www.bol.ucla.edu/~ofattal/Circulation10282000.htm)

Proper sizing for the patient is important. If the airway is too large, it may push the epiglottis against the larynx leading to airway obstruction. If the airway is too small, the tongue may not be sufficiently moved away from the soft palate leading to airway obstruction by the tongue.

TABLE 5-1 Size Chart for Berman and Guedel Oropharyngeal Airways

	EXTRA LARGE ADULT	LARGE ADULT	MEDIUM ADULT	SMALL ADULT	CHILD	INFANT
Berman	110 mm	100 mm	90 mm	80 mm	60 mm	43 mm
Guedel	120 mm	110 mm	100 mm	80 mm	60, 70 mm	55 mm

INSERTION OF OROPHARYNGEAL AIRWAY

Prior to insertion of an oropharyngeal airway, ensure that the patient is sedated or unconscious. If the patient begins to gag or retch during the procedure, remove the airway immediately and reassess the necessity of an oropharyngeal airway. Sometimes the airway may be opened and maintained by repositioning of the head (e.g., head tilt-chin lift, jaw thrust).

Body fluid or isolation precautions must be observed throughout the procedure. The patient should be in a supine position, and the mouth is opened using the scissors (crosses fingers) technique. If a tongue blade is available, the tongue is depressed and the oropharyngeal airway may be inserted with the pharyngeal curvature. Some practitioners prefer to insert the airway into the patient's mouth upside down so that the distal end of the airway is facing the hard palate (roof of the patient's mouth). As the airway is inserted fully, it is turned 180° until the flange (proximal end) rests on the patient's lips or teeth (White, 2004). The correct placement of an oropharyngeal airway is shown in Figure 5-2.

Figure 5-2 The correct placement of an oropharyngeal airway. Note how the distal tip of the airway rests at the base of the tongue.

ESOPHAGEAL OBTURATOR AIRWAY (EOA)

esophageal obturator airway (EOA): An EOA has a closed (blind) distal end and it is inserted into the esophagus.

blind distal end: The far end of a tube without an opening.

Unlike an endotracheal tube, an **esophageal obturator airway (EOA)** is inserted into the esophagus. It is used as an alternative to bag and mask ventilation. The EOA is a disposable tube; its structure consists of an opening at the proximal (top) end, many small holes near the upper end, and a **blind distal end.** Near the distal end is a large cuff that is inflated during use. The inflated cuff prevents air from entering the stomach and subsequent regurgitation and aspiration. A mask fits over the tube to prevent leaks around the patient's face during ventilation (Burton et al., 1997; White, 2004). Figure 5-3 shows an esophageal obturator airway.

The opening at the proximal end of the tube attaches to a ventilation bag. The small holes at the hypopharyngeal level allow ventilation to the lungs. The closed distal end of the EOA prevents aspiration or removal of air or gastric contents from the stomach. Since an EOA is inserted into the esophagus, the cuff at the distal end must be inflated during use to prevent air from entering the stomach (Wilkins, 2003; White, 2004).

☑ Since an EOA is inserted into the esophagus, the cuff at the distal end must be inflated during use to prevent air from entering the stomach.

INSERTION OF EOA

The cuff of an EOA is first inflated with 20 to 30 cc of air to check for cuff integrity and leaks. The cuff is then deflated, and the proximal end of the EOA is inserted through the opening of a mask. The distal end of the tube is lubricated with a water-soluable lubricant and

Figure 5-3 An esophageal obturator airway (EOA).

TABLE 5-2   Precautions in the Use of an Esophageal Obturator Airway

An EOA should not be used in awake or semiconscious patients.

An EOA should not be used in children under 16 years of age or under 5 ft tall.

An EOA should not be used in patients with known esophageal disease.

Do not remove the EOA until the patient has regained consciousness.

then inserted into the patient's esophagus until the mask rests on the patient's face. Due to the large volume of air used to inflate the cuff, it is extremely important to check for proper tube placement before cuff inflation and ventilation. Asphyxia and tracheal damage are severe complications if the cuff is inflated while the tube is misplaced in the trachea (Wilkins, 2003; White, 2004). Table 5-2 lists other precautions during use of the EOA.

☑ The EOA is not designed to be used as an artificial airway for positive pressure ventilation.

The EOA is not designed to be used as an artificial airway for positive pressure ventilation. Since it is used as a temporary airway, it should be replaced with an endotracheal intubation as soon as feasible. With the EOA in place, endotracheal intubation is done using the standard procedure. After endotracheal intubation, bilateral breath sounds should be verified as the endotracheal tube may follow the EOA and enter the esophagus. After ascertaining correct placement, the endotracheal tube is secured prior to removal of the EOA. Suction setup should be ready in case of vomiting during removal of the EOA.

ESOPHAGEAL GASTRIC TUBE AIRWAY (EGTA)

esophageal gastric tube airway: A tube used in esophageal intubation. It has a patent distal end to relieve gastric distention.

The **esophageal gastric tube airway (EGTA)** is similar in design to the EOA. Whereas the EOA has a closed distal end, the EGTA has an opening at the distal end (Figure 5-4). The opening allows removal or aspiration of air and gastric contents from the stomach via a gastric tube. The advantage of this design is the relief of gastric distention that may occur during bag to mask ventilation (Wilkins et al., 2003; White, 2004).

☑ There are two ports on the EGTA mask. The resuscitation bag must be attached to the ventilation port.

With an EGTA, the ventilation holes along the proximal end of the tube are absent. Ventilation is provided through the mask by a traditional manual resuscitation bag. Since there are two ports on the mask, the resuscitation bag must be attached to the ventilation port. Table 5-3 outlines the distinct features of the EOA and the EGTA.

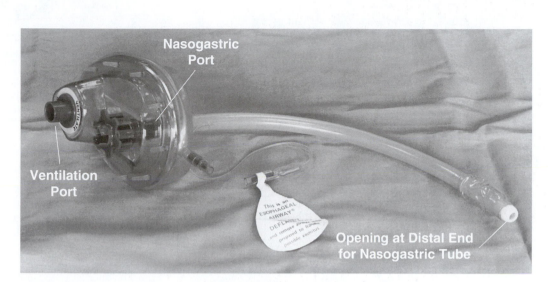

Figure 5-4 An esophageal gastric tube airway (EGTA).

TABLE 5-3 Distinct Features of the EOA and the EGTA

ESOPHAGEAL OBTURATOR AIRWAY	ESOPHAGEAL GASTRIC TUBE AIRWAY
Esophageal intubation	Esophageal intubation
Ventilation holes along tube	No ventilation holes along tube
Blind distal end	Patent distal end
One port on mask for ventilation	Two ports on mask (ventilation/gastric tube)

laryngeal mask airway: A tube with a small cushioned mask on the distal end that provides a seal over the laryngeal opening.

☑ With proper care and sterilization, LMA can be reused up to 40 times.

LARYNGEAL MASK AIRWAY (LMA)

The **laryngeal mask airway (LMA)** resembles a short endotracheal tube with a small cushioned, oblong-shaped mask on the distal end (Figure 5-5) (Brain et al., 1997; Brimacombe et al., 1998; Verghese et al., 1998). It was invented in England in 1981 by anesthesiologist Archie Brain and was available commercially in 1988. In 1991, this airway device was approved by the Food and Drug Administration for clinical use in the United States (Ferson et al., 1997). The original LMA (LMA-Classic) is a reusable device, made primarily of medical-grade silicone rubber and is latex free. With proper care and sterilization, it can be reused up to 40 times.

Figure 5-5 The components of the laryngeal mask airway (LMA). (Courtesy of LMA North America, Inc.)

USE AND APPLICATION OF LMA

☑ The cushioned mask of the LMA provides a seal over the laryngeal opening. It is not necessary for the LMA to enter the larynx or trachea.

The LMA fills a niche as an airway management tool between a face mask and an endotracheal tube (Brimacombe & Berry, 1996; Fetzer, 1998). When the cushioned mask of the LMA is inflated, it provides a seal over the laryngeal opening. It is not necessary therefore for the LMA to enter the larynx or trachea. Figure 5-6 shows the dorsal view of the position of the LMA in relation to the pharyngeal anatomy. After proper placement, spontaneous ventilation or low-level (up to 20 cm H_2O) positive pressure ventilation is possible without an endotracheal tube (LMA North America, Inc., 1999).

☑ LMA should be considered when tracheal intubation is precluded by lack of expertise or equipment or when attempts at endotracheal intubation have failed.

The LMA is also indicated as a method of establishing a patent airway during resuscitation in the profoundly unconscious patient with absent glossopharyngeal and laryngeal reflexes who may need assisted ventilation. The LMA should be considered when tracheal intubation is precluded by lack of expertise or equipment or when attempts at endotracheal intubation have failed (LMA North America, Inc., 1999). Other uses and application of the LMA are outlined in Table 5-4.

CONTRAINDICATIONS FOR LMA

☑ The LMA does not protect an airway from the effects of regurgitation and aspiration.

The design of the LMA does not protect an airway from the effects of regurgitation and aspiration. For this reason, the LMA should not be used in patients who have not fasted or those with hiatal hernia. Since the seal provided by the LMA may not withhold pressures over 20 cm H_2O, a leak may occur during high airway pressure situations. Patients with low lung compliance should use a traditional endotracheal tube instead of an LMA. In addition, the LMA should not be used in patients who are not profoundly unconscious and in those with severe oropharyngeal trauma.

Figure 5-6 Dorsal view of the LMA showing position in relation to pharyngeal anatomy. (Courtesy of LMA North America, Inc.)

TABLE 5-4   Uses and Application of a Laryngeal Mask Airway

Establishes airway in proven difficult intubations

Provides spontaneous and controlled ventilation in infants and children

Serves as a bridge to more secured airways

Provides complete survey of the larynx and trachea prior to thoracotomy

Provides lower work of breathing than endotracheal tube

Provides less hemodynamic response during surgical procedures

Provides less airway reaction

Offers benefit of shorter stay in hospital due to avoidance of endotracheal intubation

(Data from Ferson et al., 1997; Fukutome et al., 1998; Joo & Rose, 1998; Joshi et al., 1998; Kim & Bishop, 1999; Lopez-Gil, Brimacombe & Alvarez, 1996; Marietta et al., 1998; Parmet et al., 1998; Stanwood, 1997; Webster et al., 1999; Zerafa et al., 1999.)

TABLE 5-5   Selection of Laryngeal Mask Airway and Maximum Cuff Inflation Volume

SIZE	PATIENT GROUP	MAXIMUM CUFF VOLUME
1	Neonates and infants up to 5 kg	Up to 4 mL
1.5	Infants between 5 and 10 kg	Up to 7 mL
2	Infants and children between 10 and 20 kg	Up to 10 mL
2.5	Children between 20 and 30 kg	Up to 14 mL
3	Children over 30 kg and small adults	Up to 20 mL
4	Normal and large adults	Up to 30 mL
5	Larger adults	Up to 40 mL

(Data from LMA North America, Inc., 1999.)

☑ The LMA may not withhold airway pressures greater than 20 cm H_2O.

☑ For most adults, size 4 should be used for females and size 5 for males.

SELECTION OF LMA

The LMA is either reusable (silicone-based) or disposable (polyvinyl chloride). The disposable LMA-Unique performs similarly to the reusable LMA in clinical situations (Verghese et al., 1998). For most adult females, size 4 should be used and size 5 should be used for most adult males (Asai et al., 1998). The standard cuff pressure is 60 cm H_2O (Berry et al., 1998), but the air in the cuff should be adjusted to the minimal effective volume so as to decrease intracuff pressure, pressure on the pharynx (Asai et al., 1998), and incidence of sore throat (Nott et al., 1998). Table 5-5 provides the suggested LMA size for patients ranging from neonates to large adults and the maximal cuff inflation volume (LMA North America, Inc., 1999).

INSERTION OF LMA

Prior to insertion of the LMA, the patient is in a supine position, and the head is advanced slightly. The chin is depressed to open the mouth. With the cuff completely deflated or partially inflated (Dingley & Asai, 1996), the LMA is inserted blindly without a laryngoscope through the mouth and advanced along the hard palate. It is then further advanced to the posterior pharynx and turned toward the trachea and larynx. At this point, the LMA may be guided with fingers to ascertain that it makes the proper turn (Watson et al., 1999). Figure 5-7(A)–(G) show the standard insertion technique of the LMA.

☑ The LMA may be removed safely when the patient is anesthetized or awake.

REMOVAL OF LMA

The LMA may be discontinued when an upper airway is no longer needed for ventilation and oxygenation. Removal can be done safely when the patient is anesthetized or awake. During removal of the

Figure 5-7(A) Method for holding the LMA for insertion. (Courtesy of LMA North America, Inc.)

Figure 5-7(B) With the head extended and the neck flexed, carefully flatten the LMA tip against the hard palate. (Courtesy of LMA North America, Inc.)

Figure 5-7(C) To facilitate LMA introduction into the oral cavity, gently press the middle finger down on the jaw. (Courtesy of LMA North America, Inc.)

Figure 5-7(D) The index finger pushes the LMA in a cranial direction following the contours of the hard and soft palates. (Courtesy of LMA North America, Inc.)

Figure 5-7(E) Maintaining pressure with the finger on the tube in the cranial direction, advance the mask until definite resistance is felt at the base of the hypopharynx. (Courtesy of LMA North America, Inc.)

Figure 5-7(F) Gently maintain cranial pressure with the nondominant hand while removing the index finger. (Courtesy of LMA North America, Inc.)

Figure 5-7(G) Inflation without holding the tube allows the mask to seat itself optimally. (Courtesy of LMA North America, Inc.)

LMA, the patient must be monitored carefully for complications such as regurgitation, laryngeal spasm, bronchospasm, coughing, retching, excessive salivation, and oxygen desaturation (Nunez et al., 1998; Samarkandi, 1998).

LIMITATIONS OF LMA

Due to the unique position of its mask, rotation or turning of the LMA may cause misplacement of the mask and result in gastric insufflation and air leakage from the mask seal (Latorre et al., 1998). For this reason, the patient's head position and alignment of the LMA should be checked frequently to ensure adequate ventilation. Positive pressure ventilation may be provided via the LMA at peak inspiratory pressure of up to 20 cm H_2O. For patients with low compliance or high air flow resistance, the LMA may not be able to withstand the pressure and air leaks may develop. When high peak inspiratory pressure is anticipated, the LMA should be replaced with an endotracheal tube (LMA North America, Inc., 1999).

The LMA is not a secured airway and it does not protect the lower airway from aspiration. The esophagus, which lies posterior to the LMA, has complete access to the larynx, and thus regurgitation or aspiration is a potential complication (Norton et al., 1998).

The LMA may be disposable or reusable. The reusable version of the LMA is handmade, thus the cost is rather significant. With proper sterilization by steam **autoclave** and careful handling, it can be reused up to 40 times as long as the mask is not damaged during use, handling, and steam autoclaving. Table 5-6 outlines the limitations of the LMA.

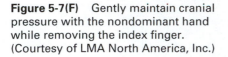 The LMA is sterilized by steam autoclave.

autoclave: A method of sterilization using steam pressure, usually at 250°F (121°C) for a specific length of time.

TABLE 5-6   Limitations of the Laryngeal Mask Airway

Rotation of the LMA may cause misplacement of mask, gastric inflation, and air leaks.

Cuff does not provide seal at pressures greater than 20 cm H_2O.

The LMA does not protect the lower airway from aspiration.

Reusable version is costly but it can be reused after cleaning and sterilization.

Steam autoclaving is the only recommended method of sterilization for reusable LMA.

---

pharyngealtracheal lumen airway:
A tube that may be inserted into the trachea or esophagus.

✓ The PTLA is inserted blindly either into the trachea or esophagus.

✓ Both lumens on the PTLA can be used to provide ventilation. Lumen 1 is used when the tube enters the esophagus and lumen 2 is used when it is in the trachea.

PHARYNGEALTRACHEAL LUMEN AIRWAY (PTLA)

The **pharyngealtracheal lumen airway (PTLA),** also called esophageal-tracheal airway, is a combination of esophageal and endotracheal tube in one unit (e.g., Combitube, by Kendall-Sheridan Corporation, Argyle, NY). Due to its design, ventilation is possible when the PTLA is inserted blindly either into the trachea or esophagus (Liao & Shalit, 1996). The PTLA can be inserted easily by unskilled personnel (Yardy, Hancox & Strang, 1999), and it has been used successfully as an alternate artificial airway in patients outside the hospital (Blostein, Koestner & Hoak, 1998; Hoak & Koestner, 1997; Rumball & MacDonald, 1997). Ventilation is provided via a 15-mm airway connector at the proximal end of the PTLA.

There are two cuffs on the PTLA, a proximal latex pharyngeal cuff (100 cc) and a PVC cuff (15 cc) near the distal end of the tube (Figure 5-8). Both lumens on the PTLA can be used to provide ventilation. Lumen 1 is used when the tube enters the esophagus and the distal cuff seals off the

Openings

Figure 5-8   A pharyngealtracheal lumen airway (PTLA).

Figure 5-9 After placement of the pharyngealtracheal lumen airway, both cuffs are inflated. (A) When the tube enters the esophagus, lumen No. 1 is used to ventilate the patient via the openings between the cuffs. (B) When the tube enters the trachea, lumen No. 2 is used to provide ventilation directly into the trachea.

esophagus. Lumen 2 is used when it is in the trachea and the proximal cuff seals off the trachea. Figure 5-9 shows the relative positions of the PTLA when it enters the esophagus or trachea.

INSERTION AND USE OF PTLA

The PTLA can be inserted with or without a laryngoscope. The tube is properly inserted once the black rings lie opposite the front teeth. After insertion, both cuffs are inflated immediately. Since the PTLA is designed to provide ventilation when the tube is in the trachea or esophagus, it does not matter whether the tube enters the esophagus or trachea.

During **blind intubation,** the PTLA is more likely to go into the esophagus. Therefore, ventilation through the PTLA should be done via lumen 1 first. When the distal end of the PTLA is in the esophagus, air goes through the side ports, becomes trapped between the cuffs, and is forced into the trachea. If ventilation via lumen 1 is poor, lumen 2 should be used to provide ventilation as the distal end of the PTLA may be in the trachea.

If ventilation is poor with lumens 1 and 2, a cuff leak may be present. This problem may be corrected by inflating the proximal cuff with more air. Try lumen 1 again and check for adequacy of ventilation. If ventilation is still poor, the entire procedure described earlier can be repeated after preoxygenating the patient.

blind intubation:
Insertion of an
artificial airway
without use of
visual aid.

✔ Following blind intubation with a pharyngealtracheal lumen airway (PTLA), ventilation should be attempted initially through lumen 1 of the PTLA.

COMPLICATIONS WITH USE OF PTLA

Cases of complications associated with the use of the PTLA have been reported. These complications are related to either hemodynamic stress or air leaks. In one report, the hemodynamic and catecholamine stress response after insertion of the PTLA were significantly higher compared to laryngeal mask airway or endotracheal intubation. This observation might be attributed to the pressure of the pharyngeal cuff of the PTLA (Oczenski et al., 1999). In another report, different types of air leak (subcutaneous emphysema, pneumomediastinum, and pneumoperitoneum) were observed as a result of using the PTLA. Esophageal laceration appears to be the cause of these air leaks (Richards, 1998; Vézina et al., 1998).

DOUBLE-LUMEN ENDOBRONCHIAL TUBE (DLT)

double-lumen endobronchial tube: A special airway for independent lung ventilation. It has two separate lumens, two cuffs, and two pilot balloons.

The **double-lumen endobronchial tube (DLT)** has two separate lumens (tracheal and bronchial), two cuffs (tracheal and bronchial), and two pilot balloons (tracheal and bronchial). It is also known as double-lumen tracheobronchial tube and may be either a left- or right-sided tube.

The left-sided tube is more commonly used than the right-sided tube. This is because precise placement of the right-sided tube is more difficult as the right upper lobe bronchus is only about 2 cm from the carina of an adult. Should the distal end of the right-sided tube pass the right upper lobe bronchus, there would have no ventilation to the right upper lobe. Figure 5-10 shows a left-sided DLT in its working position with both cuffs inflated.

INDICATIONS

☑ Independent lung ventilation is done via a DLT to facilitate lung isolation, surgical procedure, and bronchopleural/bronchocutaneous fistulas.

There are three main uses of DLTs. They are used to provide independent lung ventilation where isolation of the lungs is desirable in order to prevent lung-to-lung spillage of blood or pus. They are also used to provide one-lung ventilation so that the nonventilated lung may undergo surgical procedure on the thoracic structures with minimal movement. In disease conditions such as bronchopleural and bronchocutaneous fistulas, DLTs can provide ventilation by overcoming the persistent air leak through the fistulas (Barash, 2001).

SELECTION OF DLT

☑ Adult-sized DLTs range from 35 to 41.

It is essential to use the largest DLT appropriate for the patient since most complications associated with DLTs result from using small tubes. Recognizing the diameter of the bronchus (usually the left) is a

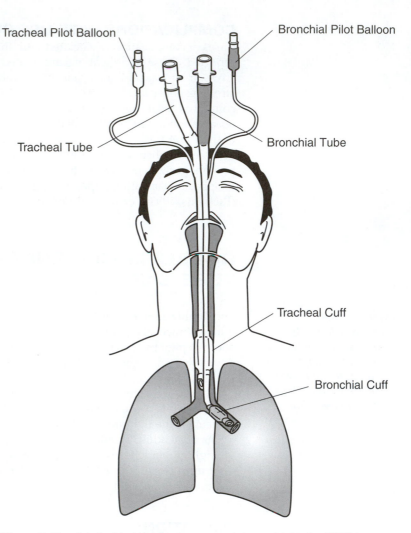

Tracheal Pilot Balloon

Bronchial Pilot Balloon

Tracheal Tube

Bronchial Tube

Tracheal Cuff

Bronchial Cuff

Figure 5-10 A left-sided double-lumen endobronchial tube (DLT) in working position with the tracheal and bronchial cuffs inflated.

crucial determinant of success in the use of a DLT. On a typical posterior-anterior (PA) chest radiography, the air bronchogram is enlarged by 10% as the bronchi are about 15 cm from the plate (Russell, 2004). If the bronchi are not visible on the chest radiography, the diameter of the left bronchus may be estimated by using 68% of the tracheal diameter. Table 5-7 shows the guidelines for choosing a left-sided DLT. In general, 28 and 32 French (Fr) DLTs are suitable for small children; 35 Fr for large children or small adults; and 37, 39, and 41 Fr for adults (Brodsky, 1997).

TABLE 5-7 Guidelines for Choosing an Adult Left-Sided DLT

MEASURED TRACHEAL WIDTH (mm)	PREDICTED LEFT BRONCHUS WIDTH (mm)	DOUBLE-LUMEN TUBE SIZE	OUTER DIAMETER (mm)	
			MAIN BODY	LEFT LUMEN
>18	>12.2	41 Fr	14–15	10.6
16.1–18	10.9–12.1	39 Fr	13–14	10.1
15.1–16	10.2–10.8	37 Fr	13–14	10.0
<15	9.5–10.1	35 Fr	12–13	9.5

Note: Tracheal width as measured from the PA chest radiography. Predicted left bronchus width is 68% of the measured tracheal width. (Brodsky, 1997).

INSERTION OF DLT

✔ The stylet should be removed as soon as the DLT has passed the vocal cords.

After the patient is anaesthetized and paralyzed, the DLT is inserted into the trachea using direct laryngoscopy until the tracheal cuff is just below the vocal cords. At this point, the DLT is about 6 cm from the final position. If a stylet is used to guide the DLT, it should be removed as soon as the DLT has passed the vocal cords. This maneuver minimizes the incidence of airway trauma caused by the stylet.

The bronchial cuff is then inflated in the trachea until the air leak stops on inflation. The bronchial adaptor is connected to the ventilator circuit and both lungs of the patients are ventilated via the bronchial tube (Figure 5-11A).

With each breath, the tube is advanced into the trachea until the bronchial segment plugs the bronchus. The endpoint signs are (1) resistance to advancement (even with low compliance lungs), (2) unilateral ventilation by observation and auscultation, and (3) reduction in compliance (e.g., ↑ PIP in volume-controlled ventilation). At this point, the tube is about 2.5 to 3 cm (bronchial cuff length plus 1 cm) from its final position (Figure 5-11B).

✔ Proper positioning of the DLT can be verified by auscultation or fiberoptic bronchoscopy.

Once the bronchial plugging point has been identified, the bronchial cuff is deflated and the tube inserted another 2.5 to 3 cm (bronchial cuff length plus 1 cm). The final bronchial cuff volume needed to seal should be small, about 1 to 2 mL. The patient connection is now changed to the tracheal connection. The tracheal cuff is inflated until a seal is made in the trachea (Figure 5-11C). Proper positioning of the DLT can be verified by auscultation or fiberoptic bronchoscopy (Klein et al., 1998).

If the tube goes right, turning the head 90° so that the chin is on the right shoulder and rotating the tube on its axis to restore the bronchial tube to point laterally to the left can usually achieve insertion into the left main bronchus (Russell, 2004).

RISK FACTORS FOR AIRWAY RUPTURE

✔ The most severe form of airway injuries caused by DLTs is airway rupture.

Use of DLTs may lead to airway injuries (Campos, 2000), and the most severe form of airway injuries is *airway rupture*. The incidence of airway rupture is higher when large and medium size red rubber

Bronchial Tube

Tracheal Tube

A

B

C

Figure 5-11 (A) A left double lumen endobronchial tube (DLT) with the bronchial cuff inflated firmly in the trachea. Both lungs are ventilated via the bronchial tube. (B) The overinflated bronchial cuff plugging the left main stem bronchus. (C) The DLT in its final position resting in the left-main bronchus with both cuffs inflated. In this final position, ventilation of the right lung is possible via the tracheal tube (as shown). The left lung may be ventilated by using the bronchial tube. (Courtesy of Dr. W. John Russell. Used with permission)

TABLE 5-8   Risk Factors for Airway Rupture

RISK FACTOR	EXAMPLES
Direct trauma	Forceful insertion
	Tube too large for the bronchus
	Tube advanced with stylet in place (questionable)
	Movement of tube while both cuffs are inflated
	Carinal hook damage
Cuff overinflation	Too rapid an inflation
	Too large a volume
	Nitrous oxide distention
Preexisting airway pathology	Congenital airway wall abnormalities
	Airway wall weakness from tumor infiltration or infection
	Airway distortion from mediastinal lymph nodes or tumor

DLTs are used. In contrast, small polyvinyl-chloride (PVC) DLTs have been associated with airway rupture (Akhtar, 1999). Some risk factors for airway rupture are listed in Table 5-8.

Some recommendations for the safe placement of a DLT (Fitzmaurice, 1999) include (1) choose the largest PVC DLT that is appropriate for the patient, (2) remove the bronchial stylet once the tip of the tube is past the vocal cords, (3) never overinflate either cuff and use 3 mL syringe to inflate the bronchial cuff, (4) when nitrous oxide is used measure the cuff pressures intermittently and keep the bronchial pressure <30 cm H_2O, (5) deflate the bronchial cuff when lung isolation is not required.

SUMMARY

Special airways discussed in this chapter are useful in situations where bag/mask ventilation is inadequate, endotracheal intubation is not readily achievable, or independent lung ventilation is required. A respiratory care practitioner should be knowledgeable and proficient in the use of these airways in different patient and clinical situations.

Self-Assessment Questions

1. As you are providing bag/mask ventilation to a 70-kg patient, you encounter a great deal of air flow resistance during inspiration. You would select an oropharyngeal airway with a length that equals to the distance from the:

   A. center of the mouth to the angle of the jaw.   C. tip of the nose to the earlobe.
   B. corner of the mouth to the angle of the jaw.   D. ridge of the nose to the earlobe.

2. An esophageal obturator airway (EOA) has a(n) _____ distal end and it is inserted into the _____.

    A. open, trachea   C. closed, trachea
    B. open, esophagus   D. closed, esophagus

3. Since an EOA is inserted into the _____, the cuff at the distal end must be _____ before ventilation is initiated.

    A. tracheal, deflated   C. esophagus, deflated
    B. trachea, inflated   D. esophagus, inflated

4. Since there are two ports on the mask of the _____, the resuscitation bag must be attached to the ventilation port.

    A. esophageal obturator airway   C. esophageal gastric tube airway
    B. laryngeal mask airway   D. pharyngealtracheal lumen airway

5. The silicone-based laryngeal mask airway may be reused up to _____ times with proper handling and _____.

    A. 40, chemical sterilization   C. 100, chemical sterilization
    B. 40, steam autoclaving   D. 100, steam autoclaving

6. Since the cushioned mask of a laryngeal mask airway (LMA) provides a seal over the _____, it is not necessary for the LMA to enter the larynx or trachea.

    A. tracheal opening   C. esophageal opening
    B. laryngeal opening   D. vocal cords

7. Which of the following is *not* true concerning the laryngeal mask airway (LMA)?

    A. LMA does not protect an airway from   C. Size 4 and size 5 LMAs are suitable
       regurgitation and aspiration.   for most adults.
    B. LMA is sterilized by steam autoclave.   D. LMA may withhold airway pressures
                                    up to 40 cm H_2O.

8. A pharyngealtracheal lumen airway (PTLA) is inserted into the:

    A. trachea.   C. trachea or esophagus.
    B. esophagus.   D. esophagus or larynx.

9. Both lumens on the PTLA can be used to provide ventilation. Lumen 1 is used when the tube enters the _____ and lumen 2 is used when it is in the _____.

    A. trachea, esophagus   C. trachea, larynx
    B. esophagus, trachea   D. esophagus, larynx

10. Following blind intubation with a PTLA, ventilation should be attempted initially through lumen 1 of the PTLA because:

    A. an airway usually goes into the trachea during blind intubation.

    B. an airway usually goes into the esophagus during blind intubation.

    C. lumen 1 has a closed distal end.

    D. lumen 2 has a closed distal end.

11. Clinical conditions that may require independent lung ventilation include all of the following *except:*

    A. antibiotic resistant left lung infection.

    B. respiratory distress syndrome.

    C. bronchopleural fistula.

    D. right lung lobectomy.

12. Following proper insertion and placement of a double-lumen endobronchial tube,

    A. only the bronchial cuff is inflated.

    B. only the tracheal cuff is inflated.

    C. both cuffs are inflated.

    D. both cuffs are deflated.

Answers to Self-Assessment Questions

1. A. center of the mouth to the angle of the jaw.

2. D. closed, esophagus

3. D. esophagus, inflated

4. C. esophageal gastric tube airway

5. B. 40, steam autoclaving

6. B. laryngeal opening

7. D. LMA may withhold airway pressures up to 40 cm H_2O.

8. C. trachea or esophagus.

9. B. esophagus, trachea

10. B. an airway usually goes into the esophagus during blind intubation.

11. B. respiratory distress syndrome.

12. C. both cuffs are inflated.

References

Akhtar, M. J. (1999). Double lumen tubes & airway rupture (myths exploded)! *J Cardiothora Vasc Anesth, 13*(3).

Asai, T., Howell, T. K., Koga, K., et al. (1998). Appropriate size and inflation of the laryngeal mask airway. *Br J Anaesth, 80*(4), 470–474.

Barash, P. G., et al. (2001). *Clinical anesthesia* (4th ed.). Philadelphia: Lippincott Williams & Wilkins.

Berry, A. M., Brimacombe, J. R., McManus, K. F., et al. (1998). An evaluation of the factors influencing selection of the optimal size of laryngeal mask airway in normal adults. *Anaesthesia, 53*(6), 565–570.

Blostein, P. A., Koestner, A. J., & Hoak, S. (1998). Failed rapid sequence intubation in trauma patients: Esophageal tracheal combitube is a useful adjunct. *J Trauma, 44*(3), 534–537.

Brain, A. I., Verghese, C., Addy, E. V., et al. (1997). The intubating laryngeal mask. I: Development of a new device for intubation of the trachea. *Br J Anaesth, 79*(6), 699–703.

Brimacombe, J., & Berry, A. (1996). The laryngeal mask airway—anatomical and physiological implications. *Acta Anaesthesiol Scand, 40*(2), 201–209.

Brimacombe, J., Keller, C., Morris, R., et al. (1998). A comparison of the disposable versus the reusable laryngeal mask airway in paralyzed adult patients. *Anesth Analg, 87*(4), 921–924.

Brodsky, J. B., et al. (1997). Selecting the correct size left double-lumen tube. *J Cardiothorac Vasc Anesth, 11*(7), 924–925.

Burton, G. G., et al. (1997). *Respiratory care: A guide to clinical practice* (4th ed.). Baltimore, MD: Lippincott Williams & Wilkins.

Campos, J. H., et al. (2000). The incidence of right upper-lobe collapse when comparing a right-sided double-lumen tube versus a modified left double-lumen tube for left-sided thoracic surgery. *Anesth Analg, 90*(3), 535–540.

Dingley, J., & Asai, T. (1996). Insertion methods of the laryngeal mask airway. A survey of current practice in Wales. *Anaesthesia, 51*(6), 596–599.

Ferson, D. Z., Nesbitt, J. C., Nesbitt, K., et al. (1997). The laryngeal mask airway: A new standard for airway evaluation in thoracic surgery. *Ann Thorac Surg, 63*(3), 768–772.

Fetzer, S. J. (1998). Laryngeal mask airway: Indications and management for critical care. *Crit Care Nurse, 18*(1), 83–87.

Fitzmaurice, B., et al. (1999). Airway rupture from double-lumen tubes. *J Cardiothorac Vasc Anesth, 15*(3), 322–9.

Fukutome, T., Amaha, K., Nakazawa, K., et al. (1998). Tracheal intubation through the intubating laryngeal mask airway (LMA-Fastrach) in patients with difficult airways. *Anaesth Intensive Care, 26*(4), 387–391.

Hoak, S., & Koestner, A. (1997). Esophageal tracheal Combitube in the emergency department. *J Emerg Nurs, 23*(4), 347–350.

Joo, H., & Rose, K. (1998). Fastrach—a new intubating laryngeal mask airway. Successful use in patients with difficult airways. *Can J Anaesth, 45*(3), 253–256.

Joshi, G. P., Morrison, S. G., White, P. F., et al. (1998). Work of breathing in anesthetized patients: Laryngeal mask airway versus tracheal tube. *J Clin Anesth, 10*(4), 268–271.

Kim, E. S., & Bishop, M. J. (1999). Endotracheal intubation, but not laryngeal mask airway insertion, produces reversible bronchoconstriction. *Anesthesiology, 90*(2), 391–394.

Klein, U., et al. (1998). Role of fiberoptic bronchoscopy in conjunction with the use of double-lumen tubes for thoracic anesthesia: A prospective study. *Anesthesiology, 89*(5), 1282–1283.

Latorre, F., Eberle, B., Weiler, N., et al. (1998). Laryngeal mask airway position and the risk of gastric insufflation. *Anesth Analg, 86*(4), 867–871.

Liao, D., & Shalit, M. (1996). Successful intubation with the Combitube in acute asthmatic respiratory distress by a Paramedic. *J Emerg Med, 14*(5), 561–563.

LMA North America, Inc. (1999). *Instruction Manual LMA-Classic/LMA-Flexible.* San Diego, CA.

Lopez-Gil, M., Brimacombe, J., & Alvarez, M. (1996). Safety and efficacy of the laryngeal mask airway. A prospective survey of 1400 children. *Anaesthesia, 51*(10), 969–972.

Marietta, D. R., Lunn, J. K., Ruby, E. I., et al. (1998). Cardiovascular stability during carotid endarterectomy: Endotracheal intubation versus laryngeal mask airway. *J Clin Anesth, 10*(1), 54–57.

Norton, A., Germonpré, J., & Semple, T. (1998). Pulmonary aspiration of blood following traumatic laryngeal mask airway insertion. *Anaesth Intensive Care, 26*(2), 213–215.

Nott, M. R., Noble, P. D., & Parmar, M. (1998). Reducing the incidence of sore throat with the laryngeal mask airway. *Eur J Anaesthesiol, 15*(2), 153–157.

Nunez, J., Hughes, J., Wareham, K., et al. (1998). Timing of removal of the laryngeal mask airway. *Anaesthesia, 53*(2), 126–130.

Oczenski, W., Krenn, H., Dahaba, A. A., et al. (1999). Hemodynamic and catecholamine stress responses to insertion of the Combitube, laryngeal mask airway or tracheal intubation. *Anesth Analg, 88*(6), 1389–1394.

Parmet, J. L., Colonna-Romano, P., Horrow, J. C., et al. (1998). The laryngeal mask airway reliably provides rescue ventilation in cases of unanticipated difficult tracheal intubation along with difficult mask ventilation. *Anesth Analg, 87*(3), 661–665.

Richards, C. F. (1998). Piriform sinus perforation during Esophageal-Tracheal Combitube placement. *J Emerg Med, 16*(1), 37–39.

Rumball, C. J., & MacDonald, D. (1997). The PTL, Combitube, laryngeal mask, and oral airway: A randomized prehospital comparative study of ventilatory. *Prehosp Emerg Care, 1*(1), 1–10.

Russell, W. J. (2000). Insertion of a double lumen tube. Retrieved May 10, 2004, from http://www.usyd.edu.au/su/anaes/lectures/dlt.html.

Samarkandi, A. H. (1998). Awake removal of the laryngeal mask airway is safe in paediatric patients. *Can J Anaesth, 45*(2), 150–152.

Stanwood, P. L. (1997). The laryngeal mask airway and the emergency airway. *AANA J, 65*(4), 364–370.

Verghese, C., Berlet, J., Kapila, A., et al. (1998). Clinical assessment of the single use laryngeal mask airway—the LMA-unique. *Br J Anaesth, 80*(5), 677–679.

Vézina, D., Lessard, M. R., Bussières, J., et al. (1998). Complications associated with the use of the Esophageal-Tracheal Combitube. *Can J Anaesth, 45*(1), 76–80.

Watson, N. C., Hokanson, M., Maltby, J. R., et al. (1999). The intubating laryngeal mask airway in failed fibreoptic intubation. *Can J Anaesth, 46*(4), 376–378.

Webster, A. C., Morley-Forster, P. K., Janzen, V., et al. (1999). Anesthesia for intranasal surgery: A comparison between tracheal intubation and the flexible reinforced laryngeal mask airway. *Anesth Analg, 88*(2), 421–425.

White, G. C. (2004). *Equipment theory for respiratory care* (4th ed.), Clifton Park, NY: Thomson Delmar Learning.

Wilkins, R. L., et al. (2003). *Egan's fundamentals of respiratory care* (8th ed.). St. Louis, MO: Mosby.

Yardy, N., Hancox, D., & Strang, T. (1999). A comparison of two airway aids for emergency use by unskilled personnel. The Combitube and laryngeal mask. *Anaesthesia, 54*(2), 181–183.

Zerafa, M., Baulch, S., Elliott, M. J., et al. (1999). Use of the laryngeal mask airway during repair of atrial septal defect in children. *Paediatr Anaesth, 9*(3), 257–259.

Suggested Reading

American Society of Anesthesiologists (1993). Practice guidelines for management of the difficult airway—a report by the American Society of Anesthesiologists Task Force on management of the difficult airway, *Chest 78*, 597–602.

(A list of the articles used to develop the above guidelines is available by writing to the American Society of Anesthesiologists, 520 North Northwest Highway, Park Ridge, Illinois 60068-2573)

CHAPTER SIX

AIRWAY MANAGEMENT IN MECHANICAL VENTILATION

David W. Chang

OUTLINE

KEY TERMS

- carina
- endotracheal tube
- laryngoscope
- Magill forceps
- Mallampati classification
- pilot balloon
- radiopaque
- rapid sequence intubation

- sniffing position
- speaking valve
- stylet
- tracheostomy tube
- unplanned extubation
- vagus nerve
- vallecula
- vocal cords

INTRODUCTION

In mechanical ventilation, artificial airways provide a vital link between the ventilator and the patient. Two common artificial airways used in conjunction with mechanical ventilators are the endotracheal (ET) and tracheostomy tubes. For these airways to work properly and efficiently, they must be used and maintained correctly. This chapter provides a practical presentation on oral and nasal intubation, suctioning, and extubation. Supplies commonly used for intubation and suctioning are also included.

INTUBATION

☑ The surgical procedure that creates an opening at the trachea is called *tracheotomy*.

tracheostomy tube: An artificial airway inside the trachea that is inserted through a surgical opening at the trachea.

Endotracheal (ET) intubation is the placement of an ET tube inside the trachea through the mouth or nostril. It is estimated that 15 million patients undergo ET intubation annually (Coppolo et al., 1990).

ET intubation is a simpler procedure than tracheotomy—a surgical procedure that creates an airway opening by cutting into the trachea. Compared to an ET tube (Figure 6-1), a **tracheostomy tube** (Figure 6-2) is much shorter and it provides closer access to the lower airways. It has a lower mechanical deadspace volume than an ET tube. It also ventilates the patient more efficiently and enhances secretion removal. In spite of many advantages of a tracheostomy tube, ET intubation is preferred as the initial means of establishing an artificial airway.

Oral and nasal intubations are commonly done by respiratory care practitioners. When these two routes are not accessible or when the need for a long-term artificial airway is expected, a tracheotomy is done by a physician who is proficient in this surgical procedure.

Figure 6-1   Two adult endotracheal tubes (8.0 mm ID). Note that one's cuff is inflated and the other's is not. Also note the markings visible on the tubes.

Figure 6-2   An adult tracheostomy tube with a disposable inner cannula that may be replaced as required to maintain patency.

Table 6-1   Indications for Using Artificial Airway

INDICATION	EXAMPLES
Relief of airway obstruction	Epiglottitis Facial burns and smoke inhalation Vocal cord edema
Protection of the airway	Prevention of aspiration Absence of coordinated swallow
Facilitation of suctioning	Excessive secretions Inadequate cough
Support of ventilation	Ventilatory failure / respiratory arrest Chest trauma Postanesthesia recovery Hyperventilation to ↓ intracranial pressure

(Data from Shapiro et al., 1991; White, 2002; Whitten, 1997.)

INDICATIONS

The decision to perform ET intubation versus tracheotomy is based on the expected duration of need. In general, if the patient requires an artificial airway for a brief period (e.g., 10 days or less) and full recovery is expected, an ET tube is used. On the other hand, if the patient's condition is critical and recovery is not expected any time soon (e.g., more than 21 days), a tracheostomy tube is preferred (Shapiro et al., 1991).

Choosing when to intubate is also a difficult clinical decision because delayed intubation may lead to hypoventilation, hypoxemia, and hypoxia. The timing of intubation can be based on four indications: (1) relief of airway obstruction, (2) protection of the airway, (3) facilitation of suctioning, and (4) support of ventilation (Shapiro et al., 1991). Some examples for each of these indications are listed in Table 6-1.

COMMON ARTIFICIAL AIRWAYS IN MECHANICAL VENTILATION

☑ Oral intubation is easy to perform and is often done in emergency situations.

An ET tube may be inserted orally (oral intubation) or nasally (nasal intubation) through the larynx and into the trachea. Oral intubation is easy to perform and it is often done in emergency situations. Nasal intubation is more time-consuming and it is more suitable in elective intubations.

☑ An oral route of intubation allows the passage of a larger ET tube than nasal intubation.

ORAL ENDOTRACHEAL TUBE

Intubation through the mouth is the preferred method of establishing an artificial airway (Figure 6-3). An oral route allows the passage of a

Figure 6-3 This illustration shows how an inflated cuff seals the trachea.

✓ A larger ET tube lowers the peak, plateau, and mean airway pressures.

larger ET tube than nasal intubation. A larger tube has less air flow resistance, and it lowers the airway pressure requirements. However, oral intubation is less comfortable to the patient and may cause gagging and excessive secretion production. Agitated patients may bite down on the tube and cause air flow obstruction.

NASAL ENDOTRACHEAL TUBE

✓ Disadvantages of nasal intubation include difficulty to insert, use of a smaller ET tube, and potential development of sinusitis.

Intubation through the nostril is better tolerated by the patient. It provides an ideal access to the lower airway in conditions where oral access is limited (e.g., oral trauma). The disadvantages of nasal intubation include difficulty to insert, use of a smaller ET tube, and potential development of sinusitis.

TRACHEOSTOMY TUBE

✓ The decision to change from an ET tube to a tracheostomy tube is based on the patient's condition and prognosis.

A tracheostomy tube is inserted through a surgical opening into the trachea. In long-term mechanical ventilation, it is used to replace the ET tube that has been in place for 21 days or longer (Shapiro et al., 1991).

The tracheostomy tube bypasses the upper airway and the glottis and therefore avoids any potential injury in these areas and offers lower air flow resistance. It is also easier to maintain, stabilize, and suction. In addition, the patient can eat and drink with the tracheostomy cuff properly inflated (Shapiro et al., 1991).

✓ Sterile technique must be followed during tracheostomy tube care and suctioning.

Tracheostomy tubes are not without drawbacks. Since a tracheostomy tube is inserted through a surgical opening, infection and trauma to the surgical site are always a threat. To reduce the potential complications of tracheostomy, sterile and aseptic techniques must be followed during tracheostomy care and suctioning (White, 2002).

INTUBATION PROCEDURE

Mallampati classification: A method to evaluate the degree of difficulty in intubation.

laryngoscope: An instrument that is used to displace the tongue and soft tissues, and visualize the larynx and vocal cords during endotracheal intubation.

stylet: A flexible but semirigid wire placed inside an endotracheal tube to provide it with a desired curvature.

Magill forceps: Special forceps used to perform nasal intubation under direct vision.

Intubation is a fairly simple procedure. In order to become proficient in this procedure one may need to exercise good organization and frequent practice. The procedure described below provides the basics and it may vary somewhat depending on the preference of an individual and existing protocol of the respiratory therapy department.

PREINTUBATION ASSESSMENT

Prior to intubation, the patient must be assessed to rule out any potential contraindications to include head injury, cervical spine injury, airway burns, and facial trauma (Finucane & Santora, 2003). Anesthesia consultation is advised in cases of unfamiliarity or difficult intubation.

The degree of difficulty in intubation due to anatomical structures can be evaluated by using the **Mallampati classification** method (Figure 6-4). This method is based on the anatomical structures visible with the mouth wide open and tongue protruded in a sitting position. Ease of oral intubation ranges from Class 1—easiest—to Class 4—most difficult—(Table 6-2) (Finucane & Santora, 2003).

SUPPLIES

The minimum supplies needed for ET intubation include (1) **laryngoscope** handle, (2) blade, (3) ET tube, (4) 10-cc syringe, (5) water-soluble lubricant, (6) tape, and (7) stethoscope. Optional supplies for ET intubation include (8) **stylet**, (9) topical anesthetic, and (10) **Magill forceps**.

In addition to the intubation supplies, proper airway management also requires oral airway, nasal airway, oxygen supply, and resuscitation bag/mask system.

Class 1   Class 2   Class 3   Class 4

Figure 6-4   Mallampati classification.

TABLE 6-2   Mallampati Classification and Interventions

MALLAMPATI	ABLE TO SEE	INTERVENTION
Class 1	Soft palate, fauces, uvula, anterior, and posterior tonsillar pillars	Conscious sedation
Class 2	Soft palate, fauces, and uvula	Conscious sedation
Class 3	Soft palate and base of uvula	Seek anesthesia consultation
Class 4	Soft palate only	Seek anesthesia consultation

✓ The laryngo-scope handle is held by the left hand.

✓ Common laryngoscope blades range from size 0 (neonates) to 4 (adults).

✓ A straight blade lifts the tongue *and* epiglottis upward to expose the vocal cord and related structures.

✓ A curved blade lifts the tongue only.

vallecula: An area between the base of the tongue and epiglottis; an anatomical landmark for the placement of the curved blade.

✓ A straight blade works better in patients with short necks, high or rigid larynxes, or obesity.

Laryngoscope Handle.   The laryngoscope handle contains batteries and it allows attachment of the blade and manipulation of the blade during intubation. Figure 6-5 shows a laryngoscope handle with a Miller blade.

The laryngoscope handle is held in the left hand since all standard blades attached to the handle are designed for right-hand intubations.

Blade.   The laryngoscope blade attaches its flange onto the post of the handle (Figure 6-6). Once snapped into position, the built-in light source at the distal end of the blade comes on. A laryngoscope blade is either straight or curved and ranges from size 0 (neonates) to 4 (adults). Size 3 and size 4 blades are intended for small and large adults, respectively. The straight (Miller) blade is used to pick up the epiglottis during intubation. The curved (MacIntosh) blade is placed in an area called **vallecula,** and indirectly moves the epiglottis out of the way.

Figure 6-5   A conventional laryngoscope with a Miller blade attached.

Indentation

Bar

Blade

Figure 6-6 Attaching the laryngoscope blade to the handle. The blade locks into place when it is properly engaged.

The basic technique of intubation is the same no matter which type of blade is used. The primary difference between these two blades is that a straight blade lifts the tongue *and* epiglottis upward to expose the vocal cords and related structures (Figure 6-7). The epiglottis is not visible when a straight blade is placed properly. The tip of a curved blade rests at the vallecula (between base of tongue and epiglottis) and lifts the tongue only (Figure 6-8). The epiglottis may be seen through the mouth when a curved blade is used properly.

Patients with short necks, high larynxes, or who are obese often need straight blades to displace the tongue and attached soft tissues upward. A straight blade also works better in patients with rigid larynxes due to scar formation or trauma (Whitten, 1997).

A curved blade is easy to learn to use as it can be easily positioned by advancing to the base of the tongue. Once the tongue is lifted upward, the epiglottis moves upward with the attached soft tissues thus exposing the **vocal cords.**

Despite one's training and preference, it is essential to gain experience and proficiency in using both types of laryngoscope blades, since in some emergency situations, the preferred type of blade may not be readily available.

Endotracheal Tube.   **Endotracheal tubes** come in sizes ranging from 2 to 10. The size refers to the internal diameter (ID) of the tube in millimeters (mm) and it comes in 0.5-mm increments. To reduce

vocal cords: *Two thin, almost parallel folds of tissue within the larynx that vibrate as air passes between them; an important landmark as the entry point to the trachea during intubation.*

endotracheal tube: *An artificial airway inside the trachea that is inserted through the mouth or nostril.*

Figure 6-7 Proper placement of a straight (Miller) blade during intubation. The blade lifts up the epiglottis anteriorly to expose the glottic opening and vocal cords. (From Finucane, B. T., & Santora, A. H. (2003), *Principles of airway management* (3rd ed.). New York: Springer-Verlag. Used with permission.)

Figure 6-8 Proper placement of a curved (McIntosh) blade during intubation. The tip of blade is in the vallecula (between base of tongue and epiglottis). The epiglottis is elevated by using a forward-upward lift to expose the glottic opening and vocal cords. (From Finucane, B. T., & Santora, A. H. (2003), *Principles of airway management* (3rd ed.). New York: Springer-Verlag. Used with permission.)

radiopaque: *Impenetrable to X-rays or other forms of radiation. It appears as a light area on the radiograph.*

pilot balloon: *The small balloon on the proximal end of an endotracheal or tracheostomy tube. It is used to regulate the volume of air in the cuff and to serve as an* indicator *of air volume in the cuff.*

☑ For adult ET tubes, the syringe used to inflate the cuff should have a capacity of 10 cc or larger.

☑ Use only a water-soluble lubricant on the distal end of an ET tube.

☑ Petroleum or oil-based lubricants must not be used as they can cause adverse reactions to the lungs.

☑ If the ET tube is not secured properly, inadvertent extubation or main-stem intubation may result.

☑ A stylet is not required for successful oral intubation and it is not used in nasal intubation.

air flow resistance, the largest size appropriate to a patient should be used.

The proximal end of an ET tube has a 15-mm adapter that fits all standard ventilator circuits and aerosol therapy adapters. Along the body of the tube, a **radiopaque** line runs lengthwise for the verification of tube location by chest radiograph. Markings in centimeters (cm) are also shown along the tube for easy determination of the depth of intubation. The volume of air in the cuff at the distal end of the ET tube is controlled by using a large (10 cc or larger) syringe via the **pilot balloon.**

The ET tube is normally held in the right hand with the curvature facing forward. When intubating a spontaneously breathing patient, the tube is advanced into the trachea during spontaneous inspiratory efforts (when the vocal cords are opened wide). During expiration, the ET tube may bounce off the closed vocal cords and enter the esophagus.

10-cc Syringe. A syringe with a capacity of 10 cc or larger is used to test the pilot balloon and ET tube cuff before intubation and to inflate the cuff after intubation. After testing the integrity of the pilot balloon and cuff, air is withdrawn from the cuff to the syringe. The air-filled syringe may be left attached to the pilot balloon for rapid inflation of the cuff immediately after intubation.

Water-Soluble Lubricant. A water-soluble lubricant is used to lubricate the distal end of the ET tube for easy insertion into the trachea. Petroleum or oil-based lubricants must *not* be used in ET intubation. Once entering the lungs, they can cause adverse reactions to the airways and lung parenchyma.

Tape. Tape is used to secure the ET tube so that the tube will not move too high causing inadvertent extubation, or too low leading to main-stem intubation. Benzoin or other commercially available solutions may be effective in making the tape more adhesive to the damp skin. Zinc oxide base tape (by Hy Tape Corporation, New York) also sticks well to the skin when it is exposed to moisture.

Stethoscope. A stethoscope is needed to auscultate bilateral breath sounds immediately after intubation.

Stylet. A flexible stylet wire guide is placed inside the ET tube to form a desired curvature and make it more rigid for ease of intubation. Use of a stylet is not required for successful oral intubation. A stylet is not used in nasal intubation.

When a stylet is used, make certain that its end does not extend below the tip of the ET tube because the stylet can traumatize the tracheal wall. As a standard practice, the portion of stylet extending from the proximal end of the ET tube (outside the patient's mouth) is bent before intubation to prevent it from slipping deep inside the ET tube.

Topical Anesthetic. A mild, topical anesthetic may be used to numb the mucosal membrane that may come in contact with the blade or ET tube. Use of a topical anesthetic is not feasible in emergency intubation or necessary in unconscious patients. It is useful to reduce the incidence of bronchospasm and vomiting when elective intubation is done in conscious and alert patients.

Magill Forceps. Magill forceps are used to perform nasal intubation. After the ET tube has been inserted through the nostril and becomes visible through the mouth, the laryngoscope blade and Magill forceps are used together to guide the ET tube into the trachea under direct vision.

SELECTION OF ENDOTRACHEAL TUBE

The size of an ET tube should be the largest one appropriate to a patient. Comparing to a smaller ET tube, a larger one offers lower airway resistance, and lower (peak, plateau, mean) airway pressures. A larger ET tube also improves dynamic compliance and facilitates secretion removal.

Table 6-3 shows the estimated size of the ET tube based on body size. In addition to the body weight or body size, final selection of an ET tube should be based on the clinical condition and tolerance of the patient.

VENTILATION AND OXYGENATION

Before each intubation attempt, the patient must be adequately ventilated and oxygenated. If the patient is not breathing spontaneously, a resuscitation bag/mask system is used to provide ventilation and oxygenation (Figure 6-9).

If an intubation attempt is not successful after 30 sec, the ET tube and laryngoscope blade should be removed immediately and the

☑ Select the *largest* tube that is appropriate to the patient.

☑ Mentally count from 1 to 30 when you begin the intubation attempt.

☑ Intubation attempts lasting longer than 30 sec may cause hypoxia and arrhythmias.

☑ For an 8-year-old, the calculated ET tube size would be 4.5 + (8/4) = 4.5 + 2 = 6.5 mm ID

TABLE 6-3   Estimation of ET Tube Size

PATIENT		ESTIMATED SIZE*
Neonate	<1000	2.5 mm ID
Neonate	1000 to 2000	3.0 mm ID
Neonate	2000 to 3000	3.5 mm ID
Neonate	>3000	4.0 mm ID
Child	1 to 2 years	4.5 mm ID
Child	2 to 12 years	4.5 + (age/4) mm ID
Average adult female		7.5 to 8.5 mm ID
Average adult male		8.0 to 9.0 mm ID

*<size 6 uncuffed, size 6 cuffed or uncuffed, >size 6 cuffed (Graber, 2004).

Figure 6-9 Correct use of a mask to manually ventilate a patient.

patient ventilated with a bag/mask system and 100% oxygen. Ventilation and oxygenation should continue for at least 30 sec or until the pulse oximetry (SpO_2) reading returns to the baseline level or in the 90s.

ORAL INTUBATION
The sequence outlined in Table 6-4 provides a general procedure for oral intubation. It should be modified to suit individual situations and to comply with existing protocols.

NASAL INTUBATION
The procedure for nasal intubation is similar to that for oral intubation. In nasal intubation, the ET tube is inserted through the nostril and then guided by the Magill forceps into the trachea (Table 6-5).

Blind Intubation.   In alert and cooperative patients who are breathing spontaneously, "blind" nasal intubation may be done by inserting the ET tube into a nostril and advancing it slowly during inspiratory efforts. When the distal end of the ET tube approaches the trachea, air movement can be heard through the ET tube. The general depth of

✓ "Blind" nasal intubation is done by advancing the ET tube slowly during spontaneous inspiratory efforts by listening for air movement through the ET tube.

TABLE 6-4   Procedure for Oral Intubation

1. Assemble and test supplies (e.g., check light source, lubricate ET tube cuff).
2. Lubricate the deflated cuff with a water-soluble lubricant.
3. Explain procedure to patient.
4. Ventilate and preoxygenate patient with 100% oxygen.
5. Tilt the head back and place in the **sniffing position** (Figure 6-10).
6. Hold laryngoscope handle with left hand.
7. Open mouth and insert blade into the right side of mouth.
8. Slide blade to the base of tongue and sweep blade to the left.
9. Maneuver the tip of straight blade underneath the epiglottis or the tip of curved blade at the vallecula.
10. Lift handle and blade up anteriorly to displace the tongue and attached soft tissues (Figure 6-11).
11. Locate the (epiglottis [curve blade only]), larynx, and vocal cords (Figure 6-12).
12. Insert ET tube through the vocal cords under direct vision.
13. For adults, the centimeter marking on the ET tube should initially be placed at the lips or incisors at 21 to 23 cm.
14. Inflate cuff and check for bilateral breath sounds.
15. Confirm proper depth of ET tube placement with chest radiograph.

TABLE 6-5   Procedure for Nasal Intubation

1. Assemble and test supplies (e.g., check light source, lubricate ET tube cuff).
2. Lubricate the deflated cuff with a water-soluble lubricant.
3. Explain procedure to patient.
4. Ventilate and preoxygenate patient with 100% oxygen.
5. Tilt the head back and place in the sniffing position.
6. Insert ET tube into a nostril and advance slowly until the distal end is near the tongue.
7. Open mouth and insert blade into the right side of mouth.
8. Slide blade to the base of tongue and sweep blade to the left.
9. Lift handle and blade up anteriorly to displace the tongue and attached soft tissues.
10. Locate the epiglottis, larynx, and vocal cords.
11. Use right hand to insert Magill forceps into mouth and guide ET tube through the vocal cord under direct vision.
12. For adults, the centimeter marking on the ET tube should initially be placed at the nares at 24 to 26 cm.
13. Inflate cuff and check for bilateral breath sounds.
14. Confirm proper depth of ET tube placement with chest radiograph.

sniffing position: An ideal head position for endotracheal intubation. It is done by tilting the forehead back slightly and moving the mandible anteriorly to the patient.

Figure 6-10 The head tilt (sniffing) position is done by tilting the forehead back slightly and moving the mandible anteriorly to the patient.

Figure 6-11 Anatomy of the upper airway as viewed with a laryngoscope in place.

Figure 6-12   Anatomical structures seen during direct laryngoscopy.

nasal intubation is guided by the distance marking (e.g., 25 cm) on the ET tube. Breath sounds and a chest radiograph are then assessed to confirm proper placement of the ET tube.

COMMON ERRORS

Errors can occur when intubation is done in a hurried fashion. They are also more likely to occur when it is done by someone who is not proficient or experienced with the intubation procedure. By staying calm during an intubation attempt and updating the intubation skills in a controlled setting (e.g., in operating room), errors can be minimized or avoided.

Table 6-6 outlines some problems that may be encountered during an intubation attempt. The potential cause and solution to each problem are provided.

SIGNS OF ENDOTRACHEAL INTUBATION

After intubation and inflation of the cuff, correct placement of the ET tube in the trachea must be checked immediately. If the patient is breathing spontaneously, bilateral breath sounds should be heard. Speech will not be possible since the vocal cords are bypassed by the ET tube and no longer receive air flow for making sound. In addition, air flow may be felt over the ET tube opening. Moisture or condensation will form inside the ET tube on exhalation. A carbon dioxide (CO_2)

TABLE 6-6   Common Problems During Intubation

PROBLEM (POTENTIAL CAUSE)	SOLUTION
Difficult to put blade or tube in mouth (Improper head position)	Use "sniffing" position by (1) tilting head back slightly and (2) moving chin anteriorly.
Trauma to teeth and soft tissues (Improper use of handle and blade)	Open mouth wider. Do not pivot on teeth to lift blade and tongue.
Unable to see epiglottis, larynx, or vocal cords (Blade is inside esophagus)	Withdraw *curved* blade until it reaches the vallecula (between base of tongue and epiglottis). Withdraw *straight* blade until it reaches the epiglottis.
Unable to advance ET tube when straight blade is used (ET tube is blocked by the light bulb on the right side of straight blade)	Rotate blade slightly counterclockwise (top of handle to left) to move light bulb out of the way.
Esophageal intubation, vomiting, and aspiration (Inserting the ET tube into *any* "opening" hoping it is the tracheal opening)	Find vocal cords and insert the ET tube through the cords under direct vision.
Arrhythmias (Hypoxia caused by prolonged intubation attempt)	Stop intubation. Ventilate and oxygenate.

☑ Rising SpO_2 presence of bilateral breath sounds, air flow, condensations on ET tube, and CO_2 are signs of successful ET intubation.

carina: The point at the lower end of the trachea separating openings of the main-stem bronchi.

☑ For adult patients, the tip of an ET tube should be about 1.5 in. above the carina.

indicator or end-tidal CO_2 monitor may be attached to the end of the ET tube to detect CO_2 in the expired gas sample.

The CO_2 detection device contains a chemical that changes color in the presence of carbon dioxide. After intubation, the detection device is attached to the endotracheal tube and the color on the device is observed. If the color turns from purple to yellow, it is an indication of successful endotracheal intubation since expired air from the lungs contains approximately 5% carbon dioxide.

If the patient is not breathing spontaneously, bilateral breath sounds should be checked by manual ventilation with a resuscitation bag. The placement of the stethoscope diaphragm should be along the midaxillary line. When the ET tube is properly placed (about 1.5 in. above the **carina**), the chest should expand and the abdomen should not have a gurgling sound during manual ventilation. Breath sounds heard on one side of the chest may suggest main-stem intubation. In the absence of obvious lung pathology (e.g., atelectasis), borderline main-stem intubation produces uneven bilateral breath sounds.

Finally, the definitive confirmation of correct placement of the ET tube is done by a chest radiograph. For adult patients, the depth of intubation may be adjusted accordingly so that the distal end of the ET tube is about 1.5 in. above the carina (Tasota et al., 1987). This distance from the carina is considered ideal as the ET tube may move *down* by an average of about 1 in. (1.9 cm) with neck flexion (Conrady et al., 1976).

SIGNS OF ESOPHAGEAL INTUBATION

☑ Do not check breath sounds at anterior chest locations close to the trachea since air flow in the *esophagus* can give false "breath sounds" in neonates and thin adults.

Placing an ET tube into the esophagus is a grave error. Hypoventilation, tissue and cerebral hypoxia are certain and immediate following esophageal intubation of an apneic patient. Furthermore, manual ventilation via an ET tube that has been placed in the esophagus may lead to aspiration of stomach contents and make subsequent intubations extremely difficult. Signs of esophageal intubation include oxygen desaturation ($\downarrow$SpO$_2$), deteriorating vital signs, cyanosis, stomach distention, and aspiration.

☑ In the absence of obvious lung pathology, uneven bilateral breath sounds may suggest mainstem intubation.

In almost all instances, esophageal intubation can be avoided by confirming that the ET tube passes through the vocal cords under *direct vision*. If the vocal cords are not seen or cannot be identified, the ET tube *must not* be inserted. Another experienced physician or practitioner should attempt to reintubate. Valuable time must not be wasted when a difficult intubation is encountered.

☑ Esophageal intubation can be avoided by inserting the ET tube through the vocal cords under *direct vision*.

Esophageal Detection Device. The esophageal detection device (EDD) is a sensitive and specific tool to detect esophageal intubation in the emergency setting (Kasper & Deem, 1998). This device provides a negative-pressure test using a compressible and self-inflating bulb with two openings. The upper end contains a one-way valve to allow air to escape from the bulb. The lower end has an adaptor that connects to the endotracheal tube. After intubation, the bulb is attached to the endotracheal tube and then compressed. With tracheal placement, the bulb draws air from the trachea and should reinflate to its original shape within 10 sec. With esophageal placement, the bulb receives little or no air from the constricted esophagus and it remains deflated (Wilkins et al., 2003). Since false positive and false negative results have been reported, the EDD test results should be used in conjunction with other clinical signs following an intubation attempt.

RAPID SEQUENCE INTUBATION

rapid sequence intubation (RSI): Intubation with an endotracheal tube under controlled settings.

Rapid sequence intubation (RSI) describes an urgent need to gain control of a patient's airway. It has been done safely and successful in both adult and pediatric patients (Davis et al., 2002; Dufour et al., 1995; Sagarin et al., 2002). RSI is done using an endotracheal tube under controlled settings to optimize the intubation conditions, to protect the airway against aspiration, and to facilitate ventilation and oxygenation.

TABLE 6-7   Indications for Rapid Sequence Intubation

INDICATION	NOTES
Airway obstruction	Inability to maintain patent airway with other devices (e.g., oropharyngeal airway, laryngeal mask airway)
Severe brain injury	Glasgow coma scale of 8 or less
Severe hypoxemia	PaO_2/F_IO_2 ratio <250
Abnormal respiratory rate	Spontaneous respiratory rate <10/ min or >30/min
Hemodynamic instability	Deteriorating hemodynamic values (e.g., vital signs, CVP, PAP, PCWP)

Modified from http://www.traumaburn.com. Retrieved April 21, 2004.

INDICATIONS AND CONTRAINDICATIONS

Indications for rapid sequence intubation include airway obstruction, severe brain injury, severe hypoxemia, abnormal respiratory rate, and hemodynamic instability (Table 6-7).

RSI should not be performed if a patient is able to sustain adequate ventilation and oxygenation while breathing spontaneously. It should not be attempted if the provider is unfamiliar with the proper procedure, intubation supplies, and drugs used in RSI. Following unsuccessful RSI attempts, surgical approach should be considered in special circumstances such as airway trauma or difficult anatomy.

PRACTICE GUIDELINES

The procedure for RSI varies among different protocols. However, each protocol typically consists of the following elements: preparation, pre-RSI medications, cricoid pressure, intubation, and post-RSI stabilization (Figure 6-13). (Bergen et al., 1997; Robinson et al., 2001; Sokolove et al., 2000; Smith et al., 2000).

In preparing for RSI, the following equipment and supplies should be readily available: cardiac monitor, intravenous access for pre-RSI medications, pulse oximeter, oxygen, drugs for advanced cardiac life support (ACLS), and cricothyrotomy tray for unsuccessful RSI attempts (Tayal, 1999).

Sedation and muscle paralysis facilitate RSI. Different drugs are available for RSI, and they should be chosen based on the patient's condition, indications, and contraindications. Common pre-RSI medications include etomidate (Amidate) for sedation (Guldner et al., 2003; Smith et al., 2000) and succinylcholine (Stewart, 2003; Walker, 1993) for neuromuscular paralysis. For adult patients, 20 mg of etomidate may be given intravenously over 30 to 60 sec. Succinylcholine may not be necessary if etomidate alone provides adequate sedation and results in successful intubation. If succinylcholine is needed, 100 mg or 1.5 mg/kg should be adequate. Since

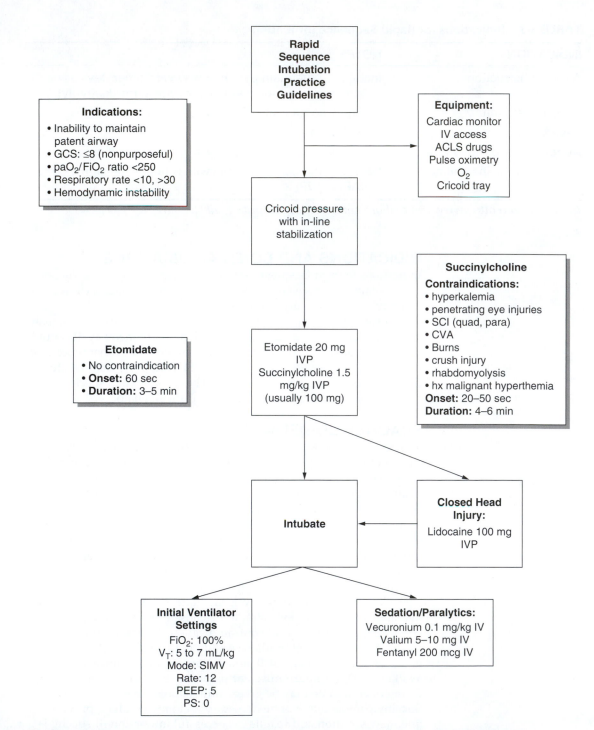

Figure 6-13   Rapid sequence intubation practice guideline. (Vanderbilt University Medical Center, Division of Trauma and Burns. Used with permission.)

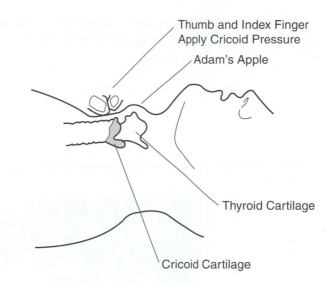

Thumb and Index Finger
Apply Cricoid Pressure

Adam's Apple

Thyroid Cartilage

Cricoid Cartilage

Figure 6-14   Sellick's (cricoid pressure) maneuver

☑ Pre-RSI medications should be chosen based on the patient's condition, indications, and contraindications.

☑ Common pre-RSI medications for adults include 20 mg of etomidate (Amidate) for sedation and 100 mg of succinylcholine.

☑ Cricoid pressure is applied to close off the esophagus and to minimize aspiration.

the onset of etomidate and succinylcholine is about 60 sec, intubation should be ready to proceed prior to administration of pre-RSI medications. Cricoid pressure using the Sellick's maneuver (Figure 6-14) should be done to close off the esophagus and to minimize aspiration.

After sedation and relaxation of respiratory muscles are achieved, oral intubation is done using traditional method as described earlier in this chapter. If post-RSI paralysis and sedation are desired, vecuronium (Norcuron, a steroidal-based nondepolarizing neuromuscular blocking agent), diazepam (Valium, an antianxiety agent) and fentanyl (Sublimaze, a synthetic opiate analgesic) may be used. The suggested adult IV dosages for vecuronium, diazepam, and fentanyl are 0.1 mg/kg, 5 to 10 mg, and 200 µg, respectively.

MANAGEMENT OF ENDOTRACHEAL AND TRACHEOSTOMY TUBES

Once the patient is successfully intubated with an artificial airway, it must be managed properly to prevent complications. Failure to secure the airway may lead to inadvertent or self-extubation. Excessive cuff pressures may lead to tracheal mucosal tissue injuries. Finally, failure to humidify the secretions makes removal of secretions from the artificial airway difficult and this condition may lead to pneumonia and atelectasis.

SECURING ENDOTRACHEAL AND TRACHEOSTOMY TUBES

The ET tube can be secured by using adhesive tape or commercially made harness. As shown in Figure 6-15A (oral intubation) and 6-15B (nasal intubation) they are used around the base of the head or neck for maximal security. Caution must be exercised as this technique may cause facial swelling and injuries to the lips when applied around the neck too tightly.

Since moisture often gathers between the tape and skin, tapes that can withstand moisture are more desirable. Zinc oxide base tape (by

Figure 6-15 (A) Use of a commercially made harness to secure an oral endotracheal tube. (B) One method of securing the tube of a nasally intubated patient.

Hy Tape Corporation, New York) is one that sticks well to the skin when exposed to moisture.

Tracheostomy tubes are secured by tying a string to the two openings on the collar. The string goes around the neck for good fit and security.

CUFF PRESSURE

> ☑ The ET tube cuff pressure should be 25 cm H$_2$O or less to minimize pressure-induced injuries to the trachea.

The estimated capillary perfusion pressure in the trachea is about 30 cm H$_2$O. If the cuff pressure is greater than the capillary perfusion pressure, ischemic injury and tissue necrosis may occur.

The ET tube cuff pressure should be 25 cm H$_2$O or less to allow adequate capillary perfusion in the trachea. For patients with hypotension, the cuff pressure should be kept even lower to compensate for the reduced capillary flow due to hypotension. Figure 6-16 shows the use of a pressure manometer and syringe to adjust the ET tube cuff pressure. Figure 6-17 shows a photograph of the Posey Cufflator with a built-in manometer. Air may be added to the ET tube cuff by pumping the bulb on the cufflator. Air may be removed from the ET tube cuff by opening the release valve on the cufflator.

MINIMAL OCCLUSION VOLUME AND MINIMAL LEAK TECHNIQUE

If a cuff pressure manometer is not readily available, the minimal occlusion volume or minimal leak technique may be used to reduce the likelihood of pressure-induced injuries to the trachea caused by excessive cuff pressure.

Pilot Balloon

Figure 6-16 (A) When the stop cock points toward the syringe, the manometer measures the cuff pressure. (B) When the stop cock points toward the manometer, the syringe may be used to fill or withdraw air from the cuff.

Figure 6-17　The Posey Cufflator.

☑ The minimal occlusion volume is obtained by inflating the cuff to a point at which no air leak is heard at end-inspiration.

☑ The minimal leak technique is done by inflating the cuff until the leak stops and then removing a small amount of air until a *slight* audible leak can be heard at end-inspiration.

The minimal occlusion volume is obtained by inflating the cuff to a point at which no air leak is heard at end-inspiration. The air leak around the cuff can be heard by placing the stethoscope diaphragm on the trachea, as close to the location of the cuff as possible. The end-inspiration point is used because the trachea reaches its maximal diameter at end-inspiration.

The minimal leak technique is done by inflating the cuff until the leak stops and then removing a small amount of air until a *slight* audible leak can be heard at end-inspiration (Chang, 1995).

IRRIGATION AND SUCTION

Intubated patients are at risk for secretion retention because the ET tube and ventilator attachments form a closed system and do not allow removal of secretions. Secretions must be removed by way of ET suctioning. However, frequent and inappropriate ET suctioning can cause mucosal damage and increase the incidence of suction-induced hypoxemia and arrhythmias. Therefore, ET suctioning should not be done on a preset sechedule, it should be done only when indicated.

The size of a suction catheter should be large enough for removal of secretions. However, an oversized suction catheter may impede airflow through the ET tube. As a rule of thumb, the outside diameter of the suction catheter should not exceed 50% of the inside diameter of the ET tube. A quick way to select the suitable suction catheter is to multiply the ET tube size by 2 and use the next smaller size of catheter (Wilkins et al., 2003). For example, a size 14 Fr suction

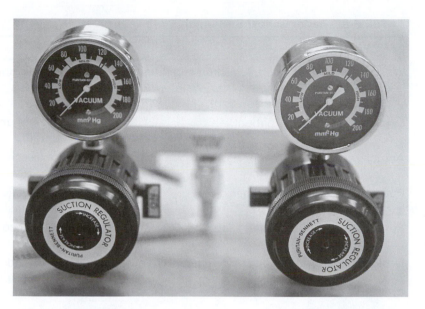

Figure 6-18   A Puritan-Bennett suction regulator with vacuum pressures ranging from 0 to 200 mm Hg.

catheter should be used for a size 8 ET tube since 2 × 8 = 16 and the next smaller size is 14.

The level of vacuum pressure should be kept below 100 mm Hg for adults and less than that for infants and children (Figure 6-18). The effectiveness of suction (based on the amount of secretion removed) is optimal at this vacuum pressure. Pressures higher than 100 mm Hg are not more effective but more likely to cause damage to the tracheal wall (Kuzenski, 1978).

Suction-induced hypoxemia may be avoided by preoxygenating the patient with 100% oxygen and limiting the duration of suctioning to less than 15 sec (Belknap et al., 1980; Stone et al., 1989). A closed in-line suction system (e.g., Ballard) may be useful to suction patients who have copious amounts of secretions. This system allows frequent suctioning without the need to disconnect the ventilator circuit. Since it is a closed system, the PEEP level as well as other ventilation and oxygenation settings on the ventilator may be maintained throughout the suctioning period (Rodenhizer, 2004). As an added financial benefit over the traditional disposable suction catheters, the in-line suction system does not require routine daily changes (Koleff et al., 1997).

Adult endotracheal tubes with a small dorsal lumen above the cuff are available to allow removal of subglottic secretions with a vacuum pressure of 20 mm Hg or less. Since the vacuum pressure is relatively low, obstruction or blockage of the dorsal lumen may occur. Patency of this lumen may be restored by injecting a small amount of air through the lumen (Tyco Healthcare, 2004). In one study, intermittent

☑ To avoid suction-induced hypoxemia, preoxygenate the patient and keep the duration of suction to less than 15 sec.

TABLE 6-8   Endotracheal Suctioning

PROCEDURE	RATIONALE
Wash hands and gather all suction supplies (catheter, sterile gloves, water, water container, and saline solution).	Avoid need to obtain other supplies once sterile gloves have been put on hands.
Explain procedure to patient.	Assure patient understanding and cooperation.
Adjust vacuum to 100 mm Hg.	Prevent excessive vacuum and mucosal damage.
Put sterile water in container.	For testing suction device and flushing secretions inside catheter.
Put on sterile gloves using aseptic technique.	Minimize nosocomial infection.
Designate "sterile" and "contaminated" hands.	Use sterile hand to handle all supplies requiring aseptic technique (i.e., suction catheter).
	Use contaminated hand to handle all other supplies (e.g., ET tube adapter, suction tubing).
Attach suction catheter (sterile hand) to suction tubing (contaminated hand).	Ensure sterile and aseptic techniques.
Test vacuum and suction with sterile water.	Ensure proper function of suction setup.
Remove ET tube adapter and irrigate with 5 cc of sterile saline if necessary (contaminated hand).	Loosen secretions.
Manually hyperinflate the patient's lungs with resuscitation bag.	Ensure adequate ventilation and oxygenation. Seek help if necessary.
Insert catheter into ET tube (sterile hand) and advance until resistance is met. Withdraw catheter slightly.	Avoid suctioning the tracheal wall and minimize mucosal damage.
Activate suction (contaminated hand) and withdraw catheter (sterile hand) by rotating the catheter.	Increase removal of secretions.
Limit the duration of suction to less than 15 sec.	Prevent suction-induced hypoxia and arrhythmias.
Auscultate chest and repeat suction if necessary.	Avoid unnecessary suctioning.

(Data from Barnes, 1986; Belknap et al., 1980; Chulay, 1988; Stone, et al.,1989.)

drainage of subglottic secretion has been shown to reduce the incidence of ventilator-associated pneumonia in patients receiving mechanical ventilation (Smulders et al., 2002).

The sequence outlined in Table 6-8 provides a general procedure for ET suctioning. It should be modified to suit individual situations and to comply with existing protocols. For example, irrigation of the ET tube and lungs with saline solution before suctioning is a controversial practice (Bostick et al., 1987; Shekleton et al., 1987).

speaking valve: *A one-way valve attachment to the tracheostomy tube that allows the user to talk.*

☑ Speaking valves block the exhaled air through the tracheostomy tube and direct it through the vocal cords making phonation possible.

☑ Contraindications for using speaking valve include laryngeal stenosis, vocal cord paralysis, and severe tracheal stenosis.

SPEAKING VALVES

Fenestrated tracheostomy tubes have been in use for many years to facilitate weaning of tracheostomy tube and to allow phonation (Mallinckrodt, 2004). With the opening of a fenestrated tracheostomy tube blocked, the fenestrated openings allow the patient to move air through the vocal cords making phonation possible (Figure 6-19).

A **speaking valve** is a newer device which consists of a one-way valve that fits on a traditional or fenestrated tracheostomy tube over a 15-mm connection. The one-way valve allows the patient to breathe in, but exhaled air is blocked and diverted around the deflated cuff or fenestrations. The air moves through the vocal cords making phonation possible (Figure 6-20). Some common speaking valves are the Passy-Muir (Passy-Muir Inc., Irvine, CA), the Phonate (Mallinckrodt, 2004), and the Montgomery and Ventrach speaking valves (Boston Medical Products, 2004).

CONTRAINDICATIONS

Contraindications for using a speaking valve include laryngeal stenosis, vocal cord paralysis, and severe tracheal stenosis. These conditions impede air flow making ventilation and phonation difficult (Mallinckrodt, 2004).

Figure 6-19 Uncuffed fenestrated tracheostomy tube.

A   **B**

Figure 6-20   (A) Speaking valve. (B) The one-way valve dose not allow exhalation through the tracheostomy. The exhaled air is directed toward the vocal cords making phonation possible. (Copyright 2003 AARC Times Magazine, a publication of the American Association for Respiratory Care. Reprinted with permission.)

☑ The design of the speaking valve allows only inhalation through the tracheostomy tube, but not exhalation.

☑ Before the speaking valve is placed on a fenestrated tracheostomy tube, the fenestrations must be opened by removing the non-fenestrated inner cannula or using a fenestrated inner cannula.

SAFETY REQUIREMENTS

Before the speaking valve is placed on a cuffed tracheostomy tube, the cuff must first be deflated. An inflated cuff would make exhalation through the tracheostomy tube impossible because the design of the speaking valve allows only inhalation, but not exhalation. A deflated cuff would allow the patient to exhale around the tracheostomy tube, through the vocal cords and the mouth or nose.

Before the speaking valve is placed on a fenestrated tracheostomy tube, the fenestrations must be opened by removing the non-fenestrated inner cannula or using a fenestrated inner cannula. The cuff of the fenestrated tracheostomy tube may be inflated or deflated. This technique allows the exhaled air to move toward the vocal cords and the mouth or nose (Pruit, 2003). Table 6-9 summarizes the safety requirements in using a speaking valve on a tracheostomy tube.

TABLE 6-9 Safety Requirements in Using a Speaking Valve

TYPE OF TRACHEOSTOMY TUBE	REQUIREMENT
Traditional	Cuff must be deflated.

Fenestrated	Fenestrations must be opened by:
	    removing the nonfenestrated inner cannula, or
	    using a fenestrated inner cannula.
	Cuff may be inflated only when fenestrations are open.

POSITIVE-PRESSURE VENTILATION

Air leak is common when using a speaking valve. For patients who are breathing spontaneously, the amount of air leak is of no concern. In mechanically ventilated patients, the air leak may require careful and periodical adjustments of the tidal volume, PEEP, and alarm settings (Pruitt, 2003). To ensure adequate ventilation and oxygenation, the vital signs and pulse oximetry of the patient must be closely monitored. Deteriorating vital signs and oxygen desaturation are signs of speaking valve malfunction, severe air flow obstruction, or air leak.

EXTUBATION

Extubation should be done as soon as feasible. Early extubation not only provides immediate relief to the patient, but also shortens the duration of a hospital stay, reduces health care costs, and conserves resources (Cheng, 1995; Lichtenthal et al., 1995; Velasco, 1995). In one study of patients undergoing coronary artery bypass grafting, the average saving per patient was $6,000 in the early extubation group (Arom, 1995).

PREDICTORS OF SUCCESSFUL EXTUBATION

A patient is ready for extubation after regaining airway reflexes and showing no signs of cardiopulmonary distress. The general criteria for assessing a patient's readiness to be extubated may include the rapid shallow breathing index, occlusion pressure/maximal inspiratory pressure ratio, blood gases, muscle strength, and general cardiopulmonary signs.

☑ The patient should be allowed to breathe spontaneously for at least three minutes before taking measurements. Otherwise, the f/V_T index may not reflect the patient's actual condition.

Rapid Shallow Breathing Index. The rapid shallow breathing (f/V_T) index can be obtained easily by measuring the breathing frequency and minute volume during 1 min of spontaneous breathing (Epstein, 1995; Yang et al., 1991). f/V_T is calculated by dividing the spontaneous breathing frequency per minute by the average tidal volume in liters. A value of less than 100/min/L is highly predictive of successful extubation outcome.

TABLE 6-10   General Criteria for Extubation

CRITERIA	METHODS OF ASSESSMENT
Rapid shallow breathing index	f/V_T less than 100/min/L
Blood gases	Acceptable blood gases on F_IO_2 less than 40% and spontaneous minute ventilation less than 10 L/min PaO_2/F_IO_2 more than 250 mm Hg
Ventilatory reserve	Maximal inspiratory pressure >-20 cm H_2O Vital capacity >15 mL/kg
Cardiopulmonary assessment	Absence of cardiopulmonary problems (e.g., CHF, pulmonary edema, pneumonia, tachycardia, arrhythmia, chest retractions, distended stomach)

(Data from Capdevila et al., 1995; Epstein, 1995; Listello et al., 1994; Whelan et al., 1994; White, 2002; Whitten, 1997.)

Other Common Indicators.   Acceptable blood gases, ventilatory reserve, general cardiopulmonary signs, infrequent need for suctioning (>4 hours), being alert, and SpO_2 $>95\%$ are other useful indicators that may be used to guide the extubation decision (Pronovost, 2002). These criteria and the rapid shallow breathing index are very simple and easy to use. They are summarized in Table 6-10 along with their respective methods of assessment.

☑ P0.1/MIP ratio of 0.9 or lower is predictive of successful extubation outcome.

P0.1/MIP Ratio.   The occlusion pressure at 0.1 sec to maximal inspiratory pressure (P0.1/MIP) ratio is a more complicated procedure than the preceding criteria. A special manometer is needed to measure the airway occlusion pressure at 0.1 sec from the onset of inspiration, with the airway occluded at the functional residual capacity (Capdevila et al., 1995; Whitelaw et al., 1993). Since P0.1 is measured at zero flow, it is independent of the compliance and resistance characteristics of the respiratory system. P0.1 reflects the neuromuscular drive to breathe—a prerequisite for successful extubation and adequate spontaneous breathing. The MIP reflects the respiratory muscle strength and ventilatory reserve. A P0.1/MIP ratio of 0.9 or lower has great predictive value of successful extubation (Capdevila et al., 1995).

☑ Competent personnel and intubation supplies must be readily available during extubation.

PROCEDURE

There should be no disagreement that extubation is easier than intubation. Nevertheless, the person who is doing the extubation must be proficient in intubation as well. Since the criteria used for the extubation decision cannot predict a successful outcome every time, one must anticipate the need for reintubation on short notice. Intubation supplies must also be readily available during extubation.

Before extubation, the procedure is explained to the patient and the patient is positioned in a Fowler's (semisitting) position. Hyperinflation

Figure 6-21   Use of a flow-inflating manual resuscitator, suction catheter, and a syringe during extubation.

✓ The cuff must be deflated before extubation.

and oxygenation are provided to the patient with a manual resuscitator via the ET tube. The ET tube is then suctioned.

If the patient has an adequate vital capacity and cough reflex, the cuff is deflated completely and the ET tube is removed. Encourage the patient to breathe deeply and cough, and use a Yankaur (rigid tonsil tip) suction device to remove excess secretions in the patient's oropharynx.

If the patient does not have an adequate vital capacity and cough reflex, the suction catheter may be left extending from the distal end of the ET tube and continuous suction is applied while the ET tube is being removed. An alternate method is to leave the suction catheter in the oropharynx with continuous suction while the ET tube is being removed. Either method may be used to remove secretions from the patient's airway or oropharynx (Figure 6-21).

✓ Aspiration, laryngospasm, hoarseness, and laryngeal and subglottic edema are some complications immediately after extubation.

Vital signs, blood gases, and signs of tissue damage should be assessed carefully after extubation. Some immediate postextubation complications include aspiration, laryngospasm, hoarseness, and laryngeal and subglottic edema. Other more severe complications that may not be immediately apparent are mucosal injuries, laryngeal stenosis, tracheal inflammation, dilation or stenosis, and vocal cord paralysis (Young et al., 1995).

UNPLANNED EXTUBATION

unplanned extubation: Unexpected removal of an endotracheal or tracheostomy tube before the patient is ready for extubation.

Unplanned extubation or inadvertent extubation (self-inflicted or accidental) accounts for about 8% to 10% of all extubations in ICU patients (Listello et al., 1994). For patients who self-extubate the

TABLE 6-11   Clinical Predictors for Reintubation

UNFAVORABLE CLINICAL PREDICTOR*	RATIONALES
(1) SIMV or AC rate >6/min	Patient is dependent on the ventilator.
(2) Most recent pH ≥7.45	Oxyhemoglobin saturation curve shifts to left ($\uparrow O_2$ affinity and $\downarrow O_2$ release to tissues).
(3) Most recent PaO_2/F_IO_2 <250 mm Hg	Poor oxygenation status.
(4) Highest heart rate in the past 24° >120/min	Cardiac compensation for poor perfusion or oxygenation.
(5) Presence of ≥3 medical disorders	Potential of medical complications.
(6) Not alert	Poor mental status; blunted drive for breathing.
(7) Reason for intubation other than preoperative	Presence of medical problems and potential complications.

Presence of four or more predictors favors reintubation. Presence of three or less predictors indicates no need for reintubation.

endotracheal tube, about 50% of them do not need to be reintubated (Betbese, 1998; Chevron, 1998). Whether or not to reintubate the patient can be a difficult decision. Delayed reintubation may lead to adverse outcomes such as hypoventilation, hypoxemia, and hypoxia. In general, the decision to reintubate may be based on clinical observations and the criteria for extubation (i.e., rapid shallow breathing index, blood gases, ventilatory reserve, and general cardiopulmonary signs). However, these measurements may not have been done immediately before extubation since the extubation is not planned.

To avoid this problem, other criteria based on routinely available patient information have been identified and used for the reintubation decision. They are summarized in Table 6-11. In the model set, the presence of four or more factors indicates the need for reintubation and the presence of three or fewer factors reflects a satisfactory patient outcome without reintubation (Listello et al., 1994).

COMPLICATIONS OF ENDOTRACHEAL AIRWAY

Endotracheal intubation is an extremely useful procedure in the establishment of an artificial airway but it also carries many potential complications. As shown in Table 6-12, complications may develop at different stages of intubation and extubation. Some conditions are life-threatening (e.g., esophageal intubation, bradycardia) while others

TABLE 6-12   Complications Related to Use of Endotracheal Tube

SEQUENCE OF EVENTS	COMPLICATIONS
During intubation	Trauma to teeth and soft tissues Esophageal intubation Vomiting and aspiration Hypoxia due to prolonged intubation attempt Arrhythmias Bradycardia due to vagal stimulation
While intubated	Obstruction by secretions Pneumonia and atelectasis Kinking of ET tube Aspiration (from feeding and ineffective cuff) Mucosal injuries Laryngeal damage Improper tube position (too high, too low) Pressure sores around ET tube Inadvertent extubation Sinusitis (nasal intubation)
Immediately after extubation	Aspiration Laryngospasm Hoarseness Laryngeal and subglottic edema
Following extubation	Mucosal injuries Laryngeal stenosis Tracheal inflammation, dilation, stenosis Vocal cord paralysis

(Data from Chang, 1995; Dillier, 2004; White, 2002; Whitten, 1997; Young et al., 1995.)

are minor and often reversible (e.g., pressure sores, hoarseness). It is essential to understand and recognize the potential complications so that appropriate steps may be taken to avert harmful outcomes.

DURING INTUBATION

☑ Trauma to the teeth and soft tissues can occur during intubation.

☑ Esophageal intubation is commonly done by inexperienced practitioners.

Trauma to the teeth and soft tissues can occur during intubation since ET intubation is often done in emergency situations. Difficult intubations compound the problem and lead to injuries when the patient has one or more of these conditions: obesity, receding chin, overbite, rigid or short neck, or blood or vomitus in oropharynx.

Esophageal intubation is the most dangerous complication. It may occur when it is performed by an inexperienced practitioner or under awkward patient positions (e.g., patient lies on the floor). Esophageal intubation frequently leads to vomiting and aspiration, thus making subsequent intubation attempts more difficult or nearly impossible.

vagus nerve: The pneumogastric or tenth cranial nerve. Its superior and recurrent laryngeal nerves and their branches adjoin the upper end of trachea and are sensitive to stimulation by the endotracheal tube or suction catheter.

Prolonged intubation attempt leads to hypoxia and if uncorrected, dangerous arrhythmias may occur. Excessive stimulation of the **vagus nerve** can cause bradycardia. Arrhythmias induced by hypoxia and bradycardia caused by vagal stimulation may be reversed by removing the ET tube and oxygenating the patient until a normal sinus rhythm returns.

WHILE INTUBATED

Complications that occur while the patient is intubated vary greatly according to the duration of ET tube placement and the airway management techniques. As a general rule, the longer an ET tube is in place, the more likely that complications will occur while the patient is intubated.

✓ Failure to remove retained secretions could lead to pneumonia and atelectasis.

Since normal mucocillary functions of the mucosal membrane and the cough reflex are lost with an ET tube in place, retention of secretions must be removed promptly. If secretions are thick, irrigation with saline solution or acetylcysteine (Mucomyst®) should be done before suctioning. Failure to remove retained secretions may lead to pneumonia and atelectasis (Chang, 1995).

Kinking of an ET tube may be easily corrected by repositioning the connection between the ET tube and the ventilator circuit. Inadvertent extubation may be prevented by properly sedating the patient or by using restraints on the extremities.

✓ The distance marking on the ET tube is made in reference to the patient's lips or nares (e.g., 22 cm at the lips).

The position of the ET tube should be checked frequently by chest auscultation and concurrently when a routine chest radiograph is done. Once the ET tube is properly placed, the distance marking on the ET tube (centimeter mark) should be noted on the ventilator flow sheet. This reference number provides a quick reference point but should not be used as a substitute for routine assessment of the ET tube position.

IMMEDIATELY AFTER EXTUBATION

✓ Extubation of a semiconscious patient may stimulate the vocal cords and lead to reflex spasm.

Laryngospasm usually occurs as a result of extubation when the patient is semiconscious. Extubation during this excitement stage tends to stimulate the vocal cords and lead to reflex protective spasm. For this reason, extubation should be done when the patient is either deeply anesthetized or preferably, fully awake (Whitten, 1997).

✓ Stridor is the harsh or high-pitched sound heard during spontaneous respiration.

Stridor is heard when laryngospasm or laryngeal and subglottic edema occur. In minor cases of stridor, use of cool aerosol and 0.25 to 0.5 cc of 2.25% racemic epinephrine in 5 cc of saline may be helpful. Dexamethasone at 0.15 mg/kg may help prevent worsening laryngeal and subglottic edema. In severe cases of laryngospasm, airway obstruction may have developed and reintubation is often required (Whitten, 1997).

FOLLOWING EXTUBATION

Mucosal injuries, laryngeal stenosis, tracheal damages (inflammation, dilation, and stenosis), and vocal cord paralysis are some long-term complications following extubation. The best way to avoid these complications is to practice proper airway care while the patient is intubated.

SUMMARY

The most important element of airway management is intubation. Esophageal intubation can be deadly and it must not be done under any circumstance (e.g., secretions in the airway, poor view, or awkward patient position). The golden rule for endotracheal intubation is "If you don't see it (the vocal cords or related structures), don't do it."

Use of artificial airways also requires proper and routine maintenance to prevent complications. Humidification, suctioning, cuff pressure, and unplanned extubation are some important aspects in airway management during mechanical ventilation. Since the artificial airway is inside the patient's mouth and trachea and is not readily visible, practitioners must have a keen sense of observation and timely clinical judgement to detect any complications or potential troubles.

Self-Assessment Questions

1. The decision to intubate a patient is based on all of the following indications with the *exception* of:

A. airway obstruction.   C. mechanical ventilation.
B. hypoxemia.   D. removal of secretions.

2–5. Match the indications for using an artificial airway with the respective examples.

Indication	Examples
2. Relief of airway obstruction	A. Absence of coordinated swallow
3. Protection of the airway	B. Ventilatory failure
4. Facilitation of suctioning	C. Excessive secretions
5. Support of ventilation	D. Epiglottitis

6. You are getting ready to intubate a patient who has been classified as Class 3 using the Mallampati method. You would _____ because the _____ are seen during assessment.

    A. provide conscious sedation, soft palate and base of uvula.
    B. provide conscious sedation, fauces, uvula, and tonsillar pillars.
    C. seek anesthesia consultation, soft palate, and base of uvula.
    D. seek anesthesia consultation, fauces, uvula, and tonsillar pillars.

7. As you are preparing to intubate a 49-year-old, 60-kg (132-lb) patient, you notice that there are two endotracheal tubes, size 7 and size 8. You would use the _____ tube because it offers _____ than the other ET tube.

    A. size 8, lower air flow resistance
    B. size 8, higher air flow resistance
    C. size 7, lower air flow resistance
    D. size 7, higher air flow resistance

8. You are called to intubate a patient in the dialysis unit. Since there are no crash cart and intubation equipment nearby, you are asked to bring along the minimal supplies needed for intubation. In addition to the laryngoscope handle, blade, and endotracheal tube, which of the following supplies is the most essential item for intubation and ventilation?

    A. water-soluble lubricant
    B. tape
    C. stylet
    D. 10-cc syringe

9. You are getting ready to perform an elective intubation on a 32-year-old, 78-kg (172-lb), 5 ft 2 in. patient in the intensive care unit. Based on the patient's physical characteristics, you would ask for a size _____, _____ laryngoscope blade.

    A. 2, Miller
    B. 3, Miller
    C. 4, MacIntosh
    D. 5, MacIntosh

10. When you intubate the patient in the preceding question, you would place the tip of the blade just under the _____ and use the laryngoscope handle to _____.

    A. tongue, pry the mouth open
    B. tongue, lift up anteriorly
    C. epiglottis, pry the mouth open
    D. epiglottis, lift up anteriorly

11. As you are intubating an apneic patient, you notice on the cardiac monitor that the patient has developed arrhythmias during the procedure. You would remove the blade and endotracheal tube immediately and provide:

    A. cardiac defibrillation and ventilation.
    B. 100% oxygen via a nonrebreathing mask.
    C. 100% oxygen via manual resuscitation bag/mask system.
    D. chest compression and ventilation.

12. The best approach to avoid esophageal intubation is to ensure that the endotracheal tube goes through the _____ under direct vision.

    A. underside of tongue   C. vocal cords
    B. pharynx   D. epiglottis

13. Trauma done to the teeth of a patient undergoing an intubation procedure is most likely caused by using:

    A. a straight blade.   C. an oversized endotracheal tube.
    B. a curved blade.   D. pivoting action to lift blade and tongue.

14. After intubating a spontaneously breathing 40-kg (88-lb) patient, all of the following signs may be used to assess correct placement of the endotracheal tube *except*:

    A. presence of breath sounds at the sternum.   C. air movement over the ET tube opening.
    B. loss of speech.   D. formation of moisture inside the ET tube.

15. The onset time for etomidate and succinylcholine used in rapid sequence intubation is about _____ min and these drugs last about _____ min.

    A. 1, 1   C. 5, 10
    B. 1, 5   D. 5, 20

16. In order to avoid mucosal injuries of the trachea, the cuff of an endotracheal tube may be managed by any one of the following techniques *except*:

    A. minimal occlusion volume.   C. cuff pressure less than 25 cm H_2O.
    B. periodic deflation for 20 minutes q 4°.   D. minimal leak technique.

17. A speaking valve that is attached to a cuffed tracheostomy tube does not allow the patient to _____ through the valve. For this reason, the cuff must be _____.

    A. exhale, inflated   C. exhale, deflated
    B. inhale and exhale, inflated   D. inhale and exhale, deflated

18. A physician asks you to evaluate Mr. King, a postabdominal surgical patient, for possible extubation. Based on the information below, you would recommend to the physician that the patient be a candidate for extubation because he meets all criteria for extubation with the *exception* of:

    A. rapid shallow breathing (f/V_T) index of 150/min/L.   C. maximal inspiratory pressure of -38 cm H_2O.
    B. PaO_2/F_IO_2 of 280 mm Hg.   D. F_IO_2 of 35%.

19. A 25-year-old postappendectomy patient extubated herself and you are asked by the physician to evaluate this patient for possible reintubation. Based on the following list of clinical predictors for reintubation, you would recommend that the patient _____ since she has met _____ of the predictors.

Unfavorable Clinical Predictor
(1) SIMV rate = 8/min
(2) Most recent pH = 7.42
(3) Most recent PaO_2/F_IO_2 = 210 mm Hg
(4) Highest heart rate in the past 24° = 110/min
(5) Patient diagnosis is appendicitis
(6) Patient is alert
(7) Patient is in postoperative recovery

A. be reintubated, 2
B. be reintubated, 4

C. not be reintubated, 2
D. not be reintubated, 4

20. A patient develops bradycardia during an intubation attempt. You would stop intubation immediately and _____ the patient since this condition is likely caused by _____.

A. rest, vagal stimulation
B. ventilate, hypoventilation

C. oxygenate, hypoxia
D. defibrillate, impending cardiac arrest

21. Several hours after endotracheal intubation, a 35-year-old patient becomes restless in spite of using sedatives and analgesics. The physician is concerned that the ET tube may move down the main bronchus because of excessive head movement. You would recommend that _____ be done and the tip of the ET tube be positioned about _____ in. from the carina.

A. auscultation, 0.5
B. auscultation, 1.5

C. chest radiograph, 0.5
D. chest radiograph, 1.5

Answers to Self-Assessment Questions

1. B. hypoxemia.

2. D. Epiglottitis

3. A. Absence of coordinated swallow

4. C. Excessive secretions

5. B. Ventilatory failure

6. C. seek anesthesia consultation, soft palate and base of uvula.

7. A. size 8, lower air flow resistance

8. D. 10-cc syringe

9. B. 3, Miller

10. D. epiglottis, lift up anteriorly

11. C. 100% oxygen via manual resuscitation bag/mask system

12. C. vocal cords

13. D. pivoting action to lift blade and tongue

14. A. presence of breath sounds at the sternum.

15. B. 1, 5

16. B. periodic deflation for 20 min q 4

17. C. exhale, deflated

18. A. rapid shallow breathing (f/V_T) index of 150/min/L.

19. C. not be reintubated, 2

20. A. rest, vagal stimulation

21. D. chest radiograph, 1.5

References

Arom, K. V. (1995). Cost-effectiveness and predictors of early extubation. *Ann of Thorac Surg, 60*(1), 127–132.

Barnes, C. A. (1986). Minimizing hypoxemia due to endotracheal suctioning: A review of the literature. *Heart Lung, 15*, 164–172.

Belknap, J. D., et al. (1980). The effects of preoxygenation technique on arterial blood gases in the mechanically ventilated patient. *Am Rev Respir Dis, 121*(Suppl.), 210.

Bergen, J. M., et al. (1997). A review of etomidate for rapid sequence intubation in the emergency department. *J Emerg Med, 15*(2), 221–230.

Betbese, A. J., et al. (1998). A prospective study of unplanned endotracheal extubation in intensive care unit patients. *Crit Care Med, 26*, 1180–1186.

Bostick, J., et al. (1987). Normal saline installation as part of the suctioning procedure: Effects on PaO_2 and amount of secretions. *Heart Lung, 16*, 532–537.

Boston Medical Products. (2004). Montgomery tracheostomy speaking valve and Ventrach speaking valve. Retrieved April 26, 2004 from http://www.bosmed.com/tracheostomy.htm

Capdevila, X. J., et al. (1995). Occlusion pressure and its ratio to maximum inspiratory pressure are useful predictors for successful extubation following T-piece weaning trail. *Chest, 108*, 482–489.

Chang, V. M. (1995). Protocol for prevention of complications of endotracheal intubation. *Crit Care Nurse, 15*, 19–27.

Cheng, D. C. H. (1995). Pro-Early extubation after cardiac-surgery decreases intensive-care unit stay and cost. *J Cardiothorac Vas Anes, 9*(4), 460–464.

Chevron, V., et al. (1998). Unplanned extubation: risk factors of development and predictive criteria for reintubation. *Crit Care Med, 26,* 1049–1053.

Chulay, M. (1988). Arterial blood gas changes with a hyperinflation and hyperoxygenation suctioning intervention in critically ill patients. *Heart Lung, 17*, 654–661.

Conrady, P. A., et al. (1976). Alteration of endotracheal tube position: flexion and extension of the neck. *Crit Care Med, 4*, 7–12.

Coppolo, D. P., et al. (1990). Self-extubation: a twelve-month experience. *Chest, 98*, 165–169.

Davis, B. D., et al. (2002). Role of rapid sequence induction for intubation in the prehospital setting: helpful or harmful? *Curr Opin Crit Care, 8*(6), 571–577.

Dillier, C. M., et al. (2004). Laryngeal damage due to an unexpectedly large and inappropriately designed cuffed pediatric tracheal tube in a 13-month-old child. *J Anaesth, 51*(1), 72–75.

Dufour, D. G., et al. (1995). Rapid sequence intubation in the emergency department. *J Emerg Med, 13*(5), 705–710.

Epstein, S. K. (1995). Etiology of extubation failure and the predictive value of the rapid breathing index. *Am J Respir Crit Care Med, 152*, 545–549.

Finucane, B. T., & Santora, A. H. (2003). *Principles of airway management* (3rd ed). New York: Springer-Verlag.

Graber, M. A. (2004). Resuscitation, airway management, and acute arrhythmias: Table 1-1: endotracheal tube sizes for children. Retrieved April 29, 2004, from http://www.vh.org/pediatric/provider/pediatrics/familypracticehandbook/table/1-1.html

Guldner, G., et al. (2003). Etomidate for rapid-sequence intubation in young children: hemo-dynamic effects and adverse events. *Acad Emerg Med*, *10*(2), 134–139.

Kasper, C. L., & Deem, S. (1998). The self-inflating bulb to detect esophageal intubation during emergency airway management. *Anesthesiology, 88*(4), 898–902.

Kollef, M. H., et al. (1997). Mechanical ventilation with or without daily changes of in-line suction catheters. *Am J Respir Crit Care Med*, *156*(2 Pt. 1), 466–472.

Kuzenski, B. M. (1978). Effect of negative pressure on tracheobronchial trauma. *Nurs Res, 28*, 260–273.

Lichtenthal, P. R., et al. (1995). Perioperative cardiac anesthesia and early extubation keys to decreasing costs in the cardiac-surgery ICU. *Anesthesiology, 83*(3A), A1093.

Listello, D., et al. (1994). Unplanned extubation—Clinical predictors for reintubation. *Chest, 105*, 1496–1503.

Mallinckrodt Inc. (2004). Tracheostomy tube adult home care guide. Retrieved April 26, 2004, from http://edcenter.mallinckrodt.com/Courses/c23/AdultHCG.pdf

Martinez, A., et al. (2003). Minute ventilation recovery time - a predictor of extubation outcome. *Chest, 123,* 1214–1221.

Marvez-Valls, E., et al. (2002). Protocol for rapid sequence intubation in pediatric patients – a four-year study. *Med Sci Monit*, *8*(4), CR229–234.

Passy-Muir tracheostomy and ventilator speaking valves (Instruction booklet). Irvine, CA: Passy-Muir.

Pronovost, P. J., et al. (2002). Reducing failed extubations in the intensive care unit. *Jt Comm J Qual Improv*, *28*(11), 595–604.

Pruitt, W. C. (2003, September). Caring for the patient with a tracheostomy: Speaking, plug-ging, and decannulation. *AARC Times, 9,* 48–54.

Rodenhizer, K. (2004). Ballard trach care closed suction system summary of benefits and associated literature. Retrieved April 26, 2004, from http://www.xmission.com/%7Egastown/herpmed/closed.htm

Robinson, N., et al. (2001). In patients with head injury undergoing rapid sequence intuba-tion, does pretreatment with intravenous lignocaine/lidocaine lead to an improved neuro-logic outcome? *Emerg Med J*, *18*(6), 453–457.

Sagarin M. J., et al. (2002). Rapid sequence intubation for pediatric emergency airway management. *Pediatr Emerg Care*, *18*(6), 417–423.

Shapiro, B. A., et al. (1991). *Clinical application of respiratory care* (4th ed.). St. Louis, MO: Mosby.

Shekleton, M. E., et al. (1987). Ineffective airway clearance related to artificial airway. *Nurs Clin North Am, 22*, 167–178.

Smith, D. C., et al. (2000). A trial of etomidate for rapid sequence intubation in the emergency department. *J Emerg Med, 18*(1), 13–16.

Smulders, K., et al. (2002). A randomized clinical trial of intermittent subglottic secretion drainage in patients receiving mechanical ventilation. *Chest*, 121, 858–862.

Sokolove, P. E., at al. (2000). The safety of etomidate for emergency rapid sequence intubation of pediatric patients. *Pediatr Emerg Care, 16*(1), 18–21.

Stewart C. E. (2003). Airway Management with rapid sequence intubation: Part 1. Retrieved April 23, 2004, from http://www.emsmagazine.com/articles/airwayart.html

Stone, K. S., et al. (1989). Endotracheal suctioning. *Annu Res Nur Res, 7*, 27–47.

Tasota, F. J., et al. (1987). Evaluation of two methods used to stabilize oral endotracheal tubes. *Heart Lung, 16*, 140–145.

Tayal, V. S., et al. (1999). Rapid-sequence intubation at an emergency medicine residency: success rate and adverse events during a two-year period. *Acad Emerg Med, 6*(1), 31–37.

Tyco Healthcare (2004). Intensive Care Tracheal Tubes. Retrieved May 12, 2004, from http://www.tycohealth-ece.com/files/d0001/ty_1lrohc.pdf

Velasco, F. T. (1995). Economic rationale for early extubation. *J Cardiothorac Vas Anes, 9*(5), 2–9.

Walker, L. A. (1993). Rapid sequence intubation. *Emerg Med Reports, 14*(15), 127–132.

White, G. C. (2002). *Basic clinical lab competencies for respiratory care—An integrated approach* (4th ed.). Clifton Park, New York: Thomson Delmar Learning.

Whitelaw, W. A., et al. (1993). Airway occlusion pressure. *J Appl Physiol, 74*, 1475–1483.

Whitten, C. E. (1997). *Anyone can intubate—A practical, step-by-step guide for health professionals* (3rd ed.). San Diego: KWP Publications.

Wilkins, R. L., et al.(2003). *Egan's fundamentals of respiratory care* (8th ed.). St. Louis, MO: Mosby.

Yang, K. L., et al. (1991). A prospective study of indexes predicting the outcome of trials of weaning from mechanical ventilation. *N Engl J Med, 324*, 1445–1450.

Young, A., et al. (1995). Laryngospasm following extubation in children. *Anesthesia, 50*(9), 827.

Suggested Reading

Airway Management

American Society of Anesthesiologists (1993). Practice guidelines for management of the difficult airway - a report by the American Society of Anesthesiologists Task Force on management of the difficult airway, *Chest 78*, 597–602.
(A list of the articles used to develop the above guidelines is available by writing to the American Society of Anesthesiologists, 520 North Northwest Highway, Park Ridge, Illinois 60068-2573)

Sale, M. L., et al. (2003). A multisite survey of suctioning techniques and airway management practices. *Am J Crit Care*, *12*(3), 220–230.

Whelan, J., et al. (1994). Unplanned extubation—Predictors of successful termination of mechanical ventilatory support. *Chest, 105,* 1808–1812.

Extubation

Martinez, A., et al. (2003). Minute ventilation recovery time: A predictor of extubation outcome. *Chest, 123* (4), 1214–1221.

CHAPTER SEVEN

NONINVASIVE POSITIVE PRESSURE VENTILATION

David W. Chang

OUTLINE

KEY TERMS

- apnea index
- apnea-hypopnea index
- bilevel positive airway pressure (bilevel PAP)
- BiPAP™
- continuous positive airway pressure (CPAP)
- desaturation index
- expiratory positive airway pressure (EPAP)

- facial mask
- hypopnea index
- inspiratory positive airway pressure (IPAP)
- nasal mask
- Nasal Pillows™
- noninvasive positive pressure ventilation (NPPV)
- obstructive sleep apnea (OSA)
- positive end-expiratory pressure (PEEP)

INTRODUCTION

Noninvasive positive pressure ventilation (NPPV) is a technique of providing ventilation without the use of an artificial airway. It has been used successfully in the management of airflow obstruction in sleep apnea (Guilleminault, Philip & Robinson, 1998) and in the reduction of respiratory workload in gross obesity (Pankow et al., 1997). More recently NPPV has been used in the management of acute respiratory failure. In selected patients with acute ventilatory failure, NPPV is as effective as conventional mechanical ventilation in improving gas exchange (Abou-Shala & Meduri, 1996). Since an artificial airway is not required in the use of NPPV, fewer complications and a shorter stay in an acute care setting are two additional benefits of NPPV (Antonelli et al., 1998).

noninvasive positive pressure ventilation (NPPV): NPPV provides assisted ventilation without an artificial airway.

✔ NPPV may be used to assist patients with obstructive sleep apnea and acute ventilatory failure.

During the polio epidemics, negative pressure ventilators (i.e., iron lungs) were used to provide ventilation by generating a pressure gradient between the atmosphere and lungs. Air flows into the lungs and ventilation occurs when the pressure in the lungs becomes sub-atmospheric. Disadvantages of negative pressure ventilators include upper airway obstruction and lack of access for patient care. Modern ventilators generate the pressure gradient between the atmosphere and lungs by positive pressure. With positive pressure ventilation, the pressure in the airway opening is higher than that in the lungs. Some of the disadvantages of positive pressure ventilators are tracheal injury, infection, ventilator-associated pneumonia, barotrauma, and prolonged hospital stay (Antonelli et al., 1998; Diaz et al., 1997; Keenan et al., 1997; Kramer et al., 1995).

NPPV provides ventilation via the patient's nose or mouth without an artificial airway. For this reason, many complications of negative and positive pressure ventilation are minimized or eliminated.

TABLE 7-1 Terms Used in NPPV

ABBREVIATION	TERM	NOTES
NPPV	Noninvasive positive pressure ventilation	(1) Ventilation without an artificial airway (2) May be used as CPAP or bilevel PAP
CPAP	Continuous positive airway pressure	(1) Positive airway pressure during spontaneous breaths (2) No mechanical breaths (3) CPAP is active when IPAP = EPAP
Bilevel PAP	Bilevel positive airway pressure	(1) Provides IPAP and EPAP (2) CPAP is active when IPAP = EPAP (3) Also known as BiPAP
IPAP	Inspiratory positive airway pressure	(1) Controls peak inspiratory pressure during inspiration
EPAP	Expiratory positive airway pressure	(1) Controls end-expiratory pressure (2) Used as CPAP when IPAP = EPAP (3) Used as PEEP when IPAP > EPAP
PEEP	Positive end-expiratory pressure	(1) Positive airway pressure at end-expiratory phase (2) With mechanical breaths

TERMINOLOGY

In noninvasive positive pressure ventilation, the meanings of some terms are slightly different from traditional usage. These terms, abbreviations, and a brief description for each term are outlined in Table 7-1.

PHYSIOLOGIC EFFECTS OF NPPV

inspiratory positive airway pressure (IPAP): level of airway pressure during inspiratory phase only.

As in traditional positive pressure ventilation, NPPV has two primary pressure settings. One pressure setting is used during the inspiratory phase and the other during the expiratory phase.

During the inspiratory phase, the **inspiratory positive airway pressure (IPAP)** works like any other positive pressure breathing (ventilation) device. The IPAP level is similar to the peak airway *expiratory positive airway pressure (EPAP): level of airway pressure during expiratory phase only.*

pressure in traditional mechanical ventilation. In general, the degree of ventilation is directly related to the IPAP level. A higher IPAP level would result in a larger tidal volume and minute ventilation. The **expiratory positive airway pressure (EPAP)** is the same as PEEP during mechanical ventilation or CPAP during spontaneous breathing. In addition to its ability to improve oxygenation by increasing the functional residual capacity, EPAP also relieves upper airway obstruction with its splinting action.

The level of IPAP and EPAP can be titrated according to a patient's oxygenation and ventilation needs. Since two benefits of NPPV are improvement of PO_2 and PCO_2 (Brown et al., 1998; Nicholson et al., 1998), these two parameters can be used as titration endpoints. If arterial blood gas results are available, oxygenation (PaO_2) and ventilation ($PaCO_2$) endpoints can be easily assessed. Alternatively, pulse oximetry (SpO_2) and capnography ($P_{ET}CO_2$) may be used for the titration of appropriate IPAP and EPAP levels.

☑ PaO_2, $PaCO_2$, SpO_2, and $P_{ET}CO_2$ may be used for titration of IPAP and EPAP.

USE OF CONTINUOUS POSITIVE AIRWAY PRESSURE (CPAP)

continuous positive airway pressure (CPAP): CPAP does not include any mechanical breaths.

Continuous positive airway pressure (CPAP) provides positive airway pressure during the entire spontaneous breath and it does not include any mechanical breaths. For this reason, the work of breathing is entirely assumed by the patient. CPAP is discussed in this chapter because it shares many similar characteristics with other strategies of NPPV (e.g., lack of artificial airway, use of nasal or facial mask, use of airway pressures). In fact, when the inspiratory pressure and expiratory pressure of a bilevel positive airway pressure device are set at the same level, the effect is similar to that of CPAP.

☑ CPAP is the treatment of choice for obstructive sleep apnea without significant CO_2 retention.

CPAP is the treatment of choice for obstructive sleep apnea without significant carbon dioxide retention (Henderson & Strollo, 1999; Rosenthal, Nykamp & Guido et al., 1998). CPAP should be used with care and close monitoring of the patient as it is not effective in apnea due to neuromuscular causes. Table 7-2 outlines the indication and contraindications for CPAP therapy.

OBSTRUCTIVE SLEEP APNEA

obstructive sleep apnea (OSA): OSA is caused by severe air flow obstruction during sleep.

Sleep apnea is defined as a temporary pause in breathing that lasts at least 10 sec during sleep (Wilkins & Dexter, 1998). Sleep apnea may be caused by air flow obstruction (obstructive sleep apnea), loss of neurologic breathing effort (central sleep apnea), or a combination of these two conditions (mixed sleep apnea). **Obstructive sleep apnea (OSA)**

TABLE 7-2   Indication and Contraindications for Continuous Positive Airway Pressure

INDICATION	CONTRAINDICATION
Obstructive sleep apnea	Apnea due to neuromuscular causes
	Progressive hypoventilation
	Fatigue of respiratory muscles
	Facial trauma
	Claustrophobia

apnea index:
average number of apneas in each hour of sleep during a test.

hypopnea:
reduction in airflow for 10 or more seconds that is at least 50% below an estimated baseline amplitude, usually associated with an oxygen desaturation or a pulse alteration.

apnea-hypopnea index: *average number of apnea and hypopnea in each hour of sleep during a test.*

desaturation index:
average number of oxygen desaturations of 4% or more from baseline in each hour of sleep during a test.

is diagnosed by nocturnal polysomnography and the severity is determined by the apnea and desaturation index (Arai et al., 1998; Redline & Strohl, 1998; Waite, 1998).

The severity of OSA is quantified by the **apnea index** (respiratory disturbance index). The apnea index represents the average number of apneas in each hour of sleep during a test. For example, if a patient slept for 8 hours during a test and had 160 apneas, the apnea index would be 20. **Apnea-hypopnea index** refers to the average number of apnea or **hypopnea** in each hour of sleep during a test. **Desaturation index** describes the average number of oxygen desaturations of 4% or more from baseline (measured by pulse oximeter) in each hour of sleep during a test (Mooe et al., 2000).

Approximately 40 million Americans have chronic sleep disorders and the number of persons affected by OSA ranges from 2% to 4% of middle-aged adults. The distribution between genders is 4% to 9% in men and 1% to 2% in women. The incidence of OSA among morbidly obese patients is 12 to 30 times higher (Kyzer & Charuzi, 1998; Piccirillo et al., 1998; Skomro & Kryger, 1999).

Risk factors for OSA include history of snoring and witnessed apneas, obesity, increased neck circumference, hypertension, and family history of OSA (Skomro & Kryger, 1999). In patients with OSA, the major clinical signs and symptoms are snoring, daytime sleepiness, restless sleep, morning fatigue, and headaches. If untreated, OSA can lead to hypertension, left and right ventricular hypertrophy, sudden cardiovascular death, and increased risk for brain infarction (Kyzer & Charuzi, 1998).

Treatments for OSA include oral applications such as prosthetic mandibular advancement (Ishida et al., 1998; Millman, Rosenberg & Kramer, 1998), surgical interventions such as tonsillectomy and uvulopalatopharyngoplasty for upper obstructions (Miyazaki, Itasaka & Tada et al., 1998; Powell, Riley & Robinson, 1998), and weight reduction gastric surgery for morbidly obese patients (Kyzer & Charuzi, 1998). Conservative therapies such as weight loss and patient positioning have been disappointing. CPAP has become the treatment of choice for the vast majority of patients with moderate to severe OSA (Henderson & Strollo,

1999; Rosenthal et al., 1998; Wilkins & Dexter, 1998). The procedure to titrate CPAP level is discussed later in this chapter.

USE OF BILEVEL POSITIVE AIRWAY PRESSURE (BILEVEL PAP)

bilevel positive airway pressure (bilevel PAP): Bilevel PAP has two pressure levels, whereas CPAP has only one.

positive end-expiratory pressure (PEEP): An airway pressure that is above 0 cm H_2O at end-expiration.

☑ Two indications for bilevel PAP are acute respiratory failure and acute hypercapnic exacerbations of COPD.

Bilevel positive airway pressure (bilevel PAP) differs from CPAP in that bilevel PAP has two pressure levels, whereas CPAP has only one. Bilevel PAP has an inspiratory positive airway pressure (IPAP) setting that provides mechanical breaths and an expiratory positive airway pressure (EPAP) level that functions as **positive end-expiratory pressure (PEEP).** When bilevel PAP is used as an adjunct to provide mechanical ventilation, the two major indications are acute respiratory failure (Abou-Shala & Meduri, 1996; Jasmer, Luce & Matthay, 1997; Keenan et al., 1997; Kramer et al., 1995; Wysocki et al., 1995) and acute hypercapnic exacerbations of COPD (Diaz et al., 1997; Girault et al., 1997). The most common criteria for the determination of acute respiratory failure are blood gas results. Typical results may show partially compensated respiratory acidosis with moderate hypoxemia (e.g., pH < 7.35, $PaCO_2$ > 50 mm Hg, PO_2 < 55 mm Hg). For patients with hypoxemic respiratory failure, refractory hypoxemia may be present in addition to increasing PCO_2. PaO_2/F_IO_2 ratio of less than 200 suggests presence of refractory hypoxemia (low PaO_2 at high F_IO_2).

Patients who are unable to use or tolerate a nasal or facial mask are not candidates for NPPV (CPAP or bilevel PAP). These patients include those with facial trauma and claustrophobia. Inability to handle secretions is also a contraindication for NPPV. NPPV should not be used in apneic patients. For apneic patients, traditional mechanical ventilation is indicated. Furthermore, patients who have acute respiratory distress requiring hospital admission should not be treated with NPPV, as this strategy may delay endotracheal intubation and initiation of mechanical ventilation and may lead to poor patient outcome (Wood et al., 1998). Table 7-3 outlines the common indications and contraindications for NPPV.

TABLE 7-3   Indications and Contraindications for Noninvasive Positive Pressure Ventilation

INDICATION	CONTRAINDICATION
Reduction of respiratory workload in obesity	Apnea
Acute respiratory failure	Unable to handle secretions
Acute hypercapnic exacerbations of COPD	Facial trauma
	Claustrophobia

Foam Spacer

Mask
Swivel

Gel
Cushion

Optional
Support Ring

Pressure
Monitoring
Port

A

B

Figure 7-1 (A) Structure of a nasal mask; (B) Nasal mask in use. (Copyright 2004, Respironics, Inc., and its affiliates, Murraysville, PA. All rights reserved.)

COMMON INTERFACES FOR CPAP AND BILEVEL PAP

✔ Nasal mask, facial mask, and nasal pillows are interfaces for NPPV.

Since CPAP or NPPV is done without an artificial airway, the interface between the patient and ventilator is typically an external device connecting the ventilator tubing to the patient's nose, mouth, or face. Some common NPPV devices are nasal mask, facial mask, and nasal pillows.

NASAL MASK

nasal mask: A mask that covers only the nose. It is used in noninvasive positive pressure ventilation.

The **nasal mask** is the most common interface used in NPPV. A typical nasal mask has a soft cushion that surrounds and makes contact with the patient's nasal area. The soft cushion provides comfort to the patient while maintaining a seal to keep gas from leaking. While a tight seal is desirable, a minor leak is acceptable as it is not likely to compromise the effectiveness of NPPV. A common error is selecting a nasal mask that is too large for the patient. There are many nasal masks available. For patient comfort and compliance, it is a good practice to let the patient try out different sizes for maximal comfort and minimal leakage. Figure 7-1 shows the structure of a typical nasal mask and when it is in use.

✔ A minor leak is acceptable when using a nasal mask. A facial mask should be considered when the leak is significant.

Since a nasal mask does not cover the mouth, leakage through the mouth is a common problem. This is particularly true when PPV is provided at high positive pressures. A minor leak is acceptable as long as ventilation and oxygenation are not hindered. However, a facial mask should be considered when the leak is significant. During initial set up of a nasal mask, pulse oximetry may be used to check for improvement in oxygenation and adequacy of oxygen saturation. Soon after stabilization of the patient, blood gases should be done to fine-tune settings on the ventilator so as to verify proper oxygenation, ventilation, and acid-base balance. Table 7-4 shows the advantages and disadvantages of the nasal mask.

FACIAL MASK

facial mask: A mask that covers the nose and mouth. It is used in noninvasive positive pressure ventilation.

The function of a **facial mask** (Figure 7-2) is essentially the same as a nasal mask. It has a soft cushion that surrounds and makes contact with the patient's nasal and oral area. As does the nasal mask, the soft cushion provides comfort to the patient while maintaining a seal to keep gas from leaking. With a facial mask, a tight seal is easier to maintain than with a nasal mask because both the nose and mouth are covered. However, because the mouth is covered, regurgitation and aspiration can be potential problems with the use of a facial mask. Asphyxiation can also occur in the event of ventilator failure, or electrical or gas source disconnection. Proper disconnection alarms and patient monitors must be functional during use

✔ Regurgitation and aspiration can be a potential problem when a facial mask is used.

TABLE 7-4   Advantages and Disadvantages of the Nasal Mask

ADVANTAGE	DISADVANTAGE
Comfort	Gas leaks
Patient compliance	Nasal dryness or drainage

☑ With a facial mask, asphyxiation can also be a problem in the event of ventilator failure, or electrical or gas source disconnection.

Nasal Pillows™: *Nasal Pillows are a small interface commonly used during CPAP therapy.*

☑ A chin strap to close the mouth or a facial mask should be considered when gas leak through the mouth is significant.

of NPPV via a facial mask. Table 7-5 shows the advantages and disadvantages of the facial mask.

NASAL PILLOWS™

Nasal pillows™ resemble nasal masks but are smaller. Nasal pillows are more commonly used during CPAP therapy. This interface consists of two small cushions that fit under the nose. Since it has a pressure range of 3 to 20 cm H_2O, nasal pillows are not as effective as the larger nasal and facial masks when they are used in the bilevel PAP mode. Figure 7-3 shows the structure of nasal pillows and Figure 7-4 shows the insertion, placement, and adjustment of this interface.

Nasal Pillows™ are more comfortable than facial masks but gas leak is a potential problem. If significant gas leaks occur through the mouth, a chin strap may be used to close the mouth or a facial mask should be considered.

Figure 7-2   A facial mask in use. (Copyright 2004, Respironics, Inc. and its affiliates, Murraysville, PA. All rights reserved.)

TABLE 7-5   Advantages and Disadvantages of the Facial Mask

ADVANTAGE	DISADVANTAGE
Good seal	Claustrophobia
	Patient noncompliance
	Regurgitation and aspiration
	Asphyxiation in power or gas outage
	Alarm and monitor may be necessary

Figure 7-3   Structure of a nasal pillows interface. (A) Nasal Pillows™; (B) Plenum shell; (C) Vent-hole insert; (D) Wing knob (to adjust the angle of plenum shell); (E) Hose; (F) Hose guide; (G) Outrigger; (H) Spine; (I) Swivel adapter; (J) Cradle; (K) Side straps. (Reprinted by permission of Mallinckrodt, Inc.)

Figure 7-4 Use of a nasal pillows interface. (A) Insert the Nasal Pillows™ into nostrils; (B) Place the cradle (back pad) below the curve at the back of head; (C) For a comfortable fit, adjust the following points: (a) height of the cradle; (b) length of unit; (c) height of plenum shell; (d) angle of plenum shell. (Reprinted by permission of Mallinckrodt, Inc.)

TABLE 7-6   Troubleshooting Potential Problems with Interfaces

POTENTIAL PROBLEM	SUGGESTED SOLUTIONS
Air leaks	Adjust headgear Try chin strap Try spacers or foam pads Try another size or a different mask
Pressure points, sore or dry eyes	Adjust headgear Change spacers or foam pads Try another size or a different mask
Nasal congestion/discharge	Adjust positive pressure setting Add filter Add humidity
Nasal airway drying	Increase fluid intake Increase room humidity Try nasal saline or water-based lubricant
Skin breakdown/irritation	Adjust or try another headgear Use spacers, foam pads, or topical ointments Try another size or a different mask Resize mask Change to a different cleaning solution
Sensitive front teeth	Adjust headgear Try smaller or different mask
Headgear problem	Try disposable headgear with more stretch Try different or larger headgear

(Modified from An interface for every face, *from Mallinckrodt, Inc. Used with permission.)*

POTENTIAL PROBLEMS WITH INTERFACES

Since patients are different in size and facial structure, the selection of an interface must be done on an individual basis. Following selection of an interface, a trial period usually is required for the patient to get used to the interface and to identify problems with it. Table 7-6 outlines the potential problems with CPAP/NPPV interface and the possible solutions.

inspiratory positive airway pressure:
An airway pressure that is above 0 cm H₂O during inspiration.

TITRATION OF CONTINUOUS POSITIVE AIRWAY PRESSURE

When positive airway pressure is used to treat or relieve OSA, the appropriate CPAP level is done by setting the CPAP level or by adjusting the **inspiratory positive airway pressure (IPAP)** and

expiratory positive airway pressure:
An airway pressure that is above 0 cm H_2O at end-expiration.

☑ The initial CPAP is started at 4 cm H_2O, and titrated to a desired endpoint.

expiratory positive airway pressure (EPAP) at the same level, initially at 4 cm H_2O. After setting up the machine and placing the interface on the patient, pulse oximetry readings and number of apnea episodes during polysomnography are used to fine-tune the CPAP level.

AUTOTITRATION

Autotitration (autoadjusting) CPAP equipment are available for long-term home treatment to improve effectiveness by ensuring that the pressure is near optimal to the patient's needs. The working mechanism by which these equipment titrate pressures varies greatly. Some equipment detects snoring while others detect inspiratory flow patterns or airway vibration. In patients with uncomplicated OSA, unattended autotitration of CPAP may be suitable for the relief of airway obstruction. Autotitration should be used following thorough medical screening and complete patient education on the use of the prescribed CPAP device (Berthon-Jones et al., 1996; Teschler et al., 1996).

Unattended autotitration should not be used in patients with central sleep apnea, cerebral vascular accident, prolonged hypoventilation, hypovolemia, or cardiac failure. Other potential contraindications to autotitrating CPAP equipment include uncontrolled asthma, epilepsy, angina, fluid and electrolyte disturbances, nocturnal myoclonus, epilepsy, and other parasomnias. Severe air leak around the mask should be corrected before implementing autotitrating CPAP (Teschler et al., 1998).

RAMP

Ramp is a feature in which the starting pressure (e.g., 3 cm H_2O) gradually increases over time (up to 45 min) until the desired pressure is reached. This feature is ideal for patients who may have trouble tolerating a sudden onset of high pressure.

C-FLEX™

C-Flex™ is a method of delivering CPAP for the treatment of OSA. A common complaint by patients is that they have trouble exhaling against the continuous positive pressure. This problem may result in frequent awakening during sleep, sleep fragmentation, and occasional noncompliance in the use of the equipment. C-Flex™ provides pressure relief during exhalation. This reduces the continuous pressure in which the patient must overcome during exhalation.

C-Flex™ is titrated in the same way as conventional CPAP. During use, the equipment monitors the airflow during exhalation and reduces expiratory pressure proportional to expiratory flow. The relief pressure is provided on a breath-to-breath basis, depending on the actual expiratory airflow. Prior to the end of expiration and start of inspiration, the preset CPAP level is restored. Three levels of C-Flex™ (1, 2, 3) are available and each higher level provides progressively increased pressure relief.

TITRATION OF BILEVEL POSITIVE AIRWAY PRESSURES

☑ The initial bilevel positive airway pressures are started at 8 cm H_2O (inspiratory) and 4 cm H_2O (expiratory) and titrated to a desired endpoint.

When positive airway pressure is used to treat acute respiratory failure, the IPAP and EPAP levels are set independently. Bilevel refers to the inspiratory and expiratory positive airway pressure settings. For example, a bilevel positive airway pressure setting of 8 and 4 means that the IPAP is 8 cm H_2O and the EPAP is 4 cm H_2O. The procedure for titration of IPAP and EPAP (ResMed Corp., 1998a) is outlined in Table 7-7.

BI-FLEX™

Bi-Flex™ is a method of delivering bilevel PAP in which the airflow during inhalation and exhalation is "softened." This makes breathing more natural and comfortable for the patient. This mode provides pressure relief at the end of inhalation and the start of exhalation (Figure 7-5). Three levels of patient adjustable Bi-Flex™ (1, 2, 3) are available and each higher level provides progressively increased pressure relief.

TABLE 7-7   Procedure to Titrate Bilevel Positive Airway Pressure

1. Set mode: spontaneous/timed.
2. Start the IPAP at 8 cm H_2O and the EPAP at 4 cm H_2O.
3. Set IPAP maximum time 0.15 to 0.25 sec longer than the patient's actual inspiratory time. IPAP maximum time should not be set longer than 50% of the respiratory cycle.
4. Attach mask to patient, ensure proper fit, and start machine.
5. Increase IPAP in 1 to 2 cm H_2O increments to provide more ventilatory assistance and larger tidal volume.
6. Increase EPAP in 1 to 2 cm H_2O increments to improve oxygenation or to relieve upper airway obstruction.
7. If poor synchronization occurs, check for leaks or alter IPAP maximum time to improve synchronization.
8. Use supplemental oxygen if baseline saturation remains low with appropriate IPAP and EPAP settings.
9. Do not increase IPAP or EPAP level beyond patient tolerance.

(*Modified from* ResMed VPAP II S/T Clinical Guide.)

Figure 7-5 Bi-Flex® provides pressure relief at the end of inhalation and the start of inhalation. Level 3 provides the highest level of pressure relief as indicated by the pressure drop below the baseline pressure.

SUMMARY

Noninvasive strategies of assisted breathing have been used successfully in providing sufficient ventilation and oxygenation to patients with obstructive sleep apnea (CPAP), acute ventilatory failure and impending ventilatory failure (bilevel positive airway pressure). The two advantages of NPPV are (1) an artificial airway is not necessary and (2) reduced risks associated with endotracheal intubation and traditional mechanical ventilation.

As with other noninvasive procedures applied to a potentially critical condition, close monitoring of the patient is an absolute requirement. Use of accessory muscles, changes in vital signs, and signs of hypoxia are some indications that the patient's condition is deteriorating. The patient must be assessed in a timely manner. If indicated, the patient should be intubated and mechanically ventilated if NPPV fails to stabilize or improve the patient's condition.

Self-Assessment Questions

1. Which of the following is *not* true in regard to noninvasive positive pressure ventilation (NPPV)?

   A. NPPV provides assisted ventilation with an artificial airway.

   B. NPPV can provide positive end-expiratory pressure (PEEP).

   C. NPPV may be used to assist patients with obstructive sleep apnea.

   D. NPPV may be used to assist patients with acute ventilatory failure.

2. The titration endpoints of IPAP and EPAP during bilevel PAP may include all of the following measurements *except*:

   A. SpO_2.
   B. PaO_2.

   C. PvO_2.
   D. $P_{ET}CO_2$.

3. Continuous positive airway pressure (CPAP) provides positive airway pressure during the _____ spontaneous breath, and it _____ mechanical breaths.

   A. entire, includes
   B. entire, does not include

   C. inspiratory phase of, includes
   D. inspiratory phase of, does not include

4. When CPAP is in use, the total amount of work of breathing is provided by the:

   A. patient.
   B. ventilator.

   C. patient and ventilator.
   D. pressure level of CPAP.

5. CPAP is the treatment of choice for _____ sleep apnea without significant _____.

   A. central, hypoxemia
   B. central, carbon dioxide retention

   C. obstructive, hypoxemia
   D. obstructive, carbon dioxide retention

6. All of the following clinical conditions are contraindications for CPAP *except*:

   A. fatigue of respiratory muscles.
   B. progressive hypercapnia.

   C. obesity.
   D. hypoventilation due to neuro-muscular causes.

7. Sleep apnea is defined as a temporary pause in breathing that lasts at least _____ during sleep.

   A. 5 sec
   B. 10 sec

   C. 30 sec
   D. 60 sec

8. During NPPV, mechanical breaths are provided by the _____ setting whereas the end-expiratory pressure is determined by the _____ setting.

   A. IPAP, EPAP
   B. EPAP, IPAP

   C. PEEP, IPAP
   D. PEEP, EPAP

9. The interfaces for NPPV include all of the following devices *except*:

   A. nasal mask.
   B. endotracheal tube.

   C. nasal pillows.
   D. facial mask.

10. Which of the following interfaces is *least* likely to develop a significant air leak during NPPV?

    A. nasal mask
    B. simple mask

    C. nasal pillows
    D. facial mask

11. The facial mask is the only NPPV interface that has all of the following inherited risks *except*:

    A. aspiration.
    B. asphyxiation.

    C. regurgitation.
    D. hyperventilation.

12. The initial CPAP level is started at _____ cm H_2O and titrated to a desired endpoint.

    A. 2
    B. 4

    C. 6
    D. 8

13. The initial bilevel positive airway pressures are started at _____ cm H_2O (inspiratory) and _____ cm H_2O (expiratory) and subsequently titrated to a desired endpoint.

    A. 2, 6
    B. 4, 8

    C. 6, 2
    D. 8, 4

14. During titration of bilevel positive airway pressure, the _____ is increased in 1 to 2 cm H_2O increments to provide more ventilatory assistance and larger tidal volume.

    A. PEEP
    B. CPAP

    C. IPAP
    D. EPAP

15. During titration of bilevel positive airway pressure, the _____ is increased in 1 to 2 cm H_2O increments to improve oxygenation or to relieve upper airway obstruction.

    A. IPAP
    B. EPAP

    C. peak inspiratory pressure
    D. plateau pressure

16. Ramp is a strategy used in CPAP to allow the patient to accept a gradual:

    A. increase in inspiratory pressure.
    B. increase in inspiratory flow.

    C. decrease in inspiratory pressure.
    D. decrease in inspiratory flow.

Answers to Self-Assessment Questions

1. B. NPPV cannot provide positive end-expiratory pressure (PEEP).

2. C. PvO_2.

3. B. entire, does not include

4. A. patient.

5. D. obstructive, carbon dioxide retention

6. C. obesity.

7. B. 10 sec

8. A. IPAP, EPAP

9. B. endotracheal tube

10. D. facial mask

11. D. hypoventilation

12. B. 4

13. D. 8, 4

14. C. IPAP

15. B. EPAP

16. A. increase in inspiratory pressure.

References

Abou-Shala, N., & Meduri, G. U. (1996). Noninvasive mechanical ventilation in patients with acute respiratory failure. *Crit Care Med*, *24*(4), 705–715.

Antonelli, M., Conti, G., Rocco, M., et al. (1998). A comparison of noninvasive positive-pressure ventilation & conventional mechanical ventilation in patients with acute respiratory failure. *N Engl J Med*, *339*(7), 429–435.

Arai, H, Furuta, H., Kosaka, K., et al. (1998). Changes in work performances in obstructive sleep apnea patients after dental appliance therapy. *Psychiatry Clin Neurosci, 52*(2), 224–225.

Berthon-Jones M., et al. (1996). Nasal continuous positive airway pressure treatment: Current realities & future. *Sleep, 19*(9 Suppl.), S131–5.

Brown, J. S., Meecham Jones, D. J., Mikelsons, C., et al. (1998). Using nasal intermittent positive pressure ventilation on a general respiratory ward. *J R Coll Physicians Lond, 32*(3), 219–224.

Diaz, O., Iglesia, R., Ferrer, M., et al. (1997). Effects of noninvasive ventilation on pulmonary gas exchange & hemodynamics during acute hypercapnic exacerbations of chronic obstructive pulmonary disease. *Am J Respir Crit Care Med, 156,* 1840–1845.

Girault, C., Richard, J. C., Chevron, V., et al. (1997) Comparative physiologic effects of noninvasive assist-control & pressure support ventilation in acute hypercapnic respiratory failure. *Chest, 111*(6), 1639–1648.

Guilleminault, C., Philip, P., & Robinson, A. (1998). Sleep & neuromuscular disease: Bilevel positive airway pressure by nasal mask as a treatment for sleep disordered breathing in patients with neuromuscular disease. *J Neurol Neurosurg Psychiatry, 65*(2), 225–232.

Henderson, J. H., & Strollo, P. J., Jr. (1999). Medical management of obstructive sleep apnea. *Prog Cardiovasc Dis, 41*(5), 377–386.

Ishida, M., Inoue, Y., Suto, Y., et al. (1998). Mechanism of action & therapeutic indication of prosthetic mandibular advancement in obstructive sleep apnea syndrome. *Psychiatry Clin Neurosci, 52*(2), 227–229.

Jasmer, R. M., Luce, J. M., & Matthay, M. A. (1997). Noninvasive positive pressure ventilation for acute respiratory failure—underutilized or overrated? *Chest, 111*(6), 1672–1678.

Keenan, S. P., Kernerman, P. D., Cook, D. J., et al. (1997). Effects of noninvasive positive pressure ventilation on mortality in patients admitted with acute respiratory failure: A meta-analysis. *Crit Care Med, 25*(10), 1685–1692.

Kramer, N., Myer, T. J., Meharg, J., et al. (1995). Randomized, prospective trial of non-invasive positive pressure ventilation in acute respiratory failure. *Am J Respir Crit Care Med, 151,* 1799–1806.

Kyzer, S., & Charuzi, I. (1998). Obstructive sleep apnea in the obese. *World J Surg, 22*(9), 998–1001.

Millman, R. P., Rosenberg, C. L., & Kramer, N. R. (1998). Oral appliances in the treatment of snoring & sleep apnea. *Clin Chest Med*, *19*(1), 69–75.

Miyazaki, S., Itasaka, Y., Tada, H., et al. (1998). Effectiveness of tonsillectomy in adult sleep apnea syndrome. *Psychiatry Clin Neurosci*, *52*(2), 222–223.

Mooe, T., et al. (2000). Sleep-disordered breathing & myocardial ischemia in patients with coronary artery disease. *Chest*, *117*(6), 1597–1602.

Nicholson, D., Tiep, B., Jones, R., et al. (1998). Noninvasive positive-pressure ventilation in chronic obstructive pulmonary disease. *Curr Opin Pulm Med*, *4*(2), 66–75.

Pankow, W., Hijjeh, N., Schuttler, F., et al. (1997). Influence of noninvasive positive pressure ventilation on inspiratory muscle activity in obese subjects. *Eur Respir J*, *10*(12), 2847–2852.

Piccirillo, J. F., Gates, G. A., White, D. L., et al. (1998). Obstructive sleep apnea treatment outcomes pilot study. *Otolaryngol Head Neck Surg*, *118*(6), 833–844.

Powell, N. B., Riley, R. W., Robinson, A. (1998). Surgical management of obstructive sleep apnea syndrome. *Clin Chest Med*, *19*(1), 77–86.

Redline, S., & Strohl, K. P. (1998). Recognition & consequences of obstructive sleep apnea hypopnea syndrome. *Clin Chest Med*, *19*(1), 1–19.

ResMed Corp. (1998a). *ResMed VPAP II S/T Clinical Guide*, North Ryde, Australia.

ResMed Corp. (1998b). *ResMed VPAP II S/T Clinical Manual*, North Ryde, Australia.

Rosenthal, L., Nykamp, K., Guido, P., et al. (1998). Daytime CPAP titration: A viable alternative for patients with severe obstructive sleep apnea. *Chest*, *114*(4), 1056–1060.

Skomro, R. P., & Kryger, M. H. (1999). Clinical presentations of obstructive sleep apnea syndrome. *Prog Cardiovasc Dis*, *41*(5), 331–340.

Teschler, H., et al. (1996). Automated continuous positive airway pressure titration for obstructive sleep apnea syndrome. *Am J Respir Crit Care Med*, *154*(3) Pt. 1, 734–740.

Teschler H., et al. (1998). Intelligent CPAP systems: Clinical experience. *Thorax*, *53* (Suppl. 3), S49–54.

Waite, P. D. (1998). Obstructive sleep apnea: A review of the pathophysiology & surgical management. *Oral Surg Oral Med Oral Pathol Oral Radiol Endod*, *85*(4), 352–361.

Wilkins, R. L., & Dexter, J. R. (1998). *Respiratory Disease A Case Study Approach to Patient Care* (2nd ed.). Philadelphia: F.A. Davis.

Wood, K. A., Lewis, L., Von Harz, B., et al. (1998). The use of noninvasive positive pressure ventilation in the emergency department: Results of a randomized clinical trial. *Chest*, *113*(5), 1339–1346.

Wysocki, M., Tric, L., Wolff, M. A., et al. (1995). Noninvasive pressure support ventilation in patients with acute respiratory failure. *Chest*, *107*(3), 761–768.

Suggested Reading

Corrado A., et al. (2002). Iron lung vs mask ventilation in the treatment of acute on chronic respiratory failure in COPD patients: a multicenter study. *Chest*, *121*(1), 189–195.

CHAPTER EIGHT

INITIATION OF MECHANICAL VENTILATION

James H. Hiers

OUTLINE

KEY TERMS

- acute ventilatory failure
- alveolar-arterial oxygen pressure gradient [P(A-a)O$_2$]
- circuit compressible volume
- dual control mode
- flow rate

- I:E ratio
- impending ventilatory failure
- maximum inspiratory pressure (MIP)
- medical futility
- prophylactic ventilatory support

INTRODUCTION

This chapter covers the indications, contraindications, and strategies for the initiation of mechanical ventilation. Once a decision is made to implement mechanical ventilation, the initial settings on the ventilator must be made using a systematic approach. It is important to realize that these initial settings are subject to change according to patient condition. Frequent intensive monitoring of the patient is necessary to use the ventilator properly and to improve the patient outcome.

INDICATIONS

acute ventilatory failure: *An increase of PaCO$_2$ (>50 mm Hg) with a concurrent decrease of arterial (pH <7.30).*

impending ventilatory failure: *A gradual increase of PaCO$_2$ (>50 mm Hg) caused by decreasing lung functions.*

prophylactic ventilatory support: *Early intervention of potential ventilatory failure by means of mechanical ventilation.*

Mechanical ventilation is indicated when the patient cannot maintain spontaneous ventilation to provide adequate oxygenation or carbon dioxide removal. The clinical conditions leading to mechanical ventilation can be grouped into four areas: (1) **acute ventilatory failure;** (2) **impending ventilatory failure;** (3) severe hypoxemia; and (4) **prophylactic ventilatory support** (Brown, 1994; Otto, 1986). Table 8-1 outlines the indications of mechanical ventilation.

ACUTE VENTILATORY FAILURE

The primary indication of mechanical ventilation is acute ventilatory failure. This is defined as a sudden increase in the PaCO$_2$ to greater than 50 mm Hg with an accompanying respiratory acidosis (pH <7.30). In the COPD patient, mechanical ventilatory support is indicated by an acute increase in the PaCO$_2$ above the patient's normal baseline PaCO$_2$ accompanied by a decompensating respiratory acidosis (Brown, 1994; Otto, 1986).

Other signs that may be useful in the assessment of acute ventilatory failure include apnea and severe cyanosis. However, mild to moderate hypoxemia (PaO$_2$ = 50 to 60 mm Hg or SaO$_2$ = 85% to 90%) does not by itself indicate the presence of acute ventilatory failure or the need for ventilatory support. If a hypoxemic patient is able to maintain adequate ventilation as documented by the PaCO$_2$, then the

TABLE 8-1   Indications for Mechanical Ventilation

INDICATION	EXAMPLES
1. Acute ventilatory failure	pH <7.30, $PaCO_2$ >50 mm Hg
2. Impending ventilatory failure	Progressive acidosis and hypoventilation to pH <7.30 and $PaCO_2$ >50 mm Hg
3. Severe hypoxemia	PaO_2 <40 mm Hg, SaO_2 <75%
4. Prophylactic ventilatory support	Postanesthesia recovery

☑ Mechanical ventilation is indicated when the patient cannot maintain spontaneous ventilation to provide adequate oxygenation or carbon dioxide removal.

☑ Acute ventilatory failure is defined as a sudden increase in the $PaCO_2$ to greater than 50 mm Hg with an accompanying respiratory acidosis (pH <7.30).

☑ Assessment of impending ventilatory failure relies on the measurements related to the lung functions (i.e., V_T, RR, V_E, VC, MIP).

patient may be supported with supplemental oxygen or continuous positive airway pressure (CPAP). Table 8-2 shows some common methods to assess the presence of acute ventilatory failure.

IMPENDING VENTILATORY FAILURE

Impending ventilatory failure occurs when a patient can maintain only marginally normal blood gases, but only at the expense of a significantly increased work of breathing. Depending on the pulmonary reserve and lung function of a patient, the $PaCO_2$ value may be normal or low at the beginning of impending ventilatory failure. This is because of an increase in minute ventilation in an attempt to compensate for the gas exchange deficiencies. However, if the underlying pathology is not corrected in time, ventilatory failure will ensue when muscle fatigue occurs as a result of prolonged, excessive work of breathing. At this time, the $PaCO_2$ will rise and the pH will fall.

If the early clinical signs indicate that a patient is in impending ventilatory failure, it is appropriate to initiate mechanical ventilation. Early intervention is done to correct hypoxemia and acidosis imposed on the major organs and to reduce the stress placed on the cardiopulmonary system. There are several objective measurements that can be used to determine whether the patient is in impending ventilatory failure. These measurements are discussed below.

Assessment of Impending Ventilatory Failure.   Development of impending ventilatory failure is dependent on the balance of metabolic needs and work of breathing. When metabolic needs cause excessive work of breathing, impending ventilatory failure is likely. Since the work of breathing is carried out entirely by the respiratory

TABLE 8-2   Assessment of Acute Ventilatory Failure in Non-COPD Patients

PARAMETER	LIMIT
$PaCO_2$	>50 mm Hg (higher for COPD patients)
pH	<7.30

system, assessment of impending ventilatory failure relies solely on the measurements related to the lung functions (i.e., tidal volume, respiratory rate, minute volume, vital capacity, and maximal inspiratory pressure). Table 8-3 shows the factors for the assessment of impending ventilatory failure.

Tidal volume.   A spontaneous tidal volume of less than 3 to 5 mL/kg is indicative of impending ventilatory failure.

Respiratory rate.   A spontaneous respiratory rate of greater than 25 to 35 breaths per minute (BPM) signifies impending ventilatory failure.

Minute volume.   If the patient's spontaneous minute volume is greater than 10 L/min, then impending ventilatory failure is likely. Although it may appear that an increasing minute volume is a sign of improving lung functions, in actuality the patient may not be able to sustain the increased work of breathing. Muscle fatigue can occur over time and lead to eventual ventilatory failure. In addition, an increase in minute volume achieved by an increased respiratory rate and a decreased tidal volume lead to a larger percentage of deadspace (wasted) ventilation. This condition increases the oxygen cost of breathing and carbon dioxide production, progressive hypercapnia, and hypoxemia.

Vital capacity.   If the patient's vital capacity is less than 15 mL/kg, then impending ventilatory failure is likely. An accurate measurement of vital capacity requires patient cooperation, which may be difficult to achieve during impending ventilatory failure. The maximum inspiratory pressure measurement can be used as its alternative if the patient is unable to perform the vital capacity maneuver.

Maximum inspiratory pressure.   The **maximum inspiratory pressure (MIP)** is a measure of the inspiratory muscle strength reflecting the patient's pulmonary reserves. Patients with an MIP of better than

maximum inspiratory pressure (MIP): *Also called negative inspiratory force (NIF). MIP reflects a patient's respiratory muscle strength. MIP of less than −20 cm H_2O (e.g., −10 cm H_2O) is one of the indications of impending ventilatory failure. It is obtained by measuring the maximum negative pressure during a forced inspiratory maneuver against a closed manometer.*

TABLE 8-3   Assessment of Impending Ventilatory Failure

PARAMETER	LIMIT
Tidal volume	<3 to 5 mL/kg
Respiratory rate and pattern	>25 to 35/min Labored or irregular respiratory pattern
Minute ventilation	>10 L/min
Vital capacity	<15 mL/kg
Maximum inspiratory pressure (MIP)	<−20 cm H_2O
$PaCO_2$ trend	Increasing to over 50 mm Hg
Vital signs	Increase in heart rate, blood pressure

-25 cm H_2O obtained within 20 sec can be assumed to have a vital capacity of 15 mL/kg (Shapiro et al., 1991). When MIP is less than -20 cm H_2O, it is one of the signs of impending ventilatory failure.

The MIP is obtained by measuring the maximum negative pressure that the patient can generate with a forced *inspiratory* maneuver against a negative manometer (pressure measuring device). Although the MIP maneuver can be performed using a face mask, it is easier to obtain with an endotracheal or tracheostomy tube.

MIP can be measured by using a T-piece with one port attached to the endotracheal or tracheostomy tube, one port attached to the negative pressure manometer, and one port attached to a special unidirectional valve that allows exhalation only. The patient is encouraged to exhale to residual volume and then inhale as forcefully as possible. The unidirectional valve allows the patient to exhale so that the subsequent MIP maneuvers can be performed from the residual volume level (Caruso et al., 1999).

PaCO$_2$ trend. A gradual but persistent increase of the $PaCO_2$ to more than 50 mm Hg is indicative of impending ventilatory failure. The $PaCO_2$ measurements should be done over a period of time and on an as needed basis. The $PaCO_2$ should be interpreted along with the patient's breathing pattern since progressive tachypnea is common during impending ventilatory failure.

Vital signs. Any clinical indicators that show a patient is under distress or is tiring must also be considered when assessing impending ventilatory failure. These indicators include tachycardia, arrhythmias, hypertension, tachypnea, use of accessory respiratory muscles, diaphoresis, and cyanosis.

SEVERE HYPOXEMIA

Hypoxemia is a common finding of lung diseases. When hypoxemia is severe, mechanical ventilation may be necessary to support the oxygenation requirement of the body. ARDS, pulmonary edema, and carbon monoxide poisoning are some clinical conditions that often require ventilatory support for the primary purpose of oxygenation.

Hypoxemia can be assessed by measuring the PaO_2, or the **alveolar-arterial oxygen pressure gradient [P(A-a)O$_2$].** Severe hypoxemia is present when the PaO_2 is less than 60 mm Hg on 50% or more of oxygen or less than 40 mm Hg at any F_IO_2 (Shapiro et al., 1994). $P(A-a)O_2$ is the difference of PAO_2 and PaO_2. The normal $P(A-a)O_2$ at 21% F_IO_2 should be less than 4 mm Hg for every 10 years of age. On 100% oxygen, every 50-mm Hg difference in $P(A-a)O_2$ approximates 2% shunt.

$$P(A-a)O_2 = PAO_2 - PaO_2$$

☑ Severe hypoxemia is present when the PaO_2 is less than 60 mm Hg on 50% or more of oxygen or less than 40 mm Hg at any F_IO_2.

alveolar-arterial oxygen pressure gradient [P(A-a)O$_2$]: *The difference of PAO_2 and PaO_2. A gradient over 450 mm Hg while on 100% oxygen indicates severe hypoxemia or intrapulmonary shunting.*

☑ See Appendix 1 for example.

TABLE 8-4 Indications for Prophylactic Ventilatory Support

INDICATION	EXAMPLES
Reduce risk of pulmonary complications	Prolonged shock Head injury Smoke inhalation
Reduce hypoxia of major body organs	Hypoxic brain Hypoxia of heart muscles
Reduce cardiopulmonary stress	Prolonged shock Coronary artery bypass surgery Other thoracic or abdominal surgeries

☑ $PaCO_2/0.8$ may be changed to $PaCO_2 \times 1.25$

☑ Prophylactic ventilatory support is provided in clinical conditions in which the risk of pulmonary complications, ventilatory failure, or oxygenation failure is high.

☑ Untreated tension pneumothorax is an absolute contraindication to mechanical ventilation.

PaO_2 is obtained from arterial blood gas analysis and PAO_2 can be calculated as follows:

A simplified alveolar air equation:

$$PAO_2 = (P_B-PH_2O) \times F_IO_2 - (PaCO_2/R)$$

where P_B = barometric pressure, PH_2O = water vapor pressure (47 mm Hg at 37°C), and R = respiratory quotient (estimated to be 0.8). PAO_2 is mainly affected by changes of F_IO_2, $PaCO_2$, and P_B.

PROPHYLACTIC VENTILATORY SUPPORT

Prophylactic ventilatory support is provided in clinical conditions in which the risk of pulmonary complications, ventilatory failure, or oxygenation failure is high. In addition, prophylactic or early commitment of patient to the ventilator can minimize hypoxia of the major body organs. It can also reduce the work of breathing and oxygen consumption and thus preserve and rest the cardiopulmonary system, and promote patient recovery (Otto, 1986). Indications for prophylactic ventilatory support are outlined in Table 8-4.

CONTRAINDICATIONS

Since positive pressure ventilation is contraindicated in untreated tension pneumothorax, mechanical ventilation at any positive pressure level must not be done without a functional chest tube to relieve the pleural pressure. Other contraindications to mechanical ventilation are relative in nature and deal with the condition and prognosis of the patient.

There are three considerations in which mechanical ventilation should be terminated or should not be started (Campbell et al., 1992).

medical futility: *A condition in which medical interventions are useless based on past experience.*

They are based on (1) patient's informed request, (2) **medical futility,** and (3) reduction or termination of patient pain and suffering.

A patient's informed request carries with it many legal, ethical, medical, and economical concerns. The health care facilities and professionals should be prepared to work with the patient and his family on this type of request. A protocol should be established to serve as a guide before a hasty decision is needed concerning whether ventilatory support should be started or discontinued.

Schneiderman et al. (1990) suggested that medical intervention may be futile if the physicians have concluded that intervention was useless in the last 100 similar cases. It is reasonable to infer that if medical intervention will not be effective in all *probability*, life support measures including mechanical ventilation should not be started. In this case, the physician must establish an open, honest discussion with the patient and the concerned parties about the potential outcomes for withholding ventilatory support.

Another relative contraindication to mechanical ventilation is to reduce or terminate patient pain and suffering. In probable terminal cases such as metastatic cancer and multiorgan failure, the benefit of mechanical ventilation must be weighed against the degree of pain and expected length of suffering that a patient may be subjected to. Physical restraints, painful and uncomfortable medical procedures, and psychological trauma are just a few problems that may not be completely alleviated by sedatives and analgesics (Campbell et al., 1992). Of course, medical futility would be a concurrent concern in dealing with this question.

Withdrawing ventilatory support from a patient poses a greater challenge than withholding mechanical ventilation. But this difficult decision should be based on the fact that mechanical ventilation is a supportive measure, rather than a curative procedure.

I:E ratio: *A time ratio comparing the inspiratory time and expiratory time, normally between 1:2 and 1:4 in mechanical ventilation. This ratio is regulated by the inspiratory flow rate, I time, or E time and is affected by the tidal volume and respiratory rate.*

INITIAL VENTILATOR SETTINGS

When it becomes necessary to provide mechanical ventilatory support for a patient, the following basic ventilator settings must be determined: mode, respiratory rate, tidal volume, F_IO_2, inspiratory:expiratory ratio **(I:E ratio),** inspiratory flow pattern, and various alarm limits.

These initial ventilator settings are mainly based on a patient's body size, diagnosis, pathophysiology, and laboratory results. These settings only serve as a starting point and they should be adjusted according to changes in the patient's condition and requirements.

☑ Full ventilatory support may be necesssary if the patient is not breathing spontaneously between mechanical breaths.

MODE
The first step in selecting the ventilator mode is to decide whether the patient should receive full ventilatory support (FVS) or partial ventilatory support (PVS). Full ventilatory support is achieved by any mode that assumes essentially all of the work of breathing. The

majority of ventilator patients initially require full support, with the control mode or the assist/control mode. The synchronized intermittent mandatory ventilation (SIMV) mode also provides full ventilatory support if the patient is not breathing spontaneously between mechanical breaths, and the mandatory respiratory rate is set at 12 BPM or higher.

Partial ventilatory support is achieved by any mode that provides less than the total amount of the work of breathing. Partial support would be inappropriate initially for patients with ventilatory failure, and they are more commonly used during the weaning process. Some examples are bilevel positive airway pressure (BiPAP), and pressure support ventilation (PSV). These topics are discussed elsewhere in this text.

☑ Partial ventilatory support is achieved by any mode that provides less than the total amount of the work of breathing.

DUAL-CONTROL MODE

In traditional ventilation, a single control variable is selected to achieve a desired goal. Examples of the single-variable control include volume control ventilation (VCV) and pressure control ventilation (PCV). In VCV, a desired tidal volume (a control variable) is set and the pressure changes from breath to breath depending on the characteristics of the patient-ventilator system. In PCV, the desired pressure (a control variable) is set and the delivered volume changes according to the characteristics of the patient-ventilator system (Campbell et al., 2002).

dual control mode: A combined mode between two control variables (e.g., pressure and volume) that are regulated by independent feedback loops so that the delivered breath switches between pressure control and volume control.

A **dual-control mode** combines two control variables (e.g., pressure and volume) that are regulated by independent feedback loops so that the delivered breath switches between pressure control and volume control. In short, a dual-control mode is a combined mode between two control variables. When VCV and PCV are combined, the patient receives mandatory breaths that are volume targeted, pressure limited, and time cycled (Campbell et al., 2002). Since there are many dual-control modes on the market and more are forthcoming in the future, selection of any mode of ventilation (single or dual) must be based on sound scientific basis and controlled clinical trials. Furthermore, the patient must be monitored and evaluated on a regular frequency in order to ensure the safety and effectiveness of the mode of ventilation.

RESPIRATORY RATE

The initial respiratory rate (frequency) is the number of breaths per minute that is intended to provide eucapneic ventilation ($PaCO_2$ at patient's normal). It is usually between 10 to 12 BPM. This rate, coupled with a 10 to 12 mL/kg tidal volume, usually produces a minute volume that is sufficient to normalize the patient's $PaCO_2$. Respiratory rates of 20 or more BPM during pressure support ventilation are associated with *auto-PEEP* and should be avoided (Shapiro et al., 1994).

☑ Air trapping and low inspiratory flow are also contributing factors of *auto-PEEP*.

An alternative method of selecting the initial respiratory rate is to estimate the patient's minute volume requirement and divide the estimated minute volume by the tidal volume.

$$\text{Respiratory rate} = \frac{\text{Estimated minute volume}}{\text{Tidal volume}}$$

The estimated minute volume for males is equal to 4.0 multiplied by the body surface area (BSA) and for females is equal to 3.5 multiplied by the BSA. The BSA (in square meters) can be obtained from a nomogram such as the Dubois body surface area chart (Appendix 2).

$$\text{Minute Volume (Male)} = (4)(\text{BSA})$$

$$\text{Minute Volume (Female)} = (3.5)(\text{BSA})$$

Changing the Respiratory Rate. Both of these methods of selecting the initial respiratory rate assume that both CO_2 production and physiologic deadspace are normal. If the CO_2 production is elevated (due to an increase of metabolic rate) or the physiologic deadspace is increased (due to a decrease of pulmonary perfusion), the minute volume required to normalize the $PaCO_2$ will need to be increased. Since increasing the tidal volume results in higher airway pressures on a volume-limited ventilator, it is usually more appropriate to increase the minute volume by raising the respiratory rate.

After placing the patient on a ventilator, blood gases should be obtained within 15 to 30 min after the patient has stabilized to assess both ventilation and oxygenation. Since the $PaCO_2$ varies inversely with the alveolar minute ventilation, a higher than normal $PaCO_2$ (e.g., >45 mm Hg or >50 mm Hg for patients with chronic CO_2 retention) means the patient's minute volume should be increased, usually by increasing the respiratory rate. On the other hand, a lower than normal $PaCO_2$ (e.g., <35 mm Hg or <40 mm Hg for patients with CO_2 retention) indicates that the minute volume should be decreased, usually by decreasing the respiratory rate.

☑ RR is the primary control to alter the $PaCO_2$.

☑ ↑ RR if the $PaCO_2$ is too high; ↓ RR if the $PaCO_2$ is too low.

TIDAL VOLUME

The initial tidal volume is usually set between 10 to 12 mL/kg of ideal body weight. Usually the patient's actual weight can be used for selecting the tidal volume unless the patient is significantly underweight or overweight. Table 8-5 shows a method to calculate the patient's ideal body weight.

TABLE 8-5   Calculation of Ideal Body Weight

The ideal body weight (IBW) in pounds (lb) and kilograms (kg) can be calculated as follows:

Male IBW in lb = 106 + [6 × (Height in inches − 60)]
Female IBW in lb = 105 + [5 × (Height in inches − 60)]

Convert the patient's body weight from pounds to kilograms by dividing pounds by 2.2.

The lower end of the acceptable tidal volume range (i.e., about 10 mL/kg) may be appropriate for certain patients. Tidal volumes as low as 6 mL/kg have been recommended for ARDS patients (Hall et al., 1987). The primary reason for using lower tidal volumes (i.e., permissive hypercapnia) is to minimize the airway pressures and the risk of barotrauma (Feihl et al., 1994). However, use of low tidal volume ventilation may lead to complications such as acute hypercapnia, increased work of breathing, dyspnea, severe acidosis, and lung collapse (Kallet et al., 2001a, 2001b).

✓ Decreasing the tidal volume by 100 to 200 mL in COPD patients reduces the expiratory time requirements and helps to prevent air trapping.

COPD patients may also benefit from a reduced tidal volume setting. These patients have reduced expiratory flow rates due to decreased alveolar elastic recoil. For this reason, a longer expiratory time is needed for complete exhalation. If there is not enough time for complete exhalation, air trapping, V/Q mismatch, hypoxemia, and hypercapnia may result. Decreasing the tidal volume by 100 to 200 mL in COPD patients reduces the expiratory time requirements and helps to prevent air trapping. A higher **flow rate** may also be used to shorten the inspiratory time and lengthen the expiratory time for COPD patients.

flow rate: *Peak flow during the inspiratory phase. It determines how fast the tidal volume is delivered to the patient.*

For patients with a reduction of lung volumes due to lung resection, lower tidal volumes may also become necessary. Table 8-6 lists examples of clinical conditions where lower tidal volume settings may be beneficial or necessary for the patient.

circuit compressible volume: *Expansion of the ventilator circuits during inspiration leading to a small "lost" volume of gas that does not reach the patient, but is recorded as part of the expired tidal volume.*

Gas Leakage and Circuit Compressible Volume. The tidal volume actually delivered to the patient's lungs is usually lower than the ventilator delivered tidal volume. This is mainly due to (1) gas leakage in the ventilator circuitry, (2) gas leakage at the endotracheal tube cuff, and (3) **circuit compressible volume** loss.

When significant gas leakage (>5% of ventilator tidal volume) occurs, the cause must be identified and corrected. Minor gas leakage and circuit compressible volume loss can be compensated by using a larger tidal volume. Some ventilators automatically compensate for the compressible volume loss and thus maintain a stable tidal volume. Other ventilators (e.g., Hamilton Veolar) measure the volume delivered to the patient at the airway opening. This allows detection of significant volume loss due to circuit compression factor or gas leakage.

TABLE 8-6   Conditions That May Require Lower Tidal Volumes

CONDITION	EXAMPLES
Increase of airway pressure requirement	ARDS Pulmonary edema
Increase of lung compliance	Emphysema
Decrease of lung volumes	Pneumonectomy

TABLE 8-7   Determination of Circuit Compressible Volume

(1) With the circuit warmed to an operating temperature, set the respiratory rate at 10 to 16/min and the tidal volume between 100 and 200 mL with minimal flow rate and maximum high pressure limit.

(2) Completely occlude the patient Y-connection of the ventilator circuit.

(3) Record the expired volume (mL) and the peak inspiratory pressure during Y occlusion (cm H_2O).

(4) Divide the expired volume (mL) by the peak inspiratory pressure during Y occlusion (cm H_2O); this is the circuit compression factor.

(5) Multiply the circuit compression factor (mL/cm H_2O) by the peak inspiratory pressure during mechanical ventilation (cm H_2O), or (peak inspiratory pressure–PEEP) if PEEP is used.

Example:

Expired volume = 150 mL; Peak inspiratory pressure (Y occlusion) = 50 cm H_2O;
Peak inspiratory pressure (mechanical ventilation) = 60 cm H_2O; PEEP = 10 cm H_2O.

Circuit compression factor = 150 mL/50 cm H_2O = 3 mL/cm H_2O
Circuit compression volume = 3 mL/cm $H_2O \times$ (60 – 10) cm H_2O = 3 × 50 = 150 mL

Ventilator circuits are compliant and expand during a positive pressure breath. The amount of circuit expansion results in a volume that does not reach the patient but is recorded as part of the expired tidal volume. This volume "lost" in the ventilator circuit is called the circuit compressible volume and it may be calculated by following the steps in Table 8-7 (Barnes et al., 1994; Wilkins et al., 2003).

Once the circuit compressible volume is known, the patient's corrected tidal volume can be calculated by:

✓ See Appendix 1 for example.

Corrected Tidal Volume = Expired Tidal Volume
  − Circuit Compressible Volume

F_IO_2

✓ After stabilization of the patient, the F_IO_2 is best kept below 50% to avoid oxygen-induced lung injuries.

For patients with severe hypoxemia or abnormal cardiopulmonary functions (e.g., postresuscitation, smoke inhalation, ARDS), the *initial* F_IO_2 may be set at 100%. The F_IO_2 should be evaluated by means of arterial blood gas analyses after stabilization of the patient. It should be adjusted accordingly to maintain a PaO_2 between 80 and 100 mm Hg (lower for patients with chronic CO_2 retention). After stabilization of the patient, the F_IO_2 is best kept below 50% to avoid oxygen-induced lung injuries (Shapiro, 1994).

For patients with mild hypoxemia or patients with normal cardiopulmonary functions (e.g., drug overdose, uncomplicated postoperative recovery), the initial F_1O_2 may be set at 40% or at the patient's F_1O_2 prior to mechanical ventilation. It must also be evaluated and changed accordingly by means of subsequent blood gas analyses and correlated with pulse oximetry trending.

PEEP

☑ Set the initial PEEP at 5 cm H_2O and make changes based on the patient's blood gas results, F_1O_2 requirement, tolerance of PEEP, and cardiovascular responses.

Positive end-expiratory pressure (PEEP) increases the functional residual capacity and is useful to treat refractory hypoxemia (low PaO_2 not responding to high F_1O_2). The initial PEEP level may be set at 5 cm H_2O. Subsequent changes of PEEP should be based on the patient's blood gas results, F_1O_2 requirement, tolerance of PEEP, and cardiovascular responses. For titration of optimal PEEP, see Table 12-4 in Chapter 12.

I:E RATIO

☑ Auto-PEEP is present when the end-expiratory pressure does not return to baseline pressure at the end of expiration.

The I:E ratio is the ratio of inspiratory time to expiratory time. It is usually kept in the range between 1:2 and 1:4. A larger I:E ratio (longer E ratio) may be used on patients needing additional time for exhalation because of the possibility of air trapping and auto-PEEP. Occurrence of air trapping during mechanical ventilation may be checked by occluding the expiratory port of the ventilator circuit at the end of exhalation. Auto-PEEP is present when the end-expiratory pressure does not return to baseline pressure (i.e., 0 cm H_2O or the PEEP level when PEEP is in use) at the end of expiration. This unintended end-expiratory pressure caused by incomplete exhalation is called auto-PEEP.

Inverse I:E ratios have been used to correct refractory hypoxemia in ARDS patients with very low compliance. But it should not be the initial I:E setting since reverse I:E ratio has its inherent cardiovascular complications. Inverse I:E ratio should be tried only after traditional strategies have failed to improve a patient's ventilation and oxygenation status.

Depending on the features available on the ventilator, the I:E ratio may be altered by manipulating any one or a combination of the following controls: (1) flow rate, (2) inspiratory time, (3) inspiratory time %, (4) respiratory rate, and (5) minute volume (tidal volume and respiratory rate).

Effects of Flow Rate on I:E Ratio. Adjusting the flow rate is the most common method to change an I:E ratio because the flow rate control is a feature available on almost all ventilators. Table 8-8 shows the effects of

TABLE 8-8   Effects of Flow Rate on I Time and I:E Ratio

PARAMETER CHANGE	I TIME	E TIME	I:E RATIO
Increase flow rate	Decrease	Increase	Increase
Decrease flow rate	Increase	Decrease	Decrease

TABLE 8-9   Effects of V_T on I:E Ratio

PARAMETER CHANGE	I TIME	E TIME	I:E RATIO
Increase tidal volume	Increase	Decrease	Decrease
Decrease tidal volume	Decrease	Increase	Increase

a changing flow rate on the I time and I:E ratio when the V_T and RR are kept unchanged. Note that the I time and I:E ratio are inversely related. A higher I time leads to a lower I:E ratio (Tejeda et al., 1997).

Other Ventilator Controls That Affect the I:E Ratio. Besides the flow rate control, other settings available on some ventilators may also alter the I:E ratio. Table 8-9 shows the effect of changing the tidal volume on the I:E ratio, and Table 8-10 shows the effect of changing the RR on the I:E ratio.

Changing the I:E Ratio. Since the I:E ratio may be changed by altering different settings available on selected ventilators, different methods to obtain a desired I:E ratio are provided as follows (Chang, 1999).

✔ The calculated flow in Example 1 is the *minimum* flow rate required for this I:E ratio. It is usually set 10 L/min higher to meet changing minute volume requirements.

✔ At RR of 16/min, the I time needed for an I:E ratio of 1:4 is 0.75 sec. The E time is (3.75 − 0.75) sec = 3 sec.

Example 1 Using Flow to Change the I:E Ratio

Given: Minute Volume = 12 L/min
       Desired I:E Ratio = 1:3

Calculate: The flow rate for an I:E ratio of 1:3

Solution: Flow = Minute Volume × Sum of I:E Ratio
       = 12 L/min × (1 + 3)
       = 12 L/min × 4
       = 48 L/min

Example 2 Using I Time to Change the I:E Ratio

Given: RR = 16/min
       Desired I:E Ratio = 1:4

Calculate: The I time needed for an I:E ratio of 1:4

TABLE 8-10   Effects of RR on I:E Ratio

PARAMETER CHANGE	I TIME	E TIME	I:E RATIO
Increase RR	Minimal change	Decrease	Decrease
Decrease RR	Minimal change	Increase	Increase

Solution: Since RR = 16/min, time for each breath
= 60 sec/16 or 3.75 sec

I Time = Time for Each Breath × [I Ratio / Sum of
I:E Ratio]
= 3.75 sec × [1/(1+4)]
= 3.75 sec × [1/5]
= 3.75 sec/5
= 0.75 sec

I Time % and I:E Ratio.   Some ventilators (e.g., Hamilton Veolar) permit the I:E ratio to be preset, usually by setting an I time % (percent inspiratory time). In these ventilators, the flow rate is automatically adjusted by the ventilator to maintain a constant I:E ratio regardless of changes in tidal volume or respiratory rate.

The I time % and I:E ratio equivalent are listed in Table 8-11. For other I:E ratios not listed in the table, they may be calculated by following Example 3:

Example 3   Using I Time % to Set the I:E Ratio

Given: Desired I:E Ratio = 1:3.5

☑ The I time %
needed for an
I:E ratio of 1:3.5 is
22.2%.

Calculate: The I time % needed for an I:E ratio of 1:3.5

Solution: I Time % = $\dfrac{\text{I Ratio}}{\text{Sum of I:E Ratio}}$

$= \dfrac{1}{(1 + 3.5)}$

$= \dfrac{1}{4.5}$

= 22.5%

TABLE 8-11   I Time % and I:E Ratio Equivalent

I TIME %	I:E RATIO
14.3%	1:6
16.7%	1:5
20%	1:4
25%	1:3
33.3%	1:2
50%	1:1
60%	1.5:1
66.7%	2:1

Figure 8-1 Normal flow tracing of four different flow patterns: square, accelerating, decelerating, and sine. (Courtesy of Novametrix Medical Systems, Inc.)

FLOW PATTERN

Most modern ventilators offer different inspiratory flow patterns. Although there are subtle variations, the principle flow patterns are (1) square (constant) flow pattern, (2) accelerating (ascending) flow pattern, (3) decelerating (descending) flow pattern, and (4) sine wave flow pattern. The waveforms for each of these flow patterns are shown in Figure 8-1.

The square flow pattern may be used initially upon setting up the ventilator. This flow pattern provides an even, constant peak flow during the entire inspiratory phase. The initial peak flow at the very beginning of the inspiratory phase should help to overcome the airway resistance and parenchymal elastance, and the remaining peak flow throughout the inspiratory phase should enhance gas distribution in the lungs. Adjustment of the flow pattern may be made after stabilization of the patient. Note that the constant flow pattern is the only flow pattern in which the peak flow rate equals the mean flow rate. All other flow patterns will produce a mean flow rate that is less than the peak flow.

With its increasing flow throughout the respiratory cycle, the accelerating waveform may improve the distribution of ventilation in patients with partial airway obstruction. The decelerating flow pattern typically produces a high initial inspiratory pressure and the decrease in flow may help improve distribution of tidal volume and gas exchange (Campbell et al., 2002; Sullivan et al., 1977). For patients with COPD, the decelerating flow may reduce the peak inspiratory pressure, mean airway pressures, physiologic dead space, and $PaCO_2$ (Yang et al., 2002). The sine wave is considered more physiologic because it is similar to the normal spontaneous breathing inspiratory flow pattern. The sine wave may also improve the distribution of ventilation and therefore improve gas exchange.

For ventilators that do not permit a preset inspiratory time (e.g., Puritan-Bennett 7200), the inspiratory time may increase if the patient's peak inspiratory pressure increases. This is because as the PIP increases, the pressure gradient between the ventilator and the patient's airway opening increases, resulting in an increased inspiratory time. However, on ventilators in which the inspiratory time is preset, such as the Hamilton Veolar, the inspiratory time is held constant for any flow pattern selected.

In performing calculations that involve the inspiratory flow as a variable (e.g., Resistance = Pressure/Flow), the mean inspiratory flow should be used. Since the only flow pattern in which the peak flow equals the mean inspiratory flow is the square wave pattern, the ventilator should be switched to a constant flow pattern prior to measurement.

VENTILATOR ALARM SETTINGS

Although different ventilators have different alarm systems, the following alarms should be basic to any ventilator: low exhaled volume alarm, low inspiratory pressure alarm, high inspiratory pressure alarm, apnea alarm, high respiratory rate alarm, and F_IO_2 alarm. These alarms should be backed up by a battery source to prevent malfunction in the event of electrical failure.

LOW EXHALED VOLUME ALARM

> ☑ The *low* exhaled volume alarm (low volume alarm) should be set at about 100 mL *lower* than the expired mechanical tidal volume.

The *low* exhaled volume alarm (low volume alarm) should be set at about 100 mL *lower* than the expired mechanical tidal volume. This alarm is triggered if the patient does not exhale an adequate tidal volume. This alarm is typically used to detect a system leak or circuit disconnection.

LOW INSPIRATORY PRESSURE ALARM

> ☑ The *low* inspiratory pressure alarm (low pressure alarm) should be set at 10 to 15 cm H_2O *below* the observed peak inspiratory pressure.

The *low* inspiratory pressure alarm (low pressure alarm) should be set at 10 to 15 cm H_2O *below* the observed peak inspiratory pressure. This alarm is triggered if the peak inspiratory pressure is less than the alarm setting. The low inspiratory pressure alarm complements the low exhaled volume alarm and is also used to detect system leaks or circuit disconnection.

HIGH INSPIRATORY PRESSURE ALARM

The *high* inspiratory pressure alarm (high pressure limit alarm) should be set at 10 to 15 cm H_2O *above* the observed peak inspiratory pressure. This alarm is triggered when the peak inspiratory pressure is equal to

✓ The *high* inspiratory pressure alarm (high pressure limit alarm) should be set at 10 to 15 cm H_2O *above* the observed peak inspiratory pressure.

or higher than the high pressure limit. Once the alarm is triggered, inspiration is immediately terminated and the ventilator goes into expiratory cycle.

The patient must be evaluated to determine the cause of the alarm. Common causes that trigger the high inspiratory pressure alarm include water in the ventilator circuit, kinking or biting of the endotracheal tube, secretions in the airway, bronchospasm, tension pneumothorax, decreases in lung compliance, increases in airway resistance, and coughing.

APNEA ALARM

✓ The apnea alarm should be set with a 15- to 20-sec time delay.

The apnea alarm should be set with a 15- to 20-sec time delay, with less time delay at higher respiratory rate. On some ventilators such as the Puritan-Bennett 7200, the apnea alarm also triggers an apnea ventilation mode in which the ventilator provides full ventilatory support until the alarm condition no longer exists.

HIGH RESPIRATORY RATE ALARM

✓ The *high* respiratory rate alarm (high rate alarm) should be set at 10 to 15 BPM *over* the observed respiratory rate.

The *high* respiratory rate alarm (high rate alarm) should be set at 10 to 15 BPM *over* the observed respiratory rate. This alarm is especially important in the MMV mode. The high respiratory rate alarm indicates that the patient is becoming tachypneic—a sign of respiratory distress.

HIGH AND LOW F_1O_2 ALARMS

✓ Set the low and high F_1O_2 alarms at 40% and 50%, respectively, for an F_1O_2 of 45%.

The high F_1O_2 alarm should be set at 5% to 10% over the analyzed F_1O_2 and the low F_1O_2 alarm should be set at 5% to 10% below the analyzed F_1O_2.

HAZARDS AND COMPLICATIONS

Mechanical ventilation has many potential hazards (e.g., ventilator disconnection, nosocomial infection) and complications (e.g., barotrauma, hypotension). The frequency of occurrence is directly related to the length of mechanical ventilation (Liu et al., 1991; Pierson, 1990). Patients who require mechanical ventilation for longer periods are likely to develop more complications.

This section summarizes the common hazards and complications of mechanical ventilation based on several prospective studies. Special emphasis is provided for barotrauma and decrease in cardiac output and blood pressure since the effects of these complications are more urgent to the patient's progress and outcome.

TYPES OF HAZARDS AND COMPLICATIONS

Prospective studies of patient outcome during mechanical ventilation indicate that hazards and complications are related to (1) positive pressure ventilation (e.g., barotrauma, impedance of cardiac output), (2) patient condition (e.g., organ failure), (3) ventilator and artificial airway (accidental extubation), and (4) medical professionals (e.g., nosocomial infection). Examples for each of these four areas are shown in Table 8-12.

MALFUNCTION AND MISUSE OF ALARMS

The Joint Commission on Accreditation of Healthcare Organizations (JCAHO) reviewed 23 reported deaths or injuries related to long-term mechanical ventilation and found 19 deaths and four in coma. Sixty-five percent of the deaths or injuries were related to the

TABLE 8-12   Hazards and Complications of Mechanical Ventilation

CONDITION	EXAMPLES
Related to positive pressure ventilation	Barotrauma (pneumothorax, mediastinal air leak, subcutaneous air leak) Hypotension, decrease in cardiac output Arrhythmia Oxygen toxicity Bronchopleural fistula Bronchopulmonary dysplasia (in infants) Upper gastrointestinal hemorrhage
Related to patient condition	Infection (due to reduced immunity) Physical and psychologic trauma Multiple organ failure (may be preexisting)
Related to equipment (ventilator and artificial airway)	Ventilator and alarm malfunction Ventilator circuit disconnection Accidental extubation Main bronchus intubation Postintubation stridor Endotracheal tube blockage Tissue damage Atelectasis (due to inadequate tidal volume)
Related to medical professionals	Nosocomial pneumonia (due to cross-contamination) Inappropriate ventilator settings Misadventures (due to lapses of understanding and communication)

(Data from Ventilator alarm failures, *Bourke et al., 1987; Brunner et al., 1989; Milligan, 1992; Pottie et al., 1993; Pryn et al., 1989; Slee et al., 1988;* and Other hazards and complications, *Bezzant et al., 1994; Cox et al., 1991; Liu et al., 1991; Pierson, 1990; Rivera et al., 1992.*)

malfunction or misuse of ventilator alarms. A breakdown of the causes revealed that the alarms were either turned off or set incorrectly, no alarm was available for certain disconnections, testing of alarms was not performed, and response to alarm was delayed or absent (NYSNA, 2002).

These tragedies could be prevented by implementing regular preventive maintenance and testing of alarm systems on ventilators and monitors. The alarms must also be sufficiently audible with respect to the room design, distance, and noise level of the immediate patient care area. Overdependence on alarms should be avoided and emphasis should be placed on frequent direct observation and assessment of the patient-ventilator system.

☑ Risk of baro-
trauma is high
when PIP >50 cm
H_2O, plateau pressure
>35 cm H_2O, mPaw
>30 cm H_2O, and
PEEP >10 cm H_2O.

BAROTRAUMA (VOLUTRAUMA)

Barotrauma or volutrauma is the term used to describe lung tissue injury or rupture that results from alveolar overdistention. General agreement is that in most cases, peak inspiratory pressures greater than 50 cm H_2O, plateau pressures greater than 35 cm H_2O, mean airway pressures greater than 30 cm H_2O, and PEEP greater than 10 cm H_2O may induce the development of barotrauma (Bezzant et al., 1994; Slutsky, 1994). The risk of barotrauma also increases with the duration of positive pressure ventilation.

Barotrauma can occur at mean airway pressures lower than 30 cm H_2O either due to patient susceptibility or to an uneven distribution of ventilation. COPD patients are more susceptible to barotrauma presumably due to air trapping and weakened parenchymal areas (e.g., lung blebs and bullae). Uneven distribution of ventilation may result in patients with significant airway obstruction and lung parenchymal changes. A mechanical tidal volume tends to preferentially distribute to areas of low resistance and high compliance during the early portion of inspiration. This may result in transient elevated alveolar pressures with resultant overdistention and rupture despite what would normally be accepted as a "safe" pressure.

Other lung injuries that may occur as a result of positive pressure ventilation include pulmonary interstitial emphysema, pneumomediastinum, pneumoperitoneum, pneumothorax, tension pneumothorax, and subcutaneous emphysema.

DECREASE IN CARDIAC OUTPUT
AND BLOOD PRESSURE

Positive pressure ventilation has been implicated in the development of decreased cardiac output and arterial blood pressure (Bezzant et al., 1994; Franklin et al., 1994). The reason for this is that positive airway and alveolar pressures may potentially increase the normally subatmospheric pleural pressures that surround the heart and vena cava. The increased pleural pressure tends to compress the right atrium

☑ Since positive pressure ventilation increases the CVP, the pressure gradient between the right atrium and the venous drainage will be decreased with a resultant decreased venous return to the right atrium.

☑ A competent cardiovascular system can compensate for a small drop in venous return by an increased heart rate and arterial vasoconstriction.

☑ High airway pressures are more detrimental to the cardiac output in patients with high lung compliance than those with low compliance.

and vena cava, increasing the intravascular resistance and pressures associated with these structures. The pressures in the vena cava and right atrium are approximately equal and are collectively known as the central venous pressure (CVP). The usually low central venous pressure creates an intravascular pressure gradient between the right atrium and the systemic venous drainage that augments venous blood return to the right atrium. If positive pressure ventilation increases the CVP, the pressure gradient between the right atrium and the venous drainage will be decreased with a resultant decreased venous return to the right atrium. If the venous return is significantly reduced, this can result in a decreased cardiac output and arterial hypotension.

If the patient has no preexisting cardiovascular disease and is not hypovolemic, a competent cardiovascular system can compensate for a small drop in venous return and thus maintain cardiac output and blood pressure. The two primary compensatory mechanisms include an increased heart rate and arterial vasoconstriction initiated by the cardiac baroreceptors.

The magnitude of the increase in the CVP and the resultant decrease in venous return depends on several factors, including the airway pressure, lung compliance, and chest wall compliance. Higher airway pressures will more likely result in higher pleural and central venous pressures. It is important to note that increases of the mean airway pressures tend to depress venous return more than increases of the peak inspiratory pressures.

The degree of increased pleural pressure for a given airway pressure is further affected by the patient's lung and chest wall compliance. If the patient's lung compliance is low (stiff lungs), then airway pressures are less readily transmitted into the pleural space. Therefore in patients with low lung compliance, a given airway pressure will result in a smaller increase in pleural pressure and a less dramatic decrease in venous return. This does not mean that patients with low lung compliance cannot have significant decreases in cardiac output due to positive pressure ventilation. These patients must also be closely monitored for potentially significant decreases in cardiac output and blood pressure.

Patients with more compliant lungs, such as COPD patients, tend to more readily transmit a higher airway pressure into the pleural space. Therefore in these patients, a given airway pressure will tend to result in a more dramatic decrease in venous return and cardiac output.

The effects of chest wall compliance on the transmission of airway pressure into the pleural space are exactly opposite to the effects of lung compliance. A low chest wall compliance (stiff chest wall) will tend to increase the pleural pressure more significantly for a given airway pressure than a normal chest wall compliance. Conditions in which the chest wall would be less compliant than normal include the application of tight chest wall bandages that encircle the thorax and extensive chest wall burn injuries.

All ventilator patients must be monitored for signs of cardiovascular instability. However, because ventilator patients with suspected or known preexisting cardiovascular disease are more likely to suffer clinically significant decreases in cardiac output and blood pressure, these patients must be monitored with an extra measure of vigilance.

SUMMARY

Initiation of mechanical ventilation requires many decisions, ranging from the mode of ventilation to the level of PEEP. Nevertheless, this process can be simplified by following a set of established guidelines. Under most clinical conditions, the initial settings on the ventilator will satisfy the immediate requirement of most patients.

It is essential to remember that the initial settings are just that; subsequent changes to these settings must be made based on the ever-changing condition of the patient. In summary, Table 8-13 outlines the indications for mechanical ventilation and Table 8-14 provides an overview of the initial ventilator settings for an adult patient.

TABLE 8-13   Indications for Mechanical Ventilation

INDICATION	PARAMETERS
Acute ventilatory failure	$PaCO_2$ >50 mm Hg (Higher for COPD) pH <7.30 Apnea
Impending ventilatory failure	Tidal volume <3 to 5 mL/kg Respiratory rate >25 to 35/min Minute ventilation >10 L/min Vital capacity <15 mL/kg MIP <−20 cm H_2O Rising $PaCO_2$ >50 mm Hg
Severe hypoxemia	PaO_2 <60 mm Hg at F_IO_2 >50%, or PaO_2 <40 mm Hg at any F_IO_2 Severe cyanosis

Prophylactic ventilatory support	Reduce risk of pulmonary complications
	    Prolonged shock
	    Head injury
	    Smoke inhalation
	Reduce hypoxia of major body organs
	    Hypoxic brain
	    Hypoxia of heart muscles
	Reduce cardiopulmonary stress
	    Prolonged shock
	    Coronary artery bypass surgery
	    Other thoracic or abdominal surgeries

TABLE 8-14   Initial Ventilator Settings

PARAMETER	SETTING	NOTES
Mode	Assist/Control or SIMV	Provide ventilatory support.
RR	10 to 12/min	Primary control to alter ventilation and $PaCO_2$.
V_T	10 to 15 mL/kg	Peak inspiratory pressure is *directly* related to the V_T setting. Use lower V_T to reduce risk of pressure-related lung injuries.
F_IO_2	100% for severe hypoxemia or compromised cardiopulmonary status	40% for mild hypoxemia or normal cardiopulmonary status.
PEEP	5 cm H_2O for refractory hypoxemia	Monitor patient and note cardio-vascular adverse effects.
I:E	1:2 to 1:4	1:4 for patients needing longer E time due to air trapping.
Flow pattern	Square	Other flow patterns for a lower peak inspiratory pressure (manometer) and better gas distribution (breath sounds).

Self-Assessment Questions

1. Which of the following is *not* an indication for mechanical ventilation?

   A. acute ventilatory failure   C. severe hypoxemia
   B. impending ventilatory failure   D. airway obstruction

2. A patient has an admitting diagnosis of acute ventilatory failure. This condition is character-ized by a $PaCO_2$ of _____ mm Hg or greater with an accompanying respiratory _____.

   A. 20, acidosis   C. 50, acidosis
   B. 20, alkalosis   D. 50, alkalosis

3. Impending ventilatory failure may be confirmed by trending a patient's:

   A. lung functions.   C. $PaCO_2$.
   B. PaO_2.   D. pH.

4. Among other criteria of assessment, impending ventilatory failure may be present when the patient's minute ventilation is _____ 10 L/min and maximum inspiratory pressure is less than _____.

A. more than, 20 cm H_2O

B. more than, -20 cm H_2O

C. less than, 20 cm H_2O

D. less than, -20 cm H_2O

5. The primary purposes of prophylactic mechanical ventilation include all of the following *except*:

A. to minimize the risk of pulmonary complications.

B. to reduce prolonged hypoxia of major body organs.

C. to reduce the work of the cardiopulmonary system.

D. to monitor the arterial blood gases and vital signs.

6. A physician asks you to set up a volume-limited ventilator for a 35-year-old postoperative male patient who weighs 132 lb (60 kg). You would select an initial tidal volume of _____ and respiratory rate of _____.

A. 500 mL, 12/min

B. 800 mL, 20/min

C. 500 mL, 20/min

D. 800 mL, 12/min

7. As you are measuring the compressible volume of a new ventilator circuit, you notice that the observed expired volume (mL) and peak inspiratory pressure (cm H_2O) are 150 mL and 30 cm H_2O, respectively. The circuit compressible volume is therefore:

A. 2 mL/cm H_2O.

B. 3 mL/cm H_2O.

C. 4.5 mL/cm H_2O.

D. 5 mL/cm H_2O.

8. With a circuit compressible volume of 3 mL/cm H_2O, what would be the actual tidal volume delivered to the patient if the expired tidal volume is 800 mL and the peak inspiratory pressure is 50 cm H_2O?

A. 500 mL

B. 650 mL

C. 750 mL

D. 950 mL

9. Positive end-expiratory pressure (PEEP) is indicated in patients who have a decreased _____ and _____.

A. tidal volume, chronic hypercapnia

B. functional residual capacity, refractory hypoxemia

C. vital capacity, acute hypercapnia

D. tidal volume, refractory hypoxemia

10. At constant tidal volume and respiratory rate, increasing the inspiratory flow rate will lead to a _____ inspiratory time (I time) and _____ expiratory time (E time).

A. longer, longer

B. longer, shorter

C. shorter, longer

D. shorter, shorter

11. What should be the *minimum* flow rate for a minute volume of 12 L/min. and an I:E ratio of 1:4?

     A. 40 L/min   C. 60 L/min
     B. 50 L/min   D. 70 L/min

12. If the desired I:E ratio is 1:2.5, what should be the I time %?

     A. 29%   C. 45%
     B. 40%   D. 60%

13. The _____ and _____ are two alarms that are useful to detect circuit disconnection.

     A. low pressure, high pressure   C. low volume, low PEEP
     B. high PEEP, high volume   D. low pressure, low volume

14. Which of the following is *not* a common potential complication of positive pressure ventilation?

     A. hypertension   C. accidental patient disconnection
     B. decrease in cardiac output   D. barotrauma

15 to 18. Match the conditions of mechanical ventilation with the examples of the hazards and complications that might occur during mechanical ventilation.

CONDITION	EXAMPLES
15. Related to positive pressure ventilation	A. Ventilator circuit disconnect
16. Related to patient condition	B. Barotrauma
17. Related to equipment	C. Inappropriate ventilator settings
18. Related to medical professionals	D. Physical and psychologic trauma

Answers to Self-Assessment Questions

1. D. airway obstruction

2. C. 50, acidosis

3. A. lung functions.

4. B. more than, −20 cm H_2O

5. D. to monitor the arterial blood gases and vital signs.

6. D. 800 mL, 12/min

7. D. 5 mL/cm H_2O

8. B. 650 mL

9. B. functional residual capacity, refractory hypoxemia

10. C. shorter, longer

11. C. 60 L/min

12. A. 29%

13. D. low pressure, low volume

14. A. hypertension

15. B. Barotrauma

16. D. Physical and psychologic trauma

17. A. Ventilator circuit disconnect

18. C. Inappropriate ventilator settings

References

Barnes, T. A., et al. (1994). *Core textbook of respiratory care practice* (2nd ed.). St. Louis, MO: Mosby.

Bezzant, T. B., et al. (1994). Risks and hazards of mechanical ventilation: A collective review of published literature. *Dis Mon, 40*(11), 581–638.

Bourke, A. E., et al. (1987). Failure of a ventilator alarm to detect patient disconnection. *J Med Eng Technol, 11*(2), 65–67.

Brown, B. R. (1994). Understanding mechanical ventilation: Indications for and initiation of therapy. *J Okla State Med Assoc, 87,* 353–357.

Brunner, J. X., et al. (1989). Prototype ventilator and alarm algorithm for the NASA Space Station. *J Clin Monit, 5*(2), 90–99.

Campbell, M. L., et al. (1992). Terminal weaning from mechanical ventilation: Ethical and practical considerations for patient management. *Amer J Crit Care, 1*(3), 52–56.

Campbell, R. S., et al. (2002). Pressure-controlled versus volume-controlled ventilation: Does it matter? *Respir Care, 47*(4), 416–424.

Caruso, P., Friedrich, C., Denari, S. D., et al. (1999). The unidirectional valve is the best method to determine maximal respiratory pressure during weaning. *Chest, 115*(4), 1096–1101.

Chang, D. W. (1999). *Respiratory care calculations* (2nd ed.). Clifton Park, New York: Thomson Delmar Learning.

Cox, R. G., et al. (1991). Efficacy, results, and complications of mechanical ventilation in children with status asthmaticus. *Pediatr Pulmonol, 11*(2), 120–126.

Feihl, F., et al. (1994). Permissive hypercapnia. How permissive should we be? *Am J Respir Crit Care Med, 150*(6 Pt. 1), 1722–1737.

Franklin, C., et al. (1994). Life-threatening hypotension associated with emergency intubation and the initiation of mechanical ventilation. *Amer J Emerg Med, 12*(4), 425–428.

Hall, J. B., et al. (1987). Liberation of the patient from mechanical ventilation. *JAMA, 257,* 1621–1628.

Kallet, R. H., et al. (2001a). Implementation of a low tidal volume ventilation protocol for patients with acute lung injury or acute respiratory distress syndrome. *Respir Care, 46*(10), 1024–1037.

Kallet, R. H., et al. (2001b). Lung collapse during low tidal volume ventilation in acute respiratory distress syndrome. *Respir Care, 46*(1), 49–52.

Liu, Y. N., et al. (1991). Complications of mechanical ventilation: A clinical analysis of 82 cases. *Chung Hua Nei Ko Tsa Chih, 30*(11), 692–694.

Milligan, K. A. (1992). Disablement of a ventilator disconnect alarm by a heat and moisture exchanger [letter]. *Anaesthesia, 47*(3), 279.

New York State Nurses Association (2002). Nursing practice: practice alerts. Preventing ventilator-related deaths and injuries. Retrieved July 13, 2004, from http://www.nysna.org/programs/practice/alerts/ventilator_injuries.htm

Otto, C. W. (1986). Ventilatory management in the critically ill. *Emerg Med Clin North Am, 4*(4), 635–654.

Pierson, D. J. (1990). Complications associated with mechanical ventilation. *Crit Care Med, 6*(3), 711–724.

Pottie, J. C., et al. (1993). Alarm failure in the oxygen-air mixture. *Ann Fr Anesth Reanim, 12*(6), 607–608.

Pryn, S. J., et al. (1989). Ventilator disconnection alarm failures. The role of ventilator and breathing accessories. *Anaesthesia, 44*(12), 978–981.

Rivera, R., et al. (1992). Complications of endotracheal intubation and mechanical ventilation in infants and children. *Crit Care Med, 20*(2), 193–199.

Schneiderman, L. J., et al. (1990). Medical futility: Its meaning and ethical implications. *Ann Intern Med, 112,* 949–954.

Shapiro, B. A. (1994). A historical perspective on ventilator management. *New Horiz, 2*(1), 8–18.

Shapiro, B. A., et al. (1991). *Clinical application of respiratory care* (4th ed.). St. Louis, MO: Mosby.

Shapiro, B. A., et al. (1994). *Clinical application of blood gases* (5th ed.). St. Louis, MO: Mosby.

Slee, T. A., et al. (1988). Failure of low pressure alarm associated with the use of a humidifier. *Anesthesiology, 69*(5), 791–793.

Slutsky, A. S. (1994). Consensus conference on mechanical ventilation—January 28–30, 1993 at Northbrook, IL, USA, Part I. *Int Care Med, 20,* 64–79.

Sullivan, M., et al. (1977). Relationship between ventilator waveform and tidal-volume distribution. *Respir Care, 22*(4), 386–393.

Tejeda, M., Boix, J. H., Álvarez, F., et al. (1997). Comparison of pressure support ventilation and assist-control ventilation in the treatment of respiratory failure. *Chest, 111*(5), 1322–1325.

Wilkins, R. L., et al. (2003). *Egan's fundamentals of respiratory care* (8th ed.). St. Louis, MO: Mosby.

Yang, S. C., et al. (2002). Effects of inspiratory flow waveforms on lung mechanics, gas exchange, and respiratory metabolism in COPD patients during mechanical ventilation. *Chest, 122,* 2096–2104.

Suggested Reading

Tidal Volume Selection
Petrucci, N., et al. (2004). Ventilation with lower tidal volumes versus traditional tidal volumes in adults for acute lung injury and acute respiratory distress syndrome. *Cochrane Database Syst Rev, 2004*(2), CD003844.

The Acute Respiratory Distress Syndrome Network. (2000). Ventilation with lower tidal volumes as compared with traditional tidal volumes for acute lung injury and the acute respiratory distress syndrome. *N Engl J Med,* 342(18), 1301–1308.

CHAPTER NINE

MONITORING IN MECHANICAL VENTILATION

Walter C. Chop

OUTLINE

KEY TERMS

- anion gap
- cerebral perfusion pressure
- diffusion defect
- dyshemoglobins
- end-tidal carbon dioxide monitoring
- hypoventilation
- hypoxemia

- hypoxia
- intrapulmonary shunting
- oliguria
- pulse oximeter
- transcutaneous PtcCO$_2$
- transcutaneous PtcO$_2$
- ventilation/perfusion (V/Q) mismatch

INTRODUCTION

Monitoring a patient's clinical condition during mechanical ventilation is vital because clinical status often changes rapidly and unpredictably. A patient's clinical status may be affected by the underlying illness, medications, organ failure, and even the settings on the ventilator.

There are four reasons for monitoring a patient on a continuous basis: (1) baseline measurements can be used to establish the initial treatment plan and serve as a reference point for future measurements; (2) a trend can be established to document the progress or regression of a patient's condition; (3) treatment plans can be added, altered, or discontinued according to the measurements obtained; and (4) high-limit and low-limit alarms can be set on most monitors to safeguard a patient's safety.

This chapter provides an overview of monitoring techniques pertinent to ventilatory care.

VITAL SIGNS

Vital signs (heart rate, blood pressure, respiratory rate, and temperature) can provide very useful information on the overall condition of a patient. During mechanical ventilation, changes in vital signs often indicate changes in the patient's cardiopulmonary status.

HEART RATE

✓ Normal adult heart rate is between 60 and 100/min.

In the intensive care unit, heart rate assessment is readily available on the electrocardiograph (ECG) monitor. High and low alarms can be set on the monitor to warn of tachycardia and bradycardia.

hypoxemia: Deficiency of oxygen in blood; low PaO$_2$.

Tachycardia.   During mechanical ventilation, some conditions that may increase a patient's heart rate are **hypoxemia,** pain, anxiety and stress, fever, drug reactions, and myocardial infarction. Tachycardia

☑ Tachycardia may be caused by hypoxemia, pain, anxiety and stress, fever, drug reactions, and myocardial infarction.

hypoxia: Deficiency of oxygen in tissues.

can alert the clinician to blood volume or cardiac output deficits. Increase in heart rate must be looked at as part of the larger picture as it can be secondary to extreme conditions ranging from hypovolemia to anxiety.

Bradycardia.   Bradycardia and arrhythmias often occur during prolonged suctioning of the airways. Preoxygenation is necessary to minimize the occurrence of arterial desaturation during suctioning. Since arterial desaturation occurs in as little as 5 sec during suctioning, **hypoxia** and cardiac complications can happen rather rapidly. When arrhythmia or bradycardia occurs, endotracheal suctioning must be stopped and 100% oxygen should be provided to the patient immediately (Burton et al., 1997).

Bradycardia, if it appears together with a low cardiac output, can be ominous and may suggest a decrease in coronary blood flow. Table 9-1 outlines the conditions that affect the heart rate.

BLOOD PRESSURE

Continuous blood pressure monitoring in the critical patient is usually done via an indwelling arterial catheter interfaced with a pressure monitor. The most common insertion site for the catheter is the radial artery. Other sites include the brachial, femoral, popliteal, and dorsalis pedis arteries.

☑ Fluid overload, vasoconstriction, stress, anxiety, and pain may lead to hypertension.

Hypertension.   Hypertension, higher than normal blood pressure, may be caused by acute or chronic patient conditions. Acute conditions such as fluid overload, vasoconstriction, stress, anxiety, and pain may lead to hypertension. Patients who have a history of congestive heart failure, cardiovascular disease, or polycythemia may develop hypertension, which can become a complicating factor during mechanical ventilation.

TABLE 9-1   Conditions That Affect the Heart Rate

CONDITIONS THAT MAY CAUSE TACHYCARDIA	CONDITIONS THAT MAY CAUSE BRADYCARDIA
Hypoxemia	Sudden hypoxia and/or vagal stimulation during endotracheal suctioning
Hypovolemia	Inadequate coronary blood flow
Pain	Heart block
Anxiety and stress	Abnormal SA node function
Fever	Hypothermia
Drug reaction (e.g., epinephrine)	Drug reaction (e.g., morphine sulfate)
Myocardial infarction	

☑ Hypovolemia, positive pressure ventilation, and pump failure are conditions that may cause hypotension.

Hypotension. Hypotension, lower than normal blood pressure, may be due to absolute hypovolemia (blood loss), relative hypovolemia (shock), or pump failure (CHF). When hypotension occurs during mechanical ventilation, it is often associated with excessive intrathoracic pressure, peak inspiratory pressure, and lung volume. Hypotension is one of the complications of positive pressure ventilation or positive end-expiratory pressure. Table 9-2 outlines the conditions that affect the blood pressure.

RESPIRATORY RATE

hypoventilation: Below normal level of alveolar ventilation characterized by an elevated $PaCO_2$.

The normal spontaneous respiratory rate for adults is 10 to 16 breaths per minute. An increased respiratory rate (tachypnea) may be an early warning sign of **hypoventilation** or hypoxemia (Bone, 1985). If the rate exceeds 20 breaths per minute and rising, the patient should be monitored closely for an impending crisis. A sudden increase in respiratory rate may indicate acute events such as pulmonary embolism or tension pneumothorax. Rates in excess of 30 breaths per minute generally indicate respiratory distress and may lead to severe hypoxia (Bone, 1985).

Tachypnea may precede the development of respiratory failure and use of mechanical ventilation (Krieger & Ershowshy, 1994). During mechanical ventilation, tachypnea is indicative of respiratory dysfunction (Gravelyn & Weg, 1980). When tachypnea and low tidal volume are observed in a patient, successful weaning from mechanical ventilation is not likely (Tobin et al., 1986).

☑ Rapid shallow breathing is a reliable sign of ventilatory insufficiency.

Routine monitoring of a patient's spontaneous respiratory rate is a simple but very useful method to assess the pulmonary status of a ventilator patient. This is especially true during the weaning process. A sudden increase in spontaneous respiratory rate during weaning attempt is indicative of moderate or severe respiratory insufficiency or hypoxia.

TABLE 9-2   Conditions That Affect the Blood Pressure

CONDITIONS THAT MAY CAUSE HYPERTENSION	CONDITIONS THAT MAY CAUSE HYPOTENSION
Fluid overload	Decreased venous return due to positive pressure ventilation
Stress	Absolute hypovolemia (e.g., blood loss, dehydration)
Anxiety	Relative hypovolemia (e.g., sepsis, shock)
Pain	Pump failure (e.g., CHF)
Congestive heart failure	
Cardiovascular disease	
Polycythemia ($\uparrow$ blood viscosity)	

TEMPERATURE

In the intensive care unit, a patient's temperature may be measured routinely at regular intervals or monitored continuously via a rectal, esophageal, or pulmonary artery catheter probe.

☑ Hyperthermia causes a lower oxygen saturation at any PaO_2.

Hyperthermia.   Hyperthermia can occur as a result of infection, tissue necrosis, leukemia, or other conditions that increase a patient's metabolic rate and oxygen utilization. Hyperthermia also shifts the oxyhemoglobin dissociation curve to the right causing a lower oxygen saturation level at any PaO_2. This oxygen desaturation occurs because increased temperature promotes unloading of oxygen from hemoglobin to the tissues.

☑ Hypothermia lowers a person's basal metabolic rate.

Hypothermia.   Hypothermia, though seen less commonly in the critically ill patient, can occur as a result of central nervous system (CNS) problems, metabolic disorders, and from certain drugs or toxins. Hypothermia is sometimes induced in head trauma patients as a means of decreasing the patient's basal metabolic rate.

Hypothermia is also induced in patients undergoing coronary artery bypass (CAB) surgery. At this extreme low temperature, the hypothermic condition must be taken into account during management of the ventilator and patient. For example, the measured PaO_2 and $PaCO_2$ values are higher than the actual values when the sample is collected under hypothermic conditions and is analyzed at body temperature. In order to have blood gas values that accurately reflect a patient's true ventilatory and oxygenation status, corrections to the patient's core temperature must be done during blood gas analysis.

In other nonextreme hypothermic conditions ($+/- 2°C$), temperature corrections are not necessary as long as the uncorrected PaO_2 is above 60 mm Hg (Malley, 1990).

☑ Excessive cooling of the phrenic nerve during CAB surgery may cause paralysis of the hemidiaphragms.

Excessive cooling of the phrenic nerve during CAB surgery may cause paralysis of the hemidiaphragms. This condition, though temporary, may take months to resolve completely (Wilkins & Dexter, 1998). Table 9-3 outlines the conditions that affect the body temperature.

TABLE 9-3   Conditions That Affect the Body Temperature

CONDITIONS THAT MAY CAUSE HYPERTHERMIA	CONDITIONS THAT MAY CAUSE HYPOTHERMIA
Infection	CNS problem
Tissue necrosis	Metabolic disorders
Leukemia	Drugs and toxins
Increased metabolic rate	Induced
	Coronary bypass surgery
	Head injury

CHEST INSPECTION AND AUSCULTATION

Since the lungs are protected by the thoracic cage, they are not readily accessible for direct examination. Chest inspection and auscultation are two indirect methods that are useful in evaluating the condition of the lungs.

CHEST MOVEMENT

During mechanical ventilation it is important to observe the overall chest movement. One should observe the symmetrical movement of the chest with each inspiration as well as the depth and rhythm of each tidal volume cycle.

Asymmetrical movement can occur in conditions such as right bronchial intubation, atelectasis, or tension pneumothorax (Figure 9-1) (Bone, 1985). If dysynchronous motion of the chest and abdomen is noted, the patient should be evaluated for diaphragmatic fatigue or underlying pathology.

AUSCULTATION

Auscultation of a patient's breath sounds should be performed each time the practitioner assesses the patient/ventilator system. Diminished or absent breath sounds or the presence of wheezes and crackles are signs of ventilatory problems and should be recognized as causes of respiratory distress (Wilkins & Dexter, 1998). Table 9-4 shows these abnormal breath sounds and their related clinical conditions.

Figures 9-2 through 9-4 show the surface projections of lung segments and they are helpful for the correct placement of the stethoscope diaphragm. Proper identification of the lung segments involved in the disease process is essential for consistent charting and reporting, and

TABLE 9-4   Abnormal Breath Sounds and Related Conditions

BREATH SOUND	CONDITIONS
Diminished or absent	Airway obstruction
	Atelectasis
	Main-stem intubation
	Pleural effusion
	Pneumothorax
Wheezes	Airway narrowing
Inspiratory crackles	Lung consolidation
	Pulmonary edema
Coarse crackles	Excessive secretions

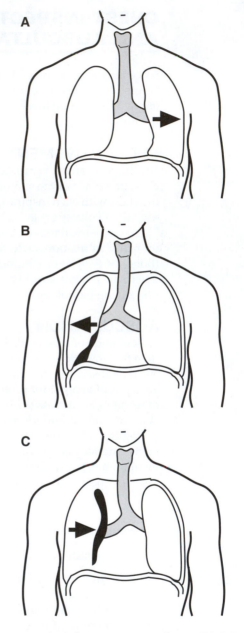

Figure 9-1 Asymmetrical chest movement due to (A) right bronchial intubation; note overinflation of the right lung and underinflation of the left lung; (B) atelectasis, the trachea and mediastinum are shifted to the affected side; (C) tension pneumothorax, the trachea and mediastinum are shifted to the opposite side.

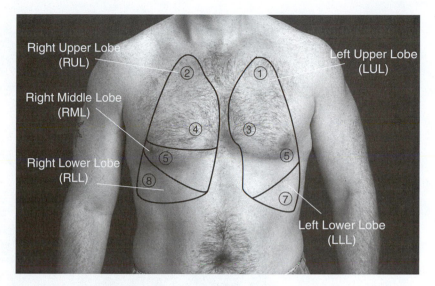

Figure 9-2 Anterior surface projection of the lung lobes and segments. Left lung: 1 LUL apical segment, 3 LUL anterior segment, 5 LUL lingula inferior and superior segments, 7 LLL anterior segment. Right lung: 2 RUL apical segment, 4 RUL anterior, 6 RML medial and lateral segments, 8 RLL anterior segment.

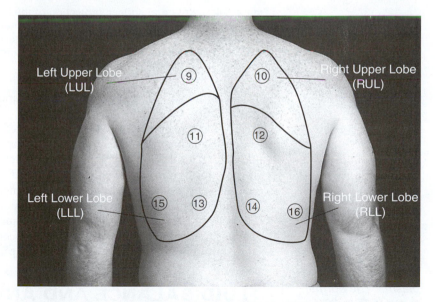

Figure 9-3 Posterior surface projection of the lung lobes and segments. Left lung: 9 LUL posterior segment, 11 LLL superior segment, 13 LLL posterior segment, 15 LLL lateral segment. Right lung: 10 RUL posterior segment, 12 RLL superior segment, 14 RLL posterior segment, 16 RLL lateral segment.

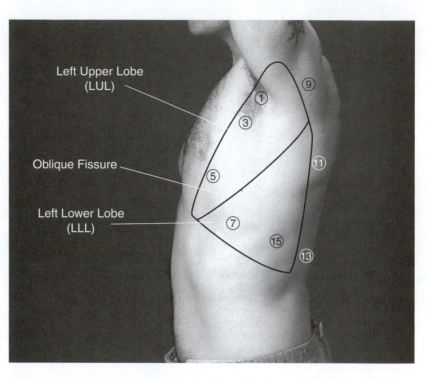

Figure 9-4 Left lateral surface projection of the lung lobes and segments. Left upper lobe: 1 LUL apical segment, 3 LUL anterior segment, 5 LUL lingula inferior and superior segments, 9 LUL posterior segment. Left lower lobe: 7 LLL anterior segment, 11 LLL superior segment, 13 LLL posterior segment, 15 LLL lateral segment.

for performing the correct chest percussion and postural drainage procedure.

The stethoscope can also be used for detection of a leaky cuff on an endotracheal or tracheostomy tube, as well as for right main-stem (bronchial) intubation. A cuff leak may be detected by placing the stethoscope diaphragm over the trachea and on top of the cuff's location. The cuff is leaking if distinct air movement can be heard toward the end of a mechanical breath. Uneven bilateral breath sounds in the absence of lung pathology (e.g., atelectasis, tension pneumothorax) may indicate main-stem intubation. The placement of an endotracheal tube should be confirmed by chest radiograph.

anion gap: *The difference between cations (positive ions) and anions (negative ions) in the plasma. The normal range is 15 to 20 when K^+ is included in the calculation (10 to 14 mEq/L when K^+ is excluded).*

FLUID BALANCE AND ANION GAP

Mechanical ventilation may affect a patient's renal function and fluid balance. Since fluid balance and electrolyte concentration are related, the **anion gap** may also be affected as a result of positive pressure ventilation. Proper fluid and electrolyte maintenance should be an integral part of mechanical ventilation to prevent these adverse outcomes.

FLUID BALANCE

Positive pressure ventilation reduces cardiac output and thus renal perfusion. Urine output is decreased due to hypoperfusion of the kidneys. Mechanical ventilation also reduces urine output as a result of an increase in antidiuretic hormone (ADH) and reduction of atrial natriuretic factor (ANF). The end result of these changes is decreased fluid output and fluid retention.

oliguria: Below normal urine output.

For these reasons, the fluid level of a ventilator patient must be monitored closely because positive pressure ventilation affects fluid balance (intake and output). Fluid intake is recorded by adding all fluids received by the patient to include fluids provided via the intravenous, oral, and nasogastric routes. Fluid output is commonly done by measuring the urine output. **Oliguria** indicates fluid inadequacy and may occur as a result of system malfunctions, decreased renal perfusion, decreased fluid intake, and decreased cardiac output. Normal urine output is 50 to 60 mL/hour. Urine output of below 20 mL/hour (or 400 mL in a 24-hour period or 160 mL in 8 hours) is indicative of fluid inadequacy (Kraus et al., 1993).

✓ Oliguria may be seen after bleeding, diarrhea, renal failure, shock, drug poisoning, deep coma, or hypertrophy of the prostate.

Reduction in cardiac output can be directly attributed to decreased venous return secondary to positive pressure ventilation and increased intrathoracic pressure. Positive pressure ventilation also causes an increase in the production of antidiuretic hormone (ADH) which further reduces the urine output.

ANION GAP

✓ Normal urine output is 50 to 60 mL/hour.

Table 9-5 shows a typical set of electrolyte parameters with their normal results. Using some of these parameters, the anion gap may be calculated and used to assess a patient's overall electrolyte balance. Anion gap is

TABLE 9-5   Normal Serum Electrolytes

CATION	CONCENTRATION (mEq/L)	ANION	CONCENTRATION (mEq/L)
Na^+	140 (138 to 142)	Cl^-	103 (101 to 105)
K^+	4 (3 to 5)	HCO_3^-	25 (23 to 27)
Ca^{++}	5 (4.5 to 5.5)	Protein	16 (14 to 18)
Mg^{++}	2 (1.5 to 2.5)	HPO_4^-, $H_2PO_4^-$	2 (1.5 to 2.5)
		SO_4^-	1 (0.8 to 1.2)
		Organic acids	4 (3.5 to 4.5)
Total cations	151	Total anions	151

the relationship of the cations (sodium [Na^+] and potassium [K^+]) to the anions (chloride [Cl^-] and bicarbonate [HCO_3^-]). The anion gap may be determined as follows:

☑ See Appendix 1 for example.

$$Anion\ gap = Na^+ - Cl^- - HCO_3^-$$
Normal range: 10 to 14 mEq/L

or

$$Anion\ gap = Na^+ + K^+ - Cl^- - HCO_3^-$$
Normal range: 15 to 20 mEq/L

☑ Metabolic acidosis in the presence of a normal anion gap is usually caused by a loss of base.

Metabolic Acidosis and Anion Gap.   Metabolic acidosis in the presence of a normal anion gap is usually caused by a loss of base. This condition is called hyperchloremic metabolic acidosis because it is usually related to excessive chloride ions in the plasma (Chang, 1999).

☑ Metabolic acidosis in the presence of an increased anion gap is usually due to increased fixed acids.

Metabolic acidosis in the presence of an increased anion gap is usually due to increased fixed acids. These acids may be produced biologically (e.g., renal failure, diabetic ketoacidosis, lactic acidosis), or they may be added from an external source (e.g., poisoning by salicylates and alcohol) (Chang, 1999).

Respiratory Compensation for Metabolic Acidosis.   In ventilator patients with adequate lung function, respiratory compensation of metabolic acidosis in the form of hyperventilation may occur. For this reason, one should not assume that respiratory insufficiency (primary alveolar hyperventilation) is present. The cause of metabolic acidosis must be identified and corrected. Furthermore, the ventilator rate must not be reduced under this condition because persistent hyperventilation by the patient will likely continue (Rooth, 1974).

☑ Severe K^+ depletion can lead to metabolic alkalosis and compensatory hypoventilation.

Metabolic Alkalosis.   It is also important to monitor a patient's potassium level during mechanical ventilation. Severe K^+ depletion can lead to metabolic alkalosis and compensatory hypoventilation (Adams & Hahn, 1982). This may prolong the weaning process when mechanical ventilation is needed to supplement the decreasing spontaneous ventilation.

ARTERIAL BLOOD GASES

Arterial blood gas (ABG) analysis provides useful information about a patient's ventilation ($PaCO_2$), oxygenation (PaO_2), and acid-base (pH) status. It is therefore an essential monitoring tool for patients

TABLE 9-6   Blood Gas Parameters and Normal Range for Adult

MONITORING FUNCTION	PARAMETER	NORMAL (P_B 760 mm Hg)	(P_B 630 mm Hg)
Ventilation	$PaCO_2$	35 to 45 mm Hg	32 to 42 mm Hg
Oxygenation	PaO_2	80 to 100 mm Hg	60 to 80 mm Hg
Acid-Base	pH HCO_3^- (calculated) B.E. (calculated)	7.35 to 7.45 22 to 26 mEq/L −2 to 2 mEq/L	7.32 to 7.42

receiving mechanical ventilation as these patients often have gas exchange and acid-base abnormalities. Table 9-6 shows the normal ABG values for adult patients.

ASSESSMENT OF VENTILATORY STATUS

Direct measurement of arterial carbon dioxide tension ($PaCO_2$) via arterial puncture or indwelling catheter is the most accurate method of assessing a patient's ventilatory status. Hypoventilation and respiratory acidosis are present when the $PaCO_2$ is increased with a concurrent decrease in pH. This condition may be corrected by increasing the rate or tidal volume on the ventilator. On the other hand, the rate or tidal volume should be reduced when hyperventilation and respiratory alkalosis occur.

When the acid-base imbalance is caused by metabolic acidosis or alkalosis, it calls for a different ventilator management strategy. The underlying metabolic problem must be corrected before changing the ventilator settings. Ventilator tidal volume or rate adjustment should not be made to "correct" metabolic acid-base abnormalities during mechanical ventilation.

Respiratory Fatigue.   The ventilator patient who develops hypercapnic respiratory failure secondary to increased carbon dioxide production (VCO_2) should be monitored closely. The VCO_2 may be increased due to a hypermetabolic state. This condition may lead to increased minute ventilation in an attempt to keep up with the increasing CO_2 production. A prolonged increase in the work of breathing may lead to respiratory muscle fatigue and ventilatory failure. It has been documented that excessive work of breathing (minute ventilation in excess of 10 L/min.) is often associated with poor outcomes when trying to wean the patient from mechanical ventilation (Stoller, 1991).

Patients with depressed central respiratory drive, elevated V_D/V_T, diminished compliance, or respiratory muscle weakness may also develop respiratory fatigue as they are unable to maintain an increased minute ventilation over an extended period of time.

ASSESSMENT OF OXYGENATION STATUS

Changes in the patient's oxygen status are commonly assessed by (1) arterial oxygen tension (PaO_2), (2) alveolar-arterial oxygen tension gradient [$P(A-a)O_2$ or $(A-a)DO_2$], (3) arterial to alveolar oxygen tension ratio (PaO_2/P_AO_2), and (4) PaO_2 to F_IO_2 ratio. A decreased PaO_2, an increased $P(A-a)O_2$, a decreased PaO_2/PAO_2 or a decreased PaO_2/F_IO_2 reflects tissue hypoxia. Table 9-7 outlines the guideline for interpretation of a patient's oxygenation status.

diffusion defect: Pathologic condition leading to impaired gas exchange through the alveolar-capillary membrane. An example is interstitial or pulmonary edema.

In general, a decrease in PaO_2 with concurrent increase in $P(A-a)O_2$ is indicative of hypoxemia due to **diffusion defect**, V/Q mismatch or shunt. A decrease in PaO_2 with little or no increase in $P(A-a)O_2$ is probably due to hypoventilation and this can be confirmed by an elevated $PaCO_2$ (Tobin, 1990).

$P(A-a)O_2$ is the difference of PAO_2 and PaO_2. It can be calculated as follows:

$$P(A-a)O_2 = PAO_2 - PaO_2$$

PaO_2 is obtained from arterial blood gas analysis and PAO_2 can be calculated by the simplified alveolar air equation, as follows:

$$PAO_2 = (P_B - PH_2O) \times F_IO_2 - \frac{(PaCO_2)}{R}$$

TABLE 9-7 Interpretation of Oxygenation Status

PARAMETERS	CRITERIA	INTERPRETATION
PaO_2	80–100 mm Hg	Normal
	60–79 mm Hg	Mild hypoxemia
	40–59 mm Hg	Moderate hypoxemia
	<40 mm Hg	Severe hypoxemia
PaO_2/F_IO_2	>200 mm Hg	Normal for critically ill patients
	<200 mm Hg	Presence of shunting likely
$P(A-a)O_2$	Room air	Should be less than 4 mm Hg for every 10 years of age, otherwise hypoxemia
	100% O_2	Every 50 mm Hg difference approximates 2% shunt
PaO_2/PAO_2	$F_IO_2 \geqslant 30\%$	>75% Normal
		<75% Hypoxemia

(Data from Girault et al., 1994; Malley, 1990; Shapiro et al., 1994.)

where P_B = barometric pressure, PH_2O = water vapor pressure (generally 47 mm Hg at 37°C), and R = respiratory quotient (estimated to be 0.8 and it may be deleted from equation when the F_IO_2 is greater than 60%). P_AO_2 is mainly affected by changes of F_IO_2, $PaCO_2$, and P_B.

Hypoventilation.   Acute hypoventilation causes CO_2 retention (increased $PaCO_2$) and respiratory acidosis. Without supplemental oxygen, hypoventilation leads to hypoxemia as well. This type of hypoxemia should not be treated with oxygen alone as the underlying condition can only be corrected by improving the alveolar ventilation.

Ventilation/Perfusion Mismatch.   When PaO_2 is decreased with little or no change in $PaCO_2$, **ventilation/perfusion (V/Q) mismatch** or intrapulmonary shunt should be suspected. Hypoxemia caused by ventilation/perfusion (V/Q) mismatch is characterized by a normal or low $PaCO_2$, and this type of hypoxemia responds well to moderate levels of supplemental oxygen.

Intrapulmonary Shunting.   Hypoxemia caused by **intrapulmonary shunting** does not respond well to high concentrations of oxygen. This is because shunted blood does not come in contact with ventilated (oxygenated) alveoli. The $PaCO_2$ is usually normal or low because the peripheral chemoreceptors respond readily to hypoxemia by increasing the minute ventilation (Bone, 1985).

Positive end-expiratory pressure (PEEP) in conjunction with oxygen are usually required to correct hypoxemia caused by intrapulmonary shunting. If hypoventilation is present as documented by an increased $PaCO_2$, ventilatory assistance may also be necessary.

Diffusion Defects.   Diffusion abnormalities can cause hypoxemia by three mechanisms: (1) low oxygen pressure gradient, (2) increased alveolar-capillary thickness, and (3) decreased alveolar surface area.

Low alveolar-arterial oxygen tension gradient is usually due to reduction in alveolar PO_2. Oxygen therapy increases the alveolar PO_2 and alveolar-arterial PO_2 tension gradient. It is therefore very effective in correcting hypoxemia caused by uncomplicated diffusion defect.

Increased alveolar-capillary thickness can be seen in conditions such as pneumonia, and pulmonary and interstitial edema. In mild and uncomplicated cases, hypoxemia may be corrected by oxygen therapy.

Decreased alveolar surface area can be seen in emphysema due to destruction of the lung tissues (Tobin, 1990). This type of structural

---

☑ Acute hypoventilation causes respiratory acidosis.

ventilation/perfusion (V/Q) mismatch: An abnormal distribution of ventilation and pulmonary blood flow. High V/Q is related to dead-space ventilation, whereas low V/Q is associated with intrapulmonary shunting.

intrapulmonary shunting: Pulmonary circulation that does not come in contact with ventilated alveoli.

☑ When the PaO_2 is decreased with little or no change in $PaCO_2$, V/Q mismatch or intrapulmonary shunt should be suspected.

☑ Hypoxemia caused by intrapulmonary shunting does not respond well to high concentrations of oxygen.

☑ PEEP and oxygen are usually required to correct hypoxemia caused by intrapulmonary shunting.

defect is not reversible, but the diffusion problem may be partially managed by oxygen therapy.

LIMITATIONS OF BLOOD GASES

Blood gas analysis and monitoring is not without its limitations. Arterial blood sampling is an invasive procedure requiring the puncture of an artery or placement of an arterial catheter. Inaccurate results can occur with introduction of air bubbles, dilution with excessive heparin, or with faulty handling of the sample itself. It is also important to keep in mind that blood gas values reflect an isolated moment in time rather than a trend. They should be used to correlate and document trends established by noninvasive monitoring devices such as pulse oximetry. Finally, arterial blood gas measurements are generally a late indicator of respiratory failure and of limited use as an early warning sign (Tobin, 1990). Nevertheless, arterial blood gases can still provide very useful information when used in conjunction with other monitoring techniques.

OXYGEN SATURATION MONITORING

pulse oximeter: A device that estimates arterial oxygen saturation (SpO_2) by emitting dual wavelengths of light through a pulsating vascular bed.

Oxygen saturation is traditionally measured by arterial blood gases. The arterial oxygen saturation (SaO_2) is not always readily available. A simple and noninvasive method to monitor the oxygen saturation is by using a **pulse oximeter.** The pulse oximetry oxygen saturation (SpO_2) is less accurate than SaO_2 but it can provide quick spot checks or a trend reflecting a patient's oxygenation status.

PULSE OXIMETRY

Pulse oximetry has become perhaps the most frequently used method of assessing a patient's oxygenation status. This noninvasive method measures the approximate oxyhemoglobin saturation (SpO_2). It is safe and easy to use. Pulse oximeters may be used intermittently to "spot check" the SpO_2 or continuously to monitor the patient's SpO_2 trend. Figure 9-5(A)–(C) show three portable pulse oximeters.

The pulse oximeter works by emitting dual wavelengths of light through a pulsating vascular field. Proper placement of the probe is necessary to obtain an accurate reading. The heart rate is also measured as the oximeter evaluates each arterial pulse (Figure 9-6). If the heart rate on the oximeter varies significantly from the actual pulse as measured by palpation or cardiac monitor, one should verify the accuracy of the SpO_2 reading. It should, however, be noted that a good match of actual and oximetry heart rates does not necessarily indicate

A

B

C

Figure 9-5   Portable pulse oximeters. [(A) Courtesy of Masimo Corporation; (B) Courtesy of Nonin Medical Inc., Plymouth, Minn.; (C) Used with permission of Minolta Konica Minolta Photo Imaging U.S.A., Inc.]

Figure 9-6   A pulse oximeter capable of monitoring SpO_2 and heart rate. (Courtesy of Datex-Engstrom, Inc.)

an accurate SpO_2 reading. The accuracy of the SpO_2 reading should be verified by periodic arterial blood gases.

ACCURACY AND CLINICAL USE OF PULSE OXIMETRY

Pulse oximetry has been used as a reliable noninvasive means of monitoring oxygenation in ventilator patients. SpO_2 of >95% has shown a strong correlation with PaO_2 of >70 mm Hg with a sensitivity of 100% (Niehoff et al., 1988).

SpO_2 can be used to facilitate F_IO_2 weaning of a ventilator patient. The F_IO_2 may be reduced to an appropriate level by use of a single arterial blood gas measurement followed by multiple pulse oximetry measurements (Rotello et al., 1992). Oxygenation of the ventilator-dependent patient can be assured when the SpO_2 is kept above 92% to 95% as this level correlates with a PaO_2 above 60 mm Hg (Jubran & Tobin, 1990). Table 9-8 outlines other clinical applications of pulse oximetry.

LIMITATIONS OF PULSE OXIMETRY

SpO_2 has good correlation with arterial oxygen saturation (SaO_2) when the SaO_2 is 95% or greater (Niehoff et al., 1988). SpO_2 becomes less

TABLE 9-8   Clinical Applications of Pulse Oximetry

CLINICAL APPLICATION	EXAMPLES
Monitor oxygenation status	Mechanical ventilation Intubation Surgery
Titrate F_IO_2	Increase F_IO_2 in hypoxemia Decrease F_IO_2 in weaning
Verify ABG accuracy	Compare O_2 saturation readings to rule out venous sample

dyshemoglobins:
Hemoglobins that do not carry oxygen (e.g., carboxyhemo-globin, methemo-globin). In the presence of dyshemo-globins, pulse oximeter reads higher than actual SaO_2.

accurate as SaO_2 decreases and overestimation of a patient's oxygenation status may result.

The accuracy of pulse oximetry can be affected by factors such as artifact and underlying patient conditions. Artifact due to motion remains a cause of inaccurate measurement despite corrective efforts (Pologe, 1987). Sunlight has been reported to give a falsely low SpO_2 measurement (Abbott, 1986). Nail polish (primarily blue, green, and black), and intravascular dyes can also give a falsely low SpO_2 reading (Welch, DeCesare & Hess, 1990). Improper placement of the oximeter probe can give a faulty SpO_2 reading as well. If a patient is wearing nail polish, the probe may be placed sideways (White, 1989).

Pathologic factors such as low perfusion states and presence of **dyshemoglobins** may lead to SpO_2 measurements that are higher than the actual SaO_2 (Schnapp & Cohen, 1990). Table 9-9 shows the factors that affect the accuracy of pulse oximetry.

TABLE 9-9   Factors That Affect the Accuracy of Pulse Oximetry

FACTORS	TYPE OF INACCURACY
Sunlight Nail polish Fluorescent light Intravenous dyes	SpO_2 measures lower than actual SaO_2.

Dyshemoglobins
   (methemoglobin, sulfahemoglobin,
   carboxyhemoglobin)
Low perfusion states
	SpO_2 measures higher than actual SaO_2.

INNOVATIONS IN PULSE OXIMETRY

A new technology for pulse oximetry has been developed to counteract common problems such as motion artifacts, low perfusion states, and low signal to noise situations (Barker & Shah, 1997; Masimo Corporation, 2001). This new innovation uses an adaptive filtering technology to separate the arterial pulse signal from nonarterial interference. Laboratory and clinical tests have shown that this new technology can provide accurate pulse oximetry readings during patient motion, low blood flow to the extremities in adults and neonates, unfavorable ambient lights, and electrical noises. These new pulse oximeters are marketed by several manufacturers (Rushworth, 1999).

END-TIDAL CARBON DIOXIDE MONITORING

end-tidal carbon dioxide monitoring: The CO_2 level measured at the end of exhalation; measured in mm Hg pressure units.

End-tidal carbon dioxide monitoring is done to monitor a patient's ventilatory status. Once a good correlation is established between $PaCO_2$ and end-tidal PCO_2 ($PetCO_2$), the number of routine blood gases may be reduced. In addition, changes of the $PetCO_2$ values and waveforms may also be obtained and interpreted for additional information about the patient/ventilator system.

CAPNOGRAPHY

Capnography is a measurement of the partial pressure of carbon dioxide in a gas sample. When the sample is collected at the end of inspiration, it is called end-tidal partial pressure of carbon dioxide ($PetCO_2$). $PetCO_2$ monitoring provides real time, noninvasive analysis of a patient's expired CO_2 trend during mechanical ventilation. Many of the newer ventilators have built-in end-tidal CO_2 monitoring capabilities. Figure 9-7 is an example of an end-tidal CO_2 monitor.

The exhaled CO_2 from the patient ventilator circuit is collected and measured by the infrared absorption technique (Hess, 1990). A mainstream sensor is placed directly onto the ventilator circuit, usually attached to an adaptor on the endotracheal tube. A sidestream sensor aspirates a sample of gas via a small tube connected to the endotracheal tube adapter. Figure 9-8 illustrates these two types of sensors.

The major advantage of mainstream analysis is the fast response time between actual CO_2 sampling and the display update. The disadvantage of the mainstream adapter is its excessive weight on the endotracheal tube as well as the additional deadspace in the ventilator/patient circuit. With mainstream sampling, water condensation

Figure 9-7 End-tidal CO_2 monitor. (Courtesy of Datex-Engstrom, Inc.)

does not affect analysis; however, secretion buildup on the cell windows can affect the accuracy. A mainstream analyzer also tends to be more frequently handled than the sidestream sensor as the clinician must disconnect it manually to suction the patient (Shelley, 1989).

A sidestream analyzer (aspirating analyzer) places the analyzing mechanism safely within the monitor and draws a sample via a tubing connected at the patient's airway (e.g., endotracheal tube). The major advantage with sidestream analysis is the ease of handling and it can be attached to other patient devices (e.g., cannula, mask). The major disadvantage is that with periodic aspiration of air samples, secretions and water can be drawn into the sampling tube and cause an occlusion. Lag time for CO_2 display is slightly (a few tenths of a second) longer than the mainstream analyzer but it is negligible. Equipment contamination may be a problem with the sidestream analyzer (Shelley, 1989).

CAPNOGRAPHY WAVEFORMS AND CLINICAL APPLICATIONS

A capnogram (Figure 9-9) shows the changes in P_ECO_2 during a complete respiratory cycle. The P_ECO_2 remains at zero during inspiration. At the beginning of expiration, the P_ECO_2 remains at zero as anatomic deadspace volume and exits the airways. The P_ECO_2 then increases dramatically as alveolar gas begins mixing with deadspace gas. Then, for

Figure 9-8 (A) Mainstream capnography sensor; (B) Sidestream capnography sensor. (Used with permission from Criticare Systems, Inc.)

Figure 9-9   The normal capnogram. (A, phase I) PCO_2 remains zero as gas exits from the anatomic deadspace; (A to B, phase II) PCO_2 rises rapidly as alveolar gas mixes with deadspace gas; (B to C, phase III) alveolar plateau shows gas flow from alveoli; Point (C) is called the end-tidal PCO_2 ($PetCO_2$). (From D. Hess (1990), Capnometry and capnography: Technical aspects, physiologic aspects, and clinical applications. *Respir Care 35*(6), 557–576. Used with permission.)

the larger part of expiration, the curve plateaus, reflecting alveolar gas. The end of the "alveolar plateau" is called the end-tidal PCO_2.

Transitory events can be examined by review of the capnographic tracing. The capnogram can be useful in determining accidental esophageal intubations, endotracheal tube cuff leaks, and airway obstructions. It can also be used to determine the synchronization of respiratory rates between the patient and ventilator. Some other clinical applications for capnography include use during weaning, cardiopulmonary resuscitation, intubation, bronchoscopy, and hypocapnic management of patients with head trauma (Carlon et al., 1988; Hess, 1990). The capnographs do not provide absolute measurements but they can be used to follow the PCO_2 changes in hemodynamically stable trauma patients (Hess, 1990). Figure 9-10 shows the representative capnograms that correlate with some common clinical conditions.

P(a-et)CO₂ GRADIENT

The correlation between $PaCO_2$ and $PetCO_2$ is excellent and the $P(a-et)CO_2$ gradient (difference) between these two measurements is about 2 mm Hg in normal individuals. For critical patients, a gradient of 5 mm Hg is considered acceptable (Niehoff et al., 1988).

The $P(a-et)CO_2$ gradient is primarily affected by alveolar deadspace ventilation (Perel & Stock, 1992), old age, presence of pulmonary disease, and changes in mechanical volume and modality.

Figure 9-10 Abnormal capnograms monitored via real time or trend screen. (A) Cardiac arrest (real time). The PetCO$_2$ values drop suddenly and proportionally. This condition indicates lung perfusion is inadequate due to a decreased cardiac output. (B) Effectiveness of external compressions can be monitored by the resultant rise in PetCO$_2$ as shown in the trend screen. (C) Kinked ET tube (trend screen). As the ET tube is obstructed (partially or completely), the PetCO$_2$ values reflect the degree of obstruction. With complete obstruction, zero PetCO$_2$ is seen. (D) Disconnection. Immediate disappearance of the PetCO$_2$ values and waveform are observed. (Used with permission from Criticare Systems, Inc.)

Table 9-10 lists some specific conditions that increase the P(a-et)CO$_2$ gradient.

Disposable ETCO$_2$ Detector.   Capnography can also be estimated via a low cost, disposable, plastic, CO$_2$ (pH) sensitive device. With this device attached to the endotracheal tube, one can quickly differentiate tracheal

TABLE 9-10   Factors That Increase the P(a-et)CO$_2$ Gradient

CLINICAL CONDITION	FACTORS
Ventilation	Increased deadspace ventilation Positive pressure ventilation
Perfusion	Decreased cardiac output Decreased pulmonary perfusion Cardiac arrest Pulmonary embolic disease
Temperature	Hyperthermia Hypothermia

End-tidal PCO_2 = 30 mm Hg

P_ACO_2 0 mm Hg

P_ACO_2 40 mm Hg

Arterial PCO_2 40 mm Hg

Obstruction

0 mm Hg

46 mm Hg

Mixed Venous PCO_2

Figure 9-11 Deadspace ventilation induced by blockage of a portion of the pulmonary blood flow (e.g., pulmonary embolism). This condition leads to a reduced $PetCO_2$ reading.

from esophageal intubation (Hess, 1990). This occurs when the pH-sensitive device on the material senses the changes in CO_2 concentration.

✓ Capnography readings reflect only changes in a patient's ventilatory status, rather than improvement or deterioration of the patient.

✓ Decreased $PetCO_2$ may not be indicative of improvement in gas exchange.

LIMITATIONS OF CAPNOGRAPHY MONITORING

Capnography readings reflect only changes in a patient's ventilatory status, rather than improvement or deterioration of the patient (Whitaker, 2001). An example of this is deadspace ventilation as seen in pulmonary embolism (Figure 9-11). A decrease in $PetCO_2$ due to physiologic deadspace ventilation does not mean that the patient's ventilatory status has improved. Lowering the ventilator rate in this situation could lead to grave consequences.

Other conditions leading to an increase in deadspace ventilation (thus a decrease in $PetCO_2$) are hypotension and high intrathoracic pressure secondary to mechanical ventilation (Whitaker, 2001). This could cause the practitioner to incorrectly assume that the decreased $PetCO_2$ indicates an improvement in gas exchange.

TRANSCUTANEOUS BLOOD GAS MONITORING

Transcutaneous blood gas monitoring involves placement of a miniature Clark (PO_2) or a Severinghaus (PCO_2) electrode on the skin via a double-sided adhesive disk. A heating coil in the electrode increases the permeability of the epidermis thus facilitating diffusion of gas from the underlying capillaries to the electrode. Transcutaneous blood gas monitoring has been used more often in neonates than in adults (Eberhard, Mint & Schafer, 1981). Figures 9-12 and 9-13 show two examples of transcutaneous O_2 and CO_2 monitors.

Figure 9-12 Transcutaneous PCO_2 and PO_2 monitor. (Courtesy of Novametrix Medical Systems, Inc.)

Figure 9-13 Transcutaneous PCO_2 and PO_2 monitor. (Courtesy of Radiometer America, Inc.)

TRANSCUTANEOUS PO₂ (PtcO₂)

In neonates, the **transcutaneous PO₂ (PtcO₂)** closely approximates the PaO_2. But in adults, the $PtcO_2$ measures lower than the actual PO_2 due to thicker skin in adults. For this reason, pulse oximetry has become the preferred method to monitor the oxygenation status of adult patients.

$PtcO_2$ also approximates the central organ PO_2 (Tremper, Waxman & Shoemaker, 1979). It has a good correlation with the cardiac output changes in a ventilator patient (Shapiro et al., 1989). In addition, a fall in $PtcO_2$ can be associated with a need for suctioning, misplaced endotracheal tube, pneumothorax, or other causes of hypoxemia (Pilbeam, 1999).

Accuracy of the $PtcO_2$ electrode is affected by skin edema, hypothermia, and capillary perfusion status.

Limitations. Accuracy of the $PtcO_2$ electrode is affected by skin edema, hypothermia, and capillary perfusion status. $PtcO_2$ is a better predictor of PaO_2 when it falls below 80 mm Hg. However, the $PtcO_2$ becomes less accurate when the PaO_2 is greater than 80 mm Hg (Palmisano & Severinghaus, 1990). When cardiac output decreases, as with the patient in shock, a disproportionate fall in $PtcO_2$ occurs.

Two other disadvantages of transcutaneous monitors are the need for frequent site changes (every 3 to 4 hours) to prevent heat damage to skin and long equilibration times after each site change.

TRANSCUTANEOUS PCO₂ (PtcCO₂)

transcutaneous **PtcCO₂:** *Measurement of PCO₂ through the skin by means of a miniature Severinghaus (PCO₂) electrode.*

Transcutaneous PCO₂ (PtcCO₂) monitoring is done to provide a means of continuous ventilatory assessment. The $PtcCO_2$ is measured by heating the underlying skin to 44°C (40°C to 42°C in neonates), which facilitates CO_2 diffusion across the skin to the CO_2 electrode.

The correlation between $PtcCO_2$ and $PaCO_2$ is good in neonates as long as perfusion is normal. This correlation in adults shows mixed results, but in general the $PtcCO_2$ may be useful as a monitoring tool once the trend has been established.

Limitations. It should be noted that $PtcCO_2$ values are usually higher than $PaCO_2$ values. This is due to increased CO_2 production as underlying tissues are heated (Marini, 1988). In addition, during shock or low perfusion states, the $PtcCO_2$ measures higher than the actual $PaCO_2$ due to increased accumulation of tissue CO_2 (Tremper & Shoemaker, 1981).

CEREBRAL PERFUSION PRESSURE

Maintenance of adequate CPP reduces mortality.

Cerebral perfusion pressure (CPP) is the pressure required to provide blood flow, oxygen, and metabolite to the brain. Under normal conditions, the brain regulates its own blood flow regardless of the systemic blood pressure and cerebral vascular resistance. This autoregulation may be lost following head trauma whereas the cerebral vascular resistance is often greatly elevated. The brain also becomes vulnerable to changing blood pressures. Depending on the degree of decrease in cerebral perfusion, effects on the brain may range from cerebral ischemia to brain death (Bouma & Muizelaar, 1990; Marion et al., 1991).

There is no class I evidence for the optimum level of CPP, but the critical threshold is believed to be from 70 to 80 mm Hg. Mortality increases about 20% for each 10 mm Hg drop in CPP. In studies involving severe head injuries, 35% reduction in mortality was achieved when the CPP was maintained above 70 mm Hg (Bouma et al., 1992; Rosner & Daughton, 1990).

CPP is the difference between the mean arterial pressure (MAP) and the intracranial pressure (ICP). The relationship is shown as follows:

$$CPP = MAP - ICP$$

Based on the relationship of MAP and ICP, a higher CPP may be maintained by raising the MAP or by lowering the ICP. In clinical practice ICP is usually controlled within normal limits (i.e., <20 mm Hg). However, it is unknown whether ICP control is necessary providing CPP is maintained above the critical threshold by raising the MAP (Changaris et al., 1987; Rosner & Daughton, 1990).

In the absence of hemorrhage, the MAP should be managed initially by maintaining an adequate fluid balance. It may then be followed by using a vasopressor such as norepinephrine or dopamine. Systemic hypotension (SBP <90 mm Hg) should be avoided and controlled as soon as possible since early hypotension is associated with increased morbidity and mortality following severe brain injury (Chesnut et al., 1993; Marmarou et al., 1991).

☑ CPP should range between 70 and 80 mm Hg.

☑ A higher CPP may be maintained by raising the MAP or by lowering the ICP.

☑ The normal ICP is 8 to 12 mm Hg; clinical practice <20 mm Hg.

☑ Systemic hypotension is associated with poor outcome in patients with severe head injuries.

SUMMARY

Monitoring in mechanical ventilation is done to provide information about the condition of the patient and the overall effectiveness of a treatment plan. The results obtained from different monitoring techniques should be used and interpreted together and should not be treated as isolated measurements. For example, a decrease in end-tidal CO_2 may indicate the presence of deadspace ventilation. But this assumption must be confirmed with other supporting evidence such as a concurrent decrease in perfusion (decrease in cardiac output or other hemodynamic values). Trending or interpreting a series of measurements is also more meaningful since the overall condition of a patient is a dynamic process, not a set of separated events.

Finally, the condition of the patient should be assessed in conjunction with the monitoring results. This is because the patient may temporarily compensate for abnormal conditions under extremely stressful settings. This erroneous "normal" measurement may not be apparent by reviewing the laboratory results alone. Therefore, careful examination of the patient should always be a vital part of monitoring in mechanical ventilation.

Self-Assessment Questions

1. A patient in the intensive care unit suddenly develops shortness of breath and the SpO_2 drops to 87%. You would anticipate all of the following vital sign measurements to increase with the *exception* of:

   A. heart rate.
   B. minute ventilation.
   C. respiratory rate.
   D. temperature.

2. Prolonged suctioning of the lungs via the endotracheal tube is not advised because this can induce:

   A. hypovolemia and shock.
   B. bradycardia and arrhythmia.
   C. hyperventilation.
   D. productive coughs.

3. One of the complications of positive pressure ventilation is that it can cause a(n) _____ venous return and _____.

   A. increased, hypertension
   B. increased, hypotension
   C. decreased, hypertension
   D. decreased, hypotension

4. A blood gas sample was collected from a hypothermic patient whose core temperature was 24°C. If the sample was analyzed at 37°C with a PO_2 of 90 mm Hg, the temperature corrected PO_2 (to patient's 24°C) would be:

   A. negligible or almost 90 mm Hg.
   B. much higher than 90 mm Hg.
   C. much lower than 90 mm Hg.
   D. dependent on the position of the oxyhemoglobin curve.

5. A physician asks you to evaluate the breath sounds of a patient who has an admitting diagnosis of pneumonia. By placing the stethoscope diaphragm next to the side of the spine below the scapula, you are listening to the breath sounds of the _____ segments of the _____ lobes.

   A. posterior, upper
   B. superior, middle
   C. posterior, middle
   D. superior, lower

6 to 9. Match the breath sounds with the conditions that may be the cause of these abnormalities. Use each answer only once.

Breath Sound	Condition
6. Diminished or absent	A. Lung consolidation
7. Wheezes	B. Airway obstruction
8. Inspiratory crackles	C. Excessive secretions
9. Coarse crackles	D. Airway narrowing

10. Excessive positive pressure or volume during mechanical ventilation may _____ the intrathoracic pressure and _____ the cardiac and urine outputs.

A. increase, increase C. decrease, increase
B. increase, decrease D. decrease, decrease

11. Metabolic acidosis (low bicarbonate) with a(n) _____ anion gap is called hyperchloremic metabolic acidosis because the excessive chloride (Cl^-) ions _____ the deficiency of bicarbonate (HCO_3^-) ions in the plasma.

A. normal, offset C. abnormal, offset
B. normal, aggravate D. abnormal, aggravate

12. A patient who has been undergoing the weaning process for mechanical ventilation suddenly stops breathing spontaneously. You would expect to see the following changes on the next set of blood gas results *except:*

A. increase in PO_2. C. decrease in pH.
B. increase in PCO_2. D. decrease in HCO_3^-.

13. In blood gas interpretation, the $PaCO_2$ is primarily used to assess a patient's _____ status and the PO_2 is useful for the _____ status.

A. ventilatory, acid-base C. acid-base, oxygenation
B. ventilatory, oxygenation D. acid-base, ventilatory

14 to 16. Match the causes of hypoxemia with the characteristics that may be used to distinguish these abnormalities. Use each answer only once.

Cause of Hypoxemia	Characteristics
14. Hypoventilation	A. Normal or low $PaCO_2$; hypoxemia does not respond to high levels of oxygen.
15. V/Q mismatch or diffusion defects	B. High $PaCO_2$; hypoxemia improves with ventilation and low levels of oxygen.
16. Intrapulmonary shunt	C. Normal or low $PaCO_2$; hypoxemia responds very well to moderate levels of oxygen.

17. A patient rescued from a house fire has an admitting diagnosis of severe smoke inhalation. She is breathing spontaneously and receiving 100% oxygen via a nonrebreathing mask. Due to her condition, pulse oximetry _____ be done because _____.

   A. should, of cost savings

   B. should, continuous monitoring is required

   C. should not, the SpO_2 reading will be higher than actual SaO_2

   D. should not, the SpO_2 reading will be lower than actual SaO_2

18. In metabolic acidosis, patients with adequate lung function are capable of compensating for this condition by _____. This would cause the end-tidal CO_2 readings to be _____ than normal.

   A. hyperventilation, higher
   B. hyperventilation, lower

   C. hypoventilation, higher
   D. hypoventilation, lower

19. Which of the following statements is *not* true regarding transcutaneous oxygen and carbon dioxide monitors?

   A. Site changes are required every 3 to 4 hours.
   B. Long equilibration time for calibration.

   C. Accurate PO_2 and PCO_2 measurements.
   D. More accurate in neonatal use.

20. In order to ensure adequate blood flow to the brain, the cerebral perfusion pressure (CPP) should be maintained between:

   A. 0 and 20 mm Hg.
   B. 30 and 50 mm Hg.

   C. 70 and 80 mm Hg.
   D. 100 and 120 mm Hg.

Answers to Self-Assessment Questions

1. D. temperature.

2. B. bradycardia and arrhythmia.

3. D. decreased, hypotension

4. C. much lower than 90 mm Hg.

5. D. superior, lower

6. B. Airway obstruction

7. D. Airway narrowing

8. A. Lung consolidation

9. C. Excessive secretions

10. B. increase, decrease

11. A. normal, offset

12. A. increase in PO_2.

13. B. ventilatory, oxygenation

14. B. High $PaCO_2$; hypoxemia improves with ventilation and low levels of oxygen.

15. C. Normal or low $PaCO_2$; hypoxemia responds very well to moderate levels of oxygen.

16. A. Normal or low $PaCO_2$; hypoxemia does not respond to high levels of oxygen.

17. C. should not, the SpO_2 reading will be higher than actual SaO_2

18. B. hyperventilation, lower

19. C. Acurate PO_2 and PCO_2 measurements.

20. C. 70 and 80 mm Hg.

References

Abbott, M. A. (1986). Monitoring oxygen saturation levels in the early recovery phase of general anesthesia. In T. P. Payne & J. W. Severinghaus (Eds.), *Pulse oximetry* (pp. 165–172). Dorchester: Springer-Verlag.

Adams, A. P., & Hahn, C. E. W. (1982). *Principles and practice of blood gas analysis.* Edinburgh: Churchill Livingstone.

Barker, S. J., & Shah, N. K. (1997). The effects of motion on the performance of pulse oximeters in volunteers. *Anesthesiology, 86,* 101–108.

Bone, R. C. (1985). Monitoring respiratory and hemodynamic function in the patient with respiratory failure. *Mechanical ventilation.* New York: Churchill Livingstone.

Bouma, G. J., & Muizelaar, J. P. (1990). Relationship between cardiac output and cerebral blood flow in patients with intact and with impaired autoregulation. *J Neurosurg, 73,* 368–374.

Bouma, G. J., Muizelaar, J. P., Bandoh, K., et al. (1992). Blood pressure and intracranial pressure-volume dynamics in severe head injury: Relationship with cerebral blood flow. *J Neurosurg, 77,* 15–19.

Burton, G. G., et al. (1997). *Respiratory care: A guide to clinical practice* (4th ed.). Baltimore: Lippincott Williams & Wilkins.

Carlon, G., Ray, C., Mordownik, S., et al. (1988). Capnography in mechanically ventilated patients. *Crit Care Med, 16,* 550–556.

Chang, D. W. (1999). *Respiratory care calculations* (2nd ed.) Clifton Park, New York: Thomson Delmar Learning.

Changaris, D. G., et al. (1987). Correlation of cerebral perfusion pressure and Glasgow Coma Scale to outcome. *J Trauma, 27,* 1007–1013.

Chesnut, R. M., et al. (1993). Early and late systemic hypotension as a frequent and fundamental source of cerebral ischaemia following severe brain injury in the Traumatic Coma Data Bank. *Acta Neurochir Suppl, 59,* 121–125.

Eberhard, P., Mindt, W., & Schafer, R. (1981). Cutaneous blood gas monitoring in the adult. *Crit Care Med, 9,* 702–705.

Girault, C., et al. (1994). Weaning criteria from mechanical ventilation. *Monaldi Arch Chest Dis, 49*(2), 118–124.

Gravelyn, T. R., & Weg, J. R. (1980). Respiratory rate as an indicator of acute respiratory dysfunction. *JAMA, 244,* 1123–1125.

Hess, D. (1990). Capnometry and capnography: Technical aspects, physiologic aspects, and clinical applications. *Resp Care, 35,* 557–573.

Jubran, A., & Tobin, M. J. (1990). Reliability for pulse oximetry in titrating supplemental oxygen therapy in ventilator-dependent patients. *Chest, 97,* 1420–1425.

Kraus, P. A. et al. (1993). Acute lung injury at Baragwanath ICU—An eight-month audit and call for consensus for other organ failure in the adult respiratory distress syndrome. *Chest, 103*(6), 1832–1836.

Krieger, B. P., & Ershowshy, P. (1994). Noninvasive detection of respiratory failure in the intensive care unit. *Chest, 2,* 254–261.

Malley, W. J. (1990). *Clinical blood gases—application & noninvasive alternatives.* Philadelphia: W.B. Saunders.

Marini, J. J. (1988). Monitoring during mechanical ventilation. *Clinics in Chest Med, 9*(1), 73–100.

Marion, D. W., et al. (1991). Acute regional cerebral blood flow changes caused by severe head injuries. *J Neurosurg, 74,* 407–414.

Marmarou, A., et al. (1991). Impact of ICP instability and hypotension on outcome in patients with severe head trauma. *J Neurosurg, 75,* S59–S66.

Masimo Corporation (2001). Masimo Signal Extraction Technology, *Technical Bulletin 1,* Irvine, CA.

Niehoff, J., Delguercio, C., LaMorte, W., et al. (1988). Efficacy of pulse oximetry and capnometry in postoperative ventilatory weaning. *Crit Care Med, 16*(7), 701–705.

Novametrix Medical Systems, Inc. (1991). *Capnograph Monitor Model 1260 User's Manual.* Wallingford, CT.

Palmisano, B. W., & Severinghaus, J. W. (1990). Transcutaneous PCO_2 and PO_2: A multi-center study of accuracy. *J Clin Monit, 6,* 189–195.

Perel, A., & Stock, M. C. (1992). *Handbook of mechanical ventilatory support.* Baltimore: Lippincott Williams & Wilkins.

Pilbeam, S. P. (1999). *Mechanical ventilation: Physiologic and clinical applications* (3rd ed). St. Louis, MO: Mosby.

Pologe, J. A. (1987). Pulse oximetry: Technical aspects. *Int Anesthiol Clin, 25,* 137–154.

Rooth, G. (1974). *Acid-base and electrolyte balance.* Chicago: Year Book Medical Publishers.

Rosner, M. J., & Daughton, S. (1990). Cerebral perfusion pressure management in head injury. *J Trauma, 30,* 933–941.

Rotello, L. C., Warren, J., Jastremski, M. S., et al. (1992). A nurse-directed protocol using pulse oximetry to wean mechanically ventilated patients from toxic oxygen concentrations. *Chest, 102,* 1833–1835.

Rushworth, G. T. (1999). Pulse oximetry: Past, present, and future. *RT, 12*(5), 53–56.

Schnapp, L. M., & Cohen, N. H. (1990). Pulse oximetry uses and abuses. *Chest, 98,* 1244–1250.

Shapiro, B. A., et al. (1989). Blood gas monitoring: Yesterday, today, and tomorrow. *Crit Care Med, 17,* 573–581.

Shapiro, B. A., et al. (1994). *Clinical application of blood gases* (5th ed.). St. Louis, MO: Mosby.

Shelley, E. J. (1989). *CSI capnography training manual.* Waukesha, WI: Criticare Systems.

Stoller, J. K. (1991). Establishing clinical unweanability. *Respir Care, 36,* 186–198.

Tobin, M. J. (1990). Respiratory monitoring during mechanical ventilation. *Crit Care Clinics, 6*(3), 679–707.

Tobin, M. J., Perez, W., et al. (1986). The pattern of breathing during successful and unsuccessful trails of weaning from mechanical ventilation. *Am Rev Respir Dis, 134,* 1111–1118.

Tremper, K., & Shoemaker, W. C. (1981). Transcutaneous oxygen monitoring of critically ill adults with and without low flow shock. *Crit Care Med, 9,* 706–709.

Tremper, K., Waxman, K., & Shoemaker, W. C. (1979). Effects of hypoxia and shock on transcutaneous PO_2 values in dogs. *Crit Care Med, 7,* 526.

Welch, J. P., DeCesare, R., & Hess, D. (1990). Pulse oximetry: Instrumentation and clinical applications. *Respir Care, 35,* 584–601.

Whitaker, K. B. (2001). *Comprehensive perinatal and pediatric respiratory care* (3rd ed.). Clifton Park, New York: Thomson Delmar Learning.

White, P. F., et al. (1989). Nail polish and oximetry. *Anesth Analg, 68,* 546–547.

Wilkins, R. L., & Dexter, J. R. (1998). *Respiratory disease—Principles of patient care* (2nd ed.). Philadelphia: F.A. Davis.

Suggested Reading

Rozycki, H. J., Sysyn, G. D., Marshall, M. K., et al. (1998). Mainstream end-tidal carbon dioxide monitoring in the neonatal intensive care unit. *Pediatrics, 101*(4 Pt. 1), 648–653.

CHAPTER TEN

HEMODYNAMIC MONITORING

David W. Chang
Gary Hamelin

─────────── OUTLINE ───────────

KEY TERMS

- afterload
- cardiac index
- cardiac output
- central venous pressure
- contractility
- hemodynamic monitoring
- impedance cardiography (ICG)

- mean arterial pressure
- preload
- pulmonary vascular resistance
- stroke volume
- systemic vascular resistance
- transducer
- venous return

INTRODUCTION

A recent advance in the management of mechanical ventilation is the use of invasive hemodynamic monitoring. This monitoring technology is not intended for every patient who requires mechanical ventilation. But for many critically ill patients, hemodynamic measurements can add valuable information to the clinical management of the patient.

In the most basic sense, hemodynamic monitoring is the measurement of the force (pressure) exerted by the blood in the blood vessels or heart chambers during systole (i.e., contraction and pumping) and diastole (i.e., relaxation and filling).

In addition to systolic and diastolic pressures in both the systemic and pulmonary circulations, hemodynamic monitoring equipment also measures cardiac output and mixed venous oxygen saturation. These and other direct measurements gathered through hemodynamic monitoring can be used to obtain other calculated values.

HEMODYNAMIC MONITORING

hemodynamic monitoring: *Measurement of the blood pressure in the vessels or heart chambers during contraction (systole) and relaxation (diastole).*

Direct **hemodynamic monitoring** requires the use of the central venous and pulmonary artery catheters. The central venous catheter measures the **central venous pressure** (right ventricular **preload**), and the pulmonary artery catheter measures the pulmonary artery pressure (right ventricular **afterload**) and the pulmonary capillary wedge pressure (left ventricular preload). Impedance cardiography is a noninvasive method to measure and calculate certain hemodynamic parameters.

TECHNICAL BACKGROUND

Measurement of hemodynamic pressures is based on the principle that liquids are noncompressible and that pressures at any given point within a liquid are transmitted equally. When a closed system is filled with liquid, the pressure exerted at one point can be measured accurately at any other point on the same level. For example, if a catheter *central venous pressure:* *Pressure measured in the vena cava or right atrium. It reflects the status of blood volume in the systemic circulation.*

preload: *The enddiastolic stretch of the muscle fiber*

afterload: *The resistance of the blood vessels into which the ventricle is pumping blood. Expressed in pressure units.*

transducer: *A device that converts one type of energy signal into another type of energy signal (e.g., a pressure signal converted into an electronic signal).*

is placed into the radial artery facing the flow of blood and then connected directly to a tubing that is filled with liquid, the pressure exerted by the blood at the tip of the catheter will be accurately transmitted to the liquid-filled tubing. This pressure signal can then be changed to an electronic signal by a **transducer** and amplified and displayed on a monitor as both a waveform and digital display.

Hemodynamic monitoring is generally done by using a combination of arterial catheter, central venous catheter, and pulmonary artery catheter. One or more of these catheters are introduced into the blood vessel, advanced to a suitable location, and then connected to a monitor at the patient's bedside. The display on the monitor is made possible by using a transducer and an amplifier between the catheter and monitor. In hemodynamic monitoring, the transducer converts a pressure signal (in the catheter) to an electronic signal (on the monitor).

To ensure accurate measurements, the transducer, catheter, and measurement site should all be at the same level. Otherwise, the force of gravity will alter the actual readings. For example, a higher reading may be obtained if the transducer and catheter are located lower than the measurement site.

As with other invasive procedures, hemodynamic monitoring should only be used when truly indicated since infection, dysrhythmia, bleeding, and trauma to blood vessels are potential complications.

UNITS OF MEASUREMENT

Hemodynamic pressure readings are measured in units of millimeters of mercury (mm Hg) in the United States and in kilopascals (kPa) in other countries using Système International (SI) units. The conversion factors in Table 10-1 may be used to change between mm Hg and kPa pressure units. Hemodynamic readings begin with the atmospheric pressure as the zero point. Since changes in atmospheric pressure are slow and insignificant, adjustments are not necessary in trending a series of measurements.

TYPES OF CATHETERS

Three different catheters are used in hemodynamic monitoring: arterial catheter, central venous catheter, and pulmonary artery catheter. The arterial catheter is used to monitor systemic arterial pressure. Venous pressure is measured by a central venous catheter in the superior vena cava or right atrium. A pulmonary artery

TABLE 10-1   Conversions of mm Hg and kilopascal (kPa)

FROM mm Hg TO kPa	FROM kPa TO mm Hg
mm Hg × 0.133 = kPa	kPa × 7.502 = mm Hg

TABLE 10-2 Insertion Sites, Location, and Uses of Hemodynamic Catheters

CATHETER	INSERTION SITES	LOCATION	COMMON USES
Arterial	Radial (first choice), brachial, femoral, or dorsalis pedis artery	Within systemic artery near insertion site	(1) Measure systemic artery pressure. (2) Collect arterial blood gas samples.
Central venous	Subclavian or internal jugular vein	Superior vena cava near right atrium or within right atrium	(1) Measure central venous pressure. (2) Administer fluid or medication.
Pulmonary artery	Subclavian or internal jugular vein	Branch of pulmonary artery	(1) Measure CVP, PAP, and PCWP. (2) Collect mixed venous blood gas samples. (3) Monitor mixed venous O_2 saturation. (4) Measure cardiac output. (5) Provide cardiac pacing.

☑ The proximal opening in the pulmonary artery catheter can also measure the right atrial pressure (i.e., CVP).

catheter (commonly known as the Swan-Ganz catheter) is used to measure the pulmonary arterial pressure and pulmonary capillary wedge pressure. The proximal opening in the pulmonary artery catheter can also measure the pressure in the right atrium. The insertion sites, location, and uses of hemodynamic catheters are summarized in Table 10-2.

ARTERIAL CATHETER

In hemodynamically unstable patients who are receiving fluid infusion or drugs to improve circulation, heart function, and blood vessel caliber, continuous and accurate blood pressure readings are essential. With an arterial catheter, most bedside monitors will display a graphic waveform as well as a digital readout of systolic pressure, diastolic pressure, and **mean arterial pressure.**

mean arterial pressure: The average blood pressure in the arterial circulation. Normal is >60 mm Hg.

INSERTION OF ARTERIAL CATHETER

Systemic arterial pressure is measured by placing an arterial catheter into the radial artery. The brachial, femoral, or dorsalis pedis arteries may also be used, but the radial artery remains the first choice because of the collateral circulation to the hand provided by the ulnar artery. The femoral artery is sometimes used to monitor left atrial pressures during cardiac surgery.

☑ Collateral circu-
lation to the
hand must be con-
firmed by doing the
Allen test before
radial artery
puncture.

Correct placement of the arterial catheter may be assessed by the appearance of an arterial waveform on the monitor (Figure 10-1). Once in place, an arterial line allows for continuous, direct measurement of systemic blood pressure as well as for convenient access to arterial blood samples for repeated blood gas analysis. Although this invasive procedure has potential risks such as bleeding, blood clot, and infection, it has advantages over noninvasive monitoring of blood pressure. Use of a sphygmomanometer (blood pressure cuff) can be simpler and safer but inaccuracies may occur in conditions of increased vascular tone and vasoconstriction (Keckeisen, 1991).

Figure 10-1 shows a normal arterial pressure waveform. The systolic upstroke (C to A) reflects the rapid increase of arterial pressure in the blood vessel during systole (ventricular contraction). The downslope or dicrotic limb (A to C) is caused by the declining pressure that occurs during diastole (ventricular relaxation). The dicrotic notch (B) is caused by the closure of the semilunar valves during diastole. The lowest point (C) of the tracing represents the arterial end-diastolic pressure.

NORMAL ARTERIAL PRESSURE AND MEAN ARTERIAL PRESSURE

The normal arterial pressure values are in the range of 100 to 140 mm Hg systolic and 60 to 90 mm Hg diastolic in most adults. From the systolic and diastolic pressures, the mean arterial pressure may be calculated as follows:

$$MAP = \frac{(P_{systolic} + 2 \times P_{diastolic})}{3}$$

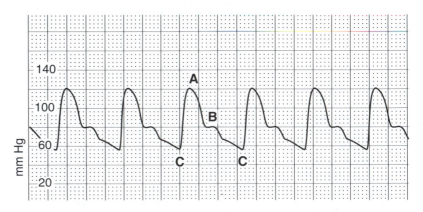

Figure 10-1 Normal arterial pressure waveform. The systolic and diastolic pressures are about 120 and 60 mm Hg, respectively. (A) Systolic peak; (B) Dicrotic notch.

A normal MAP of 60 mm Hg is considered the minimum pressure needed to maintain adequate tissue perfusion (Bustin, 1986). The diastolic value receives greater weight in this formula because the diastolic phase is about twice as long as the systolic phase. Accuracy of blood pressure readings depends on proper setup and calibration of the monitoring system.

stroke volume: *Blood volume pumped by the ventricles in one contraction.*

Since arterial pressure is the product of **stroke volume** (i.e., blood flow) and vascular resistance, changes in either parameter can affect the arterial pressure. Opposing changes of these two parameters (e.g., increase in stroke volume and decrease in vascular resistance) may present an unchanged arterial pressure or mean arterial pressure. Therefore, interpretation of arterial pressure measurements should take these two factors into consideration.

PULSE PRESSURE

Pulse pressure is the difference between arterial systolic and diastolic pressure. Since the arterial systolic and diastolic pressures are affected by stroke volume and vascular compliance, pulse pressure can be used to assess the gross changes in stroke volume and/or blood vessel compliance. High pulse pressure may occur in conditions where the stroke volume is high, blood vessel compliance is low, or heart rate is low. Low pulse pressure may occur in conditions where the stroke volume is low, blood vessel compliance is high, or heart rate is high (Christensen, 1992a, 1992b).

High Pulse Pressure. When the stroke volume is increased or the blood vessel compliance is decreased, there is a corresponding increase in systolic pressure. As long as the diastolic pressure does not increase by the same proportion, a high pulse pressure results. Bradycardia may also lead to a higher pulse pressure as a slow heart rate allows the blood volume more time for diastolic runoff and causes a lower diastolic pressure. The conditions that may lead to a high pulse pressure are summarized in Table 10-3.

Low Pulse Pressure. By the same mechanism, a decreased stroke volume or an increased blood vessel compliance leads to a corresponding decrease in systolic pressure. A low pulse pressure is seen as long as the diastolic pressure does not decrease by the same proportion.

TABLE 10-3   Conditions Leading to High Pulse Pressure

CONDITION	EXAMPLE
High stroke volume	Hypervolemia
Noncompliant blood vessel	Arteriosclerosis
Abnormal heart rate	Bradycardia

TABLE 10-4   Conditions Leading to Low Pulse Pressure

CONDITION	EXAMPLE
Low stroke volume	Hypovolemia
High compliance blood vessel	Shock
Abnormal heart rate	Tachycardia

Tachycardia may also lead to a lower pulse pressure because a high heart rate allows the blood volume less time for diastolic runoff and causes a higher diastolic pressure. The conditions leading to a low pulse pressure are summarized in Table 10-4.

POTENTIAL PROBLEMS WITH ARTERIAL CATHETER

Air bubbles and loose tubing connections can "dampen" the pressure signal. Improper leveling of the transducer and catheter can cause false high or false low readings. Inadequate pressure applied to the heparin solution bag can result in backup of blood in the tubing when the arterial pressure becomes higher than the heparin line pressure. Clotting of blood at the catheter tip or blockage of the catheter tip by the wall of the artery can interfere with the hemodynamic signal. The potential problems that are related to the arterial catheter are shown in Table 10-5.

Most intensive care units have standard procedures in place to ensure that such problems are kept to a minimum. Careful adherence to proper setup and calibration of hemodynamic monitoring equipment are essential.

TABLE 10-5   Potential Problems with Arterial Catheter

FACTORS	PROBLEM
Air bubbles in tubing Loose tubing connections	Dampens the pressure signal
Transducer and catheter placed higher than measurement site	Measurement lower than actual
Transducer and catheter placed lower than measurement site	Measurement higher than actual
Inadequate pressure applied to the heparin solution bag	Backup of blood in the tubing
Blood clot at catheter tip, catheter tip blocked by wall of artery	Inaccurate reading, signal interference

CENTRAL VENOUS CATHETER

✔ The CVP can also be monitored via the proximal port of a pulmonary artery catheter.

The central venous pressure (CVP) can be monitored through a central venous catheter placed either in the superior vena cava near the right atrium or in the right atrium. The pressure measured in the right atrium is correctly called right atrial pressure (RAP), but it is commonly called CVP.

The major advantage of the CVP in hemodynamic monitoring is to measure filling pressures in the right heart. The CVP is helpful in assessing fluid status and right heart function. However, it is often late to reflect changes in the left heart. The central venous catheter can also be used to collect "mixed" venous blood samples and for administration of medications and fluids. (Note: A true mixed venous blood sample should be obtained from the pulmonary artery via a pulmonary artery catheter.) Figure 10-2 shows the position of the catheter tip of a central venous catheter.

INSERTION OF CENTRAL VENOUS CATHETER

The central venous catheter is commonly inserted through the subclavian vein or the internal jugular vein. Correct placement of the central venous catheter may be assessed by the proper appearance of a venous pressure tracing on the monitor (Figure 10-3). Infection, bleeding, and pneumothorax are potential complications of CVP line insertion.

COMPONENTS OF CENTRAL VENOUS PRESSURE WAVEFORM

Figure 10-3 shows the tracing of a central venous (right atrial) pressure waveform and the corresponding ECG tracing. The upstroke *a* wave reflects right atrial contraction (follows the *p* wave on the ECG), *c* wave

Figure 10-2   Position of a central venous (right atrial) catheter.

Figure 10-3 Tracing of a central venous pressure waveform and its relationship to the electrocardiogram (ECG).

reflects closure of the tricuspid valve during systole (appears within the QRS complex on the ECG), x downslope occurs as the right atrium relaxes, v wave is caused by right ventricular contraction (appears at the T wave on the ECG), and y downslope reflects ventricular relaxation and rapid filling of blood from the right atrium to the right ventricle.

Abnormal Right Atrial Pressure Waveform. Since each wave or downslope on the right atrial waveform coincides with an event during systole or diastole, changes in the hemodynamic status of the heart will cause changes to certain components of the waveform, particularly the a and v waves (Schriner, 1989).

The a wave on the right atrial waveform may be elevated in conditions in which the resistance to right ventricular filling is increased. Examples include tricuspid valve stenosis, decreased right ventricular compliance due to ischemia or infarction, right ventricular volume overload or failure, pulmonic valve stenosis, and primary pulmonary hypertension. The a wave may be absent if atrial activity is absent or extremely weak.

Reflux of blood into the right atrium during contraction due to an incompetent triscupid valve will cause an elevated v wave. Elevation of a and v waves may be seen in conditions such as cardiac tamponade, volume overload, or left ventricular failure.

venous return:
Blood flow from the
systemic venous
circulation to the
right heart.

NORMAL CVP MEASUREMENT

CVP is reported as a mean pressure and its normal range in the vena cava is from 0 to 6 mm Hg. When the measurement is taken in the right atrium, the normal value range is from 2 to 7 mm Hg, slightly higher than the CVP reading (Christensen, 1992a, 1992b).

TABLE 10-6   Conditions That Affect the Central Venous Pressure

CHANGE	EXAMPLES
Decrease in CVP	Absolute hypovolemia (blood loss, dehydration)
	Relative hypovolemia (shock, vasodilation)
Increase in CVP	Positive pressure ventilation
	Increased **pulmonary vascular resistance**
	Hypervolemia
	Right ventricular failure
	Left ventricular failure (late change in CVP)

pulmonary vascular resistance: Resistance of the arterial system into which the right heart is pumping. Normal range is 50 to 150 dynes.sec/cm^5.

CHANGES IN CVP MEASUREMENT

Since **venous return** is determined by the pressure gradient between the mean arterial pressure and CVP, an increased CVP leads to a smaller pressure gradient and a lower blood return to the right heart. This condition is observed during positive pressure ventilation or as a result of right ventricular failure (e.g., reduced compliance of the ventricle after right-sided myocardial infarction). The conditions that may affect the CVP measurements are summarized in Table 10-6.

PULMONARY ARTERY CATHETER

The first pulmonary artery catheter was developed in 1953 and used in dogs by the U.S. physiologists Michael Lategola and Hermann Rahn. In the late 1960s, a more refined pulmonary artery catheter was developed and used in humans by the U.S. physicians Harold James Swan and William Ganz (Swan et al., 1970). The new pulmonary artery catheter (commonly called the Swan-Ganz catheter) is a flow-directed, balloon-tipped catheter. The addition of thermistor (for **cardiac output** measurement), and light reflective fiberoptic element (for mixed venous oxygen saturation measurement) to the catheter greatly expanded the scope and capability of hemodynamic monitoring.

cardiac output: Blood volume pumped by the heart in 1 min. Normal range is 4 to 8 L/min.

The pulmonary artery catheter is placed within the pulmonary artery, and it can measure the pulmonary arterial pressure (PAP) and the pulmonary capillary wedge pressure (PCWP). Since it is inserted at the same site as the CVP catheter, it has similar complications as well as additional ones related to balloon inflation, such as pulmonary artery hemorrhage and pulmonary infarction.

The pulmonary artery catheter (Figure 10-4) has a number of variations but typically it is 110 cm in length with three lumens (interior channels). The exterior of the catheter is marked off in 10-cm segments by thin and thick black lines to estimate the catheter tip location on insertion.

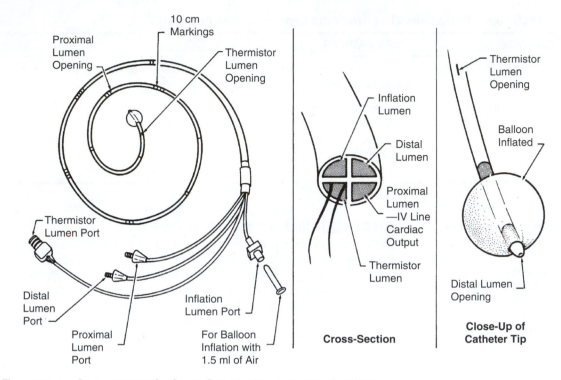

Figure 10-4 Components of a Swan-Ganz (pulmonary artery) catheter.

At the tip of the catheter there is an opening (PA distal lumen or port) connected with one lumen. About 30 cm back from the catheter tip there is another opening (proximal injectate port) connected to another lumen. When properly inserted, this proximal port is in the right atrium. Near the catheter tip is a small (1.5 cc maximum inflation volume) balloon connected to a lumen that allows for inflation of the balloon with a syringe. Also at the catheter tip is a thermistor (temperature sensing device) connected to a wire.

INSERTION OF PULMONARY ARTERY CATHETER

The pulmonary artery catheter is usually inserted into either the subclavian or internal jugular vein. From there, it is advanced to the superior vena cava and right atrium. The balloon is then inflated and the blood flow moves the catheter with its inflated balloon just as the wind moves a sail. The catheter proceeds to the right ventricle and into the pulmonary artery where it will eventually "wedge" in a smaller branch of the pulmonary artery. The balloon is then deflated and the catheter stabilized in place (Figure 10-5).

As the pulmonary artery catheter is being inserted, its movement can be followed on the bedside monitor by observing the various

Figure 10-5   Position of a pulmonary artery catheter.

pressure waveforms as the catheter passes freely from the right atrium (RA) to a wedged position in the pulmonary artery (Figure 10-6).

The balloon stays deflated and the PAP tracing remains on the monitor at all times. The balloon is inflated only when the pulmonary capillary wedge pressure is being taken.

COMPONENTS OF PULMONARY ARTERIAL PRESSURE WAVEFORM

The pulmonary arterial pressure waveform has three components: systolic phase, diastolic phase, and dicrotic notch. The dicrotic notch on the PAP waveform reflects closure of the semilunar valves at the end of contraction and prior to refilling of the ventricles. The slight elevation seen at the dicrotic notch represents the transient increase in pulmonary artery pressure due to backup of blood flow immediately following closure of the semilunar valves (Figure 10-7).

Abnormal Pulmonary Artery Waveform.   The systolic component of the pulmonary artery pressure waveform may be increased in conditions in which the pulmonary vascular resistance or pulmonary blood flow is increased. Obstruction in the left heart may also cause backup of blood flow in the pulmonary artery and an increase in pulmonary artery pressure (Schriner, 1989). An irregular pressure tracing on the pulmonary artery pressure waveform may be seen in arrhythmias due to changes in diastolic filling time and volume.

ABNORMAL PULMONARY ARTERIAL PRESSURE

Pulmonary arterial pressure (PAP) is measured when the pulmonary artery (Swan-Ganz) catheter is inside the pulmonary artery with the balloon deflated. The normal systolic PAP is about the same as the

☑ The dicrotic notch reflects closure of the semilunar valves at the end of contraction and prior to refilling of the ventricles.

☑ The systolic component of the PAP waveform may be increased in conditions in which the pulmonary vascular resistance or pulmonary blood flow is increased.

Figure 10-6 Waveform characteristics during advancement of pulmonary artery catheter. (A) Right atrium (RA) and right atrial (central venous) waveform; (B) Right ventricle (RV) and right ventricular waveform; (C) Pulmonary artery (PA) and pulmonary arterial waveform; and (D) Pulmonary capillary wedge (PCW) and pulmonary capillary wedge pressure waveform.

Figure 10-7 Pulmonary arterial pressure (PAP) waveform. (A) Beginning systole; (B) Dicrotic notch (closure of aortic valve); and (C) End-diastole.

☑ The normal
systolic PAP
ranges from 15 to
25 mm Hg. The
diastolic PAP normal
range is from 6 to 12
mm Hg.

right ventricular systolic pressure and ranges from 15 to 25 mm Hg. The normal diastolic PAP range is from 6 to 12 mm Hg.

Positive end-expiratory pressure (PEEP) can increase the PAP because overdistension of the alveoli compresses the surrounding capillaries and raises the capillary and arterial pressures (Versprille, 1990). Increase in pulmonary vascular resistance or pulmonary blood flow can also lead to an increased PAP, because the pressure measurement is directly related to the resistance and blood flow.

A higher than normal PAP may also be seen in left ventricular dysfunction such as left ventricular failure and mitral valve disease. This is because obstruction or backup of blood flow in the left heart leads to congestion in the pulmonary circulation. This is reflected as an elevated PAP.

On the other hand, the PAP may be decreased in conditions of hypovolemia or use of mechanical ventilation. When positive pressure ventilation is used on patients who have unstable hemodynamic status, it may lead to a depressed cardiac output, venous return, pulmonary circulating volume, and PAP (Versprille, 1990). The conditions that may affect the PAP are summarized in Table 10-7.

☑ Positive pres-
sure ventilation
causes a decrease
in the pulmonary
arterial pressure.

Effects of Positive Pressure Ventilation. Positive pressure ventilation causes a decrease of the pulmonary arterial pressure (Figure 10-8). This condition is due to the resultant decreased venous return to the right ventricle, lower right ventricular output, and lower blood volume (pressure) in the pulmonary arteries (Perkins et al., 1989; Versprille, 1990). In the absence of compensation by increasing the heart rate, decrease of right and left ventricular stroke volumes generally leads to a decreased cardiac output.

TABLE 10-7   Conditions That Affect the Pulmonary Arterial Pressure

PAP	CONDITIONS	EXAMPLES
Increase	Mechanical ventilation*	PEEP
	Increase in pulmonary vascular resistance	Pulmonary embolism Hypoxic vasoconstriction Primary pulmonary hypertension
	Increase in pulmonary blood flow	Hypervolemia Left to right shunt
	Left heart pathology	Left ventricular failure Mitral valve disease
Decrease	Mechanical ventilation*	Positive pressure ventilation
	Decrease in pulmonary blood flow	Hypovolemia

The effects of mechanical ventilation on the PAP are highly variable, depending on the interaction between the peak inspiratory pressure, PEEP, and patient's compliance and hemodynamic status.

☑ PCWP reflects the left ventricular preload.

PULMONARY CAPILLARY WEDGE PRESSURE

The pulmonary artery catheter is also used to measure the pulmonary capillary wedge pressure (PCWP). PCWP is measured by slowly inflating the balloon via the balloon inflation port on the pulmonary artery catheter. As the balloon inflates, the pulmonary arterial waveform on the monitor will change to the wedged pressure waveform (Figure 10-6D). Proper inflation of the balloon usually requires no more than 1.5 cc (0.75 to 1.5 cc depending on balloon size) of air. The balloon is deflated as soon as the reading of PCWP is made.

Positive Pressure Ventilation (without PEEP)
↓
Increase in Intrathoracic Pressure
↓
Decreased Venous Return
↓
Lower Right Ventricular Output
↓
Lower Blood Volume (Pressure) in the Pulmonary Artery

Note: When PEEP is used in conjunction with positive pressure ventilation, the PAP may not show a decrease because PEEP tends to increase the PAP by compressing the pulmonary vessels.

Figure 10-8   Effects of positive pressure ventilation.

☑ The PCWP reading is typically taken at end-expiration for both spontaneous breathing and mechanically ventilated patients.

The PCWP reading is typically taken at end-expiration for both spontaneous breathing and mechanically ventilated patients (Ahrens, 1991; Campbell et al., 1988). This practice should be done consistently for valid PCWP measurements and meaningful interpretation of hemodynamic data.

COMPONENTS OF PULMONARY CAPILLARY WEDGE PRESSURE WAVEFORM

The components of the PCWP waveform are similar to the CVP or right atrial waveform. When all of the components are present, the *a* wave of the PCWP waveform reflects left atrial contraction and *x* downslope represents the decrease in left atrial pressure following contraction. The *c* wave, if present, is seen along the *x* downslope and it occurs during closure of the mitral valve. The *v* wave indicates left ventricular contraction and passive atrial filling. The *y* downslope is due to the decrease in blood volume and pressure following the opening of the mitral valve (Figure 10-9).

Abnormal Pulmonary Capillary Wedge Pressure Waveform. Increased PCWP measurements are often observed in conditions where partial obstruction or excessive blood flow is present in the left heart (Schriner, 1989). Two common changes in the PCWP waveform are the *a* and *v* waves.

The *a* wave of the PCWP waveform may be increased in conditions leading to higher resistance to left ventricular filling. Some examples are mitral valve stenosis, left ventricular hypervolemia or failure, and decreased left ventricular compliance.

The *v* wave of the PCWP waveform may be increased due to mitral valve insufficiency. This condition leads to regurgitation (backward flow) of blood from the left ventricle to the left atrium through the incompetent mitral valve.

Figure 10-9 *Pulmonary capillary wedge pressure (PCWP) waveform. a wave: left atrial contraction; c wave (may be absent): closure of mitral valve; x downslope: decreased left atrial pressure following atrial contraction; v wave: left ventricular contraction and passive atrial filling; y downslope: decrease of blood volume (pressure) following the opening of mitral valve.*

ABNORMAL PULMONARY CAPILLARY WEDGE PRESSURE

✓ The normal PCWP ranges from 8 to 12 mm Hg.

The normal range for PCWP is from 8 to 12 mm Hg. Positive pressure ventilation or PEEP can affect wedge pressure readings since over-distension of the alveoli compresses the surrounding capillaries and raises the capillary and arterial pressures. A higher than normal wedge pressure may also be seen in left ventricular dysfunction. This is because left ventricular failure causes backup of blood flow in the left heart and pulmonary circulation. This is reflected as an elevated PCWP.

✓ The PCWP may be increased during positive pressure ventilation or in left ventricular dysfunction.

The PCWP measurement may be used to distinguish cardiogenic and noncardiogenic pulmonary edema. In pulmonary edema that is caused by left ventricular failure, the PCWP is usually elevated. When pulmonary edema occurs with a normal PCWP, it is probably due to an increase in capillary permeability as seen in ARDS. The conditions that may affect the PCWP measurements are outlined in Table 10-8.

VERIFICATION OF THE WEDGED POSITION

✓ Three methods may be used to confirm a properly wedged pulmonary artery catheter: PAP diastolic-PCWP gradient; postcapillary-mixed venous PO_2 gradient; and post-capillary-mixed venous O_2 saturation gradient.

Since artifact or dampened waveform may occur during inflation of the balloon, and it resembles that of a wedged pressure tracing, using the PCWP tracing alone on the monitor to verify the wedged position may not be always reliable. Three methods are available to confirm a properly wedged pulmonary artery catheter.

PAP Diastolic-PCWP Gradient. Under normal conditions, the PAP diastolic value is about 1 to 4 mm Hg higher than the average wedge pressure of the same individual (Daily et al., 1985). However, the PAP diastolic value may be lower than actual with forceful spontaneous inspiratory efforts. The PCWP may be higher than actual if there is significant downstream obstruction such as mitral valve disease (McGrath, 1986). These factors must be taken into account when

TABLE 10-8   Conditions That Affect the Pulmonary Capillary Wedge Pressure

PCWP	CONDITIONS	EXAMPLES
Increase	Increase in pulmonary blood flow	Hypervolemia
	Left heart pathology	Left ventricular failure; Mitral valve disease
	Mechanical factor	Overwedging of balloon
Decrease	Mechanical ventilation	PEEP
	Decrease in pulmonary blood flow	Hypovolemia

evaluating the pressure gradient between PAP diastolic pressure and PCWP.

Postcapillary-Mixed Venous PO₂ Gradient. The PO_2 of a blood gas sample from the distal opening of a properly wedged catheter should be at least 19 mm Hg higher than that from a systemic artery. The PCO_2 should be at least 11 mm Hg lower. These differences are expected because a properly wedged catheter does not allow mixing of shunted venous blood with the postcapillary blood. This procedure may not be feasible for a hypovolemic patient because up to 40 cc of waste (mixed venous) blood sample may be required before reaching the postcapillary blood sample (Morris et al., 1985).

Postcapillary-Mixed Venous O₂ Saturation Gradient. If the pulmonary artery catheter is capable of monitoring oxygen saturation by the oximetry method, the oxygen saturation value of a properly wedged catheter should be about 20% higher than the one recorded with the balloon deflated (Morris et al., 1985).

CARDIAC OUTPUT AND CARDIAC INDEX

☑ The normal cardiac output for an adult is from 4 to 8 L/min.

Another important value of the pulmonary artery catheter is its ability to measure cardiac output by the thermodilution technique. During cardiac output measurement, a small amount (10 mL) of iced or room temperature fluid (usually 5% dextrose in water, D5W) is injected into the proximal port of the pulmonary artery catheter. The temperature change of the blood flow is recorded as the flow passes by the thermistor at the catheter tip. This and other measurements are computed and the flow rate through the heart is displayed as cardiac output. The normal cardiac output for an adult is from 4 to 8 L/min.

*cardiac index (C.I):
A cardiac output measurement relative to a person's body size.*

☑ The cardiac index is normally 2.5 to 3.5 L/min/m².

Since cardiac output normally varies from person to person depending on the size of the individual, it is common to "index" the value by dividing cardiac output (C.O.) by body surface area (BSA). The **cardiac index** (C.I.) is normally 2.5 to 3.5 $L/min/m^2$ and it is calculated as follows:

$$C.I. = C.O. / BSA$$

SUMMARY OF PRELOADS AND AFTERLOADS

Each ventricle has its own preload and afterload measurements. Their meaning and common pathologic implications are shown in Table 10-9.

TABLE 10-9   Ventricular Preloads and Afterloads

DEVICE (MEASUREMENT)	MAIN IMPLICATION	EXAMPLES
Arterial catheter (Left ventricular afterload)	Condition of systemic arterial pressure	Arterial pressure is increased in systemic hypertension or fluid overload. Arterial pressure is decreased in systemic hypotension or fluid depletion.
Central venous catheter (Right ventricular preload)	Condition of systemic venous return	Central venous pressure (CVP) is increased in systemic hypertension or hypervolemia. CVP is decreased in systemic hypotension or hypovolemia.
Pulmonary artery catheter (Right ventricular afterload)	Condition of pulmonary artery	Pulmonary artery pressure (PAP) is increased in pulmonary hypertension or blood flow obstruction in left heart. PAP is decreased in pulmonary hypotension.
Pulmonary artery catheter (Balloon inflated) (Left ventricular preload)	Condition of left heart	Pulmonary capillary wedge pressure (PCWP) is increased in left heart blood flow obstruction. PCWP is decreased in severe hypotension or dehydration.

CALCULATED HEMODYNAMIC VALUES

From the CVP, PAP, and other related measurements, the following parameters may be calculated: stroke volume and stroke volume index, oxygen consumption and oxygen consumption index, pulmonary vascular resistance, and **systemic vascular resistance.**

systemic vascular resistance: Resistance of the arterial system into which the left heart is pumping. Normal range is 800 to 1,500 dynes.sec/cm^5.

STROKE VOLUME AND STROKE VOLUME INDEX

Stroke volume (S.V.) is calculated by dividing the cardiac output (C.O.) by the heart rate (HR). The stroke volume index is calculated by dividing the stroke volume by the body surface area (BSA).

$$S.V. = \frac{C.O.}{HR}$$

$$S.V.I. = \frac{S.V.}{BSA}$$

☑ The stroke volume is determined by three factors: contractility, preload, and afterload.

contractility: *Pumping strength of the heart. Contractility may be increased by improving the blood volume or by positive inotropic medications.*

The stroke volume is determined by three factors: **contractility,** preload, and afterload. Contractility is the pumping strength of the heart. Some conditions that may lower the contractility of the heart include extremes of myocardial compliance (too high or too low), and excessive end-diastolic volume. Preload is the end-diastolic stretch of cardiac muscle fiber, expressed in pressure units (mm Hg or cm H_2O). Hypovolemia and shock are two conditions that usually cause a decreased preload. Afterload is the tension or pressure that develops in the ventricle during systole (contraction), expressed in pressure units (mm Hg or cm H_2O). Afterload is usually increased in conditions of downstream flow obstruction or excessive volume.

OXYGEN CONSUMPTION AND OXYGEN CONSUMPTION INDEX

The oxygen consumption reflects the amount of oxygen consumed in 1 min. The oxygen consumption index is used to reflect the amount of oxygen used relative to the body size. They are calculated as follows:

$$VO_2 = Q_T \times C(a\text{--}\dot{v})O_2$$

$$VO_2 \text{ index } = \frac{VO_2}{BSA}$$

PULMONARY VASCULAR RESISTANCE

The pulmonary vascular resistance (PVR) measures the blood vessel resistance to blood flow in the pulmonary circulation. For example, PVR is elevated in pulmonary hypertension or left heart obstruction (e.g., mitral valve stenosis).

$$PVR = \frac{(PAP - PCWP) \times 80}{C.O.}$$

SYSTEMIC VASCULAR RESISTANCE

The systemic vascular resistance (SVR) measures the blood vessel resistance to blood flow in the systemic circulation. For example, SVR is elevated in systemic hypertension.

$$SVR = \frac{(MAP - RAP) \times 80}{C.O.}$$

MONITORING OF MIXED VENOUS OXYGEN SATURATION

A special version of the pulmonary artery catheter uses fiberoptic technology to enable monitoring of mixed venous oxygen saturation ($S\dot{v}O_2$). The fiberoptic central venous catheter measures the $S\dot{v}O_2$

accurately well within the clinical range (between 50% and 80%) (Fletcher, 1988). $S\dot{v}O_2$ had been used to reflect a patient's cardiac output and cardiac index status even before thermodilution cardiac output became common practice (Muir, 1970; Waller, 1982). When $S\dot{v}O_2$ is used with other monitoring capabilities of the pulmonary artery catheter, it can provide valuable data concerning oxygen delivery and consumption.

DECREASE IN MIXED VENOUS OXYGEN SATURATION

☑ The normal $S\dot{v}O_2$ is about 75%. $S\dot{v}O_2$ of less than 60% is indicative of hypoxemia, decrease in cardiac output, or increase in peripheral oxygen consumption.

For normal individuals, the measured $S\dot{v}O_2$ is between 68% and 77% with an average of 75% (McMichan, 1983). $S\dot{v}O_2$ of less than 60% is indicative of hypoxemia, decrease in cardiac output, or increase in peripheral oxygen consumption (McMichan, 1983). It reflects an imbalance between oxygen supply, oxygen demand, and use of venous oxygen reserve (Mims, 1989).

Common causes of decreased $S\dot{v}O_2$ due to poor oxygen supply include inadequate cardiac output, anemia, and hypoxic hypoxia. Causes of decreased $S\dot{v}O_2$ due to excessive oxygen use include fever, seizures, increased physical activity or work of breathing. Some conditions that may lead to a decreased $S\dot{v}O_2$ are summarized in Table 10-10.

TABLE 10-10   Conditions That Affect the $S\dot{v}O_2$ Measurement

$S\dot{v}O_2$	CONDITIONS	EXAMPLES
Decrease	Poor oxygen supply	Inadequate cardiac output Anemia Hypoxic hypoxia
	Excessive oxygen demand	Fever Seizures Increased metabolic rate Increased physical activity
	Depletion of venous oxygen reserve	Severe and prolonged hypoxia
Increase	Technical problem	Improperly wedged catheter
	Impaired oxygen utilization	Sepsis Cyanide poisoning
	Decrease in oxygen demand	Hypothermia Postanesthesia Pharmacologic paralysis

INCREASE IN MIXED VENOUS OXYGEN SATURATION

✔️ Increases in $S\dot{v}O_2$ above 75% are uncommon but may occur when the tip of the pulmonary artery catheter is improperly wedged.

Increases in $S\dot{v}O_2$ above 75% are uncommon but may occur when the tip of the pulmonary artery catheter is improperly wedged. Once in this abnormal position, the forward mixed venous blood flow is obstructed while the catheter tip senses the blood from an area with a high ventilation/perfusion ratio, and therefore a high oxygen level (Briones, 1988).

An increased $S\dot{v}O_2$ may also be observed in patients with sepsis or cyanide poisoning in which the tissues become unable to utilize oxygen (White, 1987). The mechanism of hypoxia for sepsis is due to peripheral shunting. Cyanide poisoning causes histotoxic hypoxia that renders the tissues unable to carry out aerobic metabolism. These patients may have normal PaO_2, SaO_2, CaO_2, and oxygen transport but they are often hypoxic. Lactic acidosis is a common event for these patients (Mims, 1989). Some conditions that may lead to an increased $S\dot{v}O_2$ are summarized in Table 10-10.

IMPEDANCE CARDIOGRAPHY

Impedance cardiography (ICG): a noninvasive procedure to measure or trend the hemodynamic status of a patient.

Impedance cardiography (ICG), also called thoracic electrical bioimpedance (TEB), is based on a technology originally used by NASA in the 1960s. The introduction of microprocessor and the working knowledge of echocardiography and magnetic resonance imaging make ICG possible. ICG is a noninvasive procedure to measure or trend the hemodynamic status of a patient in clinical settings ranging from critical care to out-patient care. Several noninvasive ICG devices are available and each offers different technology to measure and calculate the hemodynamic values.

The *IQ* system (Wantagh Incorporated, Bristol, MA) uses a patented signal processing technique to identify the opening and closing of the aorta valve for the precise measurement of the ventricular ejection time (VET). Another device incorporates "ensemble averaging" to estimate the VET by using the QRS of the ECG and the raw dZ/dt (change in impedance/time) waveform (SORBA Medical Systems, Inc., Brookfield, WI). A third manufacturer of ICG (BioZ System, CardioDynamics, San Diego, CA) uses digital signal processing and an R wave detection system to establish the dZ/dt. ICG has proven to be a simple and accurate method to measure and monitor a patient's hemodynamic status (Clancy et al., 1991).

THEORY OF OPERATION

✔️ ICG uses external electrodes to input a high frequency, low amplitude current and measure changes of electrical resistance (impedance) in the thorax.

ICG uses external electrodes to input a high frequency, low amplitude current and measure changes of electrical resistance (impedance) in the thorax. In a typical setup, four outer and four inner electrodes are

Figure 10-10 Typical placement of impedance cardiography (ICG) electrodes

placed on the patient as shown in Figure 10-10. The outer electrodes transmit a constant, low amplitude electrical current through the thorax. The inner electrodes measure the impedance (resistance) to the electrical signal according to the changing blood flow in the aorta.

The volume and velocity of blood flow in the ascending aorta changes with each cardiac cycle—increasing volume and velocity

Figure 10-11 Impedance cardiography waveforms. Z—pulse contour curve; dZ/dt—impedance curve; ECG—electrocardiogram curve; dZ/dt$_{max}$—maximum value of the first derivative of the impedance curve; A—opening of the aortic valve; B—maximum systolic value; X—closing of the aortic valve; C—opening of the pulmonic valve; T$_{lve}$—left ventricle ejection time.

TABLE 10-11   Hemodynamic Parameters Provided by Impedance Cardiography

MEASURED	CALCULATED
Heart rate	Stroke volume/index
Thoracic fluid content	Cardiac output/index
Mean arterial pressure[a]	Systemic vascular resistance/index
Acceleration index[b]	Left cardiac work/index
Velocity index[c]	Left stroke work/index
Pre-ejection period[d]	
Left ventricular ejection time[e]	

[a]If automatic blood pressure (oscillometric method) is used.
[b]Acceleration of blood flow in the aorta within the first 10 to 20 m/sec after the opening of the aortic valve.
[c]Peak blood flow velocity in the aorta.
[d]Time interval from the beginning of electrical stimulation of the ventricles to the opening of the aortic valve (electrical systole).
[e]Time interval from the opening to the closing of the aortic valve (mechanical systole).

✓ Since the impedance changes reflect the blood flow in the ascending aorta during systole and asystole, the changes in blood velocity are calculated and reported as values for different hemodynamic parameters.

during systole and decreasing volume and velocity during asystole. Since the impedance changes reflect the blood flow in the ascending aorta, the changes in blood velocity are calculated and reported as values for different hemodynamic parameters. Figure 10-11 shows the graphics from an ICP.

THERMODILUTION METHOD AND ICG

Thermodilution is the most commonly used invasive technique for measuring and calculating the hemodynamic values. The accuracy and reliability of this method rely on the proper (and correct) computation constant, injectate volume, injectate temperature measurement, injection technique, timing of injection, and averaging strategies (Wantagh Inc., 2004). Since the thermodilution method provides hemodynamic measurements in a limited time frame, it cannot be used to monitor the dynamic nature of the cardiovascular system.

✓ Some parameters provided by ICG include: cardiac output, cardiac index, stroke volume, stroke volume index, systemic vascular resistance, systemic vascular resistance index, contractility, and fluid status.

The noninvasive nature of ICG makes it an ideal tool to monitor a patient's hemodynamic status. Some of the measured and calculated hemodynamic parameters provided by ICG include: cardiac output, cardiac index, stroke volume, stroke volume index, systemic vascular resistance, systemic vascular resistance index, contractility, and fluid status. Table 10-11 lists some hemodynamic parameters provided by ICG.

Unlike the thermodilution method in which a pulmonary artery catheter is used, ICG cannot provide the values for pulmonary artery pressure, pulmonary artery wedge pressure, pulmonary vascular resistance, and pulmonary vascular resistance index.

☑ The correlation of cardiac output determined by ICG versus the Fick method and the thermodilution method were 0.84 and 0.80, respectively.

☑ Technical and measurement errors of ICG include: wrong placement of electrodes, abnormal body structure, tachycardia, presence of pacemaker, arrhythmias, open heart or aorta surgery, abnormal cardiac anatomy, abnormal hematocrit, and pleural effusion.

☑ ICG provides these advantages: noninvasive continuous monitoring, rapid diagnosis and assessment of cardiopulmonary status, hemodynamic response to fluids and drugs, availability outside the critical care area.

ACCURACY OF ICG

Many studies have been done to compare and validate the accuracy of ICG with other methods of hemodynamic monitoring (Drazner et al., 2002; Ziegler et al., 1999). In a study of patients with pulmonary arterial hypertension, the correlation of cardiac output determined by ICG versus the Fick method and the thermodilution method were 0.84 and 0.80, respectively (Yung et al., 2004). These correlation indices are similar to the results of other studies using different patient populations. Since ICG is less variable and more reproducible than other invasive methods, it has shown sufficient clinical usefulness to become a standard practice in noninvasive hemodynamic evaluations (Van De Water et al., 2003).

Methodology Errors. While ICP is useful in many clinical situations, there are some technical reasons and conditions that may influence the use and accuracy of ICG (Braždžionytė et al., 2004a). They include wrong placement of electrodes; abnormal body structure (cachetic or obese); tachycardia (>120/min); presence of pacemaker; arrhythmias; open heart or aorta surgery; abnormal cardiac anatomy (e.g., transpositions, aneurysms); abnormal hematocrit; and pleural effusion.

CLINICAL APPLICATIONS

With ICG, the therapeutic effects of fluid administration and resuscitation can be assessed by monitoring the stroke volume and cardiac output. ICG has also been used to evaluate the hemodynamic status of critically ill patients in the intensive care units, surgical areas, and outpatient and emergency departments (Bishop et al., 1996; Milzman et al., 1997; Shoemaker et al., 1994; Wo et al., 1995; Yancey, 2003). Evaluation and follow-up of patients with acute myocardial infarction is also possible with ICG (Braždžionytė et al., 2004b).

In subacute care, adjustment of the dosages of cardiovascular drugs can be done by monitoring the thoracic fluid status, stroke volume, and cardiac output (Franz, 1996). Since ICG monitoring is noninvasive, it can be used in outpatients as well as patients at home. The general advantages of ICG are listed in Table 10-12.

TABLE 10-12   Advantages of Impedance Cardiography

Reduces risk associated with invasive hemodynamic monitoring procedures

Provides rapid diagnosis and assessment of cardiopulmonary status

Offers continuous noninvasive hemodynamic monitoring

Monitors patient's hemodynamic response to fluids and drugs

Reduces use and risk associated with PA catheterization

Reduces cost over invasive hemodynamic monitoring procedures

Provides availability outside the hospital

SUMMARY

In order to monitor and use hemodynamic waveforms efficiently, one must remember the normal values and recognize the characteristics of normal waveforms. It is only with constant clinical practice that one may learn the intricacies and interactions of those variables that affect hemodynamic waveforms.

It is also essential to realize that monitoring of hemodynamic waveforms should be done on a continuous basis. Impedance cardiography makes this possible. Isolated and independent observations are of limited value since they do not provide a trend of changing events or patient conditions.

Self-Assessment Questions

1. In hemodynamic monitoring, the pressure measurement made inside a blood vessel is dependent on all of the following factors *except* the:

   A. blood volume.
   B. blood flow.
   C. size of blood vessel.
   D. barometric pressure.

2. During hemodynamic monitoring, the transducer, catheter, and measurement site are usually aligned at the same level. This is done to ensure that the measurements are not affected by the effect of:

   A. barometric pressure.
   B. gravity.
   C. fluid level.
   D. transducer sensitivity.

3. In the arterial pressure waveform shown, the dicrotic notch is labeled as _____ and it is caused by the _____. (See Figure 10-12.)

   A. A, opening of the aortic valve
   B. B, closure of the semilunar valves
   C. B, closure of the pulmonic valve
   D. C, closure of the semilunar valves

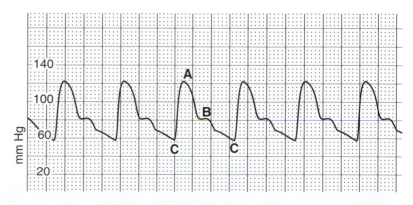

Figure 10-12 Arterial pressure waveform.

4. As you are caring for a ventilator patient, the arterial pressure waveform shows a decreasing systolic pressure and a stable diastolic pressure. Based on these two pressure measurements, the pulse pressure is _____. This condition may be caused by _____.

    A. increasing, shock
    B. increasing, hypervolemia
                              C. decreasing, bradycardia
                              D. decreasing, arteriosclerosis

5 to 7. Matching: Refer to the central venous pressure waveform (Figure 10-13) and match the wave or slope with the proper events during a cardiac cycle. Use only three of the five answers provided.

WAVE OR SLOPE	CORRESPONDING EVENT
5. *a*	A. Ventricular relaxation
6. *c*	B. Atrial contraction
7. *v*	C. Ventricular contraction
	D. Relaxation of right atrium
	E. Closure of tricuspid valve during systole

8. As you review a patient's chart, you notice that the central venous pressure readings have been decreasing from an average of 6 to 2 mm Hg. This condition may be caused by all of the following conditions *except*:

    A. positive pressure ventilation.
    B. blood or fluid depletion.
                              C. shock.
                              D. vasodilation.

9. Which of the following outlines the proper sequence for the placement of a Swan-Ganz catheter?

    A. femoral vein, left atrium, left ventricle, pulmonary artery
    B. internal jugular vein, left atrium, left ventricle, pulmonary artery
    C. femoral artery, right atrium, right ventricle, pulmonary artery
    D. subclavian vein, right atrium, right ventricle, pulmonary artery

Figure 10-13 Central venous pressure waveform.

10 to 13. Matching: Match the type of catheter with the intended hemodynamic measurements.

CATHETER	HEMODYNAMIC MEASUREMENT
10. Arterial catheter	A. Left ventricular preload
11. Central venous catheter	B. Left ventricular afterload
12. Pulmonary artery catheter with balloon deflated	C. Right ventricular preload
13. Pulmonary artery catheter with balloon inflated	D. Right ventricular afterload

14. Mr. Jones, a patient in the coronary care unit being treated for congestive heart failure, has a pulmonary artery catheter in place and the $S\dot{v}O_2$ is 55%. This $S\dot{v}O_2$ value is _____ and it may be caused by _____.

    A. too high, increase in cardiac output
    B. too high, increase in peripheral oxygen consumption
    C. too low, decrease in cardiac output
    D. too low, decrease in peripheral oxygen consumption

15. Impedance cardiography (ICP) is a noninvasive technique capable of monitoring all of the following hemodynamic values *except*:

    A. thoracic fluid volume.
    B. cardiac output.
    C. pulmonary artery pressure.
    D. systemic vascular resistance.

Answers to Self-Assessment Questions

1. D. barometric pressure.

2. B. gravity.

3. C. B, closure of the pulmonic valve

4. A. increasing, shock

5. B. Atrial contraction

6. E. Closure of tricuspid valve during systole

7. C. Ventricular contraction

8. A. positive pressure ventilation.

9. D. subclavian vein, right atrium, right ventricle, pulmonary artery

10. B. Left ventricular afterload

11. C. Right ventricular preload

12. D. Right ventricular afterload

13. A. Left ventricular preload

14. C. too low, decrease in cardiac output

15. C. pulmonary artery pressure.

References

Ahrens, T. S. (1991). Effects of mechanical ventilation on hemodynamic waveforms. *Crit Care Nurs Clin North Am, 3*, 629–639.

Bishop, M., et al. (1996). Noninvasive cardiac index monitoring in gunshot wound victims. *Acad Emerg Med, 7*, 682–688.

Braždžionytė, J., et al. (2004a). Noninvasive monitoring of central hemodynamics in acute myocardial infarction: A comparison of hemodynamic indices obtained by two different methods—impedance cardiography and transthoracic echocardiography. *Semin Cardiol, 10*(1), 25–32.

Braždžionytė, J., et al. (2004b). Routine noninvasive hemodynamic monitoring in acute myocardial infarction: Application possibilities. *Crit Care, 8*(Suppl. 1), 63.

Briones, T. L. (1988). SvO_2 monitoring: Part I. Clinical case application. *Dim Crit Care Nurs, 7*, 70–78.

Bustin, D. (1986). *Hemodynamic monitoring for critical care.* Norwalk, CT: Appleton-Century-Crofts.

Campbell, M. L., et al. (1988). Reading pulmonary artery wedge pressure at end-expiration. *Focus Crit Care, 15*, 60–63.

Christensen, B. (1992a). Hemodynamic monitoring: What it tells you and what it doesn't, Part I. *J Post Anesth Nurs, 7*(5), 330–337.

Christensen, B. (1992b). Hemodynamic monitoring: What it tells you and what it doesn't, Part II. *J Post Anesth Nurs, 7*(5), 338–345.

Clancy, T. V., et al. (1991). Cardiac output measurement in critical care patients: Thoracic electrical bioimpedance versus thermodilution. *J Trauma, 31*, 1116–1119.

Daily, E. K., et al. (1985). *Techniques in bedside hemodynamic monitoring.* St. Louis, MO: Mosby.

Drazner, M., et al. (2002). Comparison of impedance cardiography with invasive hemo-dynamic measurements in patients with heart failure secondary to ischemic or nonischemic cardiomyopathy. *Am J Cardiol, 89*(8), 993–995.

Fletcher, E. C. (1988). Accuracy of fiberoptic central venous saturation catheter below 50%. *J Appl Physiol, 64*(5), 2220–2223.

Franz, A. K. (1996). Home cardiac monitoring and technology. In Gorski L. (Ed.), *High tech home care manual* (Vol. 19, Suppl. 2, pp. 1–18), Rockville, MD: Aspen Publishing.

Keckeisen, M. (1991). Techniques for measuring arterial pressure in the postoperative cardiac surgery patient. *Crit Care Nurs Clin North Am, 3,* 699–708.

McGrath, R. B. (1986). Invasive bedside hemodynamic monitoring. *Prog Cardiovasc Dis, 29,* 129–144.

McMichan, J. C. (1983). Continuous monitoring of mixed venous oxygen saturation. In J. F. Schweiss (Ed.), *Continuous measurement of blood oxygen saturation in the high risk patient* (pp. 27–44). San Diego, CA: Beach International.

Milzman, D., et al. (1997). Continuous noninvasive cardiac output monitoring quantifies acute congestive heart failure in the emergency department. *Crit Care Med, 25,* A47.

Mims, B. C. (1989). Physiologic rationale of SvO_2 monitoring. *Crit Care Nurs Clin North Am, 1,* 619–628.

Morris, A. H., et al. (1985). Wedge pressure confirmation by aspiration of pulmonary capillary blood. *Crit Care Med, 13,* 756–759.

Muir, A. L. (1970). Mixed venous oxygen saturation in relation to cardiac output in myocardial infarction. *Br Med J, 4,* 276.

Perkins, M. W., et al. (1989). Physiologic implications of mechanical ventilation on pharma-cokinetics. *DICP, The Annals of Pharmacotherapy, 23,* 316–323.

Schriner, D. K. (1989). Using hemodynamic waveforms to assess cardiopulmonary patholo-gies. *Crit Care Nurs Clin North Am, 1,* 563–575.

Shoemaker, W. C., et al. (1994). Multicenter trial of a new thoracic electrical impedance device for cardiac output estimation. *Crit Care Med, 22,* 1907–1912.

Swan, H. J., et al. (1970). Catheterization of the heart in man with the use of a flow directed balloon-tipped catheter. *N Engl J Med, 283,* 447–451.

Van De Water, J. M., et al. (2003). Impedance cardiography: The next vital sign technology? *Chest, 123*(6), 2028–2033.

Versprille, V. (1990). The pulmonary circulation during mechanical ventilation. *Acta Anaesthesiol Scand, 34* (Suppl. 94*),* 51–62.

Waller, J. L. (1982). Clinical evaluation of a new fiberoptic catheter during cardiac surgery. *Anesth Analg, 61,* 676.

Wantagh Inc. (2005). Patented 3-dimensional signal processing. Retrieved May 19, 2005, from http://wantagh-inc.com/3d-signal.htm

White, K. M. (1987). Continuous monitoring of mixed venous oxygen saturation (SvO_2): A new assessment tool in critical care nursing—Part II. *Cardiovasc Nurs, 23,* 7–12.

Wo, C., et al. (1995). Noninvasive estimations of cardiac output and circulatory dynamics in critically ill patients. *Curr Sci, 1,* 211–218.

Yancey, C. (2003). Noninvasive hemodynamic monitoring in heart failure: Utilization of impedance cardiography. *Congest Heart Fail, 9*(5), 241–250.

Yung, G. L., et al. (2004). Comparison of impedance cardiography to direct Fick and thermodilution cardiac output determination in pulmonary arterial hypertension. *CHF, 10*(2 Suppl. 2), 7–10.

Ziegler, D., et al. (1999). Comparison of cardiac output measurements by TEB vs. intermittent bolus thermodilution in mechanical ventilated patients. *Chest, 116*(4), 281S.

CHAPTER ELEVEN

VENTILATOR WAVEFORM ANALYSIS

Frank Dennison

OUTLINE

KEY TERMS

- airway opening pressure (P_{AO})
- alveolar pressure (P_{ALV})
- constant flow waveform (CFW)
- controlled mechanical ventilation (CMV)
- descending ramp flow waveform (DRFW)
- expiratory time (T_E)
- flow-volume loop (FVL)
- lung-thorax compliance (C_{LT})
- peak alveolar pressure (Peak P_{ALV}; plateau pressure)
- peak inspiratory pressure (PIP)
- plateau pressure (Peak P_{ALV}; peak alveolar pressure)
- pressure-controlled ventilation (PCV)
- pressure-volume loop (PVL)
- inspiratory time (T_I)
- inverse ratio pressure-controlled ventilation (IRPCV)
- synchronized intermittent mandatory ventilation (SIMV)
- tidal volume (V_T)
- total cycle time (TCT)
- transairway pressure (P_{TA})
- volume-controlled ventilation (VCV)

INTRODUCTION

The advent of waveform (graphic) analysis marked the beginning of a new and exciting era in ventilator-patient management for respiratory care professionals. Waveforms give us the capacity to observe and document real-time measurements of patient-ventilator interactions.

In the past, many problematic interactions between the patient and ventilator that were suspected could not be confirmed without sophisticated equipment and time-consuming effort. Now, someone skilled at analyzing waveforms can evaluate patient-ventilator synchrony, ventilator function, pulmonary status, and appropriateness of ventilator adjustments in a matter of seconds. Also, hard copies of graphics depicting improvements in pulmonary function, ventilator management, and respiratory care can be documented. It should be common practice for practitioners to use waveforms to assist in ventilator-patient assessment and management.

To develop expertise in waveform analysis requires an in-depth understanding of the principles that govern the shape of waveforms, the characteristics of the scalars measured: flow, pressure, and volume over time, and the dynamics of the ventilator-patient interface. Skill in analysis can be developed through mathematical analysis, laboratory exercises, and clinical practice. Refer to Table 11-1 as a reference for abbreviations used in this chapter.

Prior to clinical practice, it is very helpful to observe graphics while simulating patient-ventilator interactions using training test lungs under varied conditions of lung compliance and circuit/airway resistance. Graphics should always be displayed in the ICU for observation of results when implementing adjustments and therapy to mechanically ventilated patients. This chapter provides the reader an appreciation for waveform analysis, and the knowledge necessary for improved ventilator-patient management.

TABLE 11-1 Key Abbreviations

C_{LT}	Lung-thorax compliance
CFW	Constant flow waveform
CMV	Controlled mechanical ventilation
DRFW	Descending ramp flow waveform
FVL	Flow-volume loop
IRPCV	Inverse ratio pressure-controlled ventilation
P_{ALV}	Alveolar pressure
P_{AO}	Airway opening pressure
P_{TA}	Transairway pressure
PCV	Pressure-controlled ventilation
Peak P_{ALV}	Peak alveolar pressure; plateau pressure
PIP	Peak inspiratory pressure
PVL	Pressure-volume loop
SIMV	Synchronized intermittent mandatory ventilation
T_E	Expiratory time
T_I	Inspiratory time
TCT	Total cycle time
VCV	Volume-controlled ventilation
V_T	Tidal volume

FLOW WAVES USED FOR POSITIVE PRESSURE VENTILATION

Flow, pressure, and volume are the three variables measured and displayed by graphics in real time. **Pressure-volume loops** and **flow-volume loops** are also available. Depending on conditions, modes, or manufacturers, six distinct flow patterns can be set or developed during positive-pressure ventilation (PPV). Figure 11-1 shows the **constant flow waveform (CFW),** the convex rise (dotted line) in flow; the descending ramp or concave pattern (dotted line), the ascending ramp and sine flow patterns. The CFW can present a convex pattern (dotted line) if the rise time to peak flow is slowed for patient comfort during **volume-controlled ventilation (VCV).** What is commonly called the decelerating flow waveform is more appropriately called a **descending ramp flow waveform (DRFW)** (Chatburn, 2001). Depending on the manufacturer, a ventilator may offer a "true" DRFW that descends from the initial peak flow level to zero-end-flow as presented in Figure 11-1, or one that descends to some preset end-flow level above baseline. During pressure-limited ventilation, a

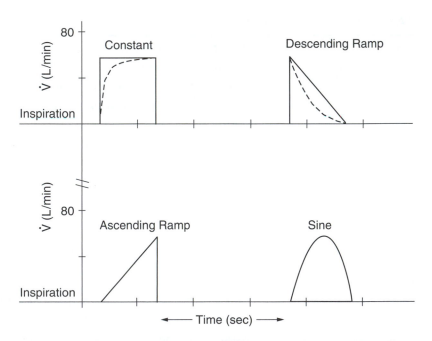

Figure 11-1 Six flow waveforms available for positive pressure ventilation: constant flow, convex constant flow pattern (dotted line), descending ramp, concave descending ramp pattern (dotted line), ascending ramp, and sine flow pattern.

DRFW may present an exponential decay or concave pattern (dotted line) depending on lung characteristics and patient demand.

The ascending ramp and sine (also called sinusoidal) waveforms are seldom used or available for PPV because the initial flow rate is not sufficient to accommodate synchronized assisted ventilation for most patients. The fast rise to peak flow offered by the CFW and DRFW patterns has proven to be superior in meeting patient flow demands in clinic and research.

The use of the sine or ascending flow waveforms may be appropriate for controlled ventilation where initial flow demand is not an issue. When a patient is heavily sedated and there is no demand for flow, the slow rise to peak flow levels may improve lung gas distribution. When there is variable resistance in diseased airways throughout the lungs, gas follows the path of lease resistance, preferentially ventilating normal lung parenchyma. Utilizing slower flow rates or rise time to peak flow levels may reduce flow resistance and improve gas distribution to the poorly ventilated areas of the lung. During assisted ventilation, however, there is a time lag between patient demand for flow (ventilator inspiratory valve opening response time) and time for gas flow to reach demand level. When the initial flow level is set higher than demanded, it will compensate for the time lag (Marini et al., 1985). Thus, during assisted ventilation with sine or ascending flow, the slower rise to peak flow may not be adequate to facilitate ventilator-patient synchrony.

EFFECTS OF CONSTANT FLOW DURING VOLUME-CONTROLLED VENTILATION

Figure 11-2 displays two theoretical sets of waveforms, a set of ideal flow and pressure (y-axis) waveforms contiguous in time (x-axis), and another set of waves with characteristic changes made for comparison. Both sets of waveforms represent mandatory breaths. Inspiration is begun (triggered), volume or flow controlled (limited), and ended (cycled) by the ventilator. The letters represent the various components and phase variables of a breath recorded by flow- and pressure-time graphics (Chatburn, 2001).

FLOW-TIME WAVEFORM

In the first flow-time waveform (Figure 11-2, left), the letters represent the four phases of the ventilatory cycle, the period of time from the beginning of one breath and the beginning of the next. Letter *a* represents the end of expiration and the beginning of inspiration where flow is either ventilator or time triggered. It is always a positive

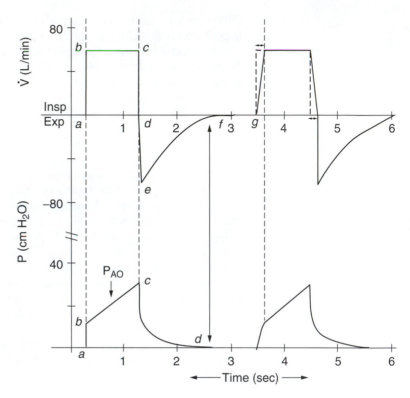

Figure 11-2 Two sets of flow- and pressure-time waveforms. The letters in the first set (left) mark the various phases of the respiratory cycle (see text). The second set (right) shows a delay in rise time to peak flow.

upward stroke on ventilator graphics. Letter *b* marks the inspiration phase with a peak and constant flow of 60 L/min.

Letter *c* marks the change from inspiration to expiration where the breath is volume or time cycled into expiration. The inspiratory flow waveforms represent conceptual or idealized waveforms. The initial flow cannot reach the peak flow level instantaneously. No ventilator can "square off" flow and pressure waveforms as they are presented in textbooks, or by ventilator graphic software. Realistic waveforms will have more rounded or slightly jagged corners and variable patterns (so-called noise) with transitive changes in flow and pressure as inspiratory and expiratory valves make rapid adjustments in flow rates. Noise, however, is mitigated by reducing the number of data sampled (measured) per second and digitized by the ventilator's hardware for graphic presentation. Approximately 30 to 50 samples of flow or pressure measurements are digitized per second, which creates smoother appearing lines, slopes, and curves for graphic representation of waveforms. Higher sampling rates would be costly. Greater attention to minor fluctuations in measurements and details is not necessary clinically, nor for graphic presentations in textbooks to learn the concepts and major principles involved with waveform analysis. Thus, minor details to graphics have been omitted for ease of presentation as well as mathematical analysis. Clinically relevant exceptions will be presented and explained.

Letter *d* depicts expiration, the fourth phase of the ventilatory cycle, which is always to the lower side of baseline or zero flow. Letter *e* represents the peak expiratory flow attained (60 L/min), which is assigned a negative value on graphics. The expiratory flow from peak end flow is normally an exponential decay pattern under passive conditions (Nunn, 1977). Letter *f* represents the end of a patient's flow as it returns to baseline, and letter *g* is the passive expiratory pause time in flow until the next breath.

PRESSURE-TIME WAVEFORM

The ideal pressure-time waveform that is created under passive conditions of CFW ventilation is a step ascending ramp. Letter *a* on the pressure waveform in Figure 11-2 indicates the beginning of inspiration and corresponds in time to the flow waveform as indicated by the dotted line connecting the two waveforms. The beginning of the pressure waveform provides information about the triggering variable of the inspiratory phase of ventilation. There is no patient effort or assist breath (Figure 11-2), which indicates that the initial flow from the ventilator is time triggered. The initial flow pushes gas from the ventilator circuit into the patient's lungs as it accelerates to peak flow level. Little volume is actually delivered to the lungs during this initial time period. Only a few milliliters of gas need to pass through the pneumotachometer at the beginning of the inspiratory limb of the circuit for the peak flow rate to be attained. In addition, some gas volume is lost (not delivered to the patient's lungs) as pressure rises in the circuit because of large bore tubing compliance (tubing expansion) and compression of gas molecules. Typically 2 to 3 mL/cm H_2O of the volume is "lost" for disposable adult circuits (MacIntyre et al., 2001).

The initial rise in pressure is mostly the result of resistance to flow through the ventilator circuit and endotracheal tube (Tobin, 1994). The back pressure resulting from impedance to ventilation (flow resistance, tubing, and lung tissue recoil pressure) is graphically recorded by a manometer at the inspiratory valve of the ventilator. Letter *b* represents the change in slope on a pressure waveform that occurs once peak flow is reached. Then the peak flow level is sustained (constant) throughout inspiration. Once flow delivery from the ventilator becomes constant, there is a relatively linear rise in the dynamic or **airway opening pressure (P_{AO}),** which parallels the linear rise in **alveolar pressure (P_{ALV})** until the **peak inspiratory pressure (PIP)** is reached at end-inspiration.

airway opening pressure (P_{AO}): Sum of transairway pressure (P_{TA}) and alveolar pressure (P_{ALV}).

alveolar pressure (P_{ALV}): Pressure required to overcome the elastic recoil property of the lungs.

peak inspiratory pressure (PIP): Highest pressure during the inspiratory phase.

Flow cannot be constant at both ends of a ventilator circuit, however, because volume is lost per unit rise in pressure as a result of tubing compliance (expansion) and gas compression. A loss in volume to the ventilator circuit equates to a loss in flow (flow = volume per time) to the lungs. There has to be some reduction in flow from the ventilator end of the circuit compared to the flow through the patient's lungs at the other end of the circuit (carina). Flow is constant on graphics as it leaves the ventilator. The flow has to be tapered at the other end of the circuit and endotracheal tube (ETT) as volume is lost per cm H_2O created during ventilation. The reduction in flow to the lungs from beginning to end-inspiration depends on tubing compliance and impedance (PIP) to ventilation. The clinical relevance of this issue has not been studied. For the presentation of CFW ventilation, P_{AO} and P_{ALV} will appear to rise linearly in parallel throughout inspiration for these ideal waveforms.

Letter c marks the PIP, the end of inspiration, and the beginning of expiration where the ventilator is time/volume cycled into expiration. The second dotted line shows that the end of inspiratory flow and rise to PIP are contiguous in time. As flow exits through the expiratory limb of the circuit, pressure is created by the resistance to flow through the circuit and measured by a manometer at the expiratory valve. Pressure subsides as gas is released into the atmosphere. Letter d marks the end of expiratory pressure being sensed by the pressure manometer. The bold, double-headed arrow shows that flow is still being recorded as gas is passing through the pneumotachometer at the expiratory valve. The manometer is not sufficiently sensitive or appropriately placed at the expiratory valve for pressure to be continuously recorded until end-expiratory flow is reached on some ventilators.

In the second flow waveform (Figure 11-2, right), the time involved (upper double-headed arrow) for the rise to peak flow is exaggerated to show a time lag between the beginning of inspiration and attainment of peak flow. This example is presented only to evaluate the idea conceptually. This delay in time corresponds to a loss in flow, and therefore volume in the initial phase of inspiration. At the end of inspiration, the volume lost initially is regained as the flow slows to zero over the same delay in time and area under the flow pattern (lower doubled-headed arrow). The peak flow could have been increased to regain the volume lost initially instead of time being extended. Thus, flow-controlled ventilation equates to volume-controlled ventilation. The concept concerning volume and the area under the flow pattern is explained in more detail in Figure 11-3. The dotted line from peak flow to the recorded pressure demonstrates that once peak flow is reached and flow remains constant, the initial rise in predominantly flow-resistive pressure changes slope and rises linearly to PIP as in the preceding example. The slope of the initial rise in pressure is lower than in the preceding vertical example because of the slower rise to peak flow.

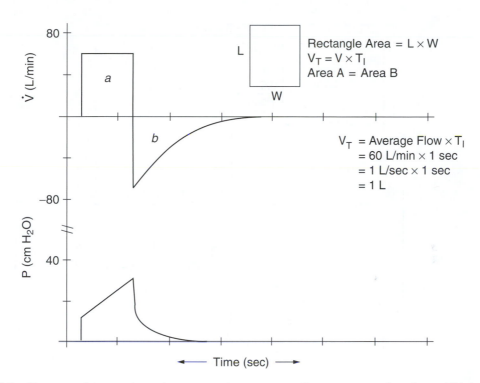

Figure 11-3 Flow waveform to show that area under a constant flow curve equals volume. Tidal volume is the product of constant flow and inspiratory time: $V_T = Flow \times T_I$.

☑ Constant Peak Flow × I Time = Tidal Volume

tidal volume (V_T): Volume delivered by ventilator during mandatory breaths.

☑ (Figure 11-3) Area *a* (inspired volume) = Area *b* (expired volume). If volume under area *b* is less than volume under area *a*, gas leak or air trapping may be present.

The basic mathematical principle demonstrated in Figure 11-3 is that area, under a flow-time curve or pattern, equals volume. We know from geometry that the area of a rectangle equals length times width (A = L × W). On the flow graph, the length side of the waveform (*y*-axis) is 60 L/min or 1 L/sec (60 L/min × 1 min/60 sec = 1 L/sec). Flow is constant for 1 sec, therefore, the width of the rectangle (*x*-axis) is 1 sec and, since length times width equals area, 1 L/sec × 1 sec = 1L **tidal volume (V_T)** delivered. Also, constant flow means there is a constant delivery of volume per unit time. For example, if 0.25 sec is used as the unit of time, a 0.25 L of gas is delivered every 0.25 sec (Volume = 1 L/sec × 0.25 sec = 0.25 L).

Since patients exhale what they inhale, it can be stated that area *b* enclosed under the expiratory flow wave equals area *a* under the CFW. If the volume enclosed by area *b* during mechanical ventilation is less than area *a*, then there must either be a leak in the circuit or some gas has not been expired or has been trapped in the patient's lungs momentarily. The pressure pattern shows a constant rise in lung pressure during the constant flow period as discussed earlier in Figure 11-2.

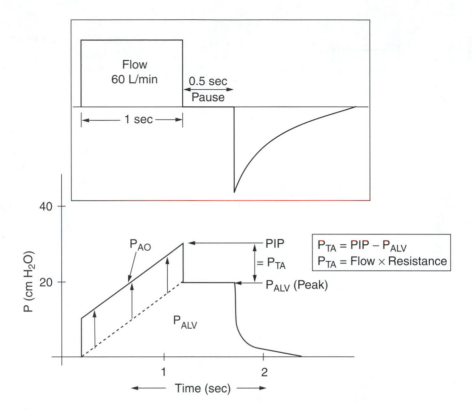

Figure 11-4 Use of end-inspiratory pause to create and measure peak alveolar pressure (peak P_{ALV} or plateau pressure) and transairway pressure (P_{TA}). Peak P_{ALV} or plateau pressure is used to calculate static compliance; P_{TA} is used to calculate airflow resistance.

inspiratory time:
Time from beginning inspiration to end of inspiration and beginning expiration.

Peak P_{ALV}: *The highest pressure recorded at the end of inspiratory pause, also known as plateau pressure.*

plateau pressure: peak alveolar pressure (peak P_{ALV}): *Pressure obtained by performing an end-inspiratory pause.*

Figure 11-4 depicts the ideal pressure waveform with details that correspond to the enclosed constant flow wave presented above it. In this example, a 0.5 sec end-inspiratory pause in delivery of flow from the ventilator has been set (prolonging **inspiratory time**). The pause in flow delivery results in a static pressure measurement being maintained at the same level for 0.5 sec, creating a plateau or pause pressure at the end of the waveform.

For the flow waveform, the double-headed arrow shows that no flow is being delivered from the ventilator for 0.5 sec. During this time period, the inspiratory and expiratory valves of the ventilator are closed to hold gas volume constant in the patient's lungs, allowing clinicians to measure lung pressure or, more importantly, alveolar pressure (P_{ALV}). Since there is no flow, the corresponding pressure created by resistance to flow dissipates immediately. Pressure drops to the **peak P_{ALV}** (**plateau pressure**) level, which can be measured because of the open communication in the ventilator circuit between the alveoli and the manometer at the ventilator. All lung pressures, not just peak P_{ALV}, is monitored during this pause in flow. However, P_{ALV} is used in the graphics and text for emphasis throughout this chapter. The extremely thin type I pneumocytes (0.5 to 2 Å) lining alveoli are more sensitive to pressure and trauma than the progressively thicker airways. P_{ALV} is a major concern and reason for performing the pause pressure measurement during ventilator management. Once peak P_{ALV} (plateau pressure) is known, circuit and airway resistance can be determined [Resistance = (PIP − peak P_{ALV})/Flow], provided a constant flow pattern is present.

Technically, calculation of circuit and airway resistance should be the pressure gradient between PIP and peak P_{ALV}. P_{pause} is intended to eliminate the contribution of the resistance to flow through the airways, and it is synonymous with peak P_{ALV} in the equation for circuit and airway resistance measurements practiced clinically. Measuring peak P_{ALV} allows for calculation of static **lung-thorax compliance (C_{LT})** (e.g., C_{LT} = Volume/Pressure, observing the graphic it can be determined that C_{LT} = 1 L/20 cm H_2O = 0.50 L/cm H_2O). The pressure-time waveform in Figure 11-4 shows, as noted earlier, that the P_{AO} represents two distinct pressures involved during inspiration with flow: the pressure caused by resistance to flow through the circuit and airways, and the elastic recoil pressure created by the airways, alveoli (P_{ALV}), and chest wall.

Under ideal conditions, there is a linear rise in P_{ALV} (dotted line) during the inspiratory cycle since there is a constant rise in volume per unit time with constant flow delivery. Flow-resistive pressure (arrows above dotted line) created by the ventilator circuit and airways is also constant, assuming flow through the respiratory system is constant. Flow resistive pressure will increase parallel to the rise in P_{ALV} during constant flow. The P_{AO} is the dynamic pressure recorded by the pressure manometer that clinicians observe at the ventilator as gas is being forced into the lungs. Another term for flow-resistive pressure during inspiration is **transairway pressure (P_{TA})**, which is the difference between P_{AO} and P_{ALV} ($P_{TA} = P_{AO} − P_{ALV}$). Thus, the P_{AO} is equal to the summation of the two distinct pressures during inspiration: P_{TA} and P_{ALV}. At end inspiration, P_{TA} equals the difference between the PIP and the peak P_{ALV} (P_{TA} = PIP − Peak P_{ALV}) during CFW ventilation. Also, P_{TA} equals flow times resistance (P_{TA} = Flow × Resistance).

CONTROLLED MECHANICAL VENTILATION

Figure 11-5 is the waveform example of **controlled mechanical ventilation (CMV).** CMV also stands for controlled or continuous mandatory ventilation. CMV is a mode that defines the specific control, phase, and conditional variables of mandatory breaths (Chatburn, 2001). The CMV waveforms demonstrate that each breath is a time-triggered mandatory breath and volume controlled because the flow

---

lung-thorax compliance (C_{LT}): The relationship of volume and pressure (V/P) that is imposed by the property of the lungs and thorax.

☑ (Figure 11-4) $P_{AO} = P_{TA} + P_{ALV}$

☑ (Figure 11-4) At end-inspiration, P_{TA} = PIP − Peak P_{ALV} during CFW ventilation.

☑ Airflow Resistance = P_{TA}/Flow

transairway pressure (P_{TA}): Flow-resistive pressure, the difference between airway opening pressure (P_{AO}) and alveolar pressure (P_{ALV}), or $P_{TA} = P_{AO} − P_{ALV}$.

controlled mechanical ventilation (CMV): Time-triggered mandatory breaths provided by the ventilator.

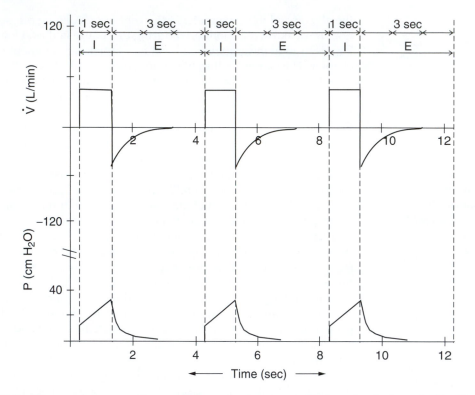

Figure 11-5 Flow- and pressure-time waveforms to show controlled mechanical ventilation. Note the absence of negative triggering pressure before the beginning of inspiration.

 Total Cycle Time (TCT) = Inspiratory time (T_I) + Expiratory time (T_E)

 Frequency (f) = 60sec/TCT

expiratory time (T_E): Time period from beginning expiration to beginning inspiration of next mechanical or spontaneous breath.

pattern is the same for each breath. Today's ventilators control flow (flow controllers), and volume is indirectly controlled. Thus, the mode is considered VCV, which means that volume and flow are held constant and pressure is allowed to fluctuate depending on lung conditions. Total respiratory cycle time is 4 sec (TCT = T_I + T_E). The frequency (f) is set at 15 (f = 60 sec/TCT = 60 sec/ 4 sec = 15). The inspiratory to expiratory (I:E) ratio is 1:3—1 sec for inspiratory time (T_I) and 3 sec for **expiratory time (T_E).**

ASSIST MANDATORY VOLUME-CONTROLLED VENTILATION

Figure 11-6 shows optimal response for two assist mandatory breaths given the same settings for the CMV mode VCV as presented in Figure 11-5. Each pressure-time waveform demonstrates that negative pressure [−2 cm H_2O (dotted line)] is created in the ventilator circuit and graphically recorded when the patient makes an effort to inspire. The dotted line connecting the first set of waveforms shows that the

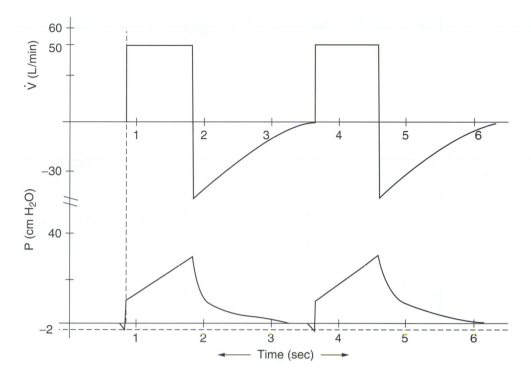

Figure 11-6 Flow- and pressure-time waveforms to show assist mechanical ventilation. Note the negative triggering pressure (-2 cm H_2O) before the beginning of inspiration.

☑ (Figure 11-6) Inspiratory flow begins as soon as the negative deflection reaches the preset sensitivity of -2 cm H_2O.

☑ (Figure 11-7) The T_I is unchanged during VCV because V_T and average flow are held constant ($T_I = V_T$/Average Flow). I:E ratios differ because of changing E time.

inspiratory flow begins as soon as the negative deflection reaches the sensitivity threshold of -2 cm H_2O set on the ventilator. When the ventilator response to patient effort is optimal, each breath is very similar to a controlled breath with the exception that there is a slight reduction (not noticed) in the P_{AO} during inspiration as the patient actively inspires in response to gas being forced into the lungs during assisted ventilation (Dick et al., 1996). When patients expand their thorax in synchrony with gas delivery from the ventilator, it relieves some of the inspiratory pressure that would build up in the circuit and lungs compared to a passive patient (sedated and paralyzed). Slight reductions (2 to 3 cm H_2O) in the P_{AO} pattern that are made apparent by the variability in PIP at end-inspiration are unremarkable. Patients commonly perform 33% to 50% of normal work loads of ventilation during optimal assist mandatory VCV breaths (Marini et al., 1985).

Figure 11-7 demonstrates the CMV mode of ventilation again. The settings are the same as in the previous examples, except that volume waveforms have been added, PEEP is being administered at 10 cm H_2O, and the patient is receiving two assist and two mandatory (nonassist) breaths. For a CFW, volume rises linearly over time as demonstrated. During expiration, volume demonstrates an exponential decay pattern

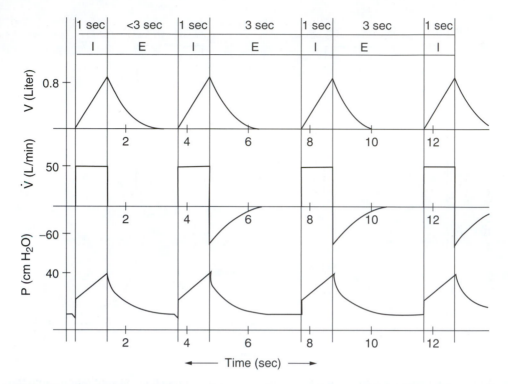

Figure 11-7 Flow-, volume-, and pressure-time waveforms to show two assist (first and second) and two controlled mechanical breaths (third and fourth). The pressure-time waveforms show 10 cm H_2O of PEEP. The sensitivity setting is about 2 cm H_2O below the PEEP level (first and second breaths).

in correspondence with the expiratory flow pattern. The I:E ratios are 1:3 for the second and third mechanical breaths as the patient expires and relaxes after the second assist breath and allows the ventilator to take control (mandatory breaths). The expiratory time for the first breath is reduced because the patient triggers a second assist breath (pressure waveform). Thus, the set I:E ratio (1:3) is reduced, because the patient triggers the second breath before the 3 sec expiratory time (T_E) has elapsed. The T_I is unchanged during VCV because V_T and average flow are held constant ($T_I = V_T$/Average Flow).

In the CMV mode, flow, V_T, and frequency (backup rate) are set, but the patient is allowed to trigger as many breaths as desired. When patients are able to trigger breaths in the CMV mode, the term *assist/control mode* is commonly used, but it is no longer recommended since it does not define a unique mode. When setting CMV, assist mandatory breaths are set unless the sensitivity is set so low that the patient cannot reach the threshold level, which is contraindicated. Patients' efforts to breathe should be supported by setting the sensitivity level appropriately.

The PEEP for the pressure-time waveforms is 10 cm H_2O and since there was no change in static compliance, the PIP was increased by 10 cm H_2O as well, when compared to Figure 11-6. For the assist breaths, it can be seen that pressure drops to 8 or 2 cm H_2O below PEEP level to trigger the first two breaths because sensitivity is set at -2 cm H_2O below baseline pressure, which is known as PEEP compensation.

☑ (Figure 11-8) During CFW ventilation, the volume rises linearly with the inspiratory time.

MATHEMATICAL ANALYSIS OF CONSTANT FLOW WAVEFORM

For better comprehension of the waveforms that develop during mechanical ventilation, respiratory care practitioners (RCPs) should be able to analyze waveforms mathematically. In Figure 11-4, it was demonstrated that once peak P_{ALV} for the pressure waveform was known, the P_{AO} could be delineated into the P_{TA} and P_{ALV} that develops throughout inspiration. Given constant flow, the P_{ALV} and P_{AO} rise linearly in parallel, and the P_{TA} remains constant. A straight line drawn from zero pressure at the beginning of inspiration to the peak P_{ALV} at the beginning of the set pause pressure should closely predict the rise in P_{ALV} throughout inspiration during CFW VCV. Figure 11-8 presents one of the mandatory volume- and pressure-time waveforms presented in Figure 11-7. The computations in Table 11-2 show the volume delivered by the CFW for each 0.25 sec unit of time under the CFW and the volume delivered for the inspiratory time elapsed throughout inspiration (1.0 sec). Table 11-3

TABLE 11-2 Calculations to Determine the Volume Delivered During CFW Ventilation (See Figure 11-8)

1. Computations necessary to find volume under the CFW:

Volume = Average Flow (L/sec) × (T_I sec)

V_T = (50 L/min × 1 min/60sec) × 1.0 sec
V_T = 0.833 L/sec × 1.0 sec
V_T = 0.833 L

Volume = 0.8333 L/sec × 0.25 sec = 0.2083 L per 0.25 sec

Volume = 0.2083 L × 2 = 0.4166 L in 0.50 sec
Volume = 0.2083 L × 3 = 0.6249 L in 0.75 sec
Volume = 0.2083 L × 4 = 0.833 L in 1.00 sec

or

Volume = 0.8333 L/sec × 0.25 sec = 0.2083 L
Volume = 0.8333 L/sec × 0.50 sec = 0.4166 L
Volume = 0.8333 L/sec × 0.75 sec = 0.6248 L
Volume = 0.8333 L/sec × 1.00 sec = 0.8333 L

V1 = 0.2083 L
V2 = 0.2083 L
V3 = 0.2083 L
V4 = 0.2083 L
V_T = V1 + V2 + V3 + V4 = 0.833 L

shows the volume computations and volume waveform, which mathematically shows that the volume rises linearly during CFW ventilation. As shown in Table 11-4, the patient's lung-thorax compliance (C_{LT}) equals 0.04166 L/cm H_2O. As shown, once C_{LT} is known, the equation for C_{LT} can be rearranged and P_{ALV} can be calculated and plotted for any number of time units throughout inspiration, assuming that static C_{LT} remains constant and the volume

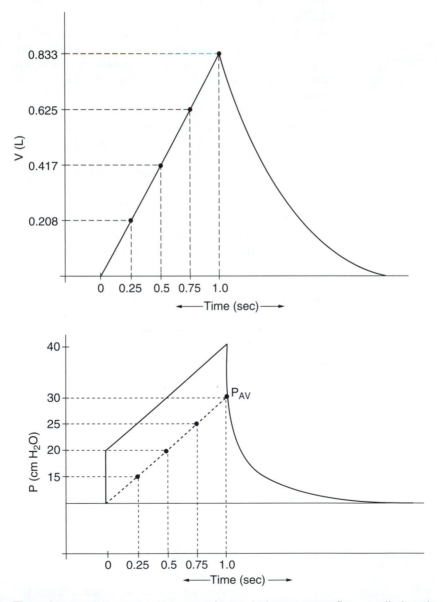

Figure 11-8 The volume- and pressure-time waveforms during constant flow ventilation show the steady increase of volume and pressure as inspiratory time progresses.

TABLE 11-3 Calculations to Determine the Inspiratory Volume Waveform that Develops during CFW Ventilation (See Figure 11-8)

1. Computations necessary to plot the volume pattern during inspiration:

Volume = Average Flow (L/sec) $\times$ T_I(sec)   Volume = 0.8333 L/sec $\times$ 0.25 sec = 0.2083 L
V_T = (50 L/min $\times$ 1 min/60sec) $\times$ 1.0 sec   Volume = 0.8333 L/sec $\times$ 0.50 sec = 0.4166 L
V_T = 0.833 L/sec $\times$ 1.0 sec   Volume = 0.8333 L/sec $\times$ 0.75 sec = 0.6249 L
V_T = 0.833 L   Volume = 0.8333 L/sec $\times$ 1.00 sec = 0.8333 L

TABLE 11-4 Calculations to Determine the P_{ALV} Pattern that Develops during CFW Ventilation (See Figure 11-8)

C_{LT} = $V_T/(P_{ALV} - PEEP)$ C_{LT} = $V_T/(P_{ALV} - PEEP)$
C_{LT} = 0.833 L/(30 cm H_2O − 10 cm H_2O) P_{ALV} = V_T/C_{LT} + PEEP
C_{LT} = 0.833 L/20 cm H_2O
C_{LT} = 0.04165 L/cm H_2O

P_{ALV} = 0.8333 L/0.04165 L/cm H_2O + 10 cm H_2O = 30 cm H_2O
P_{ALV} = 0.6249 L/0.04165 L/cm H_2O + 10 cm H_2O = 25 cm H_2O
P_{ALV} = 0.4165 L/0.04165 L/cm H_2O + 10 cm H_2O = 20 cm H_2O
P_{ALV} = 0.2083 L/0.04165 L/cm H_2O + 10 cm H_2O = 15 cm H_2O

(Figure 11-9) During SIMV, mechanical breaths may be time-triggered (controlled) arrow *a*; or patient-triggered (assisted) arrow *b*.

synchronized intermittent mandatory ventilation (SIMV): A mode of ventilation in which mechanical breaths are delivered without overlapping spontaneous breaths.

delivered for the time periods elapsed is known. Figure 11-8 demonstrates drawing a line (dotted line) through the values plotted for the volume delivered and the P_{ALV} developed over time. This demonstrates also that P_{ALV} rises linearly and in parallel to the P_{TA} throughout inspiration.

SPONTANEOUS VENTILATION DURING MECHANICAL VENTILATION

SYNCHRONIZED INTERMITTENT MANDATORY VENTILATION

Figure 11-9 shows the three types of breaths (controlled, spontaneous, and assist) offered during **synchronized intermittent mandatory ventilation (SIMV).** The first set of waveforms (Figure 11-9, left) is ideal flow- and pressure-time patterns for a volume- or flow-controlled mechanical breath. Letter *a* (arrow) beneath the first pressure waveform indicates that the breath is ventilator initiated (time triggered and controlled). The patient did not attempt to breathe

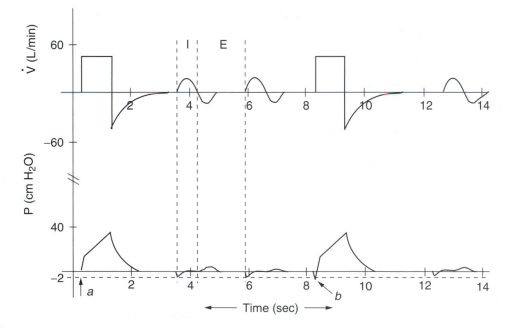

Figure 11-9 Synchronized intermittent mandatory ventilation (SIMV) waveform showing one controlled (time-triggered) mandatory breath (arrow *a*), one assist (patient-triggered) mandatory breath (arrow *b*), and three spontaneous breaths (second, third, and fifth breaths).

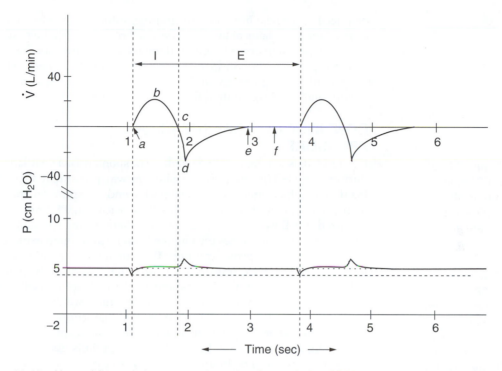

Figure 11-10   Normal flow- and pressure-time waveforms during CPAP (spontaneous breathing with PEEP). The CPAP level is 5 cm H_2O.

within the window of time (SIMV period) set up for synchronized (assist) mechanical breaths. Two sets of flow and pressure-time waveforms depicting ideal spontaneous breaths are recorded next during the time (spontaneous period) allotted for spontaneous breaths. Relative sine waves are created during spontaneous ventilation. Spontaneous breathing is accommodated on ventilators during SIMV and continuous positive airway pressure (CPAP) ventilation. During spontaneous ventilation, the patient controls flow, volume, inspiratory time, and expiratory time. The ventilator responds to the patient's effort by supplying the flow demanded. The spontaneous breaths show that the patient created a peak inspiratory flow of about 20 L/min and peak expiratory flows of about 15 L/min. The pressure waves during spontaneous breathing show a negative pressure to trigger demand flow and some positive pressure recorded in the circuit during expiration. Spontaneous breaths are explained in more detail in Figure 11-10.

The next breath in Figure 11-9 is an assist mechanical breath. Letter *b* (arrow) indicates that the patient's effort occurred to trigger the breath during the SIMV period. The manufacturer determines the amount of time allotted for synchronized mechanical and spontaneous breaths. For the next breath in the graphic, sufficient time has not elapsed for a mechanical breath to be synchronized with the patient's effort, so flow delivery is based on demand and another spontaneous breath is provided. An SIMV rate of 6/min has probably been set for the patient in this graphic with 5 to 6 sec allotted for the spontaneous breaths and 4 to 5 sec allotted for the SIMV breaths.

CONTINUOUS POSITIVE AIRWAY PRESSURE

(Figure 11-10)
In CPAP, airway pressure is above 0 cm H_2O and all breaths are spontaneous.

Figure 11-10 is a more detailed example of spontaneous ventilation during 5 cm H_2O of continuous positive airway pressure (CPAP). In the flow graphic, letter *a* (arrow) labels the end of expiration and start of inspiration; letter *b* marks the peak flow reached (20 L/min) for an idealized sine flow wave created by the patient during spontaneous breathing; letter *c* indicates the change from inspiration to expiration; letter *d* indicates the peak expiratory flow attained (20 L/min); letter *e* indicates the end of expiratory flow; and letter *f* indicates the pause following expiratory flow. The patient creates an inspiratory flow time of approximately 0.75 sec, an expiratory flow time of 1.25 sec, and an expiratory pause time of 0.75 sec. The dotted lines connecting the flow and pressure recordings in time delineate the total respiratory time into the inspiratory and total expiratory time periods. As with mechanical breaths, inspiratory effort (negative pressure recorded) triggers flow on demand (demand CPAP) once the negative pressure reaches the sensitivity threshold [−1 cm H_2O below CPAP level of 5 cm H_2O (dotted line)], or the pressure drops during a continuous flow CPAP. Ideally, gas is delivered to the patient according to the flow demands, which means that pressure will be maintained at zero throughout the inspiratory phase of ventilation. In this example, the pressure recorded during inspiration is kept near zero indicating patient flow demand is being met. During expiration, as gas is expired into the circuit, a positive pressure is momentarily recorded until the expiratory flow is too slow or the expiratory circuit and valve resistance is so low that near baseline pressure is recorded.

(Figure 11-10) In CPAP, inspiratory effort triggers and initiates flow once the negative pressure reaches the sensitivity threshold.

(Figure 11-11)
Increase in flow rate causes a higher airflow resistance and thus a corresponding increase in PIP and P_{TA}. Peak alveolar pressure (peak P_{ALV}) or plateau pressure is not affected by changes in flow rate.

EFFECTS OF FLOW, CIRCUIT, AND LUNG CHARACTERISTICS ON PRESSURE-TIME WAVEFORMS

FLOW AND TRANSAIRWAY PRESSURE

An end-inspiratory pause has been set in Figure 11-11 to delineate the P_{AO} into the two distinct pressures, P_{TA} and P_{ALV} (double-headed arrows), generated during gas flow through a ventilator circuit into a patient's lungs. For waveforms analysis, it is important to know how

Figure 11-11   Flow- and pressure-time waveforms showing the effects of flow rate on P_{TA}, P_{ALV}, and expiratory flow. Increase of inspiratory flow or airflow resistance causes an increase of P_{TA}, but no changes in peak P_{ALV} (plateau pressure) and expiratory flow.

each of these pressures is affected by changes in flow and lung characteristics. Figure 11-11 demonstrates the effects of increased inspiratory flow or airflow resistance on a pressure-time waveform, which can be compared to the effects on them created by decreased compliance (Figure 11-12). The pressure-time graphics in Figure 11-11 depict (double-headed arrows) that there has been a rise in the P_{TA} from beginning to end in the second pressure waveform because of an increase in turbulence when the constant flow was doubled from 60 to 120 L/min in the second flow wave. As gas flows through a circuit system with different twists and turns, and varied lumen sizes such as large bore tubing, humidifiers, and endotracheal tubes, turbulent flow results. In turn, the circuit system causes an exponential rise in circuit pressure with increments in flow. Conversely, an exponential decay in pressure is observed when flow is reduced (Dennsion et al., 1989). Thus, the area depicting the P_{TA} gradient ($P_{AO} - P_{ALV}$) has been more

Figure 11-12 Flow- and pressure-time waveforms showing the effects of lung-thorax compliance (C_{LT}) on P_{TA}, P_{ALV}, and expiratory flow. Decrease of C_{LT} causes an increase of P_{ALV} (plateau pressure) and peak expiratory flow, but no changes in P_{TA}.

✓ (Figure 11-12) Decrease in lung-thorax compliance causes an increase in P_{ALV} and PIP. Transairway pressure (P_{TA}) is not affected by changes in compliance.

than doubled in the second pressure waveform. Note, however, that the remarkable change in P_{AO} and PIP did not affect the peak P_{ALV} because neither the C_{LT} nor lung volume was changed. Only the rise time to peak P_{ALV} was affected because T_I was reduced by half. In this example, resistance was increased by an increase in flow. An increase in airway resistance from various lung pathologies causing bronchoconstriction and obstruction will also increase the area depicting the P_{AO} and P_{TA} gradient without a change in flow, but P_{ALV} will not be affected. Airway obstruction and bronchoconstriction will affect waveforms in other ways, but these are dealt with during discussion of using expiratory waveforms as a diagnostic tool.

COMPLIANCE AND ALVEOLAR PRESSURE

Figure 11-12 demonstrates a similar comparison between flow and pressure waveforms. PIP has substantially increased in the second example as it did in Figure 11-11. Given no change in flow or V_T to

peak alveolar pressure (peak P_{ALV}):
Pressure recorded with an end-inspiratory breath hold; reflects the elastic recoil property of the lungs; plateau pressure.

explain the increase in PIP, an end-inspiratory pause needs to be set to create the **peak alveolar pressure (peak P$_{ALV}$),** or plateau pressure for analysis. Since P$_{TA}$ remains the same for each waveform, neither the flow nor airway resistance has been changed. A decrease in total C$_{LT}$ is the only explanation for the increase in PIP, which is supported by the increase in peak P$_{ALV}$ at end-inspiration. The same peak flow, flow pattern, and volume (Area 1= Area 2) are being used for volume delivery in each example. Total C$_{LT}$ can be estimated by observing the information provided in the graphic comparison and in this example it has decreased by half. The area under the flow curve is 1 L or 1000 mL (1 L/sec $\times$ 1 sec), and total C$_{LT}$ is 50 mL/cm H$_2$O (C$_{LT}$ = 1000 mL/20 cm H$_2$O) for the first example versus 25 mL/cm H$_2$O (1000 mL/40 cm H$_2$O) in the second example.

EFFECTS OF DESCENDING RAMP FLOW WAVEFORM DURING VOLUME-CONTROLLED VENTILATION

☑ (Figure 11-13, example on left) During *time-limited* ventilation, the I time is unchanged when the flow pattern is changed from constant flow to descending ramp flow. The same volume can only be maintained if the *peak flow* of the descending ramp flow is increased.

☑ "Time-limited" usage in example: T$_I$% is set on some ventilators. TCT and T$_I$% set the I time in sec providing that the TCT and V$_T$ remain unchanged.

TIME- AND FLOW-LIMITED VENTILATION

Figure 11-13 demonstrates the changes that occur when the flow pattern on a ventilator is adjusted from a constant to a descending ramp flow waveform (DRFW) during time-limited ventilation (first example) compared to flow-limited ventilation (second example). These examples present what is known as true DRFWs (solid lines), which means that flow descends from peak level to baseline (zero-end flow).

The type of DRFW available (see Figure 11-16) for selection during VCV depends on the manufacturer. For example, the Puritan Bennett (PB) 7200ae and 840 ventilators offer a DRFW with an end flow of 5 L/min, and the Hamilton Medical Veolar provides the option of a true DRFW, or one with an end flow that is 50% of the initial peak flow, called a 50% DRFW.

The concepts presented here for Figure 11-13 are the same for the various types of DRFWs. In the first example, a DRFW is superimposed over a CFW (dotted lines) for comparison during time-limited ventilation, as offered by the Veolar in the CMV and SIMV modes. Inspiratory time (T$_I$) is held constant (time limited) when the flow waveform selection is adjusted from a CFW to a DRFW. Since the V$_T$ is set and T$_I$ is held constant, the average flow rate has to remain constant (V$_T$ = Average Flow $\times$ T$_I$). Average flow rate for a DRFW is $^1/_2$ (Peak Flow + End Flow). As demonstrated in the first comparison of flow waves example, the area enclosed by the solid and dotted line labeled *a* on the DRFW replaces the same area and, therefore, volume that was truncated from the CFW area labeled *b*. Thus, the same

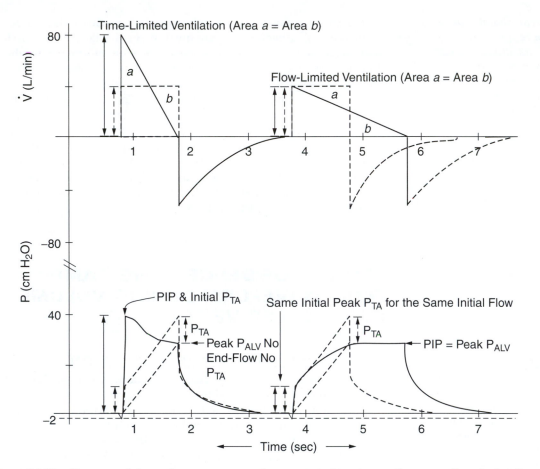

Figure 11-13 Changes of dynamic pressure waveforms created by descending ramp flow during time-limited (left) and flow-limited (right) ventilation.

volume is being delivered by either flow pattern within the same time period, and transition from a CFW to a true DRFW on a time-limited ventilator requires peak flow to be doubled.

As shown in Table 11-5, the average flow rates for the CFW and DRFW are the same (0.67 L), and given the same T_I, the V_T delivered is identical. When employing a DRFW, peak flow has to be proportionately greater as end flow is reduced if the same volume is to be delivered in the same time period.

The second example of superimposed flow wave patterns demonstrates the results of switching from a CFW to a DRFW during flow-limited ventilation. The ventilator's peak flow is held constant (flow limited) when the DRFW is selected. As the flow ramp descends, it eliminates the volume that was enclosed under area *a*. Time has to be extended until the same volume eliminated is replaced (i.e., area *b*).

TABLE 11-5 V_T Delivered by the CFW and DRFW during Time-Limited Ventilation (See Figure 11-13)

For the CFW:	For the DRFW:
PF (L/sec) = 40 L/min × min/60sec	PF (L/sec) = 80 L/min × min/60sec
PF (L/sec) = 0.67	PF (L/sec) = 1.33, EF = 0
V_T = Average Flow (L/sec) × T_I(sec)	V_T = Average Flow (L/sec) × T_I(sec)
V_T = 0.67 L/sec × 1 sec	V_T = 1/2 (PF (L/sec) + EF (L/sec) × T_I(sec)
V_T = 0.67 L	V_T = 1/2 (1.33 L/sec + 0 L/sec) × 1 sec
	V_T = 0.67 L

PF = Peak flow; EF = end flow.

✔️ (Figure 11-13, example on right) During *flow-limited* ventilation, the inspiratory peak flow is unchanged when the flow pattern is changed from constant flow to descending ramp flow. The same volume can only be maintained if the *inspiratory time* of the descending ramp flow is increased.

Given flow-limited ventilation, time fluctuates rather than peak flow to deliver the same V_T. Thus, depending on ventilator type, when flow is changed during CMV or SIMV from a CFW to DRFW, either the peak flow has to double (time-limited ventilation), or the T_I has to double (flow-limited ventilation) for the same V_T to be delivered. As shown in Table 11-6, since the initial flow rate for both flow waveforms is the same, the average flow rate for the DRFW is reduced by half compared to the CFW. The same V_T is delivered because T_I is doubled.

The pattern and level of pressure developed (Figure 11-13) during DRFW ventilation depend, as for CFW ventilation, on the peak to end-flow pattern, circuit/lung resistance, and C_{LT}. The pressure waveform examples (solid lines) for the time- and flow-limited DRFWs are superimposed over the step ascending ramp pressure waveforms (dotted lines) created by CFWs. Pressure during DRFW ventilation, depending on the peak flow level set (e.g., 80 versus 40 L/min for these examples), tends to square off compared to rising linearly as it does for CFW ventilation (see Figure 11-14). Assuming the same circuit and lung characteristics for the comparison, the

TABLE 11-6 V_T Delivered by the CFW and DRFW during Flow-Limited Ventilation (See Figure 11-13)

For the CFW:	For the DRFW:
PF (L/sec) = 40 L/min × min/60sec	PF (L/sec) = 40 L/min × min/60sec
PF (L/sec) = 0.67	PF (L/sec) = 0.67, EF = 0
V_T = Average Flow (L/sec) × T_I(sec)	V_T = Average Flow (L/sec) × T_I(sec)
V_T = 0.67 L/sec × 1 sec	V_T = 1/2 (PF (L/sec) + EF (L/sec) × T_I (sec)
V_T = 0.67 L	V_T = 1/2 (0.67 L/sec + 0 L/sec) × 2 sec
	V_T = 0.67 L

Figure 11-14 Changes of dynamic pressure and alveolar pressure (P_{ALV}) waveforms created by descending ramp flow during time-limited (left) and flow-limited (right) ventilation.

higher initial peak flow for the DRFW in the first example (80 L/min) creates a higher peak flow-resistive pressure or P_{TA} (40 cm H_2O) at the beginning of inspiration on the pressure waveform compared to flow-resistive pressure (10 cm H_2O) for the CFW. And as demonstrated, the flow-resistive pressure for DRFW decreases over time with reduction in flow, whereas the flow-resistive pressure stays constant (dotted line, double-headed arrows) for the CFW. Since the same volume is being delivered in each DRFW example and zero flow occurs at end-inspiration, the pressure at end-inspiration for both examples is the patient's peak P_{ALV}. There is no flow at end-inspiration, so no flow-resistive pressure or P_{TA} is being created. Flow-resistive pressure steadily drops to zero during inspiration for zero-end-flow ventilation. Note that PIP and peak P_{ALV} are the same for the second pressure waveform example.

In the first example, the PIP is at the beginning of inspiration because of the very high initial flow rate (80 L/min). During CFW ventilation, PIP is always the highest pressure and always at the end of inspiration because flow resistive pressure (P_{TA}) is "stacked" on top of the P_{ALV} at end-inspiration (double-headed arrows). Note also, in the second example, that initial peak flow level stays the same when switching from a constant to a DRFW during flow-limited ventilation.

Figure 11-14 delineates the DRFWs (solid lines) into their component parts of P_{TA} (open arrows) and P_{ALV} superimposed for comparison over the P_{TA} and P_{ALV} areas for CFWs (dotted lines). The P_{TA} and P_{ALV} for the CFWs rise linearly as discussed in Figure 11-4. Like CFW ventilation, the rise in P_{ALV} during DRFW ventilation is dependent on volume delivered and C_{LT}. Lung pressure rises after the initial flow period because volume accumulates in the lung, but flow-resistive pressure steadily subsides in correspondence with reduction in flow. Volume delivery (area under the flow wave) for the DRFWs decreases over time. Calculation of the volume under a true DRFW shows that 75% of the volume is delivered during the first half of inspiration. The flow waveforms in Figure 11-14 are the same as in Figure 11-13.

As shown in Tables 11-5 and 11-6, the V_T for the constant flow wave is 0.67 L (40 L/min or 0.67 L/sec), and therefore, 0.33 L is delivered in the first half of inspiration. Table 11-7 shows that the volume delivered in the first half of inspiration for the DRFW is 0.5 L.

For time-limited ventilation, greater volume being delivered in the first half of inspiration creates a faster rise in P_{ALV} in the first half of inspiration compared to the rise in P_{ALV} for the CFW, which is noted in

> ✓ (Figure 11-14) In CFW and DRFW ventilation, the rise in alveolar pressure (P_{ALV}) is directly related to the volume delivered and inversely related to the compliance.

TABLE 11-7   Volume Delivered in the First Half of Inspiration for the True DRFW Compared to the CFW (see Figure 11-14)

True DRFW Volume in the first half of inspiration:	% volume in the first half of inspiration:
Volume = Average Flow × T_I	
Volume = $1/2$ (PF L/sec + *EF L/sec) × $1/2$ T_I (sec)	80 L/min × min/60 sec = 1.33 L/sec
Volume = $1/2$ (1.33 L/sec + 0.67 L/sec) × $1/2$ (1.0 sec)	40 L/min × min/60 sec = 0.67 L/sec
Volume = $1/2$ (2 L/sec) × 0.5 sec	V_T = 0.67 L for DRFW
Volume = 0.5 L	0.5 L/0.67 L × 100 = 75%
CFW Volume in the first half of Inspiration:	% volume in the first half of inspiration:
Volume = Average Flow × $1/2$ T_I	V_T = 0.67 L for CFW
Volume = 0.67 L/sec × $1/2$ (1.0 sec)	0.33 L/0.67 L × 100 = 50%
Volume = 0.67 L/sec × 0.5 sec	
Volume = 0.33 L	

End flow for the DRFW in the first half of inspiration = 40 L/min or 0.67 L/sec the first pressure waveform. The slope of the rise in P_{ALV} for the DRFW is lower than for the CFW in the second half of inspiration because only 25% of the V_T is delivered compared to 50% of the V_T being delivered for the CFW. There can be an improvement in oxygenation using the DRFW compared to the CFW according to some research because the alveoli are more distended throughout inspiration. Thus, given the same T_I and V_T, the mean P_{ALV} is higher during DRFW compared to CFW ventilation.

The same concepts explored above can be applied to the P_{ALV} pattern for the DRFW in the second pressure waveform in Figure 11-14, but the comparison with the CFW is a little more complicated. In the second example, the comparison between flow and pressure waves is made during flow-limited ventilation. The P_{ALV} slope for the CFW is higher throughout inspiration compared to the DRFW. That is because the entire V_T is delivered by the CFW within the time period for which only 75% of the V_T is delivered by the DRFW.

As described previously, during CFW ventilation a constant volume per unit of time is delivered and therefore, a constant rise (linear) in P_{ALV} per unit time develops (assuming no change in C_{LT}). But during DRFW ventilation, there is a proportionate decrease in volume delivered per unit time, and although the summative P_{ALV} steadily rises over time, the P_{ALV} generated per unit time steadily decays during inspiration. For example, 75% of the V_T is delivered and 75% of the peak P_{ALV} is generated in the first half of inspiration. The second half of inspiration, 25% of the V_T is delivered with only a 25% increase in P_{ALV}, which is substantial reduction in P_{ALV} per unit time compared to the first half of inspiration. Thus, Figure 11-14 demonstrates that the slope for the P_{ALV} curve generated during DRFW ventilation proportionately decreases per unit time as the summative P_{ALV} increases. Consequently, a concave (progressive decay) pressure pattern is created during inspiration, consistent with the pattern of volume delivery. This issue is discussed in more detail in Figure 11-17. Note also that in Figure 11-14 as in Figure 11-13 the initial P_{TA} is higher (open arrows) when initial flow is higher.

PEAK FLOW AND TIDAL VOLUME RELATIONSHIP IN TIME-LIMITED VENTILATION

☑ (Figure 11-15) During time-limited ventilation (constant T_I), a decrease in flow causes a lower V_T, P_{TA}, and P_{ALV}.

Figure 11-15 demonstrates DRFW ventilation where T_I is maintained but flow is reduced. The first example shows that the P_{TA} is high for the set flow rate (80 L/min). Given the same lung and circuit characteristics for each set of waveforms, the second example shows the results to the pressure pattern if T_I is maintained (time-limited ventilation), but flow is reduced. Given the same T_I and a reduction in flow, the V_T is reduced (V_T = Average Flow × T_I). The consequence of the reduction in flow is that V_T is reduced as is the P_{TA} and P_{ALV} causing a change in the pattern. With the reduction in the initial P_{TA}, the

Figure 11-15 Characteristic changes of P_{TA} and P_{ALV} waveforms created by changes in peak descending ramp flow during time-limited ventilation. Decrease of peak descending ramp flow reduces the volume delivered, P_{TA}, and P_{ALV}.

pressure pattern is relatively constant and PIP is no longer at the beginning of inspiration.

EFFECTS OF END-FLOW ON TIDAL VOLUME

Figure 11-16 demonstrates the changes in P_{TA} patterns that could be expected when end flows for DRFWs are increased. In the first example, the end flow is 5 L/min (PB7200, PB840). The pressure pattern shows a slight increase in the P_{TA} above the P_{ALV} at the end of inspiration as a result of the slight resistance to end flow being above baseline. The second set of waveforms shows a 50% descending ramp flow wave where end flow is 50% of the initial peak flow set. The initial flow set is very high (100 L/min), which causes an exponential rise in initial P_{TA} (40 cm H_2O) because of turbulent flow and circuit/airway resistance. The end-P_{TA} is also relatively high from resistance to flow above the peak P_{ALV} compared to the first example since end flow is 50 L/min compared to 5 L/min. These flow and pressure patterns do

☑ (Figure 11-16) During DRFW ventilation, a higher end-flow raises the P_{TA} at end-inspiratory.

Figure 11-16   Effects of end flow on the pressure waveforms during descending ramp flow ventilation. Figure shows two end flows: 5 L/min (left) and 50% of peak inspiratory flow (right). Increase of end flow raises the transairway pressure (P_{TA}), but not the alveolar pressure (P_{ALV}).

not represent ventilation of the same patient. Peak P_{ALV} is at the same level, but V_T delivered is much greater for the second flow wave example compared to the first.

DISTRIBUTION OF DELIVERED TIDAL VOLUME

In Figure 11-17 volume-time waveforms have been added for comparison with DRFW and pressure-time waveforms. Since flow rate is highest in the beginning of inspiration for a DRFW, the slope in rise to peak volume, like P_{ALV}, is initially fast and becomes proportionately reduced over time as flow descends. In the first example, peak flow is set at 60 L/min and T_I is 1 sec, the volume delivered is 0.5 L [1/2 (60 L/min)/60 sec/min $\times$ 1 sec = 0.5 L]. The volume delivered in the first half of inspiration is 0.375 L (1/2(60 L/min Peak Flow + 30 L/min End Flow)/60 sec/min $\times$ 0.5 sec (T_1) = 0.375 L), which is 75% of 0.5 L(0.75 $\times$ 0.5 L = 0.375 L). The volume delivered in the second half of inspiration is 0.125 L(0.5 L $-$ 0.375 L = 0.125 L), which is 25% of the V_T remaining.

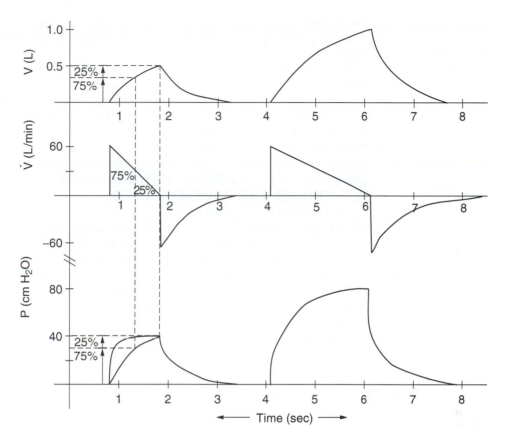

Figure 11-17 Effects of inspiratory time using descending ramp flow on the delivered tidal volume (V_T) and peak inspiratory pressure (PIP). An increase of inspiratory time from 1 (left) to 2 sec (right) raises the V_T and PIP.

The pressure-time pattern in the first example in Figure 11-17 shows the development of P_{ALV} in correspondence with delivery of the V_T. Determining the P_{ALV} curve requires knowing the volume delivered per time and the total C_{LT}. Because there is no flow at end-inspiration, there is no P_{TA} at end-inspiration, and the PIP represents the peak P_{ALV}, which is 40 cm H_2O. Total C_{LT} is 0.0125 L/cm H_2O or 12.5 mL/cm H_2O (C_{LT} = volume/P_{ALV} = 0.5 L/40 cm H_2O). If there is no change in C_{LT} during V_T delivery, P_{ALV} halfway through inspiration will depend on the volume delivered by that time. The example shows, as discussed earlier, that 75% of the V_T is delivered in the first half of inspiration, consequently 75% of the peak P_{ALV} will be attained, which is 30 cm H_2O (0.75×40 cm H_2O = 30 cm H_2O), or P_{ALV} is equal to volume calculated for that time divided by total C_{LT} (P_{ALV} = 0.375 L/0.0125 L/cm H_2O = 30 cm H_2O). The remaining 25% of the P_{ALV} is developed in the second half of inspiration (P_{ALV} = 0.25×40 cm H_2O = 10 cm H_2O, or P_{ALV} = 0.125 L/0.0125 L/cm H_2O = 10 cm H_2O). Thus, any point along

☑ When peak flow is kept constant, ↑, or ↓ in V_T, T_I, or P_{ALV} will cause like-wise changes in the other two parameters.

☑ The end flow during DRFW ventilation is zero. The alveolar pressure (P_{ALV}) or plateau pressure at this point equals the end-inspiratory pressure. End-inspiratory pause is not needed to obtain the P_{ALV}.

the P_{ALV} curve can be predicted and plotted by calculating the volume delivered per time provided total C_{LT} is known as was true for the CFW (Figure 11-8).

In the second example (Figure 11-17), peak flow is maintained at 60 L/min, but V_T is doubled [1/2(60 L/min]/60s/min × 2s = 1 L], which increases T_I to 2 sec. As a result of doubling V_T, peak P_{ALV} is doubled (P_{ALV} = 1.0 L/0/0125 L/cm H_2O = 80 cm H_2O). Note that the initial flow-resistive pressure is sustained in the second pressure waveform since the initial flow has not changed.

CMV DURING DESCENDING RAMP FLOW WAVEFORM (DRFW) VENTILATION

Figure 11-18 is an example of CMV during DRFW ventilation. The patient initiates the first two breaths and the ventilator triggers the next two breaths. During DRFW ventilation, the peak alveolar pressure (peak P_{ALV}, or plateau pressure) and C_{LT} can be calculated without the need for an end-inspiratory pause. This is because at end-inspiration, the flow is zero (i.e., similar to end-inspiratory pause) and the peak alveolar pressure remains in a plateau state.

Figure 11-18 shows DRFW ventilation with a peak flow of 60 L/min or 1 L/sec. For an inspiratory time of 0.5 sec, the tidal

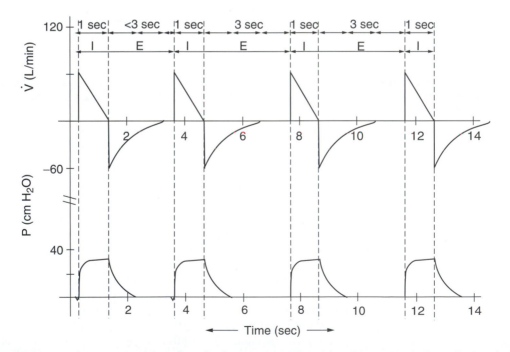

Figure 11-18 Assist (first and second) and mandatory (third and fourth) mechanical ventilation during descending ramp flow ventilation.

volume is 500 mL (1 L/sec $\times$ 0.5 sec). With an end-flow pressure of 35 cm H_2O, the calculated C_{LT} is 14.3 mL/cm H_2O (500 mL/35 cm H_2O).

WAVEFORMS DEVELOPED DURING PRESSURE-LIMITED VENTILATION

pressure-controlled ventilation (PCV): A mode of ventilation in which the peak inspiratory pressure is preset and remains stable in conditions of changing compliance and airflow resistance.

PRESSURE-CONTROLLED VENTILATION (PCV)

Figure 11-19 is an example of **pressure-controlled ventilation (PCV)**, which is a pressure-limited CMV mode where a set pressure is targeted by the ventilator. In PCV, pressure level, frequency, and I:E ratio are set by the operator. The V_T and flow rate delivered are variable, and are dependent on the pressure level and lung/airway characteristics. The ventilator is time or patient triggered and the

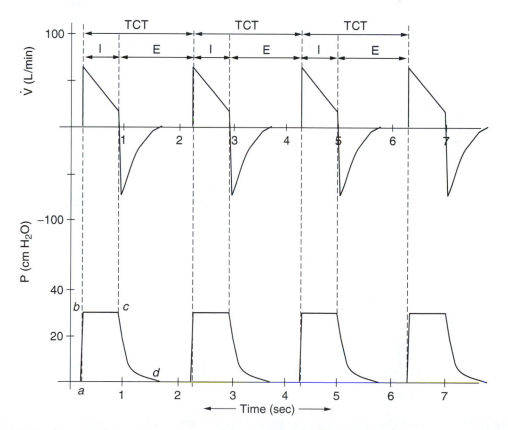

Figure 11-19 Characteristics of pressure-controlled ventilation (PCV). The pressure control level of 30 cm H_2O is set and sustained at this level throughout the inspiratory phrase. The flow patterns may vary according to the compliance and airflow characteristics.

☑ During PCV, the pressure level, rate, and I:E ratio are preset. Flow and V_T are dependent on the pressure level, patient effort, and lung/airway characteristics.

total cycle time (TCT): *Time period from beginning inspiration to the end of expiration (beginning of next inspiration).*

ventilator delivers a DRFW in a manner that will reach and sustain the set pressure level. The manufacturer may opt to establish a slow rise (convex pattern) to gradually reach the pressure limit (PB 7200ae) or a rise time % can be set for patient comfort so that there is a delay in time prior to peak flow, and therefore, the targeted pressure being reached (Figure 11-23). In Figure 11-19, the pressure level set for ventilation is 30 cm H_2O. For the letters on the pressure-time waveform, *a* marks the end of expiration and beginning of inspiration; *b* indicates the pressure control level that is set and sustained; *c* is the change from inspiration to expiration; and *d* is the end of expiration with flow. **Total cycle time (TCT)** is 2 sec and frequency is 30/min (f = 60 sec/2 sec/ breath = 30/min). T_E is twice T_I. The I:E ratio is 1:2.

Assisted Breaths during PCV. Figure 11-20 is a theoretical example of a patient who is air hungry, not relaxed, has variable flow demands, and is triggering all the breaths during PCV. By definition, PCV should sustain the pressure level set regardless of variable flow demand and lung/airway characteristics. In this example the flow pattern fluctuates with each breath, so the V_T would also be fluctuating. The PIP is set at 20 cm H_2O, and is sustained (dashed line) by the

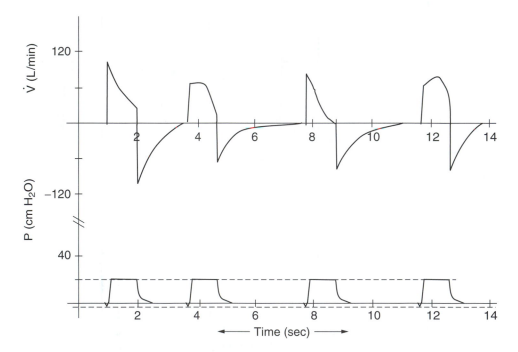

Figure 11-20 Effects of changing compliance and airflow resistance on the flow and delivered volume during PCV. The pressure waveforms remain unchanged during PCV. Flow waveforms change in response to the fluctuating compliance and airflow resistance characteristics. Since the area under each flow waveform reflects the delivered volume, the volume changes accordingly.

✓ During PCV, the flow wave patterns may fluctuate based on the patient's respiratory requirement. The V_T is dependent on the pressure level, patient effort, and lung/airway characteristics.

✓ IRPCV may be helpful in conditions of severe hypoxia and lung injury (e.g., ARDS).

ventilator. For the pressure level to be sustained, the ventilator would have to vary the flow at a highly sophisticated level to maintain the pressure set. Historically, pressure-controlled ventilation has always offered assisted breaths, but it has not offered such flexibility in flow delivery, and such variable flow demands would likely cause dyssynchrony and necessitate an increase in the pressure level set to exceed the patient's flow and volume demands. Pressure support ventilation, discussed later, demonstrates a greater capacity for accommodating variable flow demands while maintaining the pressure level of support set on the ventilator.

INVERSE RATIO PRESSURE-CONTROLLED VENTILATION (IRPCV)

Figure 11-21 demonstrates **inverse ratio pressure-controlled ventilation (IRPCV)** set at 20 cm H_2O with 10 cm H_2O of PEEP for a combined pressure (PIP) of 30 cm H_2O. IRPCV is used only under conditions of severe

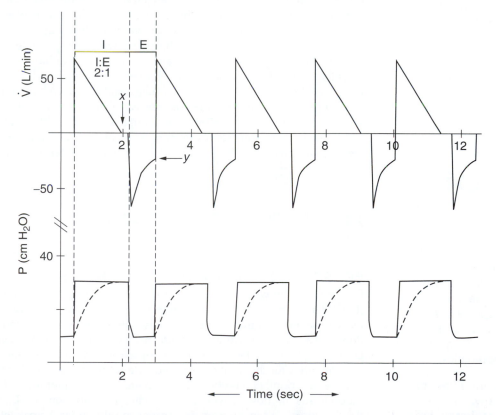

Figure 11-21 Inverse ratio pressure-controlled ventilation (IRPCV). Arrow *x* shows end of inspiratory flow because the pressure control level has been met. Arrow *y* shows incomplete exhalation, air trapping, and the potential for development of auto-PEEP.

inverse ratio pressure-controlled ventilation (IRPCV): A mode of ventilation in which the peak inspiratory pressure is preset and the I time is longer than the E time.

☑ IRPCV offers an unnatural breathing pattern and may be uncomfortable. The patient is often sedated and paralyzed to prevent patient-ventilator dyssynchrony.

hypoxemia and lung injury (ARDS). Since an inverse ratio respiratory pattern is abnormal and uncomfortable, patients are sedated and paralyzed to prevent them from "fighting" the ventilator. In this example, inspiratory flow drops to zero (arrow *x*) since the pressure target has been met. The ventilator is maintaining the set pressure level by closing the expiratory valve and curtailing flow. This process holds gas in the patient's lungs until end-inspiratory time is reached. The PIP during this no flow time period is, in effect, a pause pressure and peak P_{ALV}. The dotted lines applied to the pressure waveforms indicate the development of the P_{ALV} during inspiration and shows that peak P_{ALV} is reached when flow ends. The volume held in the patient's lungs depends on the patient's C_{LT}. If the expired V_T is monitored, the patient's lung compliance can be measured [$C_{LT} = V_T/(PIP - Total\ PEEP)$]. Total PEEP includes PEEP set plus intrinsic or auto-PEEP. Arrow *y* at the first expiratory flow wave shows that auto-PEEP is being created because the ventilator time triggers successive breaths before the exhalation is complete. Since the expiratory flow is unable to descend to the baseline, gas is trapped in the lungs. This causes elevation of the functional residual capacity and reduction of V_T delivered. During PCV, the level of auto-PEEP proportionately reduces the V_T delivered to the lungs.

Based on research, auto-PEEP should be avoided if possible, and external PEEP applied instead. A valuable advantage of having graphics is that auto-PEEP can be readily observed and prevented whenever lung conditions have changed or ventilator settings have been altered. Graphics can be observed as T_I is increased in small steps to a level that allows enough time for expiration without causing auto-PEEP. This management technique serves to increase mean P_{ALV} and improve oxygenation at lower peak P_{ALV} to reduce the potential of barotraumas.

PRESSURE SUPPORT AND SPONTANEOUS VENTILATION

PRESSURE SUPPORT VENTILATION (PSV)

☑ In PSV, only the pressure support level is preset. The V_T depends on the PS level, inspiratory effort, and patient's lung/airway characteristics.

☑ During PSV, the flow, volume, and inspiratory time are under the patient's control.

Figure 11-22 shows different features of pressure support ventilation (PSV). The first set of waveforms shows the patterns that develop for a relaxed patient breathing synchronously with the ventilator, a concave flow and a square pressure-time pattern. PSV is pressure-limited ventilation, but it is considered a spontaneous mode of ventilation. Although each breath is mechanically supported by a set pressure, each breath requires a "spontaneous effort" by the patient throughout most of inspiration to sustain flow delivery above cycling (termination) level. Thus, flow, volume, and inspiratory time are primarily under the patient's control. However, the pressure can be set high enough to limit virtually all effort by the patient except for triggering the breath.

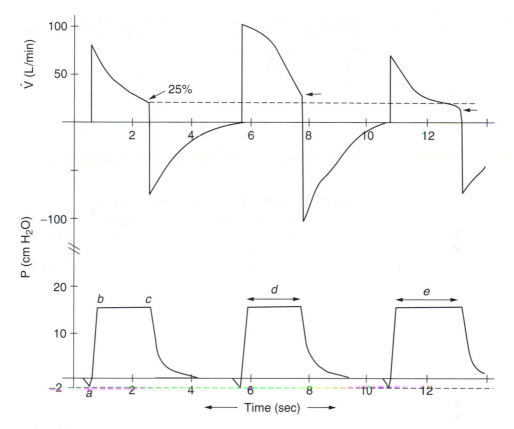

Figure 11-22 Characteristics of pressure support ventilation (PSV). The pressure support level remains constant as long as the inspiratory flow continues and is above the end flow. The inspiratory flow and inspiratory time are dependent on the patient's spontaneous breathing effort. The arrows show an end flow of 25% of the peak inspiratory flow. When the inspiratory flow reaches 25% of the peak inspiratory flow, pressure support (inspiration) ends and expiration begins.

If the patient inspires in a relaxed manner as presented in the first set of waveforms, gas accelerates to some peak flow level that results in the set pressure level to be quickly reached, but then the flow rate decays to sustain but not exceed the pressure level set. The ventilator cycles into expiration at 25% of the initial peak flow level attained, or some other manufacturer set level (e.g., 5% for the Siemens SV300).

For the first pressure waveform example, letter *a* indicates it is an assist, pressure/patient-triggered breath; letter *b* indicates that the pressure support level (15 cm H_2O) has been quickly reached; and letter *c* shows that the pressure limit has been sustained throughout inspiration. The flow wave demonstrates that the ventilator provides flow at a high level initially to meet or exceed the patient's inspiratory flow demands in order to reach the set pressure support level. The end flow per breath (dotted line) shows that each wave is flow cycled into expiration at 25% (arrows) of the initial peak flow rate. The peak and end flow may vary with each breath.

The second flow wave demonstrates that increased patient flow and volume demands are supplied, but the set pressure level is maintained. The third flow wave shows a lower, but sustained demand for flow until 25% of the initial flow is reached. The double-headed arrows (*d* and *e*) indicate the same time interval, but the inspiratory time for pressure waves *d* and *e* varies. Thus, flow, volume, and time can all vary and depend on lung/airway characteristics and the patient's breathing pattern.

ADJUSTING RISE TIME DURING PSV

Figure 11-23 demonstrates PSV at 10 cm H_2O with PEEP of 5 cm H_2O. The first set of flow and pressure waveforms is ideal. The second flow waveform demonstrates a rapid rise in initial flow that causes a spike in the initial pressure that overshoots the set pressure limit. The pressure spike at the beginning of inspiration (arrow *x*) can cause patient discomfort and increased work of breathing (Dick et al., 1996).

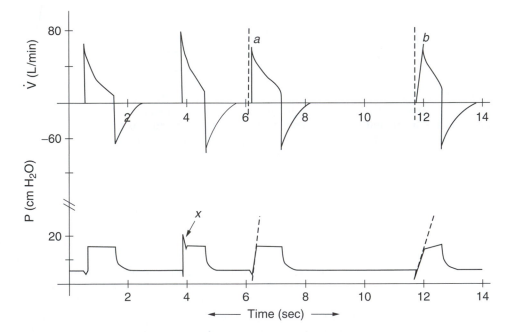

Figure 11-23 PSV at 10 cm H_2O of pressure support over 5 cm H_2O of PEEP. Arrow *x* shows a rapid rise in initial inspiratory flow generated by the patient causes a spike in the initial pressure that overshoots the pressure support level. Letters *a* and *b* show two different rise time percents. A slower rise time percent (*b*) causes a more gradual rise to the pressure support level and it provides more patient comfort.

☑ In PSV, the faster the initial rise to peak flow (short rise time), the sooner the preset PS level is reached. This may cause the ventilator to overshoot the PS limit.

☑ A slow rise time during PSV is more comfortable for the patient.

Letters *a* and *b* flow waves demonstrate a feature called rise time percent (%)—the percentage of the inspiratory cycle time required to reach the peak flow rate and the pressure limit set. The vertical dotted lines preceding the flow waveforms show that the rise to peak flow takes a progressively longer period of time. The dotted lines on the third and fourth pressure waveforms were added to show that the slope or rise to the set pressure limit is progressively slower as a result. The faster the rise in initial flow, the sooner the set pressure limit is reached. An advantage of a slower rise to the peak flow rate and set pressure levels is that greater patient comfort is provided.

SIMV (CFW) AND PSV

Figure 11-24 exemplifies the combination mode, SIMV + PSV. Two ideal CFWs and corresponding step ascending ramp pressure patterns, letters *a* and *d*, depict volume-controlled breaths, the first mandatory (*a*) and the other an assist breath (*d*). Three pressure-supported breaths, *b*, *c*, and *e*, show variable DRFWs, patient-triggered, pressure-limited (20 cm H_2O) breaths of varied flow, volume, and inspiratory time.

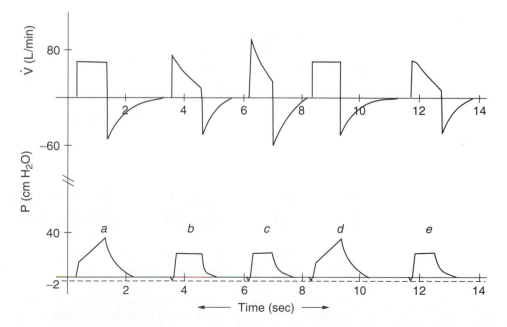

Figure 11-24 SIMV and PSV during constant flow ventilation. Mandatory breath (*a*); pressure support breaths (*b, c,* and *e*); assist breath (*d*).

Figure 11-25 SIMV and PSV during descending ramp flow ventilation. Mandatory breath (*a*); pressure support breaths (*b*, *c*, and *e*); assist breath (*d*).

SIMV (DRFW) AND PSV

Figure 11-25 depicts the combination mode, SIMV + PSV, except that DRFWs with end flows at 5 L/min have replaced the CFW used in Figure 11-24. The DRFWs for the SIMV breaths show that initial flow was set relatively high (80 L/min) resulting in PIP for pressure patterns *a* and *d* being created at the beginning of inspiration. Three pressure-supported breaths, *b*, *c*, and *e*, are displayed again for this example.

EFFECTS OF LUNG CHARACTERISTICS ON PRESSURE-LIMITED WAVEFORM

Figure 11-26 exemplifies the effect that changes in circuit/airway resistance and C_{LT} can have on waveforms, flow, and volume delivered during pressure-limited ventilation. During CMV VCV, the volume delivery is stable and the pressures (P_{TA}, P_{ALV}, or both) vary when there are changes in pulmonary mechanics. During pressure-limited ventilation, pressure is held stable and the flow and volume vary when there are changes in pulmonary mechanics.

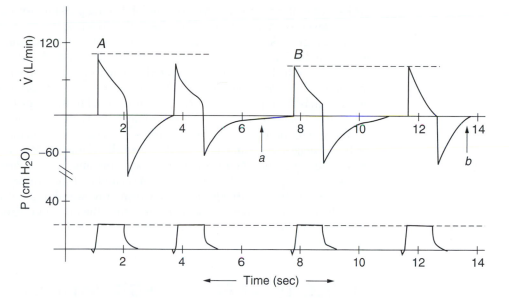

Figure 11-26 During pressure-limited ventilation, the flow and volume are dependent on the airflow and compliance characteristics of the patient/ventilator system. A higher flow and larger volume are observed in *A* and *B* (first and third breaths) than their adjacent breaths (second and fourth breaths). The waveforms show that *A* has a lower airflow resistance and *B* has a higher compliance than their adjacent breaths.

✓ During pressure-limited ventilation, an increased airflow resistance or a decreased compliance would reduce the delivered flow and tidal volume.

For each pressure-limited breath, the constant pressure waveforms under the dotted lines labeled *A* and *B* characterize different lung conditions during PCV. The peak flow and area under the inspiratory curve of the flow waveforms (first and third) are comparatively greater than the adjacent flow waveforms (second and fourth) in examples *A* and *B*. Thus, greater volume is being delivered by the first flow wave in each example.

In example *A* (first and second waveforms), given no change in C_{LT} or effort, greater airway/circuit resistance will tend to cause reduction in the initial or average flow rate, and therefore, a reduction in V_T as demonstrated by the adjacent flow waveform. A greater flow resistive pressure (P_{TA}) causes the set (target) pressure limit to be reached at a lower flow rate. A reduction in delivered V_T may be the result unless the average flow is sustained, which may be demonstrated by a reduction in initial peak flow, but an elevation in the end-flow rate. A substantial increase in airway or circuit resistance will usually result in a reduced V_T because the peak and average flows will be reduced as demonstrated in this example. Letter *a* shows that the average expiratory flow rate is reduced, causing longer T_E.

Example *B* (third and fourth waveforms) demonstrates that a reduction in the C_{LT} (i.e., ascites, ARDS) will also result in a reduction in V_T. However, the initial inspiratory flow rate is not affected since resistance to flow is not a factor. The initial driving pressure for flow, the PC level set, has not changed so the initial flow rate is sustained. However, given lower C_{LT}, more pressure is required for the same volume to be delivered, and since pressure is held constant, the result has to be a reduction in the V_T delivered. Compared to example A, less volume is delivered as shown by the area under the inspiratory flow waveform in example B. Peak flow is maintained, but the slope or descent in flow rate from peak level is greater. Thus, the average flow and V_T are reduced (V_T = Average Flow $\times$ T_I). Letter b shows that T_E is reduced since less volume is expired. The peak expiratory flow rate is about the same since the resistance to flow is the same and the driving pressure for expiratory flow, the PC level set and end-inspiratory lung pressure, was held relatively constant. During pressure-limited ventilation, the pressure remains rather constant while the flow and V_T delivered are altered with changing lung/airway characteristics.

USING WAVEFORMS FOR PATIENT AND VENTILATOR-SYSTEM ASSESSMENT

☑ Patient-ventilator dyssynchrony increases the work of breathing and prolongs weaning from mechanical ventilation.

The next objective is to describe the use of waveforms to improve ventilator-patient assessment and management. Positive pressure in the lungs is not natural. Too much volume under pressure can cause barotraumas or volutrauma. Too little volume or not enough positive end-expiratory pressure (PEEP) to keep alveoli from collapsing (derecruitment) and then reopening (recruitment) during tidal ventilation can also damage the lungs. Too little respiratory muscle use (disuse atrophy) leads to respiratory muscle weakness, and excessive imposed work of breathing (WOB) leads to respiratory muscle weakness or fatigue. Either way, weaning from mechanical ventilation is delayed.

However, no research to date suggests that patients triggering all the volume- or pressure-limited breaths in synchrony with the ventilator will develop respiratory muscle weakness from either too little or too much WOB. Conversely, volumes of research suggest that dyssynchrony during ventilator management may impose excessive WOB and prolong mechanical ventilation (Dick et al., 1996). Research also suggests lack of assisted ventilation (patient-triggered breaths) from prolonged paralysis or sedation as a reason for prolonged mechanical ventilation. The best oxygenation and ventilation should be derived at the lowest volume and least lung pressure if patients are breathing in synchrony with the ventilator, which obviates excess WOB and mitigates the potential for excessive lung pressures. Auto-PEEP can be easily observed and corrected using graphics, which reduces the potential for volume trauma. Also, patient-ventilator synchrony can be easily verified and controlled through waveform analysis.

Figure 11-27   Pressure-time waveform demonstrates response time during assist (patient-triggered) ventilation. The patient-triggered negative pressure for the first breath is enlarged to show the response time.

PATIENT-VENTILATOR DYSSYNCHRONY

☑ Dyssynchrony can occur with the assisted (patient-triggered) or controlled (time-triggered) breaths.

☑ High ventilatory demand of a patient may be fulfilled with a higher sensitivity setting, a higher peak flow, and use of flow triggering (faster response time for flow delivery).

Dyssynchrony during mechanical ventilation increases the WOB, oxygen consumption, minute ventilation, and myocardial work. Dyssynchrony can occur with the assisted (patient-triggered) or controlled (time-triggered) breaths. The first pressure waveform in Figure 11-27 depicts a detailed analysis of an assist (patient-triggered) breath. Both pressure-time waveforms depict the step ascending ramp pattern. Thus, a constant (square) flow pattern must have been set to produce these pressure waveforms. The -2 cm H_2O value below baseline (zero) represents the sensitivity threshold level setting. In the first waveform, the patient's effort to trigger the breath is exaggerated to analyze the negative pressure deflection in greater detail. The negative pressure deflection crosses the set sensitivity threshold level descending to about -4 cm H_2O before the ventilator is able to respond (deliver gas). How fast the ventilator reacts to a patient's efforts depends on the patient's respiratory drive, sensitivity level set, inspiratory valve response time, and peak flow setting. The response time is measured from the time the sensitivity threshold setting is reached to the time flow is initiated by the ventilator (short, double-headed arrow). Once flow is initiated, pressure changes from a negative to a positive direction. If a patient has a very weak or strong ventilatory drive, a greater sensitivity setting is needed (e.g., -1 instead of -3 cm H_2O), flow-triggering, or a higher peak flow setting should improve patient-ventilator synchrony.

When analyzing the patient-trigger phase of inspiratory effort, it is important to realize that the patient is always experiencing higher negative intrathoracic and intrapulmonary pressures than those recorded at the ventilator (Dick et al., 1996; Messinger et al., 1995).

There is a time lag during breathing efforts for the propagation of negative pressure created in the patient's intrapleural space to traverse the airways and respiratory circuit system, and then reach the pressure transducer in the ventilator. Research has shown that a -5 cm H_2O (versus -2 cm H_2O) sensitivity setting can increase WOB to intolerable levels (Marini et al., 1985). Thus, substantial metabolic work to breathe is required during the negative pressure time period (long, double-headed arrow). Consider, for comparison, that for normal spontaneous breathing, approximately -1 cm H_2O P_{ALV} is incurred during inspiration, and gas is flowing into alveoli throughout the inspiratory effort as the alveoli are expanding, which aids the oxygenation and ventilation process instantaneously. There is no gas movement into the alveoli during the negative deflection time period depicted in Figure 11-27. Gas is simply being decompressed and recompressed until positive pressure is recorded. Thus, during pressure triggering, the negative intrathoracic pressure is greater than the ventilator-recorded negative pressure (e.g., -10 cm H_2O intrathoracic versus -2 cm H_2O at ventilator) metabolic work (O_2 consumption) can be greatly increased. Oxygenation and ventilation are being compromised compared to normal spontaneous breathing, especially if sensitivity is set too low.

DYSSYNCHRONY DURING CONSTANT FLOW WAVEFORM (CFW) VENTILATION

(Figure 11-28) Insufficient flow (letter *a*) or insufficient tidal volume (letter *b*) may cause patient-ventilator dyssynchrony.

Signs of patient-ventilator dyssynchrony include tachypnea, agitation, use of accessory respiratory muscles, active expiration, paradoxical breathing, and respiratory alternans.

A lack of ventilator sensitivity to the patient's effort may set up the patient-ventilator dyssynchrony presented in the pressure waveform examples *a* and *b* in Figure 11-28. The graphic shows that patient-ventilator dyssynchrony occurs when increased ventilatory demands are not met by a sufficient flow or volume setting on the ventilator. Whether a particular pattern of dyssynchrony can be proven to be excessive or not is a complicated issue and beyond the scope of this chapter. Perfect waveforms are not necessary. When signs of patient-ventilator dyssynchrony are graphically displayed, decisions about ventilator management require a competent physical assessment. The first physical sign of increased WOB is tachypnea (f>20/min) and a general appearance of agitation. Other physical signs of respiratory muscle stress include accessory muscle use: neck, supra- or substernal and/or intercostal retractions, and active expiration (use of abdominal muscles). In time, depending on a patient's strength reserve and nutritional status, signs of respiratory muscle weakness or fatigue can develop, that is, a paradoxical breathing pattern and/or respiratory alternans. Unfortunately, the last signs of respiratory muscle weakness or fatigue are blood gas abnormalities showing respiratory failure (Tobin et al., 1986). For this reason, using arterial blood gas results as the primary assessment tool of competent ventilator management is a serious mistake.

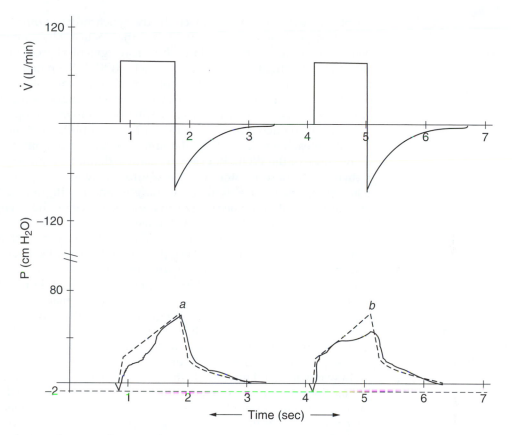

Figure 11-28 Constant flow and pressure-time waveforms showing dyssynchronous ventilation as a result of *a*, inadequate initial peak flow, or *b*, inadequate mechanical tidal volume to meet patient demand.

✓ Tachypnea and appearance of agitation may be caused by other factors such as pain and psychologic stress.

Tachypnea and general appearance of agitation may be caused by other factors such as pain and psychologic stress. Patient-ventilator synchrony may not be the problem. But if improvement in patient-ventilator synchrony eliminates the signs of physical and psychologic distress, quality patient care has been enhanced. The appropriate adjustment on the ventilator to improve synchrony is easily facilitated through waveform analysis.

The dotted line for the first pressure-time waveform *a* (Figure 11-28), exemplifies the ideal waveform for a passive patient being mechanically ventilated, that is, the ventilator is generating virtually all the pressure necessary to expand the patient's lungs. The solid line depicts patient-ventilator dyssynchrony and the corresponding waveform created during mechanical ventilation. The greater the drop in pressure and the development of irregular patterns from the ideal pattern (dyssynchrony), the less the ventilator is assisting the patient with breathing. In fact, the dyssynchrony can often impose more WOB onto the patient than that incurred by spontaneous breathing off the ventilator. Physical signs of distress indicate that the patient is enduring too much WOB. If the patient is not on the ventilator because of respiratory failure, some dyssynchrony may not pose a serious problem. Research suggests that it will compromise oxygenation and ventilation compared to optimal, which may be uncomfortable for the patient. Morbidity and mortality outcomes, however, may be the same; the patient is simply doing more of the WOB. But research shows that if patients are recovering from respiratory muscle failure, dyssynchrony can sustain respiratory muscle weakness or fatigue, and it will prolong mechanical ventilation because recovery time to regain the strength for spontaneous breathing is compromised.

☑ (Figure 11-28) Solid pressure tracing *a* shows insufficient *initial* flow (low peak flow). Solid pressure tracing *b* shows insufficient *end-inspiratory* flow (low tidal volume).

The first pressure-time waveform *a* (Figure 11-28) indicates that a higher initial flow is needed to keep pace with the patient's initial flow demands. The initial flow-resistive pressure is partially removed, so that the pressure to inflate the lungs has been transferred (imposed on) to the patient. The patient is drawing gas (flow demand) from the circuit almost as fast as the incoming gas from the ventilator. As a result, less pressure is created. Increasing the flow rate to a level greater than the patient's demand will provide assistance and restore normal pressure pattern (dotted curve).

In waveform *b* (Figure 11-28), the initial flow demand appears to be met since the initial rise in pressure is relatively normal. The drop in pressure in this example is at end-inspiration and suggests that the patient needs more flow than is being supplied. More flow delivery at the end of inspiration means more volume is being demanded than is being supplied, and the ventilator is being time cycled into expiration before that demand is met.

☑ Adjusting the peak flow, sensitivity, tidal volume; changing the mode of ventilation; or sedating the patient may restore patient-ventilator synchrony.

Sometimes, increasing the peak flow will satisfy the patient's demands in this situation because the volume is delivered sooner. This may cause the patient to relax and breathe in synchrony with the ventilator. Increasing the sensitivity may also make it easier to breathe initially, relaxing the patient and satisfying what appeared to be an inadequate peak flow or V_T setting. So experience suggests that all three methods should be attempted. No research shows that there is only one way to satisfy a particular dyssynchronous waveform pattern. These suggestions are based on knowledge, experience, and research. Sometimes only a change in mode from VCV to pressure-limited ventilation will provide patient-ventilator synchrony. And sometimes, nothing works. Some patient's breathing patterns can be so erratic that no ventilator can provide synchronous ventilation. Pain, neurologic damage, psychologic stress, or unknown reasons may be causing erratic patterns of breathing that cannot be matched by today's ventilators. Patients may have to be sedated for periods of rest under such circumstances.

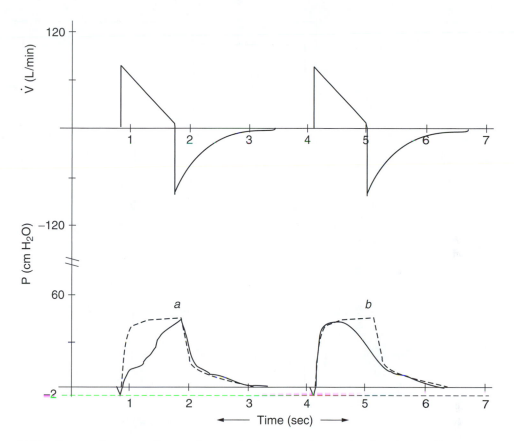

Figure 11-29 Descending ramp flow and pressure-time waveforms showing dyssynchronous ventilation as a result of *a*, inadequate initial peak flow, or *b*, inadequate mechanical tidal volume to meet patient demand.

DYSSYNCHRONY DURING DESCENDING RAMP FLOW WAVEFORM (DRFW) VENTILATION

Figure 11-29 presents the same dyssynchronous conditions depicted in Figure 11-28 except that DRFWs are being utilized. The dotted lines show the ideal pressure-time waveforms. Example *a* suggests a higher peak flow setting to meet initially high flow demands, and example *b* suggests a need for increasing the V_T. In Figures 11-28 and 11-29, signs of respiratory distress would probably result unless the patient is being sedated.

CHANGES IN PRESSURE WAVEFORMS DURING RESPIRATORY MECHANICS MEASUREMENT

Figure 11-30 shows another important benefit of graphics: assurance that the respiratory mechanics are being accurately measured. These are the same waveforms depicted in Figure 11-4 except that the dotted

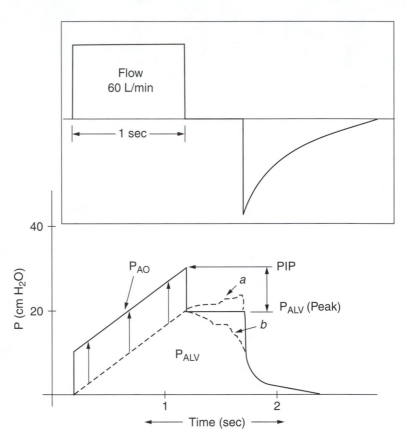

Figure 11-30 Measurements of P_{TA} and P_{ALV} can be affected by the patient's effort to breathe. Dotted line *a* shows patient's expiratory effort during the pause period. Dotted line *b* shows inspiratory effort during the pause period.

☑ Patient-ventilator dyssynchrony with *rising* airway pressure may occur when the patient moves, talks, or coughs.

lines *a* and *b* (arrows) represent possible variations in peak P_{ALV} that could result during a pause in flow. Rather than pressure remaining constant during the pause, pressure either rises above relaxed peak P_{ALV} or descends below it. Pressure rising as in example (letter *a*) often occurs when a patient tries to expire during the pause time. The procedure (pause at end-inspiration) is unnatural and patients do not always relax, and the neurologic respiratory drive to breathe may prevent it. Dyssynchronous ventilation may be occurring as well and the patient's breathing pattern does not correspond to end-inspiration in synchrony with the ventilator. There may be many reasons for an increase in pressure during this period of time. Any movement such as turning or twisting of the thorax can cause pressure to rise. Hands placed on the patient's chest while being attended by a health care provider can increase intrathoracic pressure and peak P_{ALV}. The patient trying to talk or cough will increase P_{ALV}.

☑ Patient-ventila-
  tor dyssyn-
chrony with
decreasing airway
pressure may occur
with a small leak in
the ventilator circuit.

Letter *b* (Figure 11-30) shows the patient may be trying to continue to inspire, expanding thoracic volume, decompressing gas in the system, and dropping pressure. There may be a small leak in the circuit causing pressure to drop during the pause. Using graphics, you will learn with experience that it is very difficult to obtain accurate respiratory mechanics measurements. Without graphics, errors cannot be observed and may be documented as fact. Patients have to be totally relaxed and passive during the static compliance measurement. Usually, only the CMV mode can be used during respiratory mechanics measurements. Often the minute ventilation has to be increased 10% to 15% to reduce the patient's $PaCO_2$ to apneic threshold (about 32 mm Hg) to eliminate patient's respiratory drive and induce relaxation, and to obtain valid measurements (Marini et al., 1985, 1986).

DYSSYNCHRONY DURING PRESSURE-LIMITED VENTILATION

Figure 11-31 demonstrates a pressure-support level that is set too low to comfortably satisfy patient flow or volume demand. The patient's respiratory frequency has increased well above normal (approximately

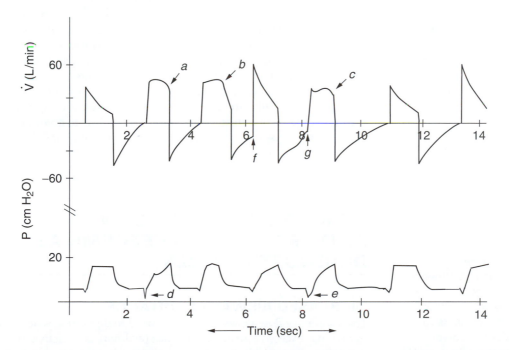

Figure 11-31 An example of pressure support ventilation in normal breaths (first, second, and fifth breaths) and in breaths where patient demands are not being met [letters *a*, *b*, and *c* (arrows)]. Letters *d* and *e* (arrows) show excessive patient triggering efforts.

✓ (Figure 11-31) Letters *a*, *b*, and *c* are examples of respiratory distress where the inspiratory flow demand is high throughout the inspiratory phase. Compare the abnormal near-constant flow patterns (*a*, *b*, and *c*) to the normal descending flow patterns (first flow wave). Letters *d* and *e* show high triggering efforts.

✓ (Figure 11-31) Letters *f* and *g* show the expiratory flow waves do not return to baseline before the next breath. Incomplete expiration may lead to air trapping.

✓ (Figure 11-32) The *solid* lines show that an increase in airflow resistance leads to higher PIP, lower expiratory flow, and longer expiratory time.

28/min) with graphic display of dyssynchrony. Physical signs of discomfort and increased work of breathing would undoubtedly accompany such a graphic display. The second, third, and fifth flow waves, *a*, *b*, and *c* (arrows), show that flow demand is high (35 to 45 L/min) throughout inspiration, sustaining near constant flow wave patterns, which are created under conditions of stress. The flow-time waves do not show a relaxed pattern as in the first flow wave, shown for comparison, where flow gradually descends to cycle the ventilator into expiration at 25% of the initial flow. Instead, flow demand is sustained (squared off) at a high level and ends abruptly, dropping quickly to zero with the patient's expiratory effort and attempts to quickly trigger another breath. The more that flow appears to square off and drop perpendicularly through the flow cycling level, the higher the flow demand, and the less the patient is relaxing during inspiration and pausing between breaths at that set level of pressure support.

The patient's high respiratory drive is also evident by evaluating the patient-triggering efforts in the pressure-time waveforms (*d* and *e* arrows). Negative pressure drops substantially below the sensitivity threshold level set below PEEP before the ventilator demand valve can respond. Gas trapping is apparent in the graphic as well, which can be seen on the third and fourth expiratory flow waves [*f* and *g* (arrows)]. Thus, expiration is not complete before the patient triggers breaths four and five. Several of the pressure waveforms are not squared off, so obviously the pressure limit set is not being sustained as should be. Increasing the pressure-support level to 15 to 20 cm H_2O would probably eliminate this patient's distress and provide adequate support for a normal level of WOB. If pressure-controlled ventilation (PCV) were being demonstrated in this example at the same pressure-limit setting, similar pressure patterns of dyssynchrony would be manifest, but fluctuations in flow to accommodate demand would be less likely. The T_I would be maintained, however, consistent with the settings for PCV.

USING EXPIRATORY FLOW AND PRESSURE WAVEFORMS AS DIAGNOSTIC TOOLS

INCREASED AIRWAY RESISTANCE

The expiratory flow waveform can be used to determine whether a patient has excessive airway resistance (asthma), obstructive, or restrictive disease (ARDS). The solid line expiratory flow wave in Figure 11-32 demonstrates excessive expiratory airway resistance. The dotted line represents a relatively normal waveform. Circuit and

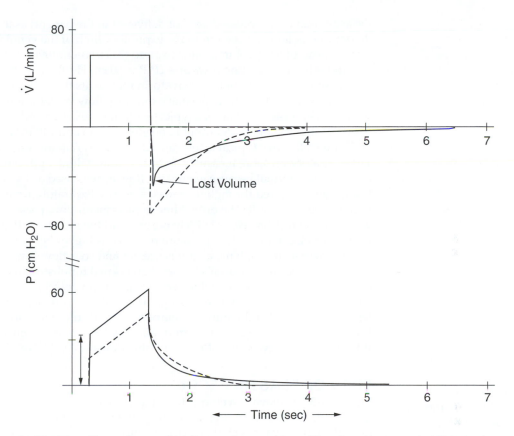

Figure 11-32 The effects of normal airflow resistance (dotted lines) and increased airflow resistance (solid lines) on the expiratory flow and pressure-time waveforms. When the airflow resistance is increased, a lower expiratory flow and a higher peak inspiratory pressure are noted.

✓ (Figure 11-32) The *solid* line in the flow-time waveform shows that an increase in airflow resistance (e.g., obstructive lung disease) prolongs the expiratory time. This condition may lead to air trapping, auto-PEEP, or volutrauma.

endotracheal tube (ETT) resistance (i.e., size 6 mm I.D. ETT) can complicate the assessment by creating a similar pattern, but RCPs can easily measure circuit resistance and eliminate it as the cause for the abnormal expiratory flow curve. Typically, circuit resistance is about 6 to 8 cm $H_2O/L/sec$ at 60 L/min with an 8 mm I.D. ETT and humidifier in line (Dennison et al., 1989), which can be subtracted from clinical measurements of airway resistance. The low peak expiratory flow, the average flow level, and abnormally long expiratory flow time (>5 sec) compared to the normal curve are obvious signs of severely elevated airway resistance in this example. High resistance will quickly reduce peak expiratory flow rate to low levels compared to normal expiratory flow waves given the same driving pressure (peak P_{ALV}) at end-inspiration. Peak P_{ALV} is usually normal for mandatory V_T (8 to 12 mL/kg ideal body weight) for most obstructive diseases other than emphysema. The spiked initial peak expiratory flow (arrow) indicates the lost volume (compressed gas not delivered to the patient) as it decompresses and is driven from the expiratory limb of the ventilator circuit ahead of lung volume being expired (Nilsestuen, 1996), because it is under high ventilating pressures (PIP = 60 cm H_2O).

The solid line pressure-time waveform represents the pattern that should be expected for the abnormal expiratory flow waveform presented in this example. This is a typical pattern for exacerbated asthma or bronchitis. The initial P_{TA} (double-headed arrow) and PIP (60 cm H_2O) are well above typical levels caused by airway/circuit resistance. The expiratory pressure measured in the expiratory limb of the circuit is lower than normal because expiratory flow is decreased as the V_T is being slowly expired through narrowed airways. Expiratory time (T_E) is increased as a result. The dotted line depicts inspiratory pressure when airway resistance is relatively normal and the P_{TA} and PIP are lower. The circuit expiratory pressure recorded is higher because expiratory flow rate through the circuit is greater and so is flow-resistive pressure as a result. Since T_E is longer than normal for obstructive diseases, there is greater potential for volutrauma from auto-PEEP, which will be readily apparent when graphics are available. A patient may have to be sedated and paralyzed temporarily to be mechanically controlled at low frequencies (6 to 8/min) and low V_T (e.g., 4 to 7 mL/kg IBW) to prevent severe auto-PEEP and lung damage (ARDSNet, 2000).

LOSS OF ELASTIC RECOIL

Figure 11-33 displays waveforms for a patient with emphysema (solid lines) compared to one with normal lung functions (dotted lines). The expiratory flow wave is similar to the example in Figure 11-32 for the asthma/bronchitic patient, but with noted changes. First, the spiked peak expiratory flow is not present because ventilating pressures for emphysema patients are typically low as in this example, where PIP is 25 cm H_2O (solid-line pressure wave) for a substantially high V_T of 1.0 L being delivered. Also, lung tissue recoil pressure (peak P_{ALV}) and the consequent expiratory flow driving pressure is reduced (approximately 15 cm H_2O in this example since initial P_{TA} is approximately 10 cm H_2O), and as a result the peak expiratory flow pattern develops more slowly and is rounded, and T_E is prolonged as demonstrated by the expiratory flow and pressure patterns.

DECREASED LUNG-THORAX COMPLIANCE (C_{LT})

When airway resistance remains constant, a decreased C_{LT} (e.g., ARDS) will increase the peak expiratory flow rate and shorten the expiratory time. In Figure 11-34, the normal expiratory flow curve (dotted) is compared to the expiratory flow curve in conditions of low C_{LT} (solid lines). The expiratory flow in conditions of low C_{LT} is generally higher and expiratory time is shorter (solid line). A shorter expiratory time correlates with faster lung emptying in conditions of low C_{LT}.

☑ (Figure 11-33) The *solid* lines show that in conditions of high compliance or loss of elastic recoil (e.g., emphysema), the peak expiratory flow is decreased (loss of the spiked peak). The PIP is also decreased because less pressure is needed to ventilate lungs with high compliance.

☑ (Figure 11-34) The *solid* expiratory flow curve shows that in conditions of low C_{LT}, the expiratory flow is generally higher and expiratory time is shorter.

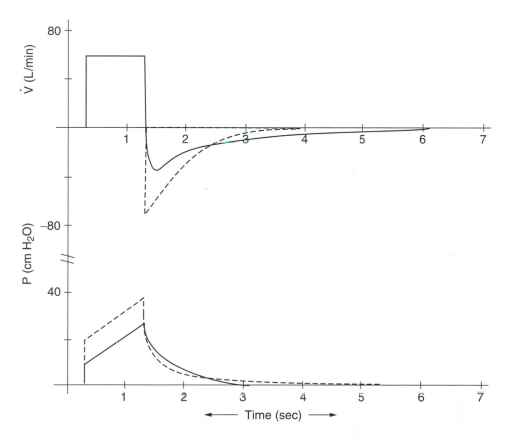

Figure 11-33 The effects of normal elastic recoil (dotted lines) and loss of elastic recoil (solid lines) on the expiratory flow and pressure-time waveforms. When the elastic recoil is decreased (i.e., low elastance or high compliance), a lower expiratory flow and a lower peak inspiratory pressure are noted.

✓ In air trapping, the expired volume is less than the inspired tidal volume for one or more breaths. The trapped air comes out with a subsequent mandatory breath resulting in a much larger expired tidal volume.

The pressure waveform (Figure 11-34) shows that the PIP (solid line) would increase as C_{LT} decreased. Note that since the flow rate is the same and airway resistance is unaffected, the initial flow resistive pressure (arrow) has not changed. Thus, the increase in PIP must be the result of a rise in peak P_{ALV} (plateau pressure). The expiratory portion of the pressure waveform (solid line) generated in the circuit on average is higher under conditions of low C_{LT} and expiratory time is shorter compared to average conditions for ventilator patients (dotted line).

GAS TRAPPING AND UNCOUNTED BREATHING EFFORTS

Gas trapping can easily be recognized by examining the volume-time waveform. In air trapping, the expired volume is less than the inspired tidal volume (i.e., the expired volume curve does not reach baseline).

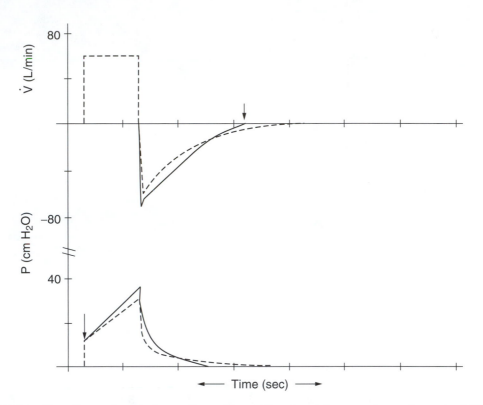

Figure 11-34 The effects of normal compliance (dotted lines) and decreased compliance (solid lines) on the expiratory flow and pressure-time waveforms. When the compliance is decreased, a higher expiratory flow, a shorter expiratory time, and a higher peak inspiratory pressure are noted.

☑ (Figure 11-35) Double arrow *a* shows that the expiratory flow is dropping rapidly (flow is near zero, parallel to baseline) with a corresponding drop in pressure. This suggests the patient is trying to *inspire* during the expiratory phase.

This observation may occur for one or more breaths. The trapped air typically comes out along with a normal tidal volume breath resulting in a larger expired tidal volume than inspired tidal volume (i.e., the expired volume curve extends below the baseline). This cycle may repeat as long as air trapping continues.

Air trapping may also be recognized by studying the expiratory flow and pressure waveforms. In Figure 11-35, the expiratory flow in the first flow wave is similar to patterns often observed in clinic for patients with obstructive airway diseases from bronchoconstriction, lesions, or severe excess in airway secretions. The first double-headed arrow *a* indicates that the expiratory flow is dropping rapidly toward zero flow. This may indicate that the patient has a high drive to breathe and is trying to "inspire" during expiration and, hence, slowing the expiratory flow and reducing expiratory pressure as pointed to (arrow *a*) on the pressure wave below it. It could also indicate that airway obstruction is slowing flow. As a result of hyperinflation or trapped gas some patients cannot expand their thorax or lungs

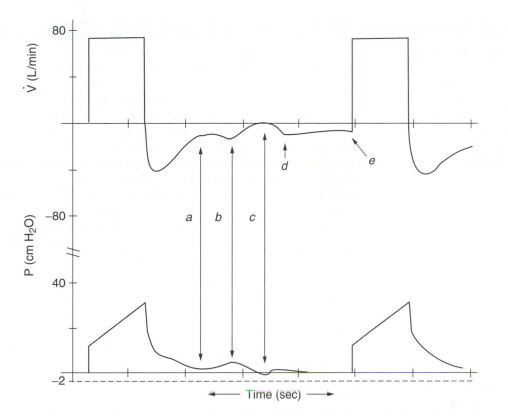

Figure 11-35 Expiratory flow and pressure waveforms during volume-controlled ventilation showing airflow obstruction, spontaneous inspiratory efforts, and auto-PEEP during the expiratory phase.

(Figure 11-35)
Double arrow *b* shows that the expiratory flow is increasing suddenly with a corresponding rise in pressure. This suggests the patient is trying to actively *expire* or sudden relief of an obstruction.

enough to create negative pressure in the ventilator-patient circuit. Their ineffective inspiratory efforts may only slow the flow of gas being released from areas of the lungs, which have longer time constants. They may be able to reduce the driving pressure (P_{ALV}), but may not be able to create sufficient negative P_{AO} to trigger a breath. The drop in flow or pressure may be obstruction to flow, which might be caused by excess secretions, structural damage to airways, or dynamic airway compression. Obstruction from a more homogeneous condition (bronchoconstriction) may present a different pattern (Figure 11-32).

The second double-headed arrow *b* points to a sudden increase in flow and corresponding expiratory pressure. This can occur if the patient attempts to actively expire or the obstruction is momentarily relieved with a change in flow dynamics and time constants.

A third double-headed arrow *c* points to an obvious inspiratory effort during expiration since flow drops momentarily to zero and an insufficient negative pressure (above sensitivity threshold) is recorded. The patient continues to expire more of the trapped gas

✓ (Figure 11-35) Double arrow *c* shows an inspiratory effort during expiration. Note that the flow momentarily drops to baseline and a negative pressure is recorded.

(arrow *d*) and flow increases and some positive pressure is recorded. A controlled mechanical breath is then time triggered before the patient has completed expiration as indicated (arrow *e*).

The patient needs to be assessed for respiratory movements whenever such patterns are observed. V_T and T_I may have to be reduced to allow more T_E, and the sensitivity threshold may have to be increased (-0.5 versus -2 cm H_2O). The respiratory effort needs to be properly documented during evaluation for weaning. Patients often trigger two or three times as many breaths as recorded by the ventilator. Inspiratory efforts during expiration can be felt by placing a hand over the patient's abdomen. Contraction of the abdominal muscles can be felt during forced expirations following the ineffective inspiratory efforts. Visual signs of chest movement, supra- or subclavicular retractions, and interruption of expiratory flow can be heard on auscultation during inspiratory efforts. The graphics can be monitored at the same time to confirm the coordination of efforts with the physical signs of respiration.

Now that the expiratory flow wave as a diagnostic tool has been discussed, refer back to Figure 11-26. Letters *a* and *b* and arrows indicate the cause for a reduction in V_T (flow × T_I) for the second and fourth waveforms. In example A, letter *a* indicates a prolonged T_E and decreased expiratory flow rate. Thus, increased airway resistance is responsible for the reduction in V_T delivery and prolonged T_E. In example B, T_E has been decreased. The peak flow is the same because the expiratory driving pressure (peak P_{ALV}) is the same, but a lower V_T is expired. Decreased C_{LT} is responsible for the reduction in V_T delivery and shortened T_E.

✓ Lack of ventilator response may be caused by dysfunction of the inspiratory valve or inappropriate sensitivity setting.

TROUBLESHOOTING VENTILATOR FUNCTION

LACK OF VENTILATOR RESPONSE

✓ (Figure 11-36) Arrow *a* shows air leak since the expiratory volume is less than the inspired tidal volume.

Another use of graphics is to check proper ventilator function. For example, inspiratory valve dysfunction (i.e., a sticking valve) or an out-of-calibration sensitivity threshold can be readily observed when the sensitivity tracing on the pressure-time waveform does not match the sensitivity setting on the ventilator (Figure 11-27).

CIRCUIT LEAKS

✓ (Figure 11-36) Arrow *b* shows that the air leak (less volume) lowers the PIP—the pressure required for volume delivery.

Volume waveforms are primarily used to ensure accurate V_T delivery. They can also be used to check for air leak (Figure 11-36). In the second volume waveform, letter *a* (arrow) demonstrates that a leak has developed since the volume never returns to the zero baseline. The ventilator still delivers the same flow pattern, but the pressure

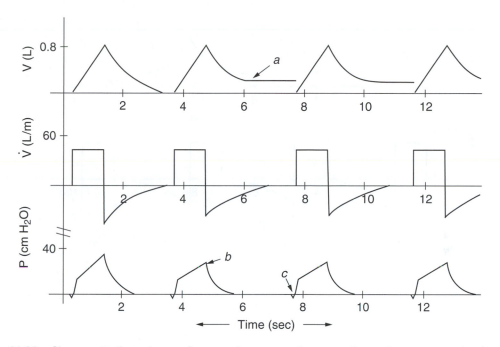

Figure 11-36   Changes to the volume-, flow-, and pressure-time waveforms demonstrate the development of an air leak. Note that the expiratory volume starting from the second breath (*a*) does not return to baseline. The peak inspiratory pressure starting from the second breath (*b*) is reduced from the previous level.

☑ (Figure 11-36) Arrow *c* shows that in air leak conditions, more negative pressure is needed to reach the preset sensitivity level.

☑ (Figure 11-37) When a circuit leak occurs in the presence of PEEP, the circuit pressure may drop to or below the preset sensitivity level (dotted lines). This causes autotriggering and rapid mechanical breaths.

waveform (*b*) shows that the PIP for ventilation has been reduced, since less volume is being delivered to the patient's lungs. Also note that the expiratory flow waves have decreased volumes expired after the leak develops. The third pressure-time waveform (*c*) is used to emphasize that the negative pressure to trigger the sensitivity threshold may appear the same (although sometimes the descent to the sensitivity threshold may be prolonged), but since negative pressure in the circuit is dependent on gas decompression, it will be more difficult for the patient to reduce pressure to the sensitivity threshold if gas can be drawn from the atmosphere.

Figure 11-37 demonstrates the same leak problem as presented in Figure 11-36. However, in this example, approximately 10 cm H_2O PEEP has been added to the circuit and patient's lungs. Again, volume does not return to zero. The PIPs and expiratory flow patterns have also been reduced for the waveforms depicted after the leak appeared. The arrow indicates that once the leak begins, pressure in the circuit starts dropping to the sensitivity setting below the PEEP level set (dotted lines). This may lead to autotriggering and go unnoticed unless respiratory rates reach extremely high levels (>25 to 30/min).

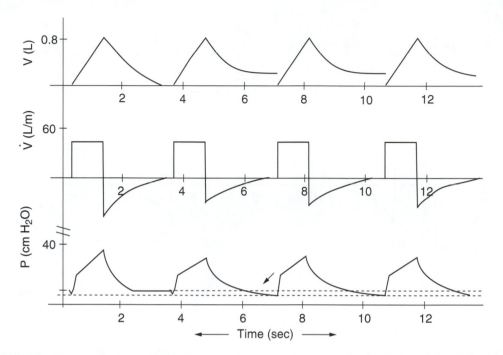

Figure 11-37 Changes to the volume-, flow-, and pressure-time waveforms demonstrate the effect of an air leak when PEEP is used. A reduced circuit pressure (due to air leak) is sufficient to drop the sensitivity level below the PEEP level, causing autotriggering and fast mechanical rate.

☑ (Figure 11-38) The double-headed arrow shows the flow-resistive pressure or transairway pressure (P_{TA}). $P_{TA} = P_{AO} - P_{ALV}$ throughout the pressure-volume loop. [Note: end-inspiratory P_{AO} = PIP, end-inspiratory P_{ALV} = peak P_{ALV} or plateau pressure. Refer to Figure 11-4 for review.]

PRESSURE-VOLUME LOOP (PVL) AND FLOW-VOLUME LOOP (FVL)

PRESSURE-VOLUME LOOP (PVL)

Another option offered by graphics software is the pressure-volume loop (PVL) presented in Figure 11-38 for an assist breath during CFW ventilation. The P_{AO} can be read from the x-axis and volume from the y-axis. The double-headed arrow indicates the flow-resistive pressure (P_{TA}) is the difference between P_{AO} and P_{ALV} (dotted line). P_{TA} remains the same throughout inspiration as it does for the step ascending ramp pressure waveform once the initial peak flow is reached and maintained during CFW ventilation. The PIP of 30 cm H_2O (dotted line) and peak P_{ALV} of 25 cm H_2O are labeled. It is assumed that the C_{LT} is unchanged in this example since P_{ALV} rises linearly with increase in volume.

EFFECTS OF LUNG-THORAX COMPLIANCE ON PVL

Figure 11-39 shows a control breath; there is no negative pressure to trigger the mechanical breath. This PVL illustrates how a reduction in C_{LT} causes the loop to move down and to the right (i.e., toward the

Figure 11-38 Characteristics of a pressure-volume loop. The dotted line within the loop is the peak alveolar pressure (P_{ALV} or plateau pressure). The transairway pressure (P_{TA} or flow resistive pressure) is the difference between the P_{ALV} and airway opening pressure (P_{AO}).

Figure 11-39 The effects of lung-thorax compliance (C_{LT}) on the pressure-volume loop during volume-controlled, constant flow ventilation. A decreased C_{LT} shifts the curve toward the pressure axis.

Figure 11-40 The effects of airflow resistance on the pressure-volume loop during volume-controlled, constant flow ventilation. An increased airflow resistance causes increase in PIP, inspiratory and expiratory P_{TA}, and P_{AO}. Note that the P_{ALV} is unchanged.

☑ (Figure 11-38) This pressure-volume loop shows that the lung-thorax compliance (C_{LT}) remains unchanged because the P_{ALV} rises linearly with increases in volume.

☑ (Figure 11-39) A decrease in C_{LT} causes the pressure-volume loop to shift to the right (toward the pressure axis).

☑ (Figure 11-39) A decrease in C_{LT} will not affect the P_{TA} because the PIP-P_{ALV} gradient (P_{TA}) remains unchanged.

☑ (Figure 11-40) In situations where the airflow resistance is increased, the P_{ALV} remains unchanged while P_{TA}, PIP, and P_{AO} are increased.

pressure axis). The increase in PIP (from 30 to 40 cm H_2O) is proportionate to the increase in P_{ALV} (from 25 to 35 cm H_2O) that is caused by the reduction in C_{LT}. The P_{TA} gradient throughout inspiration (and between PIP and peak P_{ALV}) is held constant. P_{TA} is affected by changes in resistance, not by the changes in C_{LT}.

It is essential to note that on some ventilators (e.g., Servo 300), pressure and volume may be assigned to the y- and x-axis, respectively. A reduction in C_{LT} would shift the PVL up and to the left (i.e., toward the pressure axis).

EFFECT OF AIRFLOW RESISTANCE ON PVL

Figure 11-40 shows how the PVL is affected by an increase in resistance (double-headed arrows and dotted lines). P_{ALV} remains unchanged in this example, while inspiratory and expiratory flow-resistive pressure (P_{TA}), PIP, and P_{AO} have all increased.

LOWER INFLECTION POINT ON PVL AND TITRATION OF PEEP

Figure 11-41 shows the effects on the PVL if C_{LT} changes during tidal volume delivery. The dotted line indicates that the slope of the P_{ALV}

Figure 11-41 The initial point of inflection (Ipi) shows the change in the slope from low to improved compliance. A level of PEEP slightly higher (e.g., 2 cm H₂O) than the Ipi may be used to prevent alveolar closure during expiration.

✓ (Figure 11-41) The pressure-volume (compliance) loop shows that the initial point of inflection (Ipi) is the compliance point in which the alveoli are recruited (opened) during mechanical ventilation.

✓ (Figure 11-41) In the presence of Ipi on the pressure-volume loop, PEEP may be added at or slightly above the Ipi to prevent alveoli collapse during expiration.

during V_T delivery has changed. A line has been drawn through the initial slope caused by low C_{LT}, compared to the line for the slope caused by an improvement in C_{LT}. This change in the slope from low to improved compliance is known as the initial point of inflection (Ipi) (Beydon et al., 1991). The Ipi occurs when alveoli are recruited (opened) by volume/pressure during inspiration. In this example, P_{ALV} could have been measured by adding progressively larger volumes of gas (beginning at approximately 35 mL) to the patient's lung via a large volume syringe until the V_T was reached, and then plotting the pause pressures acquired. In the presence of Ipi, some studies suggest using a PEEP level of 2 cm H_2O above the pressure at the Ipi to prevent the alveoli from closing during expiration. Other studies suggest setting PEEP above the closing P_{ALV} pressure on the expiratory side of the curve to prevent alveolar collapse during mechanical ventilation. This can be a useful strategy in the management of some ventilator patients because studies suggest that the repeated opening and closing of alveoli during mechanical ventilation causes shearing of lung parenchyma (barotraumas), which may augment ARDS and multiple organ failure. The complexity of this issue and setting the optimal PEEP level to open the lung or prevent alveolar collapse is beyond the scope of this chapter.

✓ (Figure 11-42) Overinflation of the alveoli beyond the optimal lung compliance causes the compliance to drop. The point of overinflation is called the upper inflection point (Ipu).

✓ (Figure 11-42) In the presence of Ipu on the pressure-volume loop, the tidal volume should be reduced until the Ipu (duckbill) disappears.

✓ (Figure 11-43) On a flow-volume loop, the inspiratory flow is above the horizontal axis whereas the expiratory flow is below.

✓ (Figure 11-43) Positive response to bronchodilator therapy improves the *expiratory* flow as airflow resistance is reduced. Inspiratory flow is unchanged because it is determined by the settings on the ventilator.

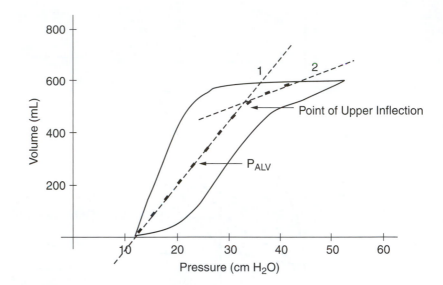

Figure 11-42   The point of upper inflection (Ipu) shows a reducing lung-thorax compliance due to hyperdistention of the alveoli. The tidal volume may be reduced until the Ipu (or duckbill) disappears.

UPPER INFLECTION POINT ON PVL AND ADJUSTMENT OF V_T

Figure 11-42 presents the PVL waveform where an upper inflection point (Ipu) exists. In this example, the P_{ALV} has been plotted as described for Figure 11-37. C_{LT} changed later during V_T delivery because of hyperdistention of the alveoli. The reduction in C_{LT} late in the inspiratory cycle is called the Ipu (Dambrosio et al., 1997). In this example, slope 1 for P_{ALV} (dotted line) is normal, and slope 2 (dotted line) shows a decrease in C_{LT} and the point of upper inflection. The appearance of the upper shape of the P_{AO} curve indicating the presence of an Ipu is known as the duckbill PVL. When a duckbill occurs, the V_T can be reduced until the duckbill vanishes (Roupe et al., 1995). A C_{LT} measurement should show improvement at that point.

EFFECTS OF AIRWAY STATUS ON FLOW-VOLUME LOOP (FVL)

Figure 11-43 shows another waveform option, the flow-volume loop (FVL). FVLs show flow measurements on the y-axis, and volume measurement on the x-axis. Inspiratory flow is above the volume measurement and expiratory flow is below. This example shows two superimposed waveforms during CFW ventilation at 40 L/min and results of pre- and postbronchodilator therapy. Following bronchodilator therapy, peak and average expiratory flow is typically improved (Gay, 1987).

Figure 11-43   The effect of airflow resistance on the flow-volume loop. A reduction in airflow resistance increases the peak expiratory flow rate.

SUMMARY

In summary, if graphics of flow-, volume- and pressure-time waveforms, pressure-volume loop, and flow-volume loop could be saved when patients were first placed on a ventilator, ventilator management of patient's progress could be studied and greatly enhanced. Follow-up graphics could be saved and superimposed over the initial copies for comparison similar to what has been done with the figures throughout this chapter. This can now be done on a minimal level on some ventilator graphics packages. Disk files or printed copies of therapeutic interventions (i.e., bronchodilators, changes in mode of ventilation, chest physical therapy etc.) and improvements could be documented. Graphic analysis could be used to facilitate discussion and be shared with colleagues and physicians. Outcome assessments of the performance of therapists and respiratory care departments in the area of ventilator management could be documented. A higher quality of ventilator-patient assessment and care is being carried out by practitioners with sufficient expertise in graphic analysis on a day-to-day basis. The sophisticated level of software needed for documentation of these improvements in practice, however, is not readily available. There have been some improvements, but much more needs to be accomplished for sophisticated analysis of patients via waveforms on a broader scale. The technology is available and it will be exciting to see the eventual changes as the professionals demand further improvements from the ventilator manufacturers. Expertise in waveform analysis at a high level is not required for professionals in respiratory care as yet, and the level of expertise is unknown. Those with knowledge and experience know that waveform analysis improves patient care and that it is a very useful tool in ventilator management. However, these improvements need to be studied and supported through research. There is still much to learn. Hopefully the knowledge you gain through study of this work will help serve that purpose.

Self-Assessment Questions

1. The accelerating and sine flow waveforms are not used for positive pressure ventilation because the initial flow rate is _____ for most patients. These two waveforms may be appropriate for _____ ventilation.

    A. too high, control
    B. too high, intermittent mandatory

    C. not sufficient, control
    D. not sufficient, intermittent mandatory

2. In flow and pressure waveforms, time in seconds is displayed along the _____ axis.

    A. x- or horizontal
    B. x- or vertical

    C. y- or horizontal
    D. y- or vertical

3. Tidal volume can be calculated or determined by measuring the _____ under a _____ waveform.

    A. slope, flow/time
    B. slope, pressure/time

    C. area, flow/time
    D. area, pressure/time

4. The area enclosed under the expiratory flow waveform should _____ the area under the inspiratory flow waveform. If the expiratory volume is less than the inspiratory volume, _____ may be present.

    A. be greater than, airflow obstruction

    B. equal to, airflow obstruction

    C. be greater than, circuit leak or gas trapping
    D. equal to, circuit leak or gas trapping

5. In assist/control mode, the I:E ratio is variable because the _____ time of a breath is dependent on the beginning of the _____ breath.

    A. inspiratory, preceding
    B. inspiratory, following

    C. expiratory, preceding
    D. expiratory, following

6. On a pressure waveform, PEEP is present when the end-expiratory pressure rests:

   A. at 0 cm H_2O. C. above 0 cm H_2O.
   B. below 0 cm H_2O. D. above 5 cm H_2O.

7. On the pressure waveform, assist effort is present when the trigger pressure reaches the _____ setting.

   A. tidal volume C. pressure limit
   B. sensitivity D. peak flow

8. In CPAP mode, there are no _____ breaths and the airway pressure is above _____ cm H_2O.

   A. mechanical, 0 C. spontaneous, 0
   B. mechanical, 5 D. spontaneous, 5

9. An increase in inspiratory flow or airflow resistance would show an unchanged _____ but increased _____. (See Figure 11-11.)

   A. P_{ALV}, PIP and P_{TA} C. P_{TA} and P_{ALV}, PIP
   B. P_{ALV} and PIP, P_{TA} D. P_{ALV}, P_{TA}

10. A decrease in total compliance (C_{LT}) would show an unchanged _____ but increased _____. (See Figure 11-12.)

    A. P_{ALV}, PIP and P_{TA} C. PIP, P_{ALV} and PIP
    B. P_{TA}, PIP and P_{ALV} D. P_{ALV}, P_{TA}

11. When the flow waveform selection is changed from constant flow to *true* descending ramp while holding inspiratory time constant, the same volume can only be maintained if the *peak flow* of the descending pattern is:

    A. increased. C. halved.
    B. decreased. D. doubled.

12. When the flow waveform selection is changed from constant flow to *true* descending ramp during *flow-limited* ventilation, the same volume can only be maintained if the *inspiratory time* of the descending pattern is:

    A. increased. C. halved.
    B. decreased. D. doubled.

13. With time-limited ventilation, the higher *initial* peak flow for the descending ramp flow wave creates a _____ initial flow resistive pressure (P_{TA}) than the P_{TA} created by the constant flow. (See Figure 11-14.)

    A. higher   C. similar

    B. lower   D. constant

14. With flow limited ventilation, the initial flow resistive pressure (P_{TA}) is the same for the _____ flow waves. The *initial* peak flow level stays the same for _____ flow during flow limited ventilation. (See Figure 11-14.)

    A. constant, constant   C. descending ramp, descending ramp

    B. constant, descending ramp   D. constant and descending ramp, constant and descending ramp

15. In constant flow and descending ramp flow ventilation, the rise in alveolar pressure (P_{ALV}) is directly related to _____ and inversely related to _____.

    A. compliance, volume delivery   C. volume delivery, compliance

    B. compliance, airflow resistance   D. volume delivery, airflow resistance

16. At constant T_I, a decreased flow leads to: (See Figure 11-15.)

    A. higher V_T and P_{ALV}.   C. lower P_{TA} and P_{ALV}.

    B. higher V_T, P_{TA}, and P_{ALV}.   D. lower V_T, P_{TA}, and P_{ALV}.

17. During descending ramp flow ventilation, a higher end flow leads to a _____ V_T and P_{TA} and it _____ affect the P_{ALV}. (See Figure 11-16.)

    A. larger, does   C. smaller, does

    B. larger, does not   D. smaller, does not

18. When peak flow is constant (square), _____ are _____ related.

    A. V_T, and P_{ALV}; directly   C. V_T, and P_{ALV}; inversely

    B. V_T T_I and P_{ALV}; directly   D. V_T, T_I and P_{ALV}; inversely

19. In pressure controlled ventilation, _____ are typically set by the operator.

    A. rate and I:E ratio   C. pressure level and rate

    B. pressure level and I:E ratio   D. pressure level, rate, and I:E ratio

20. In pressure controlled ventilation, the flow level and V_T delivered are dependent on the:

    A. pressure level set.   C. pressure level set and lung characteristics.

    B. pressure level set and patient effort.   D. pressure level set, patient effort, and lung characteristics.

21. During inverse ratio pressure controlled ventilation, the patients are usually sedated and paralyzed in order to prevent:

    A. barotrauma.
    B. dyssynchrony with the ventilator.

    C. hyperventilation.
    D. hypoxia.

22. In pressure support ventilation, only the _____ level is set and under normal condition, _____ are primarily under the patient's control.

    A. pressure support; flow, volume, and inspiratory time
    B. tidal volume; flow, volume, and inspiratory time

    C. peak inspiratory pressure; flow and volume
    D. plateau pressure; inspiratory time and volume

23. During pressure-limited ventilation, a(n) _____ airflow resistance or _____ compliance would reduce the delivered flow and tidal volume.

    A. increased, increased
    B. increased, decreased

    C. decreased, increased
    D. decreased, decreased

24. Tachypnea, agitation, accessory muscle use, active expiration, muscle fatigue, and respiratory failure are signs of:

    A. patient–ventilator dyssynchrony.
    B. hyperventilation.

    C. anxiety.
    D. decreased metabolic rate.

25. On a flow waveform, failure of the expiratory flow to return to baseline is indicative of _____ and this condition may lead to _____ and possibly auto-PEEP.

    A. incomplete inspiration, gas trapping
    B. incomplete inspiration, hypoventilation

    C. incomplete expiration, gas trapping
    D. incomplete expiration, hypoventilation

26. In the presence of excessive airway resistance, the expiratory flow is _____ and the expiratory time is _____.

    A. increased, prolonged
    B. increased, shortened

    C. decreased, prolonged
    D. decreased, shortened

27. A decreased C_{LT} leads to a higher expiratory peak flow, a _____ PIP, and a _____ expiratory time.

    A. higher, longer
    B. higher, shorter

    C. lower, longer
    D. lower, shorter

28. A delay of positive pressure waveform (i.e., lack of ventilator response) in spite of a normal negative pressure waveform (i.e., good patient effort) is indicative of:

    A. inadequate line pressure.

    B. ventilator malfunction.

    C. dysfunction of the inspiratory valve or sensitivity setting.

    D. electrical malfunction.

29. Failure of the expiratory flow to return to the zero baseline is indicative of:

    A. gas leak or air trapping.
    B. airflow obstruction.

    C. power failure.
    D. high lung compliance.

30. When circuit leak occurs in the presence of PEEP, pressure in the circuit drops to the sensitivity setting below the PEEP level and _____ develops and leads to extremely _____ mechanical breaths.

    A. auto-PEEP, slow
    B. auto-PEEP, fast

    C. autotriggering, slow
    D. autotriggering, fast

31. The difference between P_{AO} and P_{ALV} is: (See Figure 11-38.)

    A. PIP.
    B. P_{TA}.

    C. PEEP.
    D. C_{LT}.

32. On a volume pressure curve, the _____ is assumed to be stable and unchanged if P_{ALV} rises linearly with increases in volume. (See Figure 11-38.)

    A. C_{LT}
    B. PIP

    C. P_{TA}
    D. PEEP

33. On a pressure-volume loop, a reduction in C_{LT} causes the loop to move toward the: (See Figure 11-39.)

    A. y axis.
    B. volume axis.

    C. pressure axis.
    D. A and B only.

34. On a pressure-volume loop, a reduction in C_{LT} will not change the P_{TA} because the gradient between _____ remains the same. (See Figure 11-39.)

    A. P_{TA} and P_{AO}
    B. P_{AO} and P_{ALV}

    C. PIP and P_{AO}
    D. PIP and P_{ALV}

35. On a pressure-volume loop, an increase in resistance would not affect the _____ while the _____ are increased. (See Figure 11-40.)

    A. P_{ALV}; P_{TA} and PIP
    B. P_{ALV}; P_{TA}, PIP, and P_{AO}

    C. P_{TA}; PIP and P_{AO}
    D. P_{TA}; P_{AO}, PIP, and P_{ALV}

36. The initial point of inflection (Ipi) occurs when alveoli are recruited during _____. In the presence of Ipi, _____ can be added slightly above the pressure at the inflection point to prevent the alveoli from closing during expiration. (See Figure 11-41.)

    A. inspiration, PEEP   C. expiration, PEEP
    B. inspiration, tidal volume   D. expiration, tidal volume

37. Overinflation of the alveoli causes a(n) _____ in C_{LT} leading to the appearance of an upper inflection point (Ipu). The Ipu can be minimized by reducing the _____. (See Figure 11-42.)

    A. increase, PEEP   C. decrease, PEEP
    B. increase, tidal volume   D. decrease, tidal volume

38. On a flow-volume loop, the expiratory flow is _____ the horizontal axis (volume measurement) and it is usually _____ following a successful bronchodilator therapy. (See Figure 11-43.)

    A. above, increased   C. below, increased
    B. above, decreased   D. below, decreased

Answers to Self-Assessment Questions

1. C. not sufficient, control

2. A. *x-* or horizontal

3. C. area, flow/time

4. D. equal to, circuit leak or gas trapping

5. D. expiratory, following

6. C. above 0 cm H_2O

7. B. sensitivity

8. A. mechanical, 0

9. A. P_{ALV}, PIP and P_{TA}

10. B. P_{TA}, PIP and P_{ALV}

11. D. doubled.

12. D. doubled.

13. A. higher

14. D. constant and descending ramp, constant and descending ramp

15. C. volume delivery, compliance

16. D. lower V_T, P_{TA}, and P_{ALV}.

17. B. larger, does not

18. B. V_T, T_I, and P_{ALV}; directly

19. D. pressure level, rate, and I:E ratio

20. D. pressure level set, patient effort, and lung characteristics.

21. B. dyssynchrony with the ventilator.

22. A. pressure support; flow, volume, and inspiratory time

23. B. increased, decreased

24. A. patient-ventilator dyssynchrony.

25. C. incomplete expiration, gas trapping

26. C. decreased, prolonged

27. B. higher, shorter

28. C. dysfunction of the inspiratory valve or sensitivity setting

29. A. gas leak or air trapping

30. D. autotriggering, fast

31. B. P_{TA}

32. A. C_{LT}

33. C. pressure axis

34. D. PIP and P_{ALV}

35. B. P_{ALV}; P_{TA}, PIP, and P_{AO}

36. A. inspiration, PEEP

37. D. decrease, tidal volume

38. C. below, increased

References

Acute Respiratory Distress Syndrome Clinical Network (ARDSNet), (2000). Ventilation with lower tidal volumes as compared with traditional tidal volumes for acute lung injury and the acute respiratory distress syndrome. *N Engl J Med, 342,* 1301–1308.

Beydon, L., et al. (1991). Lung mechanics in ARDS: Compliance and pressure-volume curves. In Aapol, W. M., et al. (eds.) *Adult respiratory distress syndrome* (pp. 139–161). New York: Marcel Dekker.

Chatburn, R. L. (2001). A new system for understanding modes of mechanical ventilators. *Respir Care, 46*(6), 604–621.

Dambrosio, M., et al. (1997). Effects of positive end-expiratory pressure and different tidal volumes on alveolar recruitment and hyperinflation. *Anesthesiology, 87*(3), 495–503.

Dennison, F. H., et al. (1989). Analysis of resistance to gas flow in nine adult ventilator circuits. *Chest, 96,* 1374–1379.

Dick, C. R., et al. (1996). Patient–ventilator interactions. *Clini Chest Medi, 17*(3), 423–438.

Gay, P. C. (1987). Evaluation of bronchodilator responsiveness in mechanically-ventilated patients. *Am Rev Respir Dis, 136*, 880–885.

MacIntyre, N. R., et al. (2001). *Mechanical ventilation.* Philadelphia: W. B. Saunders Co.

Marini, J. J., et al. (1985). The inspiratory work of breathing during assisted mechanical ventilation. *Chest, 87*(5), 612–618.

Marini, J. J., et al. (1986). Bedside estimation of the inspiratory work of breathing during mechanical ventilation. *Chest, 89*(1), 56–63.

Messinger, G., et al. (1995). Using tracheal pressure to trigger the ventilator and control airway pressure during continuous positive airway pressure decreases work of breathing. *Chest, 108,* 509–514.

Nilsestuen, J. O., et al. (1996). Managing the patient–ventilator system using graphic analysis: An overview and introduction to graphics corner. *Resp Care, 41*(12), 1105–1120.

Nunn, J. F. (1977). *Applied respiratory physiology* (2nd ed.). Boston: Butterworths.

Roupe, E., et al. (1995). Titration of tidal volume and induced hypercapnia in acute respiratory distress syndrome. *Am J Respir Crit Care, 152*, 121–128.

Tobin, M. J. (1994). *Principles and practice of mechanical ventilation.* New York: McGraw-Hill.

Tobin, M. J., et al. (1986). The pattern of breathing during successful and unsuccessful trials of weaning from mechanical ventilation. *Am Rev Respir Dis, 134*, 1111–1118.

Suggested Reading

Flow-volume curve
Lu, Q., et al. (1999). A simple automated method for measuring pressure-volume curves during mechanical ventilation. *Am J Respir Crit Care Med, 159*(1), 275–282.

Volume-controlled and pressure-controlled ventilation
Burke, W. C., Crooke, P. S., III, Marcy, T. W., Adams, A. B., & Marini, J. J. (1993). Comparison of mathematical and mechanical models of pressure-controlled ventilation. *J Appl Physiol, 74*(2), 922–933.

Cinnella, G., Conti, G., Lofaso, F., Lorino, H., Harf, A., Lemaire, F., et al. (1996). Effects of assisted ventilation on the work of breathing: Volume-controlled versus pressure-controlled ventilation. *Am J Respir Crit Care Med, 153*(3), 1025–1033.

MacIntyre, N. R., Gropper, C., & Westfall, T. (1994). Combining pressure-limiting and volume-cycling features in a patient-interactive mechanical breath. *Crit Care Med, 22*(2), 353–357.

Munoz, J., Guerrero, J. E., Escalante, J. L., Palomino, R., & De La, C. B. (1993). Pressure-controlled ventilation versus controlled mechanical ventilation with decelerating inspiratory flow. *Crit Care Med, 21*(8), 1143–1148.

Tharratt, R. S., Allen, R. P., & Albertson, T. E. (1988). Pressure controlled inverse ratio ventilation in severe adult respiratory failure. *Chest, 94*(4), 755–762.

CHAPTER TWELVE

MANAGEMENT OF MECHANICAL VENTILATION

David W. Chang

OUTLINE

Introduction

Basic Management Strategies

Strategies to Improve Ventilation
Increase Mechanical Rate
Increase Spontaneous Tidal Volume
or Rate
Increase Mechanical Tidal Volume
Other Strategies to Improve
Ventilation
Permissive Hypercapnia

Strategies to Improve Oxygenation
Increase Inspired Oxygen Fraction
(F_IO_2)
Improve Ventilation and Reduce
Mechanical Deadspace
Improve Circulation
Maintain Normal Hemoglobin Level
Initiate Continuous Positive
Airway Pressure (CPAP)
Initiate Positive End-Expiratory
Pressure (PEEP)
Inverse Ratio Ventilation (IRV)
Extracorporeal Membrane
Oxygenation (ECMO)
High Frequency Oscillatory
Ventilation for Adults

Acid-Base Balance
Respiratory Acidosis and
Compensated Metabolic Alkalosis
Respiratory Alkalosis and
Compensated Metabolic Acidosis
Metabolic Acid-Base Abnormalities

**Troubleshooting of Common Ventilator
Alarms and Events**
Low Pressure Alarm
Low Expired Volume Alarm
High Pressure Alarm
High Respiratory Rate Alarm
Apnea/Low Respiratory Rate Alarm
High PEEP Alarm
Low PEEP Alarm
Auto-PEEP

Care of the Ventilator Circuit
Circuit Compliance
Circuit Patency
Humidity and Temperature
Frequency of Circuit Change

Care of the Artificial Airway
Patency of the Endotracheal Tube
Humidification and Removal of
Secretions
Ventilator-Associated Pneumonia

KEY TERMS

- alarm
- anion gap
- auto-PEEP
- barotrauma (volutrauma)
- brachial plexopathy
- culture and sensitivity
- extracellular fluid (ECF)
- Gram stain
- intracellular fluid (ICF)

- mechanical deadspace
- optimal PEEP
- oxygenation
- permissive hypercapnia
- prone positioning
- refractory hypoxemia
- spontaneous ventilation
- tracheal gas insufflation
- ventilator-associated pneumonia (VAP)

INTRODUCTION

The primary function of mechanical ventilation is to support the ventilatory and oxygenation requirement of a patient until such time that the patient becomes self-sufficient. During mechanical ventilation, it is essential to maintain a patient's acid-base balance, nutritional and resting needs, and fluid and electrolyte balance because these factors can affect management strategies of mechanical ventilation and patient outcome.

   This chapter discusses strategies to provide optimal ventilation and oxygenation during mechanical ventilation, as well as other methods to maintain essential physiologic functions through nutritional, fluid, and electrolyte support.

TABLE 12-1   Effects of Ventilator Setting Changes on Ventilation and Oxygenation When Changes are Indicated

SETTING	VENTILATION[*]	OXYGENATION[**]
↑ Frequency (f)	↑↑	↑
↑ Tidal volume (V_T)	↑↑	↑
↑ Fraction of inspired oxygen concentration (F_IO_2)	Unchanged or ↓	↑↑
↑ Positive end-expiratory pressure (PEEP)	Unchanged or ↓	↑↑
↑ Pressure support ventilation (PSV)	↑↑	↑
↑ Pressure gradient (ΔP) (e.g., Bilevel positive airway pressure, airway pressure release ventilation)	↑↑	↑

*   ↑ Ventilation = ↓ $PaCO_2$; ↓ Ventilation = ↑ $PaCO_2$
** ↑ Oxygenation = ↑ PaO_2, ↑ SpO_2, ↑ SaO_2

BASIC MANAGEMENT STRATEGIES

The primary goals of mechanical ventilation are to improve ventilation and oxygenation. Essentially all ventilators incorporate designs and features with these two goals in mind. Asides from the many modes of ventilation that are available, common settings that are available in most ventilators include frequency (f), tidal volume (V_T), fraction of inspired oxygenation concentration (F_IO_2), positive end-expiratory pressure (PEEP). Pressure support ventilation (PSV), and pressure gradient (ΔP). These settings and their intended effects on ventilation and oxygenation are summarized in Table 12-1.

STRATEGIES TO IMPROVE VENTILATION

☑ $PaCO_2$ >45 mm Hg is indicative of hypoventilation (the normal $PaCO_2$ for COPD patients is about 50 mm Hg).

Hypoventilation causes respiratory acidosis (ventilatory failure), and hypoxemia if supplemental oxygen is not provided to the patient. The best measure of a patient's ventilatory status is the $PaCO_2$ level. The normal $PaCO_2$ is 35 to 45 mm Hg; $PaCO_2$ greater than 45 mm Hg is indicative of hypoventilation. For COPD patients, however, the acceptable $PaCO_2$ should be the patient's normal value upon last

TABLE 12-2   Strategies to Improve Ventilation

PRIORITY	METHODS
1	Increase mechanical rate 　　Control rate in assist/control mode 　　Intermittent mandatory ventilation (IMV) rate 　　Synchronized IMV rate
2	Increase spontaneous tidal volume 　　Nutritional support and reconditioning of respiratory muscles 　　Administer bronchodilators 　　Initiate pressure support ventilation (PSV) 　　Use largest endotracheal tube possible
3	Increase mechanical tidal volume 　　Tidal volume (V_T)
4	Reduce **mechanical deadspace** 　　Use low-compliance ventilator circuit 　　Cut endotracheal tube to appropriate length 　　Perform tracheotomy
5	Consider high frequency jet or oscillatory ventilation

hospital discharge and generally it is about 50 mm Hg. When the $PaCO_2$ level goes above this value, significant hypoventilation may be present.

Strategies for improving a patient's ventilation are summarized in Table 12-2.

auto-PEEP: *Uninten-tional PEEP associ-ated with pressure support ventilation, rapid respiratory rates, slow inspira-tory flow, and air trapping.*

mechanical dead-space: *Volume of gas contained in the equipment and sup-plies (e.g., endotra-cheal tube, ventilator circuit) that does not take part in gas exchange.*

INCREASE MECHANICAL RATE

The most common approach to improve minute ventilation is to increase the respiratory rate (RR) of the ventilator. This may be the control rate in assist/control, the mandatory rate in intermittent mandatory ventilation, or other modes of ventilation that regulate the rate of the ventilator. However, the respiratory rate should not exceed 20/min as **auto-PEEP** may occur at or above this rate, espe-cially during pressure support ventilation (MacIntyre, 1986; Shapiro, 1994). The following equations show that an increase in respiratory rate causes a higher minute ventilation.

$$\uparrow \text{Minute Ventilation} = (\text{Ventilator } V_T \times \uparrow \text{Ventilator RR}) + (\text{Spontaneous } V_T \times \text{Spontaneous RR})$$

It is generally not desirable to increase the ventilator tidal volume beyond a level that is appropriate to the patient's body weight, generally 10 to 15 mL/kg (Burton et al., 1997). In volume-limited ventilators, a

✔️ The most common approach to improve minute ventilation is to increase the respiratory rate of the ventilator.

✔️ See Appendix 1 for example.

✔️ It is more advantageous for a patient to increase the spontaneous tidal volume since increasing the respiratory rate at low tidal volume promotes deadspace ventilation.

spontaneous ventilation: Volume of gas inspired by a patient. It is directly related to the patient's spontaneous tidal volume and respiratory rate.

✔️ Pressure support ventilation increases spontaneous tidal volume, and therefore the minute ventilation.

larger tidal volume requires a higher peak inspiratory pressure. This high pressure condition increases the incidence of ventilator-related lung injuries such as cardiovascular impairment and barotrauma.

To estimate the mechanical rate needed to achieve a certain $PaCO_2$, the following formula may be used, assuming the ventilator tidal volume and deadspace volume stay the same (Barnes et al., 1994; Burton et al., 1997).

$$\text{New rate} = \frac{(\text{Rate} \times \text{PaCO}_2)}{\text{Desired PaCO}_2}$$

New rate : Ventilator rate needed for a desired $PaCO_2$
Rate : Original ventilator rate
$PaCO_2$: Original arterial carbon dioxide tension
Desired $PaCO_2$: Desired arterial carbon dioxide tension

INCREASE SPONTANEOUS TIDAL VOLUME OR RATE

In most modes of mechanical ventilation, minute ventilation is the sum of the volume delivered by the ventilator and the volume achieved by a spontaneously breathing patient. For this reason, the patient can contribute to the minute ventilation by increasing either the spontaneous tidal volume or spontaneous rate.

$\uparrow$ Minute Ventilation = (Ventilator V_T × Ventilator RR) + ($\uparrow$ Spontaneous V_T × $\uparrow$ Spontaneous RR)

It is more advantageous for a patient to increase the spontaneous tidal volume since increasing the respiratory rate at low tidal volume promotes deadspace ventilation. A larger deadspace to tidal volume ratio (V_A/V_T) results because of the constant anatomic deadspace volume at a reduced tidal volume.

In some patients, the respiratory muscles are not sufficient to maintain prolonged **spontaneous ventilation** or to overcome air flow resistance imposed by the ventilator circuit and endotracheal tube. This condition may be compensated by using pressure support ventilation. The level of pressure support is usually started at 10 to 15 cm H_2O (Shapiro, 1994) and titrated until a desired spontaneous tidal volume and respiratory rate are obtained. The increase in spontaneous tidal volume improves the minute ventilation.

Low levels of pressure support ventilation (<10 cm H_2O) are titrated and used to overcome the air flow resistance of the ventilator circuit and endotracheal tube. At high levels of pressure support ventilation (>20 cm H_2O), the breathing pattern resembles pressure-limited assisted ventilation (Burton et al., 1997; Nathan et al., 1993). Pressure support ventilation increases spontaneous tidal volume, and therefore the minute ventilation.

$\uparrow$ Minute Ventilation = (Ventilator V_T × Ventilator RR) + ($\uparrow$ Spontaneous V_T × Spontaneous RR)

INCREASE MECHANICAL TIDAL VOLUME

The ventilator tidal volume is usually set according to the patient's body weight and its range available for adjustments is rather narrow. Excessive ventilator tidal volume may increase the likelihood of ventilator-related lung injuries. On the other hand, inadequate ventilator tidal volume may induce atelectasis.

Before a decision is made to increase the ventilator tidal volume, one must first consider the detrimental side effects of excessive volume and pressure. It should be implemented only when the ventilator rate is too fast and exceeds the patient's ideal breathing pattern and inspiratory-expiratory relationship.

OTHER STRATEGIES TO IMPROVE VENTILATION

Other strategies to improve the minute ventilation may involve use of ventilator circuits with low compressible volume. This helps to reduce the mechanical deadspace and volume loss due to the tubing compression factor.

The endotracheal tube is sometimes cut shorter to facilitate tube management, to clear secretions, and to reduce tubing deadspace. Tracheostomy also improves ventilation by enhancing tube management and secretion removal. In addition, it provides easier access for oral care and lower tubing deadspace than an oral endotracheal tube.

High frequency jet ventilation has been used extensively only in the infant population. It is effective to improve ventilation in infants but its use in adult patients shows mixed results.

PERMISSIVE HYPERCAPNIA

In mechanical ventilation, peak inspiratory pressure is used to create the pressure gradient and to deliver a predetermined tidal volume. Occasionally the peak inspiratory pressure can be very high in the presence of high airway resistance and low compliance. This high level of pressure and volume in the lungs may lead to ventilator-related lung injuries.

Permissive hypercapnia is a strategy to minimize the occurrence of ventilator-related lung injuries caused by positive pressure ventilation (Hickling, 2002). This is done by ventilating the patient with a small tidal volume in a range of 4 to 7 mL/kg (normally 10 to 15 mL/kg) (Feihl et al., 1994), thus making it possible to ventilate the patient with a lower peak inspiratory pressure, and to minimize potential pressure- or volume-related complications. Since the plateau pressure (i.e., end-inspiratory occlusion pressure) is the best estimate of the average peak alveolar pressure, it is often used as the target pressure when trying to avoid alveolar overdistention (Slutsky, 1994). Permissive hypercapnia using a low tidal volume (4 to 7 mL/kg) strategy is more likely to keep the plateau pressure lower than 35 cm H_2O.

permissive hypercapnia: Intentional hypoventilation of a patient by reducing the mechanical tidal volume to a range of 4 to 7 mL/kg (normally 10 to 15 mL/kg). It is used to lower the pulmonary pressures and to minimize the risk of ventilator-related lung injuries. The patient's $PaCO_2$ is significantly elevated but the acidotic pH may be neutralized by a bicarbonate IV drip.

☑ Permissive hypercapnia is a strategy to minimize the occurrence of ventilator-related lung injuries caused by positive pressure ventilation by using a *small* ventilator tidal volume (4 to 7 mL/kg).

☑ The plateau pressure should be kept below 35 cm H_2O to avoid alveolar overdistention or barotrauma.

☑ Tromethamine (THAM) lowers the carbon dioxide level and increases the bicarbonate levels. It is preferable to bicarbonate in patients who are being hypoventilated intentionally.

Small tidal volume may cause hypoventilation, CO_2 retention, and acidosis. Acidosis causes the development of central nervous dysfunction, intracranial hypertension, neuromuscular weakness, cardiovascular impairment, and increased pulmonary vascular resistance. These potential complications may be alleviated by keeping the pH within its normal range, between 7.35 to 7.45, either by renal compensation over time or by neutralizing the acid with bicarbonate or tromethamine (Marini, 1993).

Tromethamine (THAM) is a nonbicarbonate buffer that helps to compensate for metabolic acidosis. THAM decreases the hydrogen ion concentration and indirectly decreases the carbon dioxide level and increases the bicarbonate level. Because of its lowering effect on the carbon dioxide level, tromethamine may be preferable to bicarbonate in patients who are being hypoventilated intentionally (i.e., permissive hypercapnia) (Kallet et al., 2000). Dosage of 0.3 M tromethamine needed to compensate for metabolic acidosis is calculated by body weight in kilograms × base deficit in milliequivalents per liter. Side effects of tromethamine include transient hypoglycemia, respiratory depression, and hemorrhagic hepatic necrosis (Nahas et al., 1998).

By normalizing the pH, it appears that permissive hypercapnia may be a safe and beneficial strategy in the management of patients with status asthmaticus (Cox et al., 1991; Darioli et al., 1984), and adult respiratory distress syndrome (ARDS) (Feihl et al., 1994; Hickling et al., 1990; Lewandowski et al., 1992). The mechanism and physiologic changes of permissive hypercapnia are outlined in Figure 12-1.

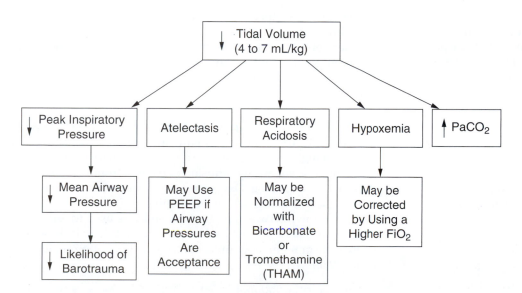

Figure 12-1   Mechanism and physiologic changes in permissive hypercapnia.

TABLE 12-3   Strategies to Improve Oxygenation

PRIORITY	METHODS
1	Increase inspired oxygen fraction (F_IO_2)
2	Improve ventilation and reduce mechanical deadspace

3	Improve circulation
	    Fluid replacement if patient is hypovolemic
	    Vasopressors if patient is in shock
	    Cardiac drugs if patient is in congestive heart failure

4	Maintain normal hemoglobin level
5	Initiate continuous positive airway pressure (CPAP) only with *adequate* spontaneous ventilation
6	Consider airway pressure release ventilation (APRV)
7	Initiate positive end-expiratory pressure (PEEP) Titrate optimum PEEP
8	Consider inverse ratio ventilation
9	Consider extracorporeal membrane oxygenation (ECMO), high-frequency ventilation, hyperbaric oxygenation, or intravascular oxygenation (IVOX) device

STRATEGIES TO IMPROVE OXYGENATION

oxygenation:
Amount of oxygen available for metabolic functions.

Oxygenation is dependent on adequate and well-balanced ventilation, diffusion, and perfusion. The strategies to improve oxygenation are therefore structured to improve the normal physiologic functions or to compensate for the abnormal functions. The prioritized methods to improve oxygenation, from simple to complex, are outlined in Table 12-3.

INCREASE INSPIRED OXYGEN FRACTION (F_IO_2)

☑ Oxygen readily corrects hypoxemia that is due to uncomplicated V/Q abnormalities.

Supplemental oxygen is most frequently used to manage hypoxemia because a high F_IO_2 increases the alveolar-capillary oxygen pressure gradient, thus enhancing diffusion of oxygen from the lungs to the pulmonary circulation. Oxygen readily corrects hypoxemia that is due to uncomplicated V/Q abnormalities.

The following two-step procedure may be used to estimate the needed F_IO_2 for a desired PaO_2 assuming that there is no severe deadspace or shunt abnormalities (Burton et al., 1997; Krider et al., 1986).

$$\text{Step 1: } P_AO_2 \text{ needed} = \frac{PaO_2 \text{ desired}}{(a/A \text{ ratio})}$$

$$\text{Step 2: } F_IO_2 = \frac{(P_AO_2 \text{ needed} + 50)}{713}$$

P_AO_2 needed : Alveolar oxygen tension needed for a desired PaO_2

PaO_2 desired : Arterial oxygen tension desired

a/A ratio : Arterial/alveolar oxygen tension ratio; (PaO_2/P_AO_2 before changes)

F_IO_2 : Inspired oxygen concentration needed to get a desired PaO_2

50 : normal $PaCO_2$/Respiratory Quotient = (40/0.8) mm Hg

713 : $P_B - PH_2O = (760 - 47)$ mm Hg

Oxygen and Ventilation.   Most patients with respiratory acidosis or ventilatory failure are also hypoxemic. Hypoxemia related to hypoventilation may be partially corrected by improving ventilation. But in most cases supplemental oxygen is also needed to treat hypoxemia. In a clinical setting, an elevated $PaCO_2$ along with hypoxemia should be treated with ventilation and oxygen.

Oxygen and PEEP.   Oxygen therapy alone may not be sufficient if the hypoxemia is caused by intrapulmonary shunting. This type of **refractory hypoxemia** requires oxygen and continuous positive airway pressure (CPAP) or positive end-expiratory pressure (PEEP).

Oxygen Toxicity.   Sufficient oxygen should be given to the patient to maintain a PaO_2 of around 80 mm Hg (lower for COPD patients). Excessive oxygen is to be avoided because of the increased likelihood of developing oxygen toxicity, ciliary impairment, lung damage, respiratory distress syndrome, and pulmonary fibrosis (Otto, 1986). Since these complications may occur within 12 to 24 hours of exposure to 100% oxygen, the general guideline is to use an F_IO_2 lower than 60% and use high levels of F_IO_2 for less than 24 hours, when possible (Winter et al., 1972).

IMPROVE VENTILATION AND REDUCE MECHANICAL DEADSPACE

Adequate ventilation is a prerequisite to oxygenation. Hypoxemia caused by hypoventilation is usually supported by supplemental oxygen during mechanical ventilation, but it must be corrected by improving alveolar ventilation. Arterial $PaCO_2$ is the best measure of a patient's ventilatory status. When $PaCO_2$ is elevated in conjunction with hypoxemia, improvement in the patient's oxygenation status may be possible by ventilation alone. The level of ventilation can be

☑ Hypoxemia related to hypoventilation may be partially corrected by improving ventilation. But in most cases, supplemental oxygen is also needed to treat hypoxemia.

refractory hypoxemia: Hypoxemia that is commonly caused by intrapulmonary shunting and does not respond well to high or increasing F_IO_2.

☑ Refractory hypoxemia responds well to supplemental oxygen when used with CPAP or PEEP.

☑ Alveolar ventilation may be improved by ↑ mechanical rate or V_T or ↑ spontaneous rate or V_T.

✓ Alveolar ventilation may be improved by ↓ the anatomic, mechanical, or alveolar deadspace.

improved by increasing the mechanical rate or tidal volume; or the patient's spontaneous tidal volume or rate.

Alveolar ventilation may also be improved by reducing the deadspace volume. Endotracheal intubation and tracheostomy are both effective in reducing the anatomic deadspace. Mechanical deadspace of an endotracheal tube may be decreased by cutting it shorter than the original length. If a high V/Q mismatch (ventilation in excess of perfusion) exists, alveolar deadspace may be reduced by improving pulmonary perfusion.

IMPROVE CIRCULATION

✓ Hypoperfusion due to congestive heart failure may be corrected by improving myocardial function.

Adequate pulmonary blood flow is necessary for proper gas exchange. If perfusion is too low relative to ventilation, deadspace ventilation (high V/Q) results. If perfusion is too high, pulmonary hypertension becomes the potential problem. In order to maintain a normal ventilation-perfusion relationship, the hemodynamic values should be monitored regularly, including systemic arterial pressure, central venous pressure, pulmonary artery pressure, and pulmonary capillary wedge pressure.

✓ In relative hypovolemia (loss of venous tone), fluid replacement should be done with extreme caution because of the potential for fluid overload when vascular tone returns to normal.

When hypovolemia occurs due to volume loss, fluid replacement is necessary. If the cause of hypovolemia is shock (relative hypovolemia; loss of venous tone), fluid replacement should be done with extreme caution because of the potential for fluid overload when vascular tone returns to normal. Vasopressors are very useful to provide quick relief from hypovolemia due to shock but the condition should be corrected by treating the cause of shock.

MAINTAIN NORMAL HEMOGLOBIN LEVEL

Monitoring of the PaO_2 alone for assessment of oxygenation status may be inadequate when a patient's hemoglobin level is below normal. This is because PaO_2 measures the amount of oxygen dissolved in the plasma whereas a vast majority (98%) of the oxygen in the blood is combined with and carried by the hemoglobins. When anemic hypoxia is suspected, the hemoglobin level should be checked for the presence of anemia (hemoglobin less than 10 g/100 mL of blood).

Treatment of anemia must be specific to the cause. For example, anemia due to excessive blood loss should be treated by stopping the blood loss and replacing the blood volume. Anemia caused by insufficient hemoglobin should be treated by replacing the red blood cells. Once the hemoglobin level is restored, the oxygen carrying capacity and oxygen content should return to normal.

✓ CPAP is only suitable for patients who have adequate respiratory mechanics and can sustain prolonged spontaneous breathing.

INITIATE CONTINUOUS POSITIVE AIRWAY PRESSURE (CPAP)

Continuous positive airway pressure (CPAP) provides positive airway pressure throughout the respiratory cycle. It increases the functional residual capacity and is therefore very useful to correct hypoxemia due to intrapulmonary shunting. Since CPAP does not provide mechanical ventilation, it is suitable only for patients who have adequate respiratory mechanics and can sustain prolonged spontaneous breathing. Adequacy of spontaneous ventilation can be documented by trending a patient's $PaCO_2$. An increasing $PaCO_2$ over time indicates that the patient is tiring and continuation of CPAP must be reevaluated.

INITIATE POSITIVE END-EXPIRATORY PRESSURE (PEEP)

✔ Like CPAP, PEEP increases the functional residual capacity and is therefore very useful to correct hypoxemia due to intrapulmonary shunting.

optimal PEEP: The lowest PEEP level leading to the best oxygenation (or compliance) status without causing cardiopulmonary side effects.

Positive end-expiratory pressure (PEEP) provides positive airway pressure at the end of the expiratory phase. It is similar to CPAP with the exception that PEEP is used in conjunction with mechanical ventilation. Spontaneous breathing is not required when PEEP is used as the patient relies on the ventilator for ventilatory support. Like CPAP, PEEP increases the functional residual capacity and is therefore very useful to correct hypoxemia due to intrapulmonary shunting.

In order to minimize the cardiovascular complications and barotrauma associated with excessive pulmonary pressures, the **optimal PEEP** should be used. Optimal PEEP may be determined by measuring many different parameters, such as PaO_2, PvO_2, compliance, and O_2 saturation. Table 12-4 shows that 10 cm H_2O is the optimal PEEP since the next level of PEEP (12 cm H_2O) causes a decrease of PaO_2 and compliance.

Weaning from PEEP. Since PEEP is used to treat refractory hypoxemia, a patient will typically be receiving high levels of oxygen. The first criterion is to reduce the F_IO_2 to nontoxic levels as quickly as the patient's condition allows. If the patient is hemodynamically stable

TABLE 12-4 Titration of Optimal PEEP Using PaO₂ and Compliance as Indicators

PEEP (cm H₂O)	PaO₂ (mm Hg)	COMPLIANCE (mL/cm H₂O)
0	43	26
5	67	33
8	77	37
10*	83	43
12	79	41

*10 cm H_2O is the optimal PEEP since the PaO₂ and compliance show a continuing upward trend with the increasing PEEP level from 0 to 10 cm H_2O. Beyond the optimal PEEP, the next PEEP setting (12 cm H_2O) causes the PaO₂ to drop from 83 to 79 mm Hg and the compliance to fall from 43 to 41 mL/cm H_2O. It is not necessary to use more than one indicator to titrate the optimal PEEP. As shown above, the PaO₂ indicator is more time-consuming and invasive than the compliance indicator.

TABLE 12-5   Weaning from PEEP and High F_IO_2

1. Maintain PEEP and decrease F_IO_2 to 40% or 50%	Keep PaO_2 >60 mm Hg or SaO_2 >90%. Monitor vital signs for acute changes.
2. Maintain F_IO_2 and decrease PEEP to about 3 cm H_2O (at 2 to 3 cm H_2O increments)	Keep PaO_2 >60 mm Hg or SaO_2 >90%. Monitor vital signs for acute changes.
3. Discontinue PEEP	Monitor vital signs for hypoxia and increased work of breathing.

☑ If the patient is hemodynamically stable and the risk of barotrauma or other PEEP complications appears minimal, it is advisable to wean the F_IO_2 to 40% prior to decreasing the PEEP.

and the risk of barotrauma or other PEEP complications appear minimal, it is advisable to wean the F_IO_2 to 0.40 prior to decreasing the PEEP. PEEP should always be decreased in small increments while the patient's oxygen saturation is closely monitored. If at all possible, the patient's saturation should not be allowed to fall below 90%. The proper sequence of weaning PEEP is outlined in Table 12-5.

INVERSE RATIO VENTILATION (IRV)

Inverse ratio ventilation (IRV) is a technique used in mechanical ventilation in which the inspiratory time is longer than the expiratory time. The inspiratory time is prolonged by decreasing the inspiratory flow rate or by increasing the inflation hold time. IRV is also observed during airway pressure release ventilation where the pressure release rate is less than 20/min (or greater than six seconds per cycle). IRV has been used to treat ARDS patients with refractory hypoxemia not responsive to conventional mechanical ventilation and PEEP (Gurevitch et al., 1986).

☑ IRV helps to improve oxygenation by (1) overcoming noncompliant lung tissue, (2) recruiting collapsed alveoli, and (3) increasing the time for gas diffusion.

The prolonged inspiratory time in IRV helps to improve oxygenation by (1) overcoming noncompliant lung tissues, (2) recruiting collapsed alveoli, and (3) increasing the time for gas diffusion. Since inspiratory time is a function of mean airway pressure, a prolonged inspiratory time can increase mean airway pressure and diminish the cardiovascular functions of a critically ill patient.

IRV can be effective in improving oxygenation in patients with ARDS. However, it should be tried on an individual basis and used as an alternative after other conventional mechanical ventilation strategies have failed to improve oxygenation.

EXTRACORPOREAL MEMBRANE OXYGENATION (ECMO)

The first use of the extracorporeal membrane oxygenator (ECMO) on an infant was done and described in 1971 (Zwischenberger et al., 1986). Since then, ECMO has been used with considerable success as an oxygenation strategy for infants with extreme hypoxemia. In adult patients, however, it has not been shown to provide better oxygenation over conventional mechanical ventilation with PEEP (Zapol et al., 1979).

HIGH FREQUENCY OSCILLATORY VENTILATION FOR ADULTS

High frequency oscillatory ventilation (HFOV) is traditionally used in neonates when conventional ventilation fails to provide adequate ventilation or oxygenation. In recent years, HFOV has been used successfully for the treatment of acute respiratory failure in adult patients based on clinical trials (Viasys Healthcare, 2005).

Unlike conventional mechanical ventilation, the $PaCO_2$ is controlled by the power (amplitude) and frequency of oscillation. In HFOV, the $PaCO_2$ decreases with a higher amplitude or a *lower* frequency and the $PaCO_2$ increases with a lower amplitude or a *higher* frequency.

Procedure. The following procedure is the suggested clinical guidelines based on the 3100B ventilator (Viasys Healthcare, Yorba Linda, CA). The actual application of HFOV must be determined by the physician and based on the patient's condition and requirement (Viasys Healthcare, 2005).

Since the mean airway pressure (mPaw) is affected by the power setting (see next paragraph), the initial mPaw should start at 5 cm H_2O above the mPaw obtained during conventional mechanical ventilation. In patients with severe hypoxia, a recruitment strategy may be used by applying a mPaw of 40 cm H_2O for 40 to 60 sec. This mPaw may be increased in 3 to 5 cm H_2O increments every 30 min until the maximum setting. When recruitment strategy is used, oxygenation may worsen in the first 30 min. A chest radiograph should be done within 4 hours to evaluate lung volume.

The power setting determines the amplitude of oscillation and thus the tidal volume. For adult patients, the power is set at 4 and rapidly increased to achieve chest wiggle. Chest wiggle is defined as visible vibration from shoulder to midthigh area. If the $PaCO_2$ rises (with a pH >7.2), the power setting is increased to achieve a change of amplitude in 10 cm H_2O increments every 30 min until it reaches the highest setting.

The initial frequency is set at 5 to 6 Hz and may be *decreased* if unable to control the elevated $PaCO_2$ with amplitude. It is important to note that a lower Hertz setting yields a higher tidal volume. The hertz setting is decreased by 1 Hz increment every 30 min until 3 Hz.

The initial inspiratory time is set at 33% and may be increased up to 50% if unable to ventilate adequately (i.e., by increasing the amplitude or decreasing the frequency). The F_IO_2 is initially set at 100%. The initial settings are summarized in Table 12-6.

Weaning from HFOV in Adults. As oxygenation improves, the F_IO_2 is weaned to 40%. Once it reaches 40%, the mPaw is reduced in 2- to 3-cm H_2O increments every 4 to 6 hours to a 22- to 24-cm H_2O range. At this point, the patients may be switched to pressure control ventilation (PCV) at a rate of 20 to 25/min, I:E of 1:1, and PEEP of 12 cm H_2O. The pressure

---

☑ In HFOV, the $PaCO_2$ decreases with a higher amplitude or a *lower* frequency.

TABLE 12-6   Initial HFOV Settings for Adults

PARAMETER	INITIAL SETTING	NOTE
Mean airway pressure	5 cm H_2O above mPaw obtained during conventional mechanical ventilation	Dependent on power setting.
Power	4	Range 1 to 10 Controls the amplitude of oscillation (ΔP) Rapidly increase power to achieve chest wiggle (i.e., visible vibration from shoulder to mid-thigh area).
Frequency (Hz)	5 to 6 Hz	A *lower* Hz setting yields a *higher* "tidal volume."
Inspiratory time	33%	If unable to ventilate, may increase inspiratory time to 50% by increasing the amplitude or by *decreasing* the frequency.
F_IO_2	100%	Titrate F_IO_2 as needed.

Initial settings from Viasys Health Care Critical Care Division (Viasys, Yorba Linda, CA)

setting during PCV is titrated to yield a delivered volume of 6 to 8 mL/kg. The plateau pressure and mPaw should be kept below 35 and 20 cm H_2O, respectively.

ACID-BASE BALANCE

When interpreted correctly, blood gas studies are very useful in the evaluation of a patient's acid-base, ventilatory, and oxygenation status. Blood gas interpretation is most accurate when it is done in conjunction with the patient's medical history and diagnosis. This section covers two pairs of blood gas abnormalities that look very similar without a closeup examination: (1) respiratory acidosis and compensated metabolic alkalosis and (2) respiratory alkalosis and compensated metabolic acidosis.

RESPIRATORY ACIDOSIS AND COMPENSATED METABOLIC ALKALOSIS

Respiratory acidosis (ventilatory failure) is caused by hypoventilation. The strategy to correct this abnormality is to improve ventilation. For specific procedures to improve ventilation, refer to the section on "Strategies to Improve Ventilation" at the beginning of this chapter.

The strategies to improve ventilation are useful only when respiratory acidosis is induced by hypoventilation. They should not be used when hypoventilation occurs as a compensatory mechanism for metabolic alkalosis. Compensated metabolic alkalosis has an elevated

☑ If hypoventilation occurs due to metabolic alkalosis, increasing mechanical ventilation may further reduce spontaneous ventilation.

TABLE 12-7   Differentiation of Compensated Respiratory Acidosis and Compensated Metabolic Alkalosis

BLOOD GAS CONDITION	pH	PaCO₂ (mm Hg)	HCO₃⁻ (mEq/L)
Primary respiratory acidosis	7.31	53	26
Compensated respiratory acidosis	7.38	52	30
Compensated metabolic alkalosis	7.43	50	32

$PaCO_2$, thus mimicking the elevated $PaCO_2$ seen in primary or compensated respiratory acidosis.

Table 12-7 compares the typical blood gases of compensated respiratory acidosis and compensated metabolic alkalosis (both show high $PaCO_2$ and high HCO_3^-). Note that in primary respiratory acidosis, the HCO_3^- is within its normal range (i.e., no renal compensation). In compensated respiratory acidosis, the pH (7.37) is on the acidotic side of its normal range (7.35 to 7.45). In compensated metabolic alkalosis, the pH (7.42) is on the alkalotic side of its normal range (7.35 to 7.45). As with other blood gas abnormalities, the patient's medical history should be used to differentiate whether the condition is a respiratory or metabolic problem.

RESPIRATORY ALKALOSIS AND COMPENSATED METABOLIC ACIDOSIS

Respiratory alkalosis is caused by alveolar hyperventilation. In general, this condition does not require mechanical ventilation intervention and it usually allows gradual weaning of the mechanical rate. However, if the hyperventilation is induced by acute hypoxia, the cause of hypoxia must be identified and treated. Otherwise, weaning the ventilator rate will cause further patient hyperventilation due to uncorrected and persistent hypoxia.

✓ If hyperventilation occurs due to acute hypoxia, weaning or use of mechanical deadspace should not be implemented.

Additional deadspace tubing between the endotracheal tube and ventilator "Y" adaptor is sometimes used to partially correct persistent respiratory alkalosis. This may be necessary when the mechanical volume and rate cannot be reduced due to the patient's tidal volume and oxygenation requirements.

It is also important to note whether the respiratory alkalosis is a compensatory mechanism for metabolic acidosis. Compensated metabolic acidosis has a decreased $PaCO_2$, thus mimicking the reduced $PaCO_2$ seen in primary or compensated respiratory alkalosis.

Table 12-8 compares the typical blood gases of compensated respiratory alkalosis and compensated metabolic acidosis (both show low $PaCO_2$ and low HCO_3^-). Note that in primary respiratory alkalosis, the HCO_3^- is within its normal range (no renal compensation). In compensated respiratory alkalosis, the pH (7.42) is on the alkalotic

TABLE 12-8 **Differentiation of Compensated Respiratory Alkalosis and Compensated Metabolic Acidosis**

BLOOD GAS CONDITION	pH	$PaCO_2$ (mm Hg)	HCO_3^- (mEq/L)
Primary respiratory alkalosis	7.50	30	23
Compensated respiratory alkalosis	7.42	27	17
Compensated metabolic acidosis	7.37	25	14

side of its normal range (7.35 to 7.45). In compensated metabolic acidosis, the pH (7.37) is on the acidotic side of its normal range (7.35 to 7.45). As with other blood gas abnormalities, the patient's medical history should be used to differentiate a respiratory or metabolic problem.

METABOLIC ACID-BASE ABNORMALITIES

✓ Ventilatory interventions by mechanical ventilation should not be done to compensate or correct primary metabolic acid-base problems.

Metabolic acid-base abnormalities should be corrected by treating their respective causes. Three major causes of metabolic acidosis are renal failure, diabetic ketoacidosis, and lactic acidosis. One of the major causes of metabolic alkalosis is hypokalemia (Shapiro et al., 1994). Ventilatory (respiratory) interventions by mechanical ventilation should not be done to compensate or correct primary metabolic acid-base problems. One should refer to a blood gas textbook for further information on the diagnosis and treatment of metabolic abnormalities.

TROUBLESHOOTING OF COMMON VENTILATOR ALARMS AND EVENTS

The type of ventilator **alarm** is easy to spot since most ventilators provide an indicator (light or sound) for each event that triggers the alarm. Once the type of alarm is identified, steps can be taken to alleviate the problem by process of elimination. This section provides the common causes for each alarm.

alarm: An absolute value of a parameter on the ventilator beyond which an alert is invoked to warn that the safety limit has been breached.

LOW PRESSURE ALARM

The low pressure limit is set to ensure that a minimum pressure is present in the ventilator circuit during each inspiratory cycle.

Low pressure alarms are triggered when the circuit pressure drops below the preset low pressure limit. If the preset low pressure limit

TABLE 12-9   Conditions That Trigger the Low Pressure/Low Volume Alarm

CONDITION	EXAMPLES
Loss of circuit pressure	Circuit disconnection Exhalation valve drive line disconnection Insufficient endotracheal tube cuff volume Loose circuit connection Loose humidifier connection
Loss of system pressure	Power failure Source gas failure or disconnection Air compressor failure
Premature termination of inspiratory phase	Excessive peak flow Insufficient inspiratory time (I time) Excessive expiratory time (E time) Inappropriate sensitivity setting (too sensitive)
Inappropriate ventilator settings	Excessive rate with insufficient peak flow Low pressure limit set too high Low tidal volume limit set too high

☑ The low pressure alarm may be triggered in (1) loss of circuit pressure (a common event), (2) loss of system pressure (an uncommon occurrence), (3) conditions leading to premature termination of inspiratory phase, and (4) inappropriate ventilator settings.

☑ The low volume alarm is usually triggered along with the low pressure alarm because loss of airway pressure usually results in loss of volume delivered.

is set at 40 cm H_2O, and the circuit pressure drops below 40 cm H_2O, the low pressure alarm will then be triggered. In all likelihood, the low volume alarm will also be triggered since pressure and volume are affected simultaneously by similar clinical conditions.

Conditions that may trigger the low pressure alarm may be grouped into four areas: (1) loss of circuit pressure (a common event), (2) loss of system pressure (an uncommon occurrence), (3) conditions leading to premature termination of inspiratory phase, and (4) inappropriate ventilator settings. These conditions and selected examples are listed in Table 12-9.

LOW EXPIRED VOLUME ALARM

The low volume limit is set to ensure that the patient receives (and exhales) a minimum volume.

The low expired volume alarm is triggered when the expired volume drops below the preset low volume limit. If the preset low expired volume limit is set at 400 mL and the expired volume drops below 400 mL, the low volume alarm will be triggered.

As mentioned before, the low volume alarm is usually triggered along with the low pressure alarm because loss of airway pressure usually results in loss of volume delivered, thus the expired volume. See Table 12-9 for examples of conditions that may trigger low volume alarm.

HIGH PRESSURE ALARM

The high pressure limit is set to control the maximum ventilator circuit pressure during a complete breathing cycle, usually during the inspiratory phase.

The high pressure alarm is triggered when the circuit pressure reaches or exceeds the preset high pressure limit. If the high pressure limit is set at 60 cm H_2O, and the circuit pressure reaches or exceeds 60 cm H_2O, the high pressure alarm will be triggered.

Conditions that trigger the high pressure alarm may be (1) increase in air flow resistance and (2) decrease in lung or chest wall compliance. These conditions and selected examples are shown in Table 12-10.

☑ The high pressure alarm may be triggered in the following conditions: (1) increase in air flow resistance and (2) decrease in lung or chest wall compliance.

HIGH RESPIRATORY RATE ALARM

The high respiratory rate limit is set to alert the practitioner that the patient has experienced tachypnea.

This alarm is triggered when the total rate exceeds the high rate limit. This condition is most likely caused by a distressed patient when the need to increase ventilation (i.e., respiratory rate) becomes necessary. When the patient consistently sets off the high respiratory rate alarm, the practitioner may need to increase the level of ventilatory support to ease the patient's work of breathing.

☑ The high rate alarm may be triggered due to (1) patient's need to increase ventilation and (2) excessive sensitivity setting.

TABLE 12-10   Conditions That Trigger the High Pressure Alarm

CONDITION	EXAMPLES

Increase in air flow resistance	Mechanical Factors
	    Kinking of circuit
	    Kinking of ET tube
	    Blocked exhalation manifold
	    Water in circuit
	    Herniated ET tube cuff
	    Main-stem bronchial intubation
	    High pressure limit set too low
	
	Patient Factors
	    Bronchospasm
	    Coughing
	    Breathing pattern out of synchronization
	        with ventilator
	    Secretions in ET tube
	    Mucus plug

Decrease in lung or chest wall compliance	Tension pneumothorax Atelectasis ARDS Pneumonia

Another cause of the high rate alarm is inappropriate sensitivity setting. When this control is set excessively sensitive to the patient's inspiratory effort, minimum inspiratory efforts or movements would cause the ventilator to initiate unwanted breaths and increase the total respiratory rate.

APNEA/LOW RESPIRATORY RATE ALARM

The apnea/low respiratory rate limit is set to ensure that a minimum number of breaths is delivered to the patient.

The apnea or low respiratory rate alarm is triggered when the total rate drops below the low rate limit. Disconnection of the ventilator circuit from the patient's endotracheal tube is the most frequent trigger of the apnea alarm, since the ventilator cannot sense any air movement (respiratory effort) from a disconnected circuit. Other triggers of the apnea/low rate alarm include patient under respiratory depressants or muscle-paralyzing agents, conditions of respiratory center dysfunction, and respiratory muscle fatigue.

✔ Disconnection of the ventilator circuit from the patient's endotracheal tube is the most frequent trigger of the apnea alarm.

Some ventilators merely alert the practitioner that the patient is having periods of apnea; the practitioner must increase ventilation to alleviate the situation. Other ventilators (e.g., Puritan-Bennett 7200) switch to a backup ventilation mode to ventilate the patient until the problem is corrected.

HIGH PEEP ALARM

The high PEEP limit is set to prevent excessive PEEP being delivered to the patient. The alarm is triggered when the actual PEEP exceeds the preset PEEP limit. Inadvertent PEEP may occur in conditions of air trapping, insufficient inspiratory flow rate (long I time), or insufficient expiratory time (short E time).

Air trapping may be reduced by decreasing the mechanical tidal volume and frequency and by using bronchodilators in patients with reversible airway obstruction. Increasing the inspiratory peak flow provides a longer E time and this may also help to reduce air trapping.

LOW PEEP ALARM

The low PEEP limit is set to ensure that the preselected PEEP is delivered to the patient. The alarm is triggered when the actual PEEP drops below the preset low PEEP limit. Failure of the ventilator circuit to hold the PEEP is usually due to leakage in the circuit or endotracheal tube cuff.

AUTO-PEEP

Auto-PEEP (intrinsic PEEP, inadvertent PEEP, occult PEEP) is the unintentional PEEP during mechanical ventilation that is associated with

✔ Auto-PEEP is associated with pressure support ventilation, significant airway obstruction, rapid respiratory rates (>20/min), insufficient inspiratory flow rates, relatively equal (about 1:1) I:E ratio, and history of air trapping.

pressure support ventilation, significant airway obstruction, rapid respiratory rates (>20/min), insufficient inspiratory flow rates, and relatively equal (about 1:1) I:E ratio. It is also more likely to occur when the patient has a history of air trapping (MacIntyre, 1986; Schuster, 1990). With auto-PEEP, the distal airway pressures in the lungs can be as high as 15 cm H_2O, while the ventilator's proximal airway pressure manometer shows zero pressure (or PEEP if PEEP is used). Auto-PEEP can be measured by occluding the expiratory port just before the next inspiration (Marini, 1988). To measure it accurately, the patient should be sedated or paralyzed.

Auto-PEEP Increases Work of Breathing.   Under normal conditions, a mechanical breath is initiated when the inspiratory negative pressure reaches the sensitivity setting of the ventilator. For example, when the normal end-expiratory pressure is 0 cm H_2O and the sensitivity is set at −2 cm H_2O, the pressure gradient (ΔP) or work of breathing to trigger a mechanical breath is 2 cm H_2O (from 0 cm to 2 cm H_2O). See Figure 12-2(A).

If auto-PEEP is present, the work of breathing is increased because the level of auto-PEEP in the lungs at end-expiratory phase must first be overcome before additional inspiratory negative pressure can be used to reach the sensitivity setting. For example, when the auto-PEEP level is 6 cm H_2O and the sensitivity is set at −2 cm H_2O, the pressure gradient (ΔP) to trigger a mechanical breath becomes 8 cm H_2O. Figure 12-2(B) shows the distribution of 8 cm H_2O of pressure (6 cm H_2O to bring auto-PEEP from 6 to 0 cm H_2O plus 2 cm H_2O to reach the preset sensitivity level).

✔ Auto-PEEP may be reduced or eliminated by (1) improving ventilation and reducing air trapping by bronchodilators and (2) prolonging the expiratory time by increasing the flow rate or reducing the tidal volume or frequency.

Strategies to Reduce Auto-PEEP.   To reduce the likelihood of auto-PEEP, the tidal volume may be reduced. The respiratory rate during pressure support ventilation should be kept less than 20 breaths per minute if possible. Auto-PEEP may also be minimized or eliminated by improving ventilation or providing a longer expiratory time. Two methods may be useful to reduce or eliminate the auto-PEEP and they are (1) improving ventilation and reducing air trapping by bronchodilators and (2) prolonging the expiratory time by increasing the flow rate or reducing the tidal volume or frequency.

Using PEEP to Reduce Effects of Auto-PEEP.   PEEP can be used to reduce the effects of auto-PEEP. The level of PEEP used to counter the effects of auto-PEEP should be kept below 85% of the measured auto-PEEP level (Wilkins et al., 2003). For example, PEEP level of up to 5 cm H_2O may be used when auto-PEEP of 6 cm H_2O is measured during mechanical ventilation. Figure 12-2(C) shows that the pressure gradient (ΔP) to trigger a mechanical breath drops to 3 cm H_2O (1 cm H_2O to bring auto-PEEP from 6 to 5 cm H_2O plus 2 cm H_2O to reach the preset sensitivity level).

Figure 12-2 (A) Without auto-PEEP, the pressure gradient (ΔP) from end-expiratory pressure to sensitivity setting is 2 cm H_2O. (B) With auto-PEEP of 6 cm H_2O, the ΔP from auto-PEEP to sensitivity setting is 8 cm H_2O. (C) With auto-PEEP of 6 cm H_2O and PEEP setting of 5 cm H_2O, the ΔP from auto-EEP to sensitivity setting is 3 cm H_2O.

CARE OF THE VENTILATOR CIRCUIT

The ventilator circuit serves as an important interface between the ventilator and the patient. Circuit compliance, circuit patency, humidity, and temperature are four essential factors to consider in the management of mechanical ventilation.

CIRCUIT COMPLIANCE

The compliance of ventilator circuits should be as low as possible. High circuit compliance leads to a higher compressible volume in the circuit during inspiration and this condition reduces the effective tidal volume delivered to the patient. For example, at a peak inspiratory pressure of 40 cm H_2O, ventilator circuit with a compliance of 5 mL/cm H_2O would expand and hold 200 mL (40 cm H_2O × 5 mL/cm H_2O) of the mechanical tidal volume. At the same peak inspiratory pressure, ventilator circuit with a compliance of 3 mL/cm H_2O would have a compressible volume of only 120 mL (40 cm H_2O × 3 mL/cm H_2O). Unless tidal volume adjustment is made to account for the circuit compliance factor, the effective tidal volume to the patient would be reduced substantially when high compliance circuits are used (Burton et al., 1997).

CIRCUIT PATENCY

Condensation imposes the most common threat to the patency of ventilator circuit. Gas temperature drops as it travels from the heated humidifier to the patient. As the temperature drops along the circuit, water vapor condenses and water collects in the tubing. This condition leads to significant airflow obstruction. Heated-wire circuit (Figure 12-3) and in-line water trap (Figure 12-4) have been used successfully to reduce condensation and the amount of water in the circuit.

Heat and Moisture Exchanger (HME).   Figure 12-5 shows a heat and moisture exchanger (HME) that may be used to replace the traditional heated humidifier. It is placed between the patient's artificial airway and the ventilator circuit. During exhalation, moisture and heat from the patient are absorbed into the honeycomb structure of the exchanger. The moisture and heat are transferred back to the patient during the next inhalation. The efficiency of HME units ranges from 70% to 90% relative humidity and 30°C to 31°C (White, 2004). Compared to the heated humidifier, ventilator circuits with a bacterial-viral filtering HME cost less to maintain and are less likely to colonize bacteria (Boots et al., 1997; Kirton et al., 1997).

HME may not be suitable for certain patients due to problems associated with adequacy of airflow, humidity, and temperature. Contraindications for HME include a thick and large amount of

Figure 12-3 A heated-wire circuit.

Figure 12-4 In-line water trap.

Figure 12-5   A photograph and a functional diagram of a heat and moisture exchanger (HME).

secretions, minute volume exceeding 10 L/min, body temperature less than 32°C, and need for aerosolized medications (Wilkins et al., 2003).

HUMIDITY AND TEMPERATURE

Since the upper airway is bypassed during mechanical ventilation, the inspired gas temperature should be kept close to the body temperature. The temperature probe for the heated humidifier should be placed inside the inspiratory limb of the ventilator circuit as close to the patient as possible. Since water vapor saturation depends on the water content as well as the temperature, the temperature setting should be adjusted for a distal temperature reading of 37°C. This ensures proper temperature and humidification to the patient (Burton et al., 1997).

FREQUENCY OF CIRCUIT CHANGE

It has been well established that the optimal interval for ventilator circuit change is once per week (Fink, Krause & Barrett, 1998; Kotilainen & Keroack, 1997; Long et al., 1996; Stamm, 1998). When compared to more frequent circuit changes, weekly circuit change does not increase the incidence of nosocomial infection, including ventilator-associated pneumonia. Weekly change also saves manpower and reduces the direct replacement cost for new ventilator circuits. (Kotilainen & Keroack, 1997).

CARE OF THE ARTIFICIAL AIRWAY

☑ Patency of the
ET tube can only
be ensured with
adequate humidifica-
tion and prompt
removal of retained
secretions.

Supplemental humidity must be provided during mechanical ventilation since the endotracheal (ET) tube does not receive humidification
normally provided by the upper airway. In addition, secretions must
be removed by suctioning if necessary because the ET tube and the
ventilator circuit are a closed system. If not removed, any secretions
coughed up by the patient are likely to stay in the ET tube. Patency
of the ET tube can only be ensured with adequate humidification and
prompt removal of retained secretions.

PATENCY OF THE ENDOTRACHEAL TUBE

In mechanical ventilation, the primary purpose of an ET tube is to
conduct air flow between the ventilator and the lungs. Since air
flow resistance is inversely related to the diameter of the tube, small
tubes cause a tremendous increase in the work of breathing. In order
to enhance air flow, the largest size ET tube that is appropriate to
the patient should be used. Mucus in the ET tube should also be
removed frequently in order to minimize air flow obstruction created by retained secretions.

Poiseuille's Law shows that when the radius of an airway is reduced
by half, the driving pressure (work of breathing) must be increased
16 times in order to maintain the same flow rate. An obstructed airway
hinders not only mechanical ventilation, but spontaneous ventilation
as well. Airway management should always be an integral part of
mechanical ventilation.

$$\text{Pressure change} = \frac{\text{Flow}}{r^4}$$

Other conditions that can affect the patency of the ET tube include
(1) kinking or bending of the tube due to poor positioning of the patient
and placement of the ventilator circuit; (2) patient biting on the ET tube
due to physical or psychologic discomfort; and (3) malfunction of the
ET tube cuff causing partial or complete blockage.

Frequent endotracheal suctioning is sometimes necessary to maintain the patency of the endotracheal tube. One of the problems with
endotracheal suctioning is hypoxia. Suction-induced hypoxia may be
minimized by preoxygenating the patient with oxygen prior to suction, limiting the total suction time to no more than 10 sec, and using
a closed in-line tracheal suction system (Wilkins et al., 2003). Since
one can perform suctioning without disconnecting the ventilator circuit, F_IO_2 and PEEP levels may be maintained. Closed in-line suction
catheters may be changed weekly (instead of daily) with no significant increase in the frequency of ventilator-associated pneumonia
(Stoller et al., 2003). Figure 12-6 shows a closed tracheal suction
system.

Figure 12-6 An example of a closed suction system manufactured by Ballard Medical, Inc.

HUMIDIFICATION AND REMOVAL OF SECRETIONS

Proper function of the ciliary blanket of the airway is dependent on adequate humidity. In mechanical ventilation, humidification of the airways and lungs is commonly provided by a heated cascade, heated wick humidifier, or heat and membrane exchanger (HME, or artificial nose). Occasionally, humidification and removal of the secretions are supplemented by use of a saline solution via a small volume nebulizer or direct endotracheal instillation.

Saline solution used in a small volume nebulizer is delivered in an aerosol form, and is thus capable of carrying pathogens into the lower airways. Instillation of saline solution directly into the trachea to facilitate endotracheal suctioning has also been implicated in the contamination of the lower airways with pathogens (Hagler et al., 1994). For these reasons, aseptic techniques for equipment handling and sterile techniques for endotracheal suctioning must be followed in order to minimize the occurrence of pulmonary contamination and ventilator-associated pneumonia (Sole et al., 2003).

ventilator-associated pneumonia (VAP): Infection of the lung parenchyma that is related to any or multiple events that the patient undergoes during mechanical ventilation.

VENTILATOR-ASSOCIATED PNEUMONIA

Patients who are intubated and on mechanical ventilation are more prone to develop nosocomial pneumonia than nonintubated patients (Craven et al., 1989). The estimated incidence of **ventilator-associated pneumonia** (VAP) ranges from 10% to 65%, with fatality rates of 13% to 55% (Kollef et al., 1994). The presence of an artificial airway bypasses the natural defense mechanism of the airway, causes local trauma and inflammation, and increases the risk of aspiration of pathogens from the oropharynx.

TABLE 12-11   Potential Sources of Ventilator-Associated Pneumonia

POTENTIAL SOURCE	LOCATIONS
Patient	Oropharynx
Health care provider	Hands
Equipment and supplies	Respiratory instruments
	Aerosol nebulizers and humidifiers
	Endotracheal tube
	Nasogastric tube
	Manual ventilation bag

✔ For the diagnosis and treatment of VAP, early microbiologic examinations contribute to appropriate use of antibiotherapy.

Gram stain: A method for staining bacteria. Gram-positive bacteria (e.g., Staphlococcus*) retain the gentian violet (purple) color and gram-negative bacteria (e.g.,* Pseudomonas*) take the red counterstain.*

culture and sensitivity: A laboratory procedure that grows the microbes in an agar plate and tests their sensitivity or resistance to different antimicrobial drugs.

✔ Gram stain is done for rapid selection of antibiotics.

In one study, 45% of the patients developed pneumonia within 3 days of intubation (Lowy et al., 1987). This condition may be caused by microbes acquired from the patient's oropharynx, respiratory instruments, health care providers (Hu, 1991), endotracheal and nasogastric tubes (Joshi et al., 1993), and manual ventilation bags (Weber et al., 1990). Table 12-11 outlines the potential sources of ventilator-associated pneumonia. Strategies to decrease ventilator-associated pneumonias include proper handwashing techniques, closed suction systems (Figure 12-6), continuous feed humidification systems, and less frequent ventilator circuit changes.

For the diagnosis and treatment of VAP, early microbiologic examinations are recommended and contribute to appropriate use of antibiotherapy. At an international conference on the diagnosis and treatment of VAP, piperacillin/tazobactam has been suggested as the preferred choice for empiric therapy, followed by a cephalosporin with antipseudomonal activity and a carbapenem. Antibiotic therapy should be started empirically, preferably within the first 12 hours of the suspicion of pneumonia and for a duration of 10 days. However, there is no consensus or established guidelines regarding the selection of antimicrobial agents or the duration of therapy (Rello et al., 2001).

Sputum Culture.   Sputum cultures should be obtained if infection of the lungs is suspected. Since the patient is intubated, the sputum sample may be obtained via an endotracheal suction setup and a sputum trap (Figure 12-7). Sputum analyses are commonly done by the **Gram stain**, and the **culture and sensitivity** methods.

The Gram stain technique is done to quickly establish the general category (gram-positive or gram-negative) of the suspected microbes so that appropriate broad-spectrum antibiotics may be administered without delay. Acid-fast sputum analysis is for pulmonary tuberculosis and silver stain is for *Pneumocystis carinii* pneumonia. Culture and sensitivity is more time-consuming but it can identify the microbes in the sputum and the most suitable antibiotics for the infection.

1.
Remove
Rubber Band.

2.
Place Tubing from
Suction Machine on
Upper Arm of Aspirating
Tube. Collect Specimen.

3.
After Specimen Collection,
Seal Aspirating Tube by
Placing Free End of Rubber
Tubing on Upper Arm.
Specimen is Ready for Lab.

Figure 12-7 Sputum collecting tube used with a suction system. The upper outlet goes to the vacuum source and the lower outlet is connected to the suction catheter.

☑ Acid-fast sputum analysis is for pulmonary tuberculosis. Silver stain is for *Pneumocystis carinii* pneumonia.

☑ Culture and sensitivity (c & s) is done to identify the microbes and effective antimicrobial agents.

extracellular fluid (ECF): *Fluid in the plasma and interstitial space. It accounts for 20% of total body water and is mainly affected by the sodium concentration in the plasma.*

intracellular fluid (ICF): *Fluid within the cells. It accounts for 40% of total body water.*

FLUID BALANCE

Fluid balance in the body is mainly affected by (1) the blood and fluid volume in the blood vessels and cells, (2) the pressure gradient between the blood vessels and the tissues around them, and (3) electrolyte concentrations.

DISTRIBUTION OF BODY WATER

Water makes up about 60% of the body weight. The distribution of this volume is 20% in the plasma and interstitial fluid (**extracellular fluid**, or **ECF**) and 40% within the cells (**intracellular fluid,** or **ICF**). Table 12-12 shows the distribution of body water.

Changes in Extracellular Fluid Distribution. The distribution of body water in the ECF and ICF compartments is not a static measurement. Depending on the physiologic needs, fluid can move into and out of any compartment along with certain electrolytes. When an excessive volume of fluid moves out of the extracellular compartment, ECF deficit occurs.

Fluid deficiency in the extracellular compartment (space) may be caused by one or a combination of these reasons: (1) inadequate intake (e.g., dehydration); (2) excessive loss (e.g., diarrhea); and (3) shifting of fluid along with the electrolytes into cells and tissues (e.g., swelling of tissues in burns).

TABLE 12-12   Distribution of Body Water

COMPARTMENT	SUBDIVISION	PERCENT OF WATER BY BODY WEIGHT
Extracellular	Plasma	5%
	Interstitial fluid	15%
Intracellular	Intracellular fluid	40%
Total		60% of body weight

CLINICAL SIGNS OF EXTRACELLULAR FLUID DEFICIT OR EXCESS

☑ When urine output drops below 20 mL/hour, it is indicative of fluid inadequacy.

Urine output is the most common method used to assess ECF abnormalities. When urine output drops below 20 mL/hour (or 400 mL in a 24-hour period, or 160 mL in 8 hours), it is called oliguria and is indicative of fluid inadequacy (Kraus et al., 1993). Excessive urine output is one of the signs of excessive ECF or excessive diuresis. Other clinical signs of ECF abnormalities include those involved with the central nervous system and the cardiovascular system. They are listed in Table 12-13.

TREATMENT OF EXTRACELLULAR FLUID ABNORMALITIES

☑ Decrease in heart rate, increase in blood pressure, and urine output are signs of improvement in ECF deficit after fluid replacement.

Treatment of ECF deficit is by fluid replacement with Ringer's lactate solution since it is similar to ECF in composition. Physiologic (0.9%) saline solution is an acceptable alternative. Success of fluid replacement therapy can be determined by reversal of those signs of ECF deficit in Table 12-13. For example, decrease in heart rate, increase in blood pressure, and urine output are signs of improvement in ECF deficit after fluid replacement.

TABLE 12-13   Signs of Extracellular Fluid (ECF) Deficit or Excess

SYSTEM	ECF DEFICIT	ECF EXCESS
CNS	Diminished sensorium	None
	Coma	
Cardiovascular	Tachycardia	Increased pulmonic P_2 heart sound
	Hypotension	Increased cardiac output
	Cold extremities	Bounding pulse
	Poor peripheral pulse	Pulmonary edema
Renal	Oliguria	Increased urine output
	Anuria (no urine)	

Excessive fluid in the extracellular space is uncommon in a clinical setting. When it occurs, pulmonary edema is a common manifestation. The treatment for excessive ECF is to withhold fluid or to give a diuretic such as furosemide (Lasix). Mannitol should not be given for diuresis as it can increase plasma volume before inducing diuresis (Eggleston, 1985).

☑ Disappearance of pulmonic P$_2$ heart sound, reduction in pulse intensity, and clearing of pulmonary edema are signs of improvement in ECF excess.

Use of diuretics will further increase the urine output. For this reason, reversal of the cardiovascular signs of ECF excess in Table 12-13 should be used to determine the success of treatment. For example, disappearance of the pulmonic P$_2$ heart sound, reduction in pulse intensity, and clearing of pulmonary edema are signs of improvement in ECF excess due to fluid restriction or diuresis. Since diuresis can affect the electrolyte composition, monitoring of electrolyte balance is essential when diuretics are used to manage ECF excess.

ELECTROLYTE BALANCE

Electrolyte balance is the difference between the cations (positively charged ions) and the anions (negatively charged ions) in the plasma. Serum cations and anions are used to calculate the anion gap and assess a patient's electrolyte balance.

NORMAL ELECTROLYTE BALANCE

Table 12-14 shows the normal values for serum electrolytes. Sodium is the major cation in the extracellular fluid compartment and it is directly related to the fluid level in the body. Potassium is the major cation in the intracellular fluid compartment and it is not related to the amount of fluid in the body.

Sodium and potassium are the two major electrolytes that must be monitored. In general, once the sodium and potassium concentrations

TABLE 12-14   Normal Serum Electrolytes

CATION	CONCENTRATION (mEq/L)	ANION	CONCENTRATION (mEq/L)
Na$^+$	140 (138 to 142)	Cl$^-$	103 (101 to 105)
K$^+$	4 (3 to 5)	HCO$_3^-$	25 (23 to 27)
Ca^{++}	5 (4.5 to 5.5)	Protein	16 (14 to 18)
Mg^{++}	2 (1.5 to 2.5)	HPO$_4^{--}$, H$_2$PO$_4^-$	2 (1.5 to 2.5)
		SO$_4^{--}$	1 (0.8 to 1.2)
		Organic acids	4 (3.5 to 4.5)
Total cations	151	Total anions	151

are properly managed and returned to normal, the chloride concentration will be corrected as well without further intervention. The following sections cover sodium and potassium abnormalities.

anion gap: The difference between cations (positive ions) and anions (negative ions) in the plasma. The normal range is 15 to 20 mEq/L when K^+ is included in the calculation (10 to 14 mEq/L when K^+ is excluded).

Anion Gap. Anion gap is the relationship of the cations [sodium (Na^+) and potassium (K^+)] to the anions [chloride (Cl^-) and bicarbonate (HCO_3^-)]. The normal range is 15 to 20 mEq/L when K^+ is included in the calculation (10 to 14 mEq/L when K^+ is excluded). When the anion gap is outside this range, electrolyte replacement may be necessary. See Chapter 9 for a discussion on the interpretation of anion gap in metabolic acidosis.

The anion gap is calculated as follows:

$$\text{Anion Gap} = Na^+ + K^+ - Cl^- - HCO_3^-$$
or
$$\text{Anion Gap} = Na^+ - Cl^- - HCO_3^-$$

☑ See Appendix 1 for example.

SODIUM ABNORMALITIES

Sodium is the major cation in the extracellular fluid (ECF) and it directly influences the ECF volume. The sodium concentration in the ECF may be higher than normal (hypernatremia) or lower than normal (hyponatremia). The clinical signs of sodium abnormalities are highlighted in Table 12-15.

☑ Hyponatremia is commonly related to ECF deficits (hypovolemia). The usual treatment is replenishment of sodium with saline solution.

Hyponatremia. Hyponatremia is a more common form of sodium abnormality than hypernatremia. It is commonly related to ECF deficit (hypovolemia). The usual treatment is replenishment of sodium with saline solution (100 to 300 mL of 2.5% or 3% saline). It is not safe to administer fluids that have no sodium as *water intoxication* may occur. Rapid movement of sodium-free fluid into the brain cells and kidney cells by the action of osmosis may cause edema and shutdown of these organs (Eggleston, 1985).

TABLE 12-15   Clinical Signs of Sodium Abnormality

SYSTEM	HYPONATREMIA	HYPERNATREMIA
Central nervous system	Muscle twitching Loss of reflexes Increased intracranial pressure	Restlessness Weakness Delirium
Cardiovascular	Blood pressure change secondary to increased intracranial pressure	Tachycardia Hypotension (if severe)
Gastrointestinal	Watery diarrhea	None
Renal	Oliguria to anuria	Oliguria

☑ Hypernatremia is an uncommon problem and it is usually related to water deficit as a result of prolonged intravenous fluid administration with sufficient sodium but no dextrose.

☑ Potassium deficiency may be caused by excessive K^+ loss (trauma, severe infection, vomiting, use of diuretics) or inadequate K^+ intake (massive or prolonged intravenous fluid infusion without supplemental potassium).

☑ Oral intake of potassium replacement is safer. If intravenous route is used, precautions must be followed to ensure patient safety.

Hypernatremia. Hypernatremia is an uncommon problem in the clinical setting. When hypernatremia occurs, it is usually related to water deficit as a result of prolonged intravenous fluid administration with sufficient sodium but no dextrose. This condition is readily reversible by a water solution supplemented with dextrose (Eggleston, 1985).

POTASSIUM ABNORMALITIES

Potassium is the major cation in the intracellular fluid (ICF), therefore it has a narrow normal range (3 to 5 mEq/L) outside the cells. The potassium concentration in the ECF may be higher than normal (hyperkalemia) or lower than normal (hypokalemia). The clinical signs of potassium abnormality are outlined in Table 12-16.

Hypokalemia. Hypokalemia is a more common form of potassium (K^+) abnormality than hyperkalemia. Potassium deficiency may be caused by excessive K^+ loss (e.g., trauma, severe infection, vomiting, use of diuretics) or inadequate K^+ intake (e.g., massive or prolonged intravenous fluid infusion without supplemental potassium). Normal breakdown of body tissue produces some potassium as a by-product, but hypokalemia may still occur if excretion exceeds production.

Deficiency of serum potassium may be corrected by oral intake or slow intravenous infusion of potassium chloride. Potassium chloride is used because hypochloremia (low chloride) usually coexists with hypokalemia and the chloride ions must be replaced at the same time.

Oral intake of potassium replacement is safer. If intravenous route is used, there are four precautions that must be followed to ensure patient safety (Eggleston, 1985): (1) Consider replacement only if the urine output is at least 40 to 50 mL/hour; (2) Never use KCl undiluted as it can cause arrhythmias and cardiac arrest; (3) Do not give more than 40 mEq of potassium in any 1 hour or more than 200 mEq in 24 hours; and (4) Concentration of potassium in the intravenous drip should not be higher than 40 mEq/L.

TABLE 12-16   Clinical Signs of Potassium Abnormality

SYSTEM	HYPOKALEMIA	HYPERKALEMIA
Neuromuscular	Decreased muscle functions	Increased neuromuscular conduction
Cardiac	Flattened T wave and depressed ST segment on ECG	Elevated T wave and depressed ST segment on ECG (mild)
	Arrhythmias	Cardiac arrest (severe)
Gastrointestinal	Decreased bowel activity	Increased bowel activity
	Diminished or absent bowel sounds	Diarrhea

☑️ Hyperkalemia may be caused by renal failure.

Hyperkalemia. Hyperkalemia is an uncommon condition in the clinical setting, but when hyperkalemia occurs it is usually caused by renal failure. Decrease in urine output (less than 200 to 300 mL/day) secondary to renal failure leads to retention of potassium ions. Therefore, the primary treatment for this form of hyperkalemia is to improve kidney function.

If hyperkalemia occurs in the presence of normal kidney function, it may be treated rapidly by using 80 mEq of sodium lactate, 100 mL of calcium gluconate, 100 mL of 50% dextrose in water, or 25 units of insulin (Eggleston, 1985).

NUTRITION

Nutritional intake should be adjusted according to a patient's requirements so inadequate intake may lead to impaired respiratory function due to reduction in the efficiency of respiratory muscles. Excessive intake may increase the patient's work of breathing due to the increased metabolic rate and carbon dioxide production.

UNDERNUTRITION

☑️ Inadequate nutritional support can lead to fatigue of respiratory muscles.

Proper nutritional support is a therapeutic necessity for patients on a mechanical ventilator. Poor nutritional status may lead to rapid depletion of cellular stores of glycogen and protein in the diaphragm (Mlynarek et al., 1987). It also leads to fatigue of the major respiratory muscles in patients with or without lung diseases and contributes to impaired pulmonary function, hypercapnia, and inability to wean (Fiaccadori & Borghetti, 1991). Risk of infection becomes more likely when a patient is undernourished because of resultant decreased cell-mediated immunity. Interstitial and pulmonary edema may develop because of severe hypoalbuminemia in which the osmotic pressure is decreased and the fluid is shifted into the interstitial space (interstitial edema), and eventually into the alveoli (pulmonary edema). Other complications of undernutrition include poor wound healing and decreased surfactant production (Table 12-17) (Ideno et al., 1995).

OVERFEEDING

☑️ High caloric enteric nutrition can cause a significant increase in oxygen consumption and carbon dioxide production. In turn, this can induce respiratory distress during weaning for patients with limited pulmonary reserve.

While undernutrition is undesirable for critically ill patients, overfeeding should be avoided. Excessive nutrition may significantly increase the work of breathing because of lipogenesis and increased carbon dioxide production. It may also lead to diminished surfactant production and fatty degeneration of the liver (Table 12-18) (Ideno et al., 1995).

High caloric enteric nutrition can cause a significant increase in oxygen consumption, carbon dioxide production, and respiratory

TABLE 12-17   Effects of Undernutrition

1. Depletion of cellular stores of glycogen and protein

2. Fatigue of respiratory muscles

3. Impaired pulmonary function

4. Decreased cell-mediated immunity

5. Interstitial or pulmonary edema

6. Poor wound healing

7. Decreased surfactant production

quotient. In turn, this can induce respiratory distress during weaning for patients with a limited pulmonary reserve.

Problems with overfeeding may also be found in total parenteral nutrition (TPN) provided via the intravenous route. Respiratory acidosis during mechanical ventilation has been reported within hours after initiation of TPN (van der Berg et al., 1988).

LOW-CARBOHYDRATE HIGH-FAT DIET

✓ A low carbohydrate high-fat diet may maximize energy intake and minimize oxygen utilization and carbon dioxide production.

Each gram of hydrous dextrose (a form of glucose) produces 3.4 kcal. For the same amount of fat emulsion, it generates 9.1 kcal. The concentrated source of energy in fat emulsion is preferred for fluid-restricted patients. A fat-based diet also reduces carbon dioxide production and ventilatory requirements (Mlynarek et al., 1987).

For this reason, an increase in fat kilocalories with a concurrent decrease in carbohydrate (dextrose) intake has been done to maximize energy intake and to minimize oxygen utilization and carbon dioxide production. The fat-based diet should contain at least 40% total fat kilocalories and it should be based on the patient's clinical status since a metabolically stressed patient may become immunosuppressed because of insufficient fat in the diet (Ideno et al., 1995).

TABLE 12-18   Effects of Overfeeding

1. Increased oxygen consumption

2. Increased carbon dioxide production

3. Increased work of breathing

4. Decreased surfactant production

5. Interstitial or pulmonary edema

6. Fatty degeneration of liver

In one study, a high-calorie diet consisting of 28% carbohydrate, 55% fat, and balanced protein resulted in significantly lower CO_2 production and arterial PCO_2 in COPD patients with hypercapnia. Furthermore, two important lung function measurements (forced vital capacity and forced expiratory volume in 1 sec) improved by 22% over baseline values with this low-carbohydrate, high-fat diet (Angelillo et al., 1985).

TOTAL CALORIC REQUIREMENTS

Energy requirements for the critically ill patient are commonly done by using the Harris-Benedict equation (Roza et al., 1984). This equation can be used to estimate a patient's resting energy expenditure (REE) and total energy expenditure (TEE).

REE is the minimum energy requirement for basic metabolic needs. TEE is the energy requirement based on a patient's disease state in which the metabolic rate is higher than normal. TEE is the product of REE and the activity/stress factors (TEE = REE × Activity × Stress Factors). These factors are used to make allowances for hypermetabolic or hypercatabolic conditions such as activity, trauma, infection, and burns. For ventilator-dependent patients, the TEE is calculated by multiplying the REE by factors ranging from 1.2 to 2.1 as shown in Table 12-19 (Askanazi et al., 1982; Roza et al., 1984).

TABLE 12-19   Calculation of Daily REE and TEE in Kilocalories

REE for men in kcal/day = 66 + 13.7 W + 5 H − 6.8 A
REE for women in kcal/day = 655 + 9.6 W + 1.85 H − 4.7 A
W = weight in kg; H = height in cm; A = age in years
TEE for men in kcal/day = REE × Activity Factor × Stress Factor
TEE for women in kcal/day = REE × Activity Factor × Stress Factor
W = Weight in kg; H = Height in cm; A = Age in year

Activity factor	
Confined to bed	×1.2
Out of bed	×1.3

Stress factor	
Minor operation	×1.20
Skeletal trauma	×1.35
Major sepsis	×1.60
Severe thermal burn	×2.10

PHOSPHATE SUPPLEMENT

In addition to the total caloric requirement, a patient's nutritional program should maintain a balanced serum phosphate level. Insufficient phosphate in a patient's diet may cause hypophosphatemia, a condition where the serum phosphate level is less than 1 mg/dL. Hypophosphatemia decreases tissue adenosine triphosphate (ATP) level, and in severe form it may cause the patient to experience confusion, muscle weakness, congestive heart failure, and respiratory failure (Mlynarek et al., 1987).

> **Hypophosphatemia** (serum phosphate level <1 mg/dL), in severe form, may cause the patient to experience confusion, muscle weakness, congestive heart failure, and respiratory failure.

ADJUNCTIVE MANAGEMENT STRATEGIES

On some occasions, the basic management strategies may not be able to maintain proper ventilation and oxygenation. In other conditions such as acute lung injury (ALI) and adult respiratory distress syndrome (ARDS), the ventilator settings may result in volume and pressure that can be inappropriate and detrimental to the patient. Under these conditions, other management strategies should be considered. They include the use of low tidal volume, prone positioning, and trachea gas insufflation.

LOW TIDAL VOLUME

Traditional tidal volume settings use 10 to 15 mL/kg of body weight and this range is often necessary to achieve normal ventilation. In one study, 48% of the critical care practitioners reported using volumes in the range of 10 to 15 mL/kg and 45% reported using 5 to 9 mL/kg (Thompson et al., 2001). In patients with ALI or ARDS, the inspiratory pressures (i.e., peak inspiratory and plateau) are often elevated due to an increased airflow resistance or/and a decreased lung compliance. The high inspiratory pressures lead to excessive distention of the normal aerated lung and may increase the incidence of **barotrauma (volutrauma).** Therefore, the traditional approach in the selection of tidal volume may exacerbate or perpetuate lung injury in patients with ALI or ARDS and increase the risk of mortality and nonpulmonary organ and system failure (Petrucci et al., 2004; The Acute Respiratory Distress Syndrome Network, 2000).

> ***barotrauma (volutrauma):*** *Air leak into the pleural space caused by excessive pressure or volume in the lung parenchyma.*

Volume Selection. In volume-targeted ventilation for patients with ALI or ARDS, the tidal volumes selected should result in a plateau pressure of <35 cm H_2O (Thompson, 2001). Plateau pressure is used as a target pressure because it reflects the condition of the lung parenchyma. For the reason of lung protection, the lowest tidal

> **The tidal volume** selected for patients with ALI or ARDS should result in a plateau pressure of <35 cm H_2O.

volume that meets the patient's minimal oxygenation and ventilation requirements should be used.

Complications.   Use of low tidal volume ventilation should be done with care as it may lead to complications such as acute hypercapnia, increased work of breathing, dyspnea, severe acidosis, and lung collapse (Kallet et al., 2001).

PRONE POSITIONING

Prone positioning (PP): Placement of the patient in a face-down position in a bed.

Prone positioning (PP) has been used to improve ventilation, oxygenation, and pulmonary perfusion in patients with acute respiratory failure and ARDS. Following PP, there is a rapid increase in oxygenation measurements (e.g., SpO_2, PaO_2, SaO_2) and improvement in lung compliance (Relvas et al., 2003). The oxygen requirement, intrapulmonary shunting, and inspiratory pressures are reduced as well (Breiburg, 2000; Fletcher et al., 2003). Table 12-20 outlines the physiologic goals of PP.

☑ PP has been used to improve ventilation, oxygenation, and pulmonary perfusion in patients with acute respiratory failure and ARDS.

While PP improves these parameters rapidly, it does not increase the survival rate of patients with acute respiratory failure or ARDS when compared to similar patients who are in the standard supine position (Gattinoni et al., 2001; Meade, 2002; Rialp et al., 2002).

☑ PP improves oxygenation parameters rapidly but it does not increase the survival rate of patients with acute respiratory failure or ARDS.

Indications and Contraindications.   The primary indication for PP is ARDS with increasing oxygen index (OI) of >30% while supine and during mechanical ventilation. OI requires measurement of the mean airway pressure (mPaw), F_IO_2, and PaO_2. See equation below and Appendix 1 for example to calculate the OI.

$$OI = \frac{(mPaw \times F_IO_2)}{PaO_2}$$

TABLE 12-20 Physiologic Goals of Prone Positioning

To improve oxygenation (e.g., SpO_2, PaO_2, SaO_2)

To improve respiratory mechanics (e.g., compliance, work of breathing)

To enhance pleural pressure gradient, alveolar inflation, and gas distribution

To reduce inspiratory pressures (e.g., peak and plateau)

To reduce atelectasis and intrapulmonary shunting

To facilitate removal of secretions

To reduce ventilator-related lung injury

(Data from Breiburg, 2000; Fletcher et al., 2003; Pelosi, 2002; Relvas et al., 2003.)

☑ After 1 hour of PP, an improvement of the OI by ≥20% of baseline value suggests beneficial response.

Contraindications for PP include increased intracranial pressure, hemodynamic instability, unstable spinal cord injury, recent abdominal or thoracic surgery, flail chest, and inability to tolerate PP.

Procedure. If no contraindication for PP exists, the patient is turned to a prone position for at least 1 hour (stabilization period). After 1 hour, the PaO_2/F_IO_2 ratio and the mPaw are measured. An improvement of the OI by ≥20% of baseline value suggests beneficial response to PP.

For optimal improvement in oxygenation and more stable improvement in the OI, pediatric patients should remain in the PP for a period longer than 12 hours. The procedure for PP (preparing the patient, placing the patient in PP and SP) has been fully described by Relvas in 2003. For adult patients, the duration of PP should be 6 hours or more depending on patient response and tolerance (Gattinoni et al., 2001; Meade, 2002).

brachial plexopathy: decreased movement or sensation in the arm and shoulder.

Complications. Complications of PP include accidental extubation, hemodynamic instability, pressure wounds or ulcers, residual obstructive and restrictive lung defects, and **brachial plexopathy** (Curley et al., 2000; Goettler, 2002; Neff, 2003; Relvas et al., 2003).

TRACHEAL GAS INSUFFLATION

Tracheal gas insufflation (TGI): Use of a small catheter to provide a continuous or phasic gas flow directly into the trachea during mechanical ventilation.

Tracheal gas insufflation (TGI) is a technique that uses a small catheter to provide a continuous or phasic gas flow directly into the endotracheal tube during mechanical ventilation. Slusky and Menon described in 1987 the use of a constant-flow device in conjunction with ventilation. Over the years, innovations have been made on similar technique. As of 2004, TGI is used only in clinical research studies and it has not been cleared for general use by the Food and Drug Administration.

☑ TGI introduces 5 to 20 L/min of oxygen or air into the endotracheal (ET) tube during mechanical ventilation.

Procedure. TGI introduces 5 to 20 L/min of oxygen or air into the endotracheal (ET) tube during mechanical ventilation. This flow is in addition to the flow provided by the ventilator. The flow provided by the TGI is regulated by a controller and is directed through a small catheter to the distal end of the ET tube. The gas exits the ET tube and arrives just above the carina (Valley Inspired Products, Burnsville, MN).

The insufflation may be continuous or phasic. In continuous flow TGI, the gas flow goes into the airway during inspiration and expiration. Some undesirable effects of continuous TGI include drying of secretions, mucosal tissue damage, increased tidal volume delivery, development of auto-PEEP, and increased effort to trigger ventilator. In phasic TGI, the gas flow goes into the airway during the last half of the expiratory phase. This phasic timing helps to flush out the ET tube with fresh gas (0% carbon dioxide) during expiration and fills the ET tube with fresh gas for the next inspiration (Figure 12-8).

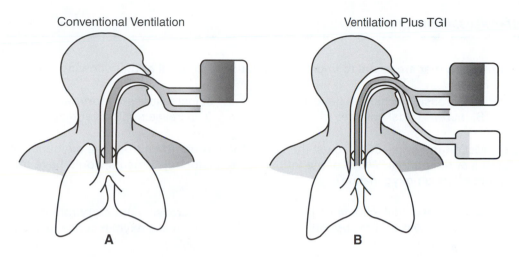

Conventional Ventilation   Ventilation Plus TGI

A   B

Figure 12-8 Conventional ventilation and tracheal gas insufflation. (A) In conventional ventilation, expired gas (~4% CO_2) remains in the endotracheal tube and goes back into the lung on the next breath. (B) With tracheal gas insufflation, the expired gas is flushed from the endotracheal tube with fresh gas (0% CO_2). This fresh gas goes into the lung on the next breath. (Courtesy of Valley Inspired Products, Burnsville, MN. Used with permission.)

☑ TGI reduces the instrumental deadspace, improves carbon dioxide clearance, and lowers the ventilation pressure and tidal volume requirements.

Potential Uses. During mechanical ventilation of newborns, TGI reduces the instrumental deadspace, improves carbon dioxide clearance, and lowers the ventilation pressure and tidal volume requirements. These effects have the potential to decrease the likelihood of secondary lung injury and chronic lung disease in newborns (Davies et al., 2002; Epstein, 2002; Kalous et al., 2003; Liu et al., 2004). TGI has also been used successfully to reduce the respiratory demand during weaning from mechanical ventilation (Hoffman et al., 2003).

TGI is a modality that has the potential to improve the management of patients with acute respiratory failure. Additional research studies and more clinical trials are necessary to make TGI an FDA-approved device for the general patient population.

SUMMARY

This chapter outlines the essential strategies that are useful in the management of patients receiving mechanical ventilation. These strategies are straightforward and can be followed by using a logical deduction process. Careful observation of the patient and ventilator must be done in order to identify the problem at hand. Once the problem has been identified, appropriate steps may be taken. It is vital to remember that no changes to ventilator settings should be made unless the reasons for doing so are safe and justifiable.

Self-Assessment Questions

1. Strategies that are useful to improve ventilation include all of the following *except*:

    A. increase mechanical deadspace.   C. increase respiratory rate.
    B. increase tidal volume.   D. increase minute ventilation.

2. Dr. McFarland asks you to adjust the ventilator in order to improve the oxygenation status of the patient. Which of the following ventilator adjustments would have the most direct effect on oxygenation?

    A. decrease tidal volume (V_T)   C. increase mandatory rate (f)
    B. decrease pressure support   D. increase oxygen concentration
       ventilation (PSV)   (F_1O_2)

3. An endotracheal tube is sometimes cut shorter because a shorter ET tube:

    A. increases the F_1O_2.   C. facilitates airway management and
    B. increases the mechanical deadspace   secretions removal.
       volume.   D. reduces the arterial pH.

4. The primary purpose of permissive hypercapnia is to reduce the patient's _____ during mechanical ventilation.

    A. tidal volume   C. pulmonary pressures
    B. pH   D. respiratory rate

5. Permissive hypercapnia is a technique in which the mechanical _____ is reduced. This leads to an increase of the patient's _____.

    A. peak airway pressure, pH   C. tidal volume, pH
    B. peak airway pressure, PaO_2 D. tidal volume, $PaCO_2$

6. CPAP and PEEP may be used to correct refractory hypoxemia caused by:

    A. deadspace ventilation.   C. intrapulmonary shunting.
    B. V/Q mismatch.   D. diffusion defect.

7. The PaO_2 of an ARDS patient has been deteriorating while on 50% oxygen. The physician asks you to suggest the best solution for this problem. You would recommend trying the following procedures in the order provided:

    A. CPAP, mechanical ventilation with   C. inverse ratio ventilation, mechanical
       PEEP, inverse ratio ventilation.   ventilation, PEEP.
    B. mechanical ventilation, CPAP, inverse D. mechanical ventilation, inverse ratio
       ratio ventilation with PEEP.   ventilation, PEEP.

8. Compensated respiratory acidosis and compensated metabolic alkalosis have similar blood gas characteristics: normal pH, high $PaCO_2$, and high HCO_3^-. One useful clue to differentiate these two conditions is that in compensated:

   A. respiratory acidosis, the pH is on the acidotic side of normal range.

   B. metabolic alkalosis, the pH is on the acidotic side of normal range.

   C. respiratory and metabolic acidosis, both pH are on the alkalotic side of normal range.

   D. respiratory and metabolic alkalosis, both pH are on the acidotic side of normal range.

9. A patient's low pressure alarm is triggered while you are performing ventilator care. The likely causes of this condition include all of the following *except*:

   A. disconnection of ventilator circuit.

   B. kinking of endotracheal tube.

   C. power failure.

   D. leakage of endotracheal tube cuff.

10. While you are looking for the cause of low pressure alarm on a ventilator, the high pressure alarm is also triggered. This condition is likely caused by:

    A. disconnection of ventilator circuit.

    B. low pressure limit set too high.

    C. loose ventilator humidifier fitting.

    D. patient coughing.

11. Analysis of sputum samples by the culture and sensitivity method is _____. It provides information on the type of _____ that the microbes are sensitive to.

    A. quick, sterilizing agents

    B. quick, antibiotics

    C. time-consuming, sterilizing agents

    D. time-consuming, antibiotics

12. The average urine output of a patient is 15 mL/hour. This output is _____ than normal and it implies that there is too _____ fluid in the extracellular fluid compartment.

    A. higher, much

    B. higher, little

    C. lower, much

    D. lower, little

13. The following electrolyte values are collected from a patient with severe sepsis who has been on a mechanical ventilator for 2 weeks. Which of the following electrolytes is out of its normal range?

Electrolyte	Value (mEq/L)
A. Na^+	138
B. K^+	1.5
C. Cl^-	105
D. HCO_3^-	25

14. In replacing fluids to a volume-depleted patient, it is not safe to administer fluids that have no sodium because _____ movement of sodium-free fluid into the brain and kidney cells may cause _____ of these organs.

    A. rapid, swelling
    B. rapid, dehydration
    C. slow, swelling
    D. slow, dehydration

15. Decreased muscle function, flattened T wave and depressed ST segment on the electrocardiogram, and diminished bowel sounds are some signs of:

    A. hyperkalemia.
    B. hypokalemia.
    C. hypernatremia.
    D. hyponatremia.

16. Proper nutrition is essential to patients receiving mechanical ventilation because undernutrition can cause:

    A. increased surfactant production.
    B. improved pulmonary function.
    C. increased metabolic rate.
    D. fatigue of respiratory muscles.

17. A diet consisting of low carbohydrate and high fat is more suitable for ventilator patients because _____ generates more calories per gram and produces less _____.

    A. fat, CO_2
    B. fat, O_2
    C. carbohydrate, CO_2
    D. carbohydrate, O_2

18. The total energy expenditure (TEE) is _____ than the resting energy expenditure (REE) because TEE _____ accounts for patient factors such as activity, trauma, and infection.

    A. higher, does
    B. higher, does not
    C. lower, does
    D. lower, does not

19. Mr. Howe, a 70-kg patient with ARDS, is being mechanically ventilated at a SIMV rate of 12/min and tidal volume of 700 mL. Over a period of 8 hours, his peak inspiratory and plateau pressures have increased to 66 and 45 mm Hg, respectively. The attending physician asks you to suggest any ventilator changes that may help to minimize the effects of rising airway pressures. You would recommend the following strategy.

    A. low respiratory rate.
    B. low tidal volume.
    C. tracheal gas insufflation.
    D. prone positioning.

Answers to Self-Assessment Questions

1. A. increase mechanical deadspace.

2. D. increase oxygen concentration (F_IO_2)

3. C. facilitates airway management and secretions removal.

4. C. pulmonary pressures

5. D. tidal volume, $PaCO_2$

6. C. intrapulmonary shunting.

7. A. CPAP, mechanical ventilation with PEEP, inverse ratio ventilation.

8. A. respiratory acidosis, the pH is on the acidotic side of normal range.

9. B. kinking of endotracheal tube.

10. D. patient coughing.

11. D. time-consuming, antibiotics

12. D. lower, little

13. B. K^+ of 1.5 mEq/L is out of normal range

14. A. rapid, swelling

15. B. hypokalemia.

16. D. fatigue of respiratory muscles.

17. A. fat, CO_2

18. A. higher, does

19. B. low tidal volume

References

Angelillo, V. A., et al. (1985). Effects of low and high carbohydrate feedings in ambulatory patients with chronic obstructive pulmonary disease and chronic hypercapnia. *Ann Intern Med, 103*(6, Pt. 1), 883–885.

Askanazi, J., et al. (1982). Nutrition and the respiratory system. *Crit Care Med, 10,* 163–172.

Barnes, T. A., et al. (1994). *Core textbook of respiratory care practice* (2nd ed.). St. Louis, MO: Mosby.

Boots, R. J., Howe, S., George, N., et al. (1997). Clinical utility of hygroscopic heat and moisture exchangers in intensive care patients. *Crit Care Med, 25*(10), 1707–1712.

Breiburg, A. N. (2000). Efficacy and safety of prone positioning for patients with acute respiratory distress syndrome. *J Adv Nur, 32*(4), 922–929.

Burton, G. G., et al. (1997). *Respiratory care: A guide to clinical practice* (4th ed.). Baltimore: Lippincott Williams & Wilkins.

Cox, R. G., et al. (1991). Efficacy, results, and complications of mechanical ventilation in children with status asthmaticus. *Pediatr Pulmonol,11*(2), 120–126.

Craven, D. E., et al. (1989). Nosocomial pneumonia in the intubated patient. New concepts on pathogenesis and prevention. *Infect Dis Clin North Am, 3*(4), 843–866.

Curley, M. A., et al. (2000). The effects of early and repeated prone positioning in pediatric patients with acute lung injury. *Chest, 118*(1), 156–163.

Darioli, R., et al. (1984). Mechanical controlled hypertension in status asthmaticus. *Am Rev Respir Dis, 129,* 385–387.

Davies, M. W., et al. (2002). Tracheal gas insufflation for the prevention of morbidity and mortality in mechanically ventilated newborn infants. *Cochrane Database Syst Rev, 2,* CD002973.

Eggleston, F. C. (1985). Simplified management of fluid and electrolyte problems. Normal balance, abnormalities and practical management. *Trop Doc, 15*(2), 55–64.

Epstein, S. K. (2002). TGIF: Tracheal gas insufflation for whom? *Chest, 122*(5), 1515–1517.

Feihl, F., et al. (1994). Permissive hypercapnia: How permissive should we be? *Am J Respir Crit Care Med, 150*(6, Pt. 1), 1722–1737.

Fiaccadori, E., & Borghetti, A. (1991). Pathophysiology of respiratory muscles in course of undernutrition. *Ann Ital Med Int (AUZ), 6*(4), 402–407.

Flink, J. D., Krause, S. A., & Barrett, J. (1998). Extending ventilator circuit change interval beyond 2 days reduces the likelihood of ventilator-associated pneumonia. *Chest, 113*(2), 405–411.

Fletcher, S. J., et al. (2003). Use of prone positioning in neurogenic pulmonary oedema. *Br J Anaesth, 90*(2), 238–240.

Gattinoni, L., et al. (2001). Effect of prone positioning on the survival of patients with acute respiratory failure. *N Eng J Med, 345*(8), 568–573.

Goettler, C. E., et al. (2002). Brachial plexopathy after prone positioning. *Crit Case, 6*(6), 540–542.

Gurevitch, M. J., et al. (1986). Improved oxygenation and lower peak airway pressure in severe adult respiratory distress syndrome: Treatment with inverse ratio ventilation. *Chest, 89,* 211.

Hagler, D. A., et al. (1994). Endotracheal saline and suction catheters: Sources of lower airway contamination. *Am J Crit Care, 3*(6), 444–447.

Hickling, K. G., et al. (1990). Low mortality associated with permissive hypercapnia in severe adult respiratory distress syndrome. *Intensive Care Med, 16,* 372–377.

Hickling, K. G. (2002). Permissive hypercapnia. *Respir Care Clin N Am*, *8*(2), 155–169.

Hoffman, L. A., et al. (2003). Effect of tracheal gas insufflation during weaning from mechanical ventilation: A preliminary study. *Am J Crit Care*, *12*(1), 31–39.

Hu, B. (1991). Lower respiratory tract flora in intubated patients. *Chung Hua I Hsueh Tsa Chih (Chinese), 71*(5), 243–245.

Ideno, K. T., et al. (1995, April/May). Managing respiratory patients' nutritional outcomes. *J Respir Care Pract,* 111–118.

Joshi, N., et al. (1993). A predictive risk index for nosocomial pneumonia in the intensive care unit. *Am J Med, 93*(2), 135–142.

Kallet, R. H., et al. (2000). The treatment of acidosis in acute lung injury with THAM. *AJRCCM, 161*(4 Pt. 1), 1149–1153.

Kallet, R. H., et al. (2001 a). Implementation of a low tidal volume ventilation protocol for patients with acute lung injury or acute respiratory distress syndrome. *Respir Care*, *46*(10), 1024–1037.

Kallet, R. H., et al. (2001 b). Lung collapse during low tidal volume ventilation in acute respiratory distress syndrome. *Respir Care*, *46*(1), 49–52.

Kalous, P., et al. (2003). Instrumental dead space in neonatology, and its elimination by continuous tracheal gas insufflation during conventional ventilation. *Acta Paediatr*, *92*(5), 518–524.

Kirton, O. C., DeHaven, B., Morgan, J., et al. (1997). A prospective, randomized comparison of an in-line heat moisture exchange filter and heated wire humidifiers: Rates of ventilator-associated early-onset (community-acquired) or late-onset (hospital-acquired) pneumonia and incidence of endotracheal tube occlusion. *Chest, 112*(4), 1055–1059.

Kollef, M. H., et al. (1994). Ventilator-associated pneumonia: Clinical considerations. *Am J Roentgen, 163,* 1031–1035.

Kotilainen, H. R., & Keroack, M. A. (1997). Cost analysis and clinical impact of weekly ventilator circuit changes in patients in intensive care unit. *Am J Infect Control, 25*(2), 117–120.

Kraus, P. A., et al. (1993). Acute lung injury at Baragwanath ICU—An eight-month audit and call for consensus for other organ failure in the adult respiratory distress syndrome. *Chest, 103*(6), 1832–1836.

Krider, T. M., et al. (1986). *Master guide for passing the Respiratory Care Credentialing Exam*. Claremont, CA: Education Resource Consortium.

Lewandowski, K., et al. (1992). Approaches to improve survival in severe ARDS. In J. L. Vincent (Ed.), *Update in intensive care and emergency medicine* (pp. 372–377). Berlin: Springer-Verlag.

Liu, Y.N., et al. (2004). Aspiration of dead space in the management of chronic obstructive pulmonary disease patients with respiratory failure. *Respir Care, 49*(3), 257–262.

Long, M. N., Wickstrom, G., Grimes, A., et al. (1996). Prospective, randomized study of ventilator-associated pneumonia in patients with one versus three ventilator circuit changes per week. *Infect Control Hosp Epidemiol, 17*(1): 14–19.

Lowy, F. D., et al. (1987). The incidence of nosocomial pneumonia following urgent endotracheal intubation. *Infect Control, 8*(6), 245–248.

MacIntyre, N. R. (1986). Pressure support ventilation. *Respir Care, 31,* 189–190.

Marini, J. J. (1988). Monitoring during mechanical ventilation. *Clin Chest Med, 9,* 73–100.

Marini, J. J. (1993). New options for the ventilatory management of acute lung injury. *New Horiz, 1*(4), 489–503.

Meade, M. (2002). Prone positioning for acute respiratory failure improved short-term oxygenation but not survival. *ACP J Club, 136*(2), 55.

Mlynarek, M., et al. (1987). Individualizing nutrition in patients with acute respiratory failure requiring mechanical ventilation. *Drug Intelligence and Clinical Pharmacy,* 21, 865–869.

Nahas, G. G., et al. (1998). Guidelines for the treatment of academia with THAM. *Drugs, 55,* 191–224.

Nathan, S. D., et al. (1993). Prediction of minimal pressure support during weaning from mechanical ventilation. *Chest, 103,* 1215–1219.

Neff, T. A., et al. (2003). Long-term assessment of lung function in survivors of ARDS. *Chest, 123*(3), 845–853.

Otto, C. W. (1986). Ventilatory management in the critically ill. *Emerg Med Clin North Am, 4*(4), 635–654.

Petrucci, N., et al. (2004). Ventilation with lower tidal volumes versus traditional tidal volumes in adults for acute lung injury and acute respiratory distress syndrome. *Cochrane Database Syst Rev, 2004*(2), CD003844.

Pielosi, P., et al. (2002). Prone positioning in acute respiratory distress syndrome. *Eur Respir J, 20*(4), 1017–1028.

Rello, J., et al. (2001). International conference for the development of consensus on the diagnosis and treatment of ventilator-associated pneumonia. *Chest, 120,* 955–970.

Relvas, M., et al. (2003). Prone positioning of pediatric patients with ARDS results in improvement in oxygenation if maintained >12 h daily. *Chest, 124,* 269–274.

Rialp, G., et al. (2002). Prone positioning in patients with acute respiratory distress syndrome. *Respir Care Clin N Am, 8*(2), 237–245, vi–vii.

Rodenhizer, K. (2004). Ballard trach care closed suction system summary of benefits and associated literature. Retrieved April 26, 2004, from http://www.xmission.com/%7Egastown/herpmed/closed.htm

Roza, A. M., et al. (1984). The Harris-Benedict equation reevaluated: Resting energy requirements and the body cell mass. *Am J Clin Nutr, 40,* 168–182.

Schuster, D. P. (1990). A physiologic approach to initiating, maintaining, and withdrawing mechanical ventilatory support during acute respiratory failure. *Am J Med, 88,* 268–278.

Shapiro, B. A., et al. (1994). *Clinical application of blood gases* (5th ed.). St. Louis, MO: Mosby.

Shapiro, B. A. (1994). A historical perspective on ventilator management. *New Horiz, 2*(1), 8–18.

Slutsky, A. S. (1994). Consensus conference on mechanical ventilation—January 28–30, 1993 at Northbrook, IL, USA, Part I. *Int Care Med, 20,* 64–79.

Slutsky, A. S., et al. (1987). Catheter position and blood gases during constant-flow ventilation. *J Appl Physiol, 62,* 513–519.

Sole, M. L., et al. (2003). A multisite survey of suctioning techniques and airway management practices. *Am J Crit Care, 12*(3), 220–232.

Stamm, A. M. (1998). Ventilator-associated pneumonia and frequency of circuit changes. *Am J Infect Control, 26*(1), 71–73.

Stoller, J. K., et al. (2003). Weekly versus daily changes of in-line suction catheters: Impact on rates of ventilator-associated pneumonia and associated costs. *Respir Care, 48*(5), 494–499.

The Acute Respiratory Distress Syndrome Network. (2000). Ventilation with lower tidal volumes as compared with traditional tidal volumes for acute lung injury and the acute respiratory distress syndrome. *N Engl J Med, 342*(18), 1301–1308.

Thompson, B. T., et al. (2001). Clinicians' approaches to mechanical ventilation in acute lung injury and ARDS. *Chest, 120,* 1622–1627.

Valley Inspired Products LLC. (2004). Tracheal gas insufflation example. Retrieved July 8, 2004, from http://www.inspiredrc.com/tgi1.htm

van der Berg, B., et al. (1988). Metabolic and respiratory effects of enteral nutrition in patients during mechanical ventilation. *Int Care Med, 14,* 206–211.

Viasys Healthcare (2005). 3100B adult HFOV when life hangs in the balance. Retrieved May 20, 2005, from http://www.viasyshealthcare.com/prod-serv/prod detail.aspx? config = ps − prod Dtl & prod ID = 62.

Weber, D. J., et al. (1990). Manual ventilation bags as a source for bacterial colonization of intubated patients. *Am Rev Respir Dis, 142*(4), 892–894.

White, G. C. (2004). *Equipment theory for respiratory care* (4th ed.). Clifton Park, New York: Thomson Delmar Learning.

Wilkins, R. L., et al. (2003). *Egan's fundamentals of respiratory care* (8th ed.). St. Louis, MO: Mosby.

Winter, P. M., et al. (1972). The toxicity of oxygen. *Anesthesiology, 37,* 210.

Zapol, W. M., et al. (1979). Extracorporeal membrane oxygenation in severe acute respiratory failure. *JAMA, 242,* 2193–2196.

Zwischenberger, J. B., et al. (1986). The role of extracorporeal membrane oxygenation in the management of respiratory failure in the newborn. *Resp Care, 31*(6).

Suggested Reading

Cartotto, R., et al. (2004). High frequency oscillatory ventilation in burn patients with the acute respiratory distress syndrome. *Burns, 30*(5), 453–463.

Mehta, S., et al. (2004). High-frequency oscillatory ventilation in adults: The Toronto experience. *Chest, 126*(2), 518–527.

Salim, A., et al. (2004). High-frequency percussive ventilation: An alternative mode of ventilation for head-injured patients with adult respiratory distress syndrome. *J Trauma, 57*(3), 542–546.

CHAPTER THIRTEEN

PROCEDURES RELATED TO MECHANICAL VENTILATION

David W. Chang

OUTLINE

KEY TERMS

- atropine sulfate
- bronchial brushing
- chest tube (thoracostomy tube)
- fiberoptic bronchoscope
- forceps biopsy
- interhospital transport
- intrahospital transport
- lidocaine

- operative tube thoracostomy
- three-chamber drainage system
- transbronchial lung biopsy (TBLB)
- transbronchial needle aspiration biopsy (TBNAB)
- transport ventilator
- trocar
- trocar tube thoracostomy

INTRODUCTION

This chapter covers three clinical topics related to mechanical ventilation: chest tube and drainage system, assisting in fiberoptic bronchoscopy, and transport of mechanically ventilated patients. A sound conceptual foundation and working knowledge of the equipment and supplies for these procedures can ensure patient safety and enhance patient care.

CHEST TUBE AND DRAINAGE SYSTEM

chest tube (thoracostomy tube): A tube that connects the pleural space and drainage system for removal of air or fluid.

Chest tube (thoracostomy tube) and vacuum drainage system are commonly used in acute care settings on patients breathing spontaneously or receiving mechanical ventilation. Respiratory care practitioners should have a good working knowledge of these devices so that hazards and complications with the chest tube setup may be recognized and corrected without delay.

INDICATIONS FOR CHEST TUBE

☑ Common indications for chest tube include large pneumothorax (>25%), hemothorax, and pleural effusion.

Common indications for chest tube include large pneumothorax (>25%), hemothorax, and pleural effusion. Causes of pneumothorax include positive pressure ventilation, ruptured bleb due to emphysema, bronchopleural fistula, leaking subpleural cyst, and chest trauma. Iatrogenic pneumothorax may be caused by invasive procedures such as thoracentesis, central vein/pulmonary artery catheterization, and bronchoscopy/transbronchial biopsy (Chen et al., 2002). Excessive pleural fluid may be caused by thoracic trauma (hemothorax), heart failure (pleural effusion), intra-abdominal infection (empyema), and blockage of lymphatic system (chylothorax) (Irwin et al., 2003).

☑ Potential compli-
cations of chest
tube placement
include hemorrhage
at insertion site,
hematoma, lacera-
tion of lung
parenchyma or
intra-abdominal
organs, and infection.

trocar: *A trocar is a*
sharply pointed
instrument for inci-
sion into the chest
cavity.

☑ The suggested
chest tube size
for teens and large
adults ranges from
28 to 40 Fr.

☑ Since clotting of
the chest tube
with blood or pleural
fluid is less likely in
pneumothoraces,
16 to 20 Fr may be
adequate for adults.

☑ To treat pneu-
mothorax, the
chest tube (16 to
20 Fr) is placed at
the second or third
intercostal space
anteriorly along the
midclavicular line or
midaxillary line.

Contraindications and Complications.   There are no absolute contraindications to chest tube placement in patients who are symptomatic from the above indications. Relative contraindications include
infection over the insertion site, and conditions that may lead to severe
bleeding during chest tube placement (Thomas, 2004).

Potential complications of chest tube placement include hemorrhage
at the insertion site, hematoma, and laceration of lung parenchyma or
intra-abdominal organs. Infection can be a late complication (Thomas,
2004).

CHEST TUBE SELECTION AND PLACEMENT

The chest tube may be straight, curved, trocar, or nontrocar. A **trocar**
is a sharply pointed instrument for incision into the chest cavity
(Figure 13-1). The suggested chest tube size for large adults ranges
from 36 to 40 French (Fr). For small adults or teens, a range from 28 to
32 Fr is adequate. For children and neonates, the appropriate chest
tube sizes are 18 and 12 to 14 Fr, respectively.

Clotting of blood inside the chest tube is a potential complication
following placement. For this reason, larger tubes are selected for
treatment of hemothorax or other thick pleural fluids (e.g., empyema).
Since clotting is less likely when the chest tube is used to treat pneumothoraces, smaller sizes (16 to 20 Fr) may be adequate for adults.

Chest Tube Placement.   Chest tubes are inserted under sterile condition at the bedside or in surgery. To treat pneumothorax, the chest
tube (16 to 20 Fr) is usually placed at the second or third intercostal
space anteriorly along the midclavicular line or midaxillary line.
For drainage of blood or other pleural fluids, a size 36 Fr (ranging
from 28 to 40 Fr) chest tube is recommended to reduce clotting.
The insertion point is from the fourth to sixth intercostal space at the

Figure 13-1   A chest tube with trocar (lower solid piece). The trocar is
placed inside the chest tube for insertion through the incision on the
chest wall.

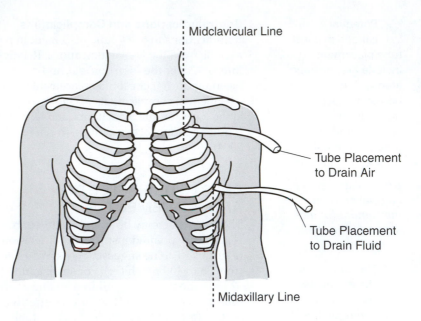

Midclavicular Line

Tube Placement
to Drain Air

Tube Placement
to Drain Fluid

Midaxillary Line

Figure 13-2   Chest tube insertion sites showing (A) second intercostal space anteriorly along the midclavicular line for relieve of pneumothorax; (B) fifth intercostal space along the midaxillary line for drainage of pleural fluid.

☑ To drain fluid, the chest tube is placed from the fourth to sixth intercostal space at the midaxillary line.

☑ The point of entry is directly over the body of the rib because arteries, veins, and intercostal nerves all lie below each rib.

operative tube thoracostomy: A technique of test tube placement by dissection into the pleura, digital inspection of the pleural space, and insertion guided with the finger and hemostat.

midaxillary line (usually a line lateral to the nipple) for optimal drainage of pleural fluid (Figure 13-2).

During chest tube placement, the point of entry is directly over the body of the rib to avoid complications. Incisions or punctures are done above the rib because arteries, veins, and intercostal nerves all lie below each rib. Figure 13-3 shows the correct placement of a chest tube entering the chest wall at the midaxillary line. The point of entry is directly over the rib.

METHODS OF PLACEMENT

Operative tube thoracostomy and trocar tube thoracostomy are two common methods to perform chest tube placement. Each method has its advantages and disadvantages (Deshpande, 2002).

Operative Tube Thoracostomy.   In **operative tube thoracostomy,** the incision is made parallel to and above the rib. It is followed by blunt dissection into the pleura. A finger is inserted into the opening for inspection of the pleural space. A chest tube is then guided into the pleural space by using a finger and hemostat or Kelly clamp (Figure 13-4). This method is safer than trocar tube thoracostomy because digital inspection eliminates the possibility of chest tube

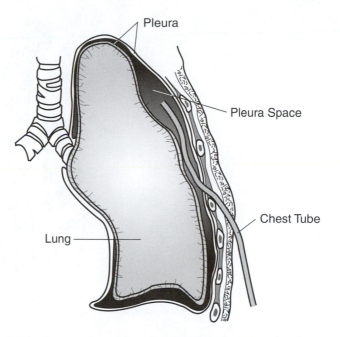

Pleura

Pleura Space

Chest Tube

Lung

Figure 13-3 Correct placement of a chest tube entering the chest wall at the midaxillary line. The point of entry is directly over the rib to avoid puncture of the arteries, veins, and intercostal nerves that lie below each rib.

Figure 13-4 The chest tube is clamped by a hemostat and both are guided into the pleural space by a finger.

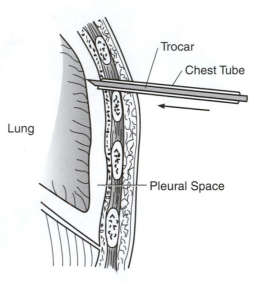

Figure 13-5 Incision is done parallel to and above the rib. The chest tube with trocar inside is inserted through the incision over the rib.

placement between the parietal pleura and the chest wall. However, it is more involved and requires a larger incision to allow the finger, chest tube, and hemostat to enter the chest wall and the pleural space.

Trocar Tube Thoracostomy.   In **trocar tube thoracostomy,** the incision is also made parallel to and above the rib. The chest tube with trocar inside is inserted through the incision (Figure 13-5). The chest tube/trocar setup should enter the chest only 1 to 2 cm, otherwise puncture of the lung is likely. Once inside the pleural space, the chest tube is advanced over the trocar—a procedure similar to the "catheter over needle" technique for artery line placement. The chest tube is clamped with a forceps before complete withdrawal of the trocar. This method requires a smaller incision and provides less tissue trauma and less patient discomfort.

Following placement, the rigid chest tube is connected to the flexible Creech tubing with a clear, ridged plastic connector flange. Since the flange has a narrow diameter, any clots from the pleural cavity may become lodged at this location. When cloth tape is used to seal and secure the connection, it should be done in a way that does not interfere with the visual inspection of any clot formation inside the connector.

The chest tube should be kept in a straight line as much as possible. If the tube is looped or kinked, the suction level will decrease and lung reexpansion may be hindered. In addition, fluid in the tube may reenter the pleural space leading to the possibility of infection.

trocar tube thoracostomy: A technique of test tube placement by incision into the pleura, insertion of trocar chest tube, and withdrawal of trocar.

☑ Kinking of the chest tube will lower the suction level, hinder lung reexpansion, and cause the fluid to enter the pleural space.

CHEST TUBE DRAINAGE SYSTEM

Following insertion and inspection of the chest tube for proper placement, the chest tube is immediately connected to a drainage system that has been previously set up. Since fluid and air are gravity dependent, all chest tube drainage systems are placed below the level of chest tube placement. There are different drainage systems for a chest tube. The most common and versatile drainage system in the hospital is the three-chamber setup such as Pleur-Evac®. Proper functioning of the drainage system must be evaluated and unusual occurrence with the drainage system must be correlated to the patient's condition and vital signs.

The one-chamber and two-chamber drainage systems are simple in design and they can be set up quickly. While these two systems do not require a vacuum source, their usefulness in the intensive care is rather limited. The **three-chamber drainage system** is the most versatile one and it requires a vacuum source to provide continuous suction. All three systems are discussed below for a clear understanding of the working mechanism of a chest tube drainage system.

three-chamber drainage system: A chest tube drainage setup that requires a vacuum source to provide continuous suction.

One-Chamber System.   In a one-chamber water-seal system [Figure 13-6(A)], the chamber initially contains 100 mL of sterile water. The short air-vent tube prevents pressure buildup in the chamber. The long tube is submerged in exactly 2 cm of water. This acts as a water seal which allows air to escape but not to return. With this system, the work of spontaneous breathing is proportional to the submersion depth of the long tube. As pleural fluid drains and accumulates in the chamber, more of the long tube is submerged and spontaneous breathing becomes more difficult.

☑ As pleural fluid drains and accumulates in the one-chamber system, more of the long tube is submerged and spontaneous breathing becomes more difficult.

Some bubbling from the long tube is normal as long as there is air in the pleural space. If there is no bubbling, either there is an obstruction or there is no more air in the pleural space.

Two-Chamber System.   The two-chamber drainage system [Figure 13-6(B)] uses chamber 1 to collect drainage or pleural fluid or evacuate pleural air. The amount of pleural drainage can be measured from chamber 1. In chamber 2, the short tube allows air to escape and prevents pressure to build up. The long tube in chamber 2 is submerged in 2 cm of water as in the one-chamber drainage system. Since chamber 1 collects all pleural fluid, the submersion depth of the long tube in chamber 2 remains unchanged. The work of spontaneous breathing is therefore unaffected by the volume of pleural fluid collected in this chamber.

☑ In a two-chamber drainage system, chamber 1 collects all pleural fluids. The fluid level in chamber 2 remains constant and the work of spontaneous breathing is unaffected.

Three-Chamber System.   The three-chamber drainage system is the most common chest tube drainage system [Figure 13-6(C)]. Chamber 1 (collection chamber) collects the pleural fluid from the patient. Chamber 2

Figure 13-6 Chest tube drainage and water seal systems. (A) One-chamber system; (B) Two-chamber system; (C) Three-chamber system. The amount of bubbling is controlled by the vacuum source and it does not indicate the level of suction applied to the pleural space. The level of suction applied to the pleural space is determined by the submersion depth of the vent tube in the suction chamber.

☑ The water level in chamber 3 (suction chamber) regulates the amount of suction in the three-chamber system.

(water seal chamber) has about 2 cm of water in it and functions as a water seal. The water level in chamber 3 (suction chamber) regulates the amount of suction in the three-chamber system. For example, a suction level of -15 cm H_2O can be achieved by adding sterile water into this chamber to a height of 15 cm H_2O. A low suction level (-10 to -20 cm H_2O) is recommended for the chest tube drainage system.

Under normal working condition, the vacuum draws air into the fluid through the venting tube in chamber 3 causing a constant slow

☑ The setting of wall vacuum and the amount of bubbling in chamber 3 do not reflect the level of suction applied to the pleural space.

☑ In a three-chamber drainage system, the amount of suction applied to the pleural space is determined by the water level and depth of submersion of the venting tube.

bubbling effect. Too much bubbling means the vacuum level is set too high. The setting of wall vacuum and the amount of bubbling do not reflect the level of suction applied to the pleural space. The level of suction applied to the pleural space is determined by the submersion depth of the venting tube in the suction chamber. For this reason, the water level in suction chamber 3 must be monitored and kept at the appropriate level in order to maintain a desired suction force (from −10 to −20 cm H_2O). Evaporation losses will lower the submersion depth and decrease the suction level.

The one- and two-column drainage systems drain fluid by gravity. If suction is desired, a three-column system must be used. Figure 13-7

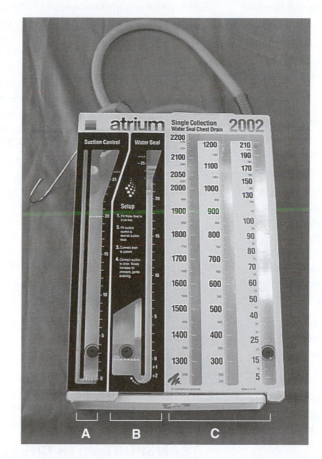

Figure 13-7   A typical chest tube drainage system that combines all three columns (collection, water seal, and suction control) in one unit. In some drainage systems, the cap for the water seal column has a pressure relief valve which is closed under normal suction and opens in case of excessive pressure caused by blocked suction source or obstructed suction tubing. This feature prevents excessive pressure being transmitted to the chest tube and pleural space.

shows a typical chest tube drainage system that combines all three chambers in one unit.

With a three-chamber drainage system, the fluid collection chamber should be inspected to note the volume and characteristics of the fluid drainage. The volume collected should decrease over time.

CARE AND REMOVAL OF CHEST TUBE

☑ If the drainage holes on the chest tube become visible, the chest tube has come out too far.

Emergencies may happen to the chest tube setup. If the drainage holes on the chest tube become visible, the physician should be notified immediately for repositioning or reinsertion. If the chest tube becomes disconnected from the patient, an occlusive dressing such as Vaseline gauze should immediately be applied over the incision opening. The physician is then notified and the patient should be monitored closely for signs of respiratory distress. If the chest tube is disconnected from the drainage unit, clamp the chest tube and reconnect it with a new drainage unit. Clamping of the chest tube should not exceed 1 min.

☑ If the chest tube becomes disconnected from the patient, an occlusive dressing such as Vaseline gauze must be applied immediately over the incision opening.

The water level in the middle (water seal) chamber normally fluctuates with respiration. This means the tube and drainage system are working properly. If a large amount of bubbling is observed in the middle chamber, air leak in the drainage system or presence of air in the pleural space may be present. The patient, connections, vacuum level, and amount of sterile water in the drainage unit should be checked for the source of air leaks.

☑ If a large amount of bubbling is observed in water seal chamber 2, air leak in the drainage system or presence of air in the pleural space may be present.

In order to maintain a desired suction level between -10 and -20 cm H_2O, the water level in the suction chamber must be kept at the appropriate level by filling it with sterile water as needed. Overfilling of water in this chamber will increase the suction level to the pleural space, whereas low water level will reduce the suction level.

The chest tube can be removed when the drainage has stopped or slowed to less than 100 mL over 24 hours; or when the pneumothorax has resolved and there is no further air leak. Air leak (bubbling in the middle chamber) may be tested by asking the patient to perform a Valsalva's maneuver or a forceful cough.

☑ Overfilling of water in suction chamber 3 will increase the suction level to the pleural space, whereas low water level will reduce the suction level.

The suture is first removed and the patient is instructed to perform a Valsalva's maneuver right before pulling out the chest tube. A petrolatum gauze and dressing are applied to the opening immediately. Follow-up chest radiography is done in 4 hours to allow proper lung reexpansion and to detect reoccurring pneumothorax (Alameda County Medical Center, 2004).

TRANSPORT WITH CHEST TUBE

On occasion, patients with a chest tube setup may need to go to another location for testing or treatment. In addition to an oxygen source, primary emergency drugs and airway equipment should be available during transport. The transport team must properly maintain the chest tube and drainage system during the entire transport process. The drainage system must be lower than the patient's chest at

TABLE 13-1   Transport with Chest Tube

1. The drainage system must be kept lower than the patient's chest at all times.
2. The chest tube must not be clamped or occluded at any time.
3. The chest tube must be connected to a functional water seal drainage system.
4. The drainage system must not be tipped or dropped.

☑ During transport, the drainage system must be kept lower than the patient's chest and the chest tube must not be clamped or occluded.

all times. The chest tube must be functional and the patient's pretransport vital signs must be monitored and maintained to ensure stable patient condition.

The chest tube must never be clamped or occluded as this action may affect mechanical or spontaneous ventilation and reverse the reexpansion of the affected lung. Furthermore, fluid flowing back into the pleural space is a source of infection. In most severe cases, a clamped chest tube may potentially convert a simple pleural air leak to life-threatening tension pneumothorax. Therefore, the chest tube must be unobstructed and connected to a functional water seal drainage system. The water seal allows air or fluid to exit the pleural space and prevents it being drawn back into the pleural space (Jacobsohn, 2004). Table 13-1 summarizes the key points to ensure proper functioning of a chest tube during patient transport.

ASSISTING IN FIBEROPTIC BRONCHOSCOPY

fiberoptic bronchoscope: An instrument that uses glass fibers to transmit images of the airway for diagnostic or therapeutic procedures under direct vision.

A **fiberoptic bronchoscope** is used to provide diagnostic and therapeutic procedures for conditions involving the airways and lungs. The insertion tube is composed of a collection of minute glass fibers that have been coated with an optical insulation to provide light and image transmission. Since its development in 1966 and introduction to the United States in 1970, it has become a common application to a variety of diagnostic and therapeutic procedures that require direct visual examination or collection of pulmonary specimens.

INDICATIONS FOR FIBEROPTIC BRONCHOSCOPY

☑ An example of diagnostic bronchoscopy is the evaluation of tumors in the airways and lungs.

Diagnostic bronchoscopy is done to gather additional information or to confirm preliminary diagnosis following history, physical, and other laboratory results (Holgate et al., 1992; Landa, 1978; Prakash et al., 1991; Prakash, 1994; Schuurmans et al., 2003). Biopsy and cytology samples are obtained for diagnostic purposes. Table 13-2 describes the techniques used in obtaining these samples. Indications for diagnostic

TABLE 13-2   Application of Flexible Bronchoscopy.

	TECHNIQUE	EXPLANATION
BIOPSY	Biopsy within visual range of the instrument	Biopsy is performed of targeted sites by forceps inserted through the bronchoscope.
	Transbronchial lung biopsy (TBLB)	Diseases appearing as diffuse shadows on chest X-rays include miliary tuberculosis, pneumoconiosis sarcoidosis, and various viral pneumonias, but it is almost impossible to obtain a definitive diagnosis based on X-ray findings only; therefore it is necessary to obtain tissue from the lung to establish a definitive diagnosis.
	Transbronchial needle aspiration biopsy (TBAB)	This method is employed when the lesion is located beyond the bronchial wall and there is no lesion in the bronchial lumen. The technique involves pressing the tip of the fiberscope lightly against the target puncture site, then firmly projecting the tip of the needle through the wall at that site. Then, while moving the tip backwards and forwards and from side to side, aspiration is performed. Then the needle is removed and the specimen is expelled on a slide by positive pressure from the syringe.
CYTOLOGY	Brushing for cytological specimens	If there is no protrusion in the bronchial lumen or if for some other reason the lesion is difficult to biopsy, a brush can be inserted through the instrument to obtain cytological material.
	Cytological brushing under fluoroscopic monitoring. This is used for the diagnosis of solitary lesions in the lung field.	First of all the related bronchi are defined by tomography or bronchography. Either forceps or a brush is inserted through the instrument channel and brought up to the target bronchus after inserting under direct endoscopic observation, thereafter bringing the forceps or brush up to the lesion under X-ray television monitoring.
	Bronchial Alveolar Lavage (BAL)	This involves wedging the tip of the flexible bronchoscope into the target segmental or subsegmental bronchus, flushing with physiologic saline solution, and then retrieving the liquid in order to examine it for cells washed from the surface of the bronchial mucosa or analysis of cellular components. Furthermore, washing of larger bronchi is referred to as bronchial lavage (BL).
	Bronchial Toilet	In cases that have undergone various thoracic surgical procedures, including cardiovascular or esophageal procedures, difficulty is often experienced in the expectoration of sputum. In such cases the flexible bronchoscope is employed routinely for the aspiration of bronchial secretions.

TABLE 13-2   Application of Flexible Bronchoscopy. (continued)

	TECHNIQUE	EXPLANATION
TREATMENT	Local administration of thrombin in cases of bloody sputum or hemoptysis	In cases of bloody sputum or hemoptysis, the bronchoscope is inserted, blood is aspirated, and if necessary, washing with physiologic saline is performed. Once the bleeding bronchus is verified the patient is placed lying on that side, to prevent aspiration of blood by the contralateral lung. Hemostasis can be achieved by insertion of a polyethylene tube and instillation of thrombin solution.
	Removal of airway foreign bodies	While some believe that the rigid bronchoscope is useful in such cases, it is possible to remove almost all airway foreign bodies by means of employing a variety of grasping forceps. Foreign bodies removal in this way include gold crowns, peanuts (frequent in children), paper clips, drug containers, and fishbone.
	Electrosurgical treatment	Joule heat caused by the electrosurgical current evaporates cells for incision and coagulation. Can be used for much of the same cases as Lasers, and treatment capability is expanded with the variety of accessories.

(Used with permission. Courtesy of Olympus America, Inc., Melville, NY)

bronchoscopy may include the evaluation of (1) tumors in the airways and lungs, (2) airway obstruction, (3) inflammation and infections such as tuberculosis and pneumonia, (4) interstitial pulmonary disease, (5) staging of lung cancer before surgery, (6) vocal cord paralysis, and (7) tissue or fluid samples collected from the airways or lungs.

☑ An example of therapeutic uses of fiberoptic bronchoscopy is the removal of secretions, mucus plugs, or polyps in the airway.

A fiberoptic bronchoscope may also be used to perform therapeutic treatments. Table 13-2 explains the techniques used in performing these treatments. Examples of therapeutic uses of fiberoptic bronchoscopy include (1) removal of secretions, mucus plugs, or polyps in the airway, (2) removal of small foreign objects (large objects are removed by rigid bronchoscope), (3) performance of difficult intubations, and (4) drainage of an abscess.

BRONCHOSCOPE AND MEDICATIONS

The main components of a fiberoptic bronchoscope are the handle and insertion tube (Figure 13-8). The handle consists of the eyepiece, bending mechanism, and channel outlet. A video scope may be fitted onto the eyepiece for video taping of the procedure. The bending mechanism allows the physician to curve the insertion tube up (180°) or down (130°) for viewing of an anatomical structure at different angles. It also helps to direct the tube toward an intended segment or subsegment. The channel outlet is used for installation of saline or topical anesthetics, suction, and for passage of biopsy forceps, cytology brush, or cannula (Olympus America, Inc.).

☑ Lidocaine, atropine sulfate, morphine sulfate, and diazepam are four common medications for bronchoscopy.

Specifications

Optical System	Field of View	120°
	Direction of View	0° (Forward Viewing)
	Depth of View	3~50 mm
Distal End	Outer Diameter	5.8 mm
Bending Section	Range of Tip Bending	Up 180°, Down 130°
Insertion Tube	Outer Diameter	5.9 mm
Working Length	–	550 mm
Total Length	–	840 mm
Instrument Channel	Inner Diameter	2.2 mm
	Minimum Visible Distance	5 mm from Distal End

Figure 13-8 An example of flexible fiberoptic bronchoscope and specifications (Olympus BF Type 40). (Used with permission. Courtesy of Olympus America, Inc., Melville, NY)

lidocaine: A medication used to reduce irritation of the mucosal membrane caused by the insertion tube.

atropine sulfate: A medication used to reduce vagal response, oral secretions, and bronchospasm during bronchoscopy.

Depending on the patient requirement and physician preference, four medications are commonly administered 30 to 90 min before the procedure. **Lidocaine** (5 to 10 mL of 1% to 4% solution) is given to the patient via aerosol 30 min before the procedure to reduce irritation of the mucosal membrane during the procedure. Before the procedure, **atropine sulfate** (0.5 to 1.0 mg) and morphine sulfate (1.5 to 10 mg) are administered intramuscularly. Atropine reduces vagal response, oral secretions, and bronchospasm. Morphine sulfate provides pain relief and suppresses coughing during the procedure. Diazepam or a suitable benzodiazepine is given intravenously in bolus to provide sedation. Table 13-3 summarizes the medications for bronchoscopy.

TABLE 13-3 Medications for Bronchoscopy

MEDICATION (ROUTE)	DOSAGE (ROUTE)	PURPOSE
Lidocaine	5 to 10 mL of 1 to 4% solution (aerosol)	Given 30 to 90 min before procedure to reduce irritation of the mucosal membrane caused by the insertion tube
Atropine sulfate	0.5 to 1.0 mg (IM)	Given before the procedure to reduce vagal response, oral secretions, and bronchospasm
Morphine sulfate	1.5 to 10 mg (IM)	Given before the procedure to provide pain relief and suppress coughing
Diazepam	2.5 to 10 mg (IV bolus) or 10 to 15 mg (oral)	Given before and during the procedure as needed to provide sedation

(Data from Ameer et al., 1989; Gompertz et al., 1997; Prakash et al., 1991; Williams et al., 1998)

INSERTION OF BRONCHOSCOPE

After testing the bronchoscope assembly, the distal end of the insertion tube is coated with a water soluble lubricant and inserted via the nare, mouth (with bit block), endotracheal tube, or tracheostomy tube. Once the insertion tube enters the trachea and reaches above the carina, the tube is directed to the intended bronchi and segments. Figure 13-9 shows the normal bronchi and segments through the bronchovideoscope.

For patients who are breathing spontaneously and without artificial airway, oxygen therapy of up to 6 L/min may be given. If the bronchoscope insertion tube is inserted via an artificial airway (endotracheal or tracheostomy tube), an aerosol setup may be used. Adequate SpO_2 may be titrated with a pulse oximeter.

☑ Hypoxia and increase in peak inspiratory pressure are common when bronchoscopy is done on patients receiving mechanical ventilation.

For patients receiving mechanical ventilation, an adaptor for the bronchoscope may be used. Minor air leak may be compensated by increasing the tidal volume. The pressure limit may need to be increased to make allowance for a larger tidal volume and insertion tube in the endotracheal tube.

TYPES OF SPECIMEN

In addition to pulmonary secretions, a flexible bronchoscope can collect other special specimens. Examples of these specimens are biopsy (forceps biopsy, transbronchial lung biopsy, and transbronchial needle aspiration biopsy) samples and bronchial brushing samples. Typically, biopsies collect tissue samples for examination whereas bronchial brushing with or without alveolar lavage collects samples for cytological

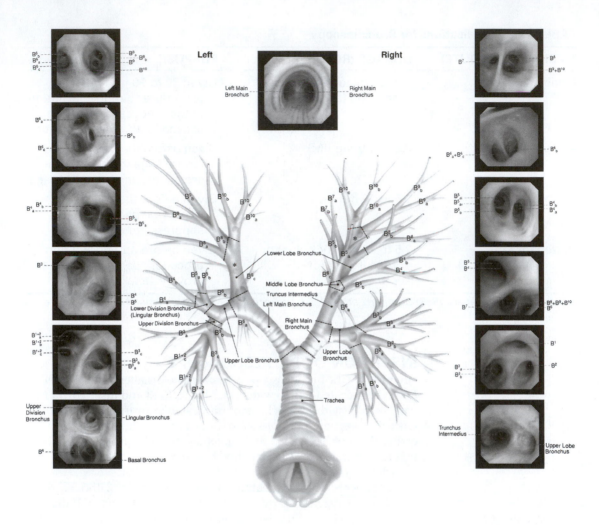

Figure 13-9 The normal bronchi and segments through the bronchovideoscope. (Used with permission. Courtesy of Olympus America, Inc., Melville, NY)

examination (Hattotuwa et al., 2002; Olympus America, Inc. 2003; Popovich et al., 1982; Rytila et al., 1999).

Secretion Collection. Pulmonary secretions are sometimes required for microscopic, culture and sensitivity, or cytology studies. These secretions are suctioned with a vacuum source and collected in a sterile sputum specimen trap. If the secretions are thick, pulmonary lavage with a saline solution may be necessary.

forceps biopsy:
Tissue specimens collected by the forceps located at the distal end of the insertion tube.

Forceps Biopsy. **Forceps biopsy** is done within the visual range of the bronchoscope. Tissue specimens are obtained by passing the biopsy forceps through the biopsy channel outlet (Figure 13-10A).

A Biopsy Forceps

B Needle

C Cytology Brush

Channel Outlet
Used for suction of phlegm, instillation of anesthetics, and for passage of biopsy forceps, cannula, etc.

Light Guide
Brilliant cold light is emitted for observation and photography

Objective Lens
Fixed focus with field of view 3–50 mm

Figure 13-10   The distal end of the insertion tube; accessories for collection of samples using a flexible bronchoscope: (A) Forceps; (B) Needle; and (C) Brush.

The razor-sharp biopsy device at the distal end of the forceps can be opened and closed by the operator using the control handle. The tissue specimen collected by the forceps is retrieved and put in a formalin solution for laboratory analysis.

transbronchial lung biopsy (TBLB):
Tissue specimens collected by the forceps during a forced exhalation maneuver.

Transbronchial Lung Biopsy.   Transbronchial lung biopsy (TBLB) is sometimes necessary to obtain a definitive diagnosis based on preliminary radiographic findings. Lung specimens are obtained by using a similar approach as in forceps biopsy. The patient is asked to inhale maximally and the opened forceps are advanced deep into the distal airway near the target site. The patient then exhales maximally causing compression of the lung tissue around the biopsy forceps. The opened forceps are then closed by force. After removal of the forceps, the specimen is retrieved for laboratory analysis.

transbronchial needle aspiration biopsy (TBNAB):
Tissue specimens collected by applying aspiration while moving the needle at the sample collection site.

Transbronchial Needle Aspiration Biopsy.   Transbronchial needle aspiration biopsy (TBNAB) is done where the lesion is located beyond the bronchial wall and there is no lesion in the bronchial lumen. This is done by pressing the tip of the bronchoscope gently against the target puncture site. The tip of the needle is then firmly projected through the mucosal wall. Aspiration (suction) is applied while moving the tip of the insertion tube of the bronchoscope back and forth and from side to side. The specimen (inside the needle) and the needle are retrieved from the bronchoscope and a syringe is used to expel the specimen from the needle (Figure 13-10B).

bronchial brushing:
Tissue or loosened
cell specimens col-
lected by a shielded
small brush using a
brushing motion.

Bronchial Brushing. Cytologic examination may be necessary when an area of pathologic change is encountered during bronchoscopy. A shielded small brush is used to brush along the bronchial mucosa and the loosened cells are adhered to the brush (Figure 13-10C). The brush is then withdrawn into the shield and the entire apparatus is removed from the channel outlet of the bronchoscope. A microscopic slide may be made by fixing it with a suitable solution. An alternative is to cut off the brush and send it for pathologic tests.

COMPLICATIONS

☑ Complications of
  bronchoscopy
include infection,
V/Q mismatch,
hemorrhage, and
pneumothorax.

In vast majority of cases, bronchoscopy is a safe procedure. However, complications do occur and they range from infection to puncture of the lungs (Credle et al., 1974; Pue et al., 1995; Suratt et al., 1976; Zavala, 1976).

Infection. There were reports of transmission and outbreak of *Mycobacterium tuberculosis* and *Pseudomonas aeruginosa* infections caused by the flexible bronchoscope (Agerton et al., 1997; Michele et al., 1997; Spach et al., 1993; Srinivasan et al., 2003). An increase in the frequency of *Pseudomonas* and other infections was also found to be associated with bronchoscopy (Hanson et al., 1991). These experiences show the need for close infection control measures in the use of bronchoscope.

Since the same bronchoscope is used to enter and explore different lung segments, the incidence of cross contamination of healthy lung segments by infected ones is a possibility. Likewise, the saline solution used for lavaging the lung segments also poses a threat of cross contamination of healthy lung segments.

Ventilation/Perfusion (V/Q) Mismatch. The bronchoscope decreases the size of the airway opening and may cause partial airflow obstruction (Matsushima et al., 1984; Shakespeare et al., 2003). Ventilation/perfusion (V/Q) mismatch and secondary hypoxemia may occur during and after bronchoscopy because of the retained lavage solution, hypoventilation from premedication, mobilized and pooled secretions, and excessive suctioning. Supplemental oxygen should be used to alleviate the problem of secondary oxygen desaturation during bronchoscopy (Yildiz, 2002). In most cases, oxygen therapy may be discontinued 4 hours after bronchoscopy.

Hemorrhage. Bleeding can occur during bronchoscopy. Most minor bleeding may be stopped by saline lavage. When substantial bleeding occurs, a vasopressor (e.g., 1 mL of 1:1000 epinephrine with 9 mL of normal saline given in 2-mL portions) can be used to control bleeding from the biopsy site. Bleeding may also be stopped by wedging the bleeding site with the distal end of the bronchoscope. If wedging cannot be done because the airway is larger than the distal end of the bronchoscope, a 6-Fr Fogarty embolectomy catheter with balloon tip may be inserted through the channel. Wedging of the bleeding site may then be done by inflating the balloon tip of the catheter. Bronchoscopes that have a built-in coagulation electrode may stop hemorrhaging by using the coagulation mode (heat-induced coagulation).

Pneumothorax.   Biopsy instruments are sharp and long enough to reach and puncture the periphery of the lung. In extremely rare cases, pneumothoraces may occur during bronchoscopy (Sun et al., 2003). Puncture of the lung while the patient is receiving mechanical ventilation may lead to tension pneumothorax. The vital signs of the patient must be monitored closely. Worsening cyanosis in spite of high oxygen concentration, diaphoresis, tachypnea, tachycardia, and thready pulse are some signs of tension pneumothorax. Chest tube is the treatment for tension pneumothorax and a complete chest tube setup should be on the bronchoscopy supplies list.

Postbronchoscopy Complications.   Incidence of serious complications and mortality associated with fiberoptic bronchoscopy is low. In one survey of over 24,000 procedures, major complications occurred in 0.08% of all cases. The mortality rate was only 0.01%, most of them secondary to hemorrhage and pneumothorax (Pue et al., 1995; Suratt et al., 1976). If sudden deterioration of the patient's condition occurs, chest radiography should be taken to rule out pneumothorax.

☑ Hypoxemia and arrhythmias are the most common complications during and after bronchoscopy.

Hypoxemia and arrhythmias are the most common complications during and after bronchoscopy (Schnapf, 1991). Oxygen therapy, proper use of topical anesthesia, and use of intermittent suction are useful techniques to minimize the occurrence of these complications. Continuous pulse oximeter should be used during the recovery period.

POSTBRONCHOSCOPY CARE
Following bronchoscopy, the patient's vital signs are monitored for at least 2 hours or until stable. During the recovery period, an aerosolized bronchodilator may be used to treat bronchospasm. Oxygen is titrated to maintain a satisfactory SpO_2 and it may be provided via nasal cannula or continuous aerosol. Food and drink are withheld from the patient until the gag reflex has returned.

Cleaning and Care of Equipment.   All equipment and supplies used in bronchoscopy must be cleaned, disinfected, or sterilized where indicated (Culver et al., 2003; Alvarado, 2000; Mehta, 1999; Weber, 2001). The bronchoscope must also be maintained on a regular basis (AORN, 2001; Mehta et al., 1990). The portion of the bronchoscope that comes in contact with the mucosal membrane must be sterilized. Bronchoscopes used in examining patients with tuberculosis or hepatitis B should also be sterilized. Ethylene oxide is used to sterilize delicate parts that cannot withstand steam autoclave. A checklist should be maintained to track delivery of equipment and supplies. Restocking of the disposables and consumables in the cart should be documented.

TRANSPORT OF MECHANICALLY VENTILATED PATIENTS

Patients receiving mechanical ventilation are critically ill or have deficiencies in the major organs or systems. They may also have difficulty in maintaining an adequate level of ventilation and oxygenation to fulfill their metabolic needs. In an intensive care setting, numerous resources are available to care for the mechanically ventilated patients. When the patients need to go from the intensive care setting to another location, some of these resources may not be readily available during transport. For this reason, a complete transport plan must be developed well in advance. The plan should include the personnel, procedure, and equipment and supplies necessary for a safe and uncomplicated transport.

INDICATIONS
The most common indication for intrahospital transport of mechanically ventilated patients is to acquire diagnostic procedures at a location other than the intensive care setting (e.g., MRI in the radiology department). For interhospital ground or air transport, it is usually done to acquire tertiary medical care or procedures (e.g., burn care, third-level nursery) that are only available at the destination facility (Ehrenwerth et al., 1986). For safety reasons, transport of mechanically ventilated patients must follow a thorough evaluation of the risk-benefit factor based on the patient's clinical condition.

CONTRAINDICATIONS

✓ A patient should not be transported when the hemodynamic status is deteriorating or unstable.

Contraindications for transport of mechanically ventilated patients include inability to provide adequate oxygenation and ventilation, inability to maintain acceptable hemodynamic status, inability to provide adequate airway control or cardiopulmonary monitoring, and lack of trained transport team members (Weg et al., 1989). A patient should not be transported when the hemodynamic status is deteriorating or unstable.

EQUIPMENT AND SUPPLIES
The availability of medical equipment and supplies during transport is rather limited and sometimes they may not be accessible. This is mainly due to limited space in the transport unit and partly due to unforeseen circumstances. This problem may be minimized by

TABLE 13-4   Respiratory Care Equipment and Supplies for Transport of Mechanically Ventilated Patients

TYPE	ITEMS*
Universal Precaution	Gloves (sterile and clean) Gowns Eye protection
Patient Assessment and Monitoring	Stethoscopes Pulse oximeter Blood pressure cuffs Cardiac or hemodynamic monitor
Airway Management	Oropharyngeal and nasopharyngeal airways Resuscitation bags and masks Intubation supplies (laryngoscope handles and blades, fresh batteries, endotracheal tubes, etc.) Cuff manometer and 10-mL syringe Suctioning devices (catheters and tonsil tip)
Oxygenation Supplies	Oxygen cylinders (full and with wrench) Oxygen tubing with adaptor
Advanced Cardiac Life Support (ACLS) Pharmacological Agents	Drugs and solutions according to current ACLS guidelines

*Some items require different sizes.

developing and using a list of equipment and supplies based on the type of transport and the characteristics of the patients. Table 13-4 shows a sample of essential respiratory care equipment and supplies for a typical transport.

TYPES OF TRANSPORT

Transport of patients who are being mechanically ventilated imposes many challenges: use of **transport ventilator** and emergency supplies, availability of a team of trained personnel, and distance of transport (Reynolds et al., 1992). When transporting a patient away from a medical care facility **(interhospital transport),** the transport team must decide which mode of transportation is most suitable. One main deciding factor is the distance between the departing facility and the destination facility. Four modes of transportation are available: ground ambulance, helicopter, propeller-drive aircraft, and jet (Rouse et al., 1992). There are advantages and disadvantages associated with each mode of transportation (Table 13-5).

Intrahospital Transport.   Transport of patients within the hospital is done for the patient to receive advanced diagnostic procedures that require use of bulky or stationary equipment (e.g., CAT scan, MRI

---

transport ventilator:
A mechanical ventilator capable of operation without piped-in gas sources or electrical connection.

interhospital transport: *Moving a patient between two hospitals.*

intrahospital transport: *Moving a patient between two locations within the hospital.*

TABLE 13-5 Modes of Transportation

MODE	RANGE	ADVANTAGE	DISADVANTAGE
Ground Ambulance	<150 miles	Low cost, safer, and more reliable than helicopter	Limited by road and traffic conditions
Helicopter	<150 miles	Not limited by road and traffic conditions	Noisy, must have landing pad at both facilities
Propeller-driven aircraft	100 to 200 miles	Faster than helicopter if landing locations are near both facilities	Reduced P_IO_2 and relative humidity since low altitude aircrafts are not pressurized
Jet	>200 miles	Fast and able to travel intercontinental distance	Low P_IO_2 and relative humidity at high altitude in non-pressurized jets

(Data from Cunningham et al., 1997; Nichols et al., 1994; Shehey, 1995; Oxer, 1975; Rouse et al., 1992.)

☑ Manual ventilation often causes inadvertent hyperventilation, varying tidal volume and rate, and fatigue of the care provider.

☑ For intrahospital transport of mechanically ventilated patients, transport ventilator is preferable to manual ventilation.

☑ In pressure control mode, the expired volume must be monitored closely. Decreasing compliance or increasing airflow resistance can lead to decreasing tidal volume.

scan). For patients who require ventilatory support for a short time (e.g., less than 30 min), manual ventilation with a resuscitation bag and oxygen may be sufficient. However, manual ventilation often causes inadvertent hyperventilation, irregular tidal volume and rate, and fatigue of the care provider (Gervais et al., 1987; Hurst et al., 1989).

For intrahospital transport of mechanically ventilated patients, transport ventilator is preferable to manual ventilation (Nakamura et al., 2003). There are a number of simple and complex transport ventilators available on the market (e.g., Avian by Viasys—Bird Products Corp, Palm Springs, CA; Crossvent by Bio-Med Devices, Inc., Guilford, CT; Esprit by Respironics, Vista, CA; LTV 1000, Pulmonetic Systems, Colton, CA; Model 740 by Mallinckrodt, Pleasanton, CA; and Uni-Vent by Impact Instrumentation, Inc. Caldwell, NJ). These FDA-approved transport ventilators are all battery powered and have similar performance and functions of the current ventilators used in the ICU (Austin et al., 2002; Miyoshi et al., 2000).

Besides the common features of a ventilator, the following capabilities are desirable on a transport ventilator: PEEP, pressure support ventilation, volume and pressure control ventilation, inverse ratio ventilation, display of expired volume, visual and audible alarms, especially for disconnection and airway pressures. For ventilators that operate with only the pressure control mode, the expired volume must be monitored closely. Decreasing compliance or increasing airflow resistance can lead to decreasing tidal volume (Rola, 2004).

Ground Ambulance and Helicopter. Interhospital transport of mechanically ventilated patients can be done safely if the patients' medical condition is optimized before departure (Reynolds et al., 2002). A ground ambulance or helicopter may be used for patient transport when the distance is less than 150 miles. Each mode of transportation has its own advantages and disadvantages (Cunningham et al., 1997; Nichols et al., 1994; Shehey, 1995). Helicopters are preferable when the traffic or terrain condition precludes a timely arrival at the destination by ground ambulances. Of course, both facilities must have a suitable landing site for helicopters.

☑ The projected total time of transport should be a factor in deciding which mode of transportation to use.

Sometimes a propeller-driven aircraft is used for a distance between 100 and 200 miles. Transporting the patient from the departure facility to the takeoff location and from the landing location to the destination facility may be time-consuming. The projected total time of transport should be a factor in deciding which mode of transportation to use.

Jet. For distances greater than 200 miles or intercontinental transport, a jet is preferred. Use of a jet is typically done for nonemergency cases since a jet involves more resources and at higher costs. The condition of patients using a jet for transport is rarely critical due to the time required for planning and long flight time. Typically, most patients use jets for transport to tertiary care facilities for advanced diagnostic procedure and therapeutic care, or from abroad to their home country (Veldman et al., 2001).

PROCEDURES FOR INTERHOSPITAL TRANSPORT

A written physician order must be obtained prior to transporting a mechanically ventilated patient. Before departure, equipment and supplies for the patient are gathered and assembled. For equipment using rechargeable batteries such as ventilator and monitor, maintain full charge with electrical power until time for departure. For other equipment such as pulse oximeter and laryngoscope handle, new batteries should be installed. Monitors are calibrated and appropriate alarm limits set based on the patient's condition. Small "E" size oxygen cylinders with wrench must be full. In the event of delay, the oxygen content should be at least twice the volume needed for a one-way transport.

☑ During transport, the patient is monitored throughout the entire period to ensure stable hemodynamic status, adequate oxygenation, and ventilation.

All tubes and lines should be secured prior to transport. During transport, the patient is monitored throughout the entire period to ensure stable hemodynamic status, adequate oxygenation, and ventilation. All ventilator parameters are checked and adjusted to ensure proper functioning. A log should be kept to document all monitoring data, adverse reactions, and interventions.

On arrival, bedside monitors and ventilators at the destination hospital are used. The position and function of the patient's endotracheal

TABLE 13-6   Potential Complications with Patient Transport and Solutions for Remediation

HAZARD AND COMPLICATION	CAUSE	SOLUTION
Hyperventilation or variable tidal volumes	Manual ventilation with resuscitation bag	Use transport ventilator
Loss of PEEP/CPAP	Inaccuracy of PEEP valve on manual resuscitation bag	Use transport ventilator
Unstable hemodynamic status	Patient condition or excessive movement of the patient	Evaluate and stabilize hemodynamic status before transport
Loss of mechanical ventilation or monitoring capability	Equipment failure	Provide manual ventilation with oxygen
Inadvertent extubation or removal of vascular access lines	Movement of patient without paying attention to arrangement of equipment/supplies	Coordinate movement of the patient and equipment/supplies
Power/gas source failure	Various causes	Use ventilator with battery capability and provide portable compressed oxygen source
Hypoxia due to high-altitude hypobaric condition.	High-altitude in non-pressurized aircraft	Monitor ventilation and SpO_2; use a higher F_IO_2; use pressurized aircraft.

(Data from Beckmann, 2004; Farmer, 1996; Dockery et al., 1999; McGough et al., 1992; Waydhas et al., 1995.)

tube are checked and documented. Pretransport ventilator settings and appropriate alarm limits are set on the ventilator after the patient has been stabilized from the transport. Finally, a verbal report is given to the therapist at the destination hospital and the written documentation is filed with the patient's medical record.

HAZARDS AND COMPLICATIONS

There are many hazards and complications associated with transport of mechanically ventilated patients. They range from hyperventilation during manual ventilation en route to a remote location to equipment failure. Table 13-6 summarizes the potential complications during transport and some solutions for remediation.

MAGNETIC RESONANCE IMAGING

Magnetic resonance imaging (MRI) produces images for detection of abnormalities in the body organs not distinctively assessable by conventional imaging techniques. The strong magnetic field generated by

☑ Transport equipment coming near the MRI scanner must be resistant to the magnetic field produced by the scanner.

the MRI scanner may draw certain metal objects toward the scanner. Steel oxygen transport cylinders and many ventilators are potential sources of a projectile risk to the patient and others. For this safety reason, only aluminum oxygen cylinders should be used (Morgan et al., 2002). All transport equipment coming near the MRI scanner must be resistant to the magnetic field produced by the scanner.

Some transport ventilators are capable of providing mechanical ventilation safely in an area where MRI is in use. Some MRI-compatible ventilators are Bio-Med Devices IC-2A® and Pneupac® Transport (Bio-Med Devices, Guilford, CT), Omni-Vent® (Allied Health Care, St. Louis, MO), and RespirTech PRO® (Vortran Medical Technologies, Sacramento, CA). When pressure control mode is used, the delivered volume may decrease in conditions of decreasing compliance or increasing airflow resistance. The expired tidal volume must therefore be monitored closely during transport.

Transport ventilators are typically smaller and have fewer features than traditional ventilators. In one report, a full-function (Servo 300) ventilator has been modified and used safely near an MRI scanner (Morgan et al., 2002).

SUMMARY

This chapter provides an overview of the essential elements of three procedures that are done to mechanically ventilated patients: chest tube and drainage system, fiberoptic bronchoscopy, and transport of mechanically ventilated patients. In a critical care setting, these procedures often involved a team of health care providers to include respiratory therapists. For this reason, respiratory therapists should be familiar with these procedures. A good working knowledge of these procedures is also essential for efficient team work and patient safety.

Self-Assessment Questions

1. Indications for chest tube placement include all of the following *except*:

    A. tension pneumothorax.　　　　C. chest trauma.
    B. pleural effusion.　　　　　　　D. hemothorax.

2. The sharp pointed instrument for incision into the chest cavity for chest tube placement is called a:

    A. trocar.　　　　　　　　　　　C. needle.
    B. chest tube.　　　　　　　　　 D. blade.

3. The ideal location of chest tube placement for drainage of pleural fluid is at the:

   A. second to third intercostal space at the midaxillary line.

   B. fourth to sixth intercostal space at the midaxillary line.

   C. second to third intercostal space at the midclavicular line.

   D. fourth to sixth intercostal space at the midclavicular line.

4. During chest tube insertion, Dr. Farland enters the chest wall by going _____ the rib because _____.

   A. above, blood vessels and nerves lie below the rib

   B. above, this location is easier to puncture

   C. below, blood vessels and nerves lie above the rib

   D. below, this location is easier to puncture

5. In a three-chamber drainage system, the amount of suction applied to the pleural space is determined by the _____ in the suction control chamber.

   A. water level and submersion depth of the venting tube

   B. amount of pleural fluid in the chamber

   C. wall vacuum level

   D. all of the above

6. A typical flexible bronchoscope may perform all of the following *except*:

   A. visual inspection of the airway.

   B. collection of specimens.

   C. suction.

   D. removal of large tumor.

7. Dr. Kingston asks you to prepare the patient for bronchoscopy and to reduce the irritation to the mucosal membrane caused by the tube. You would administer _____ via aerosol nebulizer about _____ before the procedure.

   A. atropine sulfate, 10 min

   B. atropine sulfate, 30 min

   C. lidocaine, 10 min

   D. lidocaine, 30 min

8. Atropine sulfate is used to _____ during bronchoscopy.

   A. provide pain relief

   B. reduce vagal response, oral secretions, and bronchospasm

   C. minimize irritation to the mucosal membrane

   D. provide sedation

9. During bronchoscopy, _____ may be used to collect biopsy samples.

   A. saline lavage

   B. suction catheter

   C. special needle and forceps

   D. brush

10. In order to recognize the common complications promptly during and after bronchoscopy, the patient's _____ should be monitored closely.

    A. heart rate and SpO_2

    B. blood pressure and heart rate

    C. cardiac rhythm and blood pressure

    D. SpO_2 and cardiac rhythm

11. A patient is being ready for transport to a special care hospital 100 miles away. The transport team may choose from all of the following modes of transportation *except*:

    A. ground ambulance.

    B. helicopter.

    C. jet.

    D. propeller-driven aircraft.

12. During patient transport, hyperventilation and variable tidal volumes are two common undesirable outcomes when a(n) _____ is used.

    A. anesthesia bag

    B. manual ventilation device

    C. volume control mode of ventilation

    D. pressure control mode of ventilation

Answers to Self-Assessment Questions

1. C. chest trauma.

2. A. trocar.

3. B. fourth to sixth intercostal space at the midaxillary line.

4. A. above, blood vessels and nerves lie below the rib.

5. A. water level and submersion depth of the venting tube

6. D. removal of large tumor.

7. D. lidocaine, 30 min

8. B. reduce vagal response, oral secretions, and bronchospasm

9. C. special needle and forceps

10. D. SpO_2 and cardiac rhythm

11. C. jet.

12. B. manual ventilation device

References

Agerton, T., et al. (1997). Transmission of a highly drug resistant strain (strain W1) of Mycobacterium tuberculosis: Community outbreak and nosocomial transmission via a contaminated bronchoscope. *JAMA, 278,* 1073–1077.

Alameda County Medical Center (2004). Chest tubes. Retrieved August 25, 2004, from http://www.surgery.ucsf.edu/eastbaytrauma/Protocols.

Alvarado, C. J., et al. (2000). APIC guideline for infection prevention and control in flexible endoscopy. *Am J Infect Control, 28,* 138–155.

Ameer, B., et al. (1989). Systemic absorption of topical lidocaine in elderly and young adults undergoing bronchoscopy. *Pharmacotherapy, 9,* 74–81.

Association of periOperative Registered Nurses (AORN). (2001). Recommended practices for use and care of endoscopes. *2001 standards, recommended practices and guidelines* (pp. 211–214). Denver, CO: Association of periOperative Registered Nurses.

Austin, P. N., et al. (2002). Transport ventilators. *Respir Care Clin N Am, 8*(1), 119–150.

Beckmann, U., et al. (2004). Incidents relating to the intra-hospital transfer of critically ill patients – an analysis of the reports submitted to the Australian Incident Monitoring Study in Intensive Care. *Intensive Care Med, 30*(8), 1579–1585.

Chen, K. Y., et al. (2002). Pneumothorax in the ICU: Patient outcomes and prognostic factors. *Chest, 122*(2), 678–683.

Credle, W. F., et al. (1974). Complications of fiberoptic bronchoscopy. *Am Rev Respir Dis, 109,* 67–72.

Culver, D. A., et al. (2003). Infection control in the bronchoscopy suite: A review of outbreaks and guidelines for prevention. *Am J Respir Crit Care Med, 167*(8), 1050.

Cunningham, P., et al. (1997). A comparison of the association of helicopter and ground ambulance transport with the outcome of injury in trauma patients transported from the scene. *Trauma, 43,* 940, 943.

Deshpande, K. S., et al. (2002). Is trocar guidance for chest tube insertion a disappearing art?: The advantages are speed and simplicity. *J Respir Dis, 23*(2), 96–98.

Dockery, W. K., et al. (1999). A comparison of manual and mechanical ventilation during pediatric transport. *Crit Care Med, 27*(4), 802–806.

Ehrenwerth, J., et al. (1986). Transport of critically ill adults. *Crit Care Med, 14*(6), 543–547.

Farmer, J. C. (1996). Respiratory issues in aeromedical patient transport. *Respir Care Clin N Am, 2*(3), 391–400.

Gervais, H. W., et al. (1987). Comparison of blood gases of ventilated patients during transport. *Crit Care Med, 15*(8), 761–763.

Gompertz, S., et al. (1997). Sedation in fiberoptic bronchoscopy. *Chest, 111*(4), 1142.

Hanson, P. J. V., et al. (1991). Recovery of the human immunodeficiency virus from fibreoptic bronchoscopes. *Thorax, 46,* 410–412.

Hattotuwa, K., et al. (2002). Safety of bronchoscopy, biopsy, and BAL in research patients with COPD. *Chest, 122,* 1909–1913.

Holgate, S. T., et al. (1992). New insights into airway inflammation by endobronchial biopsy. *Am Rev Respir, 145*(2, Pt. 2), S2–S6.

Hurst, J. M., et al. (1989). A comparison of blood gases during transport using two methods of ventilatory support. *J Trauma, 29*(12), 1637–1640.

Irwin, R. S., et al. (2003). *Procedures and techniques in intensive care medicine* (3rd ed.). Lippincott Williams & Wilkins: Philadelphia.

Jacobsohn, E. (2004). The management of the patient after thoracic surgery. Retrieved April 20, 2004, from http://daccx.bsd.uchicago.edu/manuals/vtmanual/postop-thorej.html

Landa, J. F. (1978). Indications for bronchoscopy. *Chest, 73* (5, Suppl.), 686–690.

Matsushima, Y., et al. (1984). Alterations in pulmonary mechanics and gas exchange during routine fiberoptic bronchoscopy. *Chest, 86,* 184–188.

McGough, E. K., et al. (1992). Variations in tidal volume with portable transport ventilators. *Respir Care, 37*(3), 233–239.

Mehta, A. C., et al. (1990). The high price of bronchoscopy: Maintenance and repair of the flexible fiberoptic bronchoscope. *Chest, 98*(2), 448–454.

Mehta, A. C., et al. (1999). Infection control in the bronchoscopy suite: A review. *Clin Chest Med, 20,* 19–32.

Michele, T. M., et al. (1997). Transmission of Mycobacterium tuberculosis by a fiberoptic bronchoscope: Identification by DNA fingerprinting. *JAMA, 278,* 1093–1095.

Miyoshi, E., et al. (2000). Performance of transport ventilator with patient-triggered ventilation. *Chest, 118*(4), 1109–1115.

Morgan, S. E., et al. (2002). Modification of a critical care ventilator for use during magnetic resonance imaging. *Respir Care, 47,* 61–68.

Nakamura, T., et al. (2003). Intrahospital transport of critically ill patients using ventilator with patient-triggering function. *Chest, 123*(1), 159–164.

Nichols, J. P., et al. (1994). A comparison of the costs and performance of an emergency helicopter and land ambulances in a rural area. *Injury, 25,* 145, 150.

Olympus America, Inc. (2003). *User manual and publications.* Melville, New York.

Oxer, H. F. (1975). Aeromedical evacuation of the seriously ill. *British Med J, 3,* 692–694.

Popovich, J., Jr., et al. (1982). Diagnostic accuracy of multiple biopsies from flexible fibreoptic bronchoscopy: A comparison of central versus peripheral carcinoma. *Am Rev Respir Dis,125,* 521–523.

Prakash, U. B. S. (Ed.), (1994). Indications for and contraindications to bronchoscopy. *Bronchoscopy* (pp. 81–89). New York: Raven Press.

Prakash, U. B. S., et al. (1991). Bronchoscopy in North America: The ACCP survey. *Chest, 100*(6), 1668–1675.

Pue, C. A., et al. (1995). Complications of fiberoptic bronchoscopy at a university hospital. *Chest, 107*, 430–432.

Reynolds, H. N., et al. (2002). Interhospital transport of the adult mechanically ventilated patient. *Respir Care Clin N Am, 8*(1), 37–50.

Reynolds, M., et al. (1992). The nuts and bolts of organizing and initiating a pediatric transport team. *Crit Care Clin, 8,* 465–479.

Rola, P. (2004). Air transport and ventilators: A review. Retrieved August 27, 2004, from http://sprojects.mmi.mcgill.ca/heart/pages/man000104r1.html

Rouse, M. J., et al. (1992). Mechanical ventilation during air medical transport: Techniques and devices. *J Air Med Transp, 11*(4), 5–8.

Rytila, P. H., et al. (1999). Comparison between bronchial biopsy and induced sputum in patients with chronic bronchitis and chronic obstructive pulmonary disease [abstract]. *Am J Respir Crit Care Med, 159,* A515.

Schnapf, B. M. (1991). Oxygen desaturation during fiberoptic bronchoscopy in pediatric patients. *Chest, 99,* 591–594.

Schuurmans, M. M., et al. (2003). Use of an ultrathin bronchoscope in the assessment of central airway obstruction. *Chest, 124*(2), 735.

Shakespeare, E., et al. (2003). The effect of flexible bronchoscopy on end-expiratory lung volumes in intubated patients on mechanical ventilation. *Chest, 124*(4), S78.

Shehey, S. (1995). Justifying the cost of your air medical transport program. *J Emergency Nursing,* 21, 564–565.

Spach, D. H., et al. (1993). Transmission of infection by gastrointestinal endoscopy and bronchoscopy. *Ann Intern Med, 118,* 117–128.

Srinivasan, A., et al. (2003). An outbreak of Pseudomonas aeruginosa infections associated with flexible bronchoscopes. *N Engl J Med, 348,* 221–227.

Sun, S. W., et al. (2003). Incidence of pneumothorax after fiberoptic bronchoscopy (FOB) in community-based hospital; are routine post-procedure chest roentgenograms necessary? *Chest, 124,* S145.

Suratt, P. M., et al. (1976). Death and complications associated with fiberoptic bronchoscopy. *Chest, 69*(6), 747–751.

Thomas, S. (2004). Chest tube placement. Retrieved April 20, 2004, from http://www.vh.org/ adult/provider/familymedicine/FPHandbook/Chapter21/Figure21-2.html

Veldman, A., et al. (2001). Proposal for a new scoring system in international interhospital air transport. *J Travel Med, 8,* 154–157.

Waydhas, C., et al. (1995). Deterioration of respiratory function after intra-hospital transport of critically ill surgical patients. *Intensive Care Med, 21*(10), 784–789.

Weber, D. J., et al. (2001). Lessons from outbreaks associated with bronchoscopy. *Infect Control Hosp Epidemiol, 22,* 403–407.

Weg, J. G., et al. (1989). Safe intrahospital transport of critically ill ventilator-dependent patients. *Chest, 96*(3), 631–635.

Williams, T., et al. (1998). The role of atropine premedication in fiberoptic bronchoscopy using intravenous midazolam sedation. *Chest, 113*(5), 1394–1398.

Yildiz, P., et al. (2002). Changes in oxygen saturation in patients undergoing fiberoptic bronchoscopy. *Chest, 121*(3), 1007–1008.

Zavala, D. C. (1976). Pulmonary hemorrhage in fiberoptic transbronchial biopsy. *Chest, 70*(5), 584–588.

Suggested Reading

Chest Tube

Carroll, P. (1996). Salvaging blood from the chest. *RN, 59*(9), 3–8.

Carroll, P. (2000). Exploring chest drain options. *RN, 63*(10), 50–58.

Carroll, P. (1995). Chest tubes made easy. *RN, 60*(12), 1–11.

Hyde, J., et al. (1997). Reducing morbidity from chest drains. *BMJ, 314,* 914–915.

O'Hanlon Nichols, T. (1996). Commonly asked questions about chest tubes. *AJN, 96*(5), 60–64.

CHAPTER FOURTEEN

PHARMACOTHERAPY FOR MECHANICAL VENTILATION

Sandra Gaviola

Luis S. Gonzalez

OUTLINE

KEY TERMS

- acetylcholine
- antiemetic
- anxiolysis
- barbiturates
- benzodiazepines
- cathartic agents
- chronotropic
- corticosteroids
- depolarizing agents

- GABA (gamma-aminobutyric acid)
- inotropic
- narcotic analgesics
- nondepolarizing agents
- parasympatholytic bronchodilators
- Ramsay Scale
- sympathomimetic bronchodilators
- xanthine bronchodilators

INTRODUCTION

Two primary purposes of drug therapy for patients using mechanical ventilation are that they (1) provide patient comfort and (2) facilitate airway management and mechanical ventilation. For example, some drugs are used to facilitate intubation (neuromuscular blockers and sedatives) and reduce air flow resistance (bronchodilators), while others are necessary to manage pain (narcotics) and induce sedation (sedatives). Proper use of drug therapy is necessary to achieve desired outcomes. A clear understanding of these drugs is also essential to avoid misuse, complications, and prolonged mechanical ventilation.

DRUGS FOR IMPROVING VENTILATION

Airway narrowing is a common complication in patients receiving mechanical ventilation. Increasing peak inspiratory pressure, wheezing, hypoxemia, and agitation are some clinical signs that indicate the presence of airway distress.

For the ventilator patient, airway distress may be caused by (1) preexisting airway disease (chronic bronchitis, asthma), (2) drug-induced bronchospasm, (3) accumulated secretions, and (4) mechanical irritation. Whatever the cause, the distress must be recognized and corrected quickly to prevent hypoxemia and further deterioration.

Along with regular endotracheal suctioning, bronchodilators and corticosteroids play a critical role in achieving optimal airway patency and constitute the majority of nebulized drugs used in respiratory care.

THE AUTONOMIC NERVOUS SYSTEM

The smooth muscles of the airway are under autonomic (involuntary) nervous control. For this reason, the patient has no control over the patency of the affected airways. When airways constrict, bronchodilators are necessary to provide airway dilation and relief.

Sympathetic and Parasympathetic Branches. The autonomic nervous system (ANS) comprises motor neurons that innervate tissues under involuntary control. Among important functions regulated by the ANS are respiration, heart rate, blood pressure, perspiration, and glandular secretions. The sympathetic and parasympathetic fibers are the basic subdivisions of the ANS and, for the most part, elicit responses in an opposing manner (at the effector sites). For example, stimulation of the sympathetic branch results in bronchodilation whereas stimulation of the parasympathetic branch causes bronchoconstriction (Tortora et al., 2002).

Adrenergic and Cholinergic Responses. The neurotransmitter substance released at the sympathetic terminal axon is epinephrine (adrenaline) and it elicits an adrenergic response.

The neurotransmitter substance released at the terminal axon of the parasympathetic fiber is acetylcholine (ACh) and it elicits a cholinergic response.

Bronchodilation can be achieved by eliciting an adrenergic response (sympathomimetic action) or by interfering with the cholinergic response (parasympatholytic action). Many bronchodilators use the sympathomimetic action **(sympathomimetic bronchodilators)** while other bronchodilators take advantage of the parasympatholytic action **(parasympatholytic bronchodilators)**. Table 14-1 shows these two pathways to achieve bronchodilation.

sympathomimetic bronchodilators:
Adrenergic agonists. Drugs that dilate the airways by stimulating the beta-2 receptors of the sympathetic nervous system. Examples are epinephrine (Adrenaline) and albuterol (Ventolin, Proventil).

parasympatholytic bronchodilators:
Anticholinergic bronchodilators. Drugs that dilate the airways by inhibiting the parasympathetic branch of the autonomic nervous system. Examples are atropine and ipratropium bromide (Atrovent).

TABLE 14-1   Two Autonomic Nervous System (ANS) Pathways for Bronchodilation

SYMPATHETIC PATHWAY	PARASYMPATHETIC PATHWAY
Stimulation of adrenergic response	Interference of cholinergic response
↓	↓
↑ Sympathomimetic activity (Stimulation of sympathetic activity)	↑ Parasympatholytic activity (Inhibition of parasympathetic activity)
↓	↓
Bronchodilation	Relative increase of sympathetic activity
	↓
	Bronchodilation

ADRENERGIC BRONCHODILATORS (SYMPATHOMIMETICS)

Adrenergic bronchodilators are agents that stimulate the adrenergic receptors via the sympathetic nerve fibers of the autonomic nervous system.

Mechanism of Action. Sympathetic adrenergic receptors are distributed throughout the body. They are identified and classified according to their response to specific neurotransmitter substances. Alpha 1, alpha 2, beta 1, and beta 2 are the types that have been identified. Some important effects associated with these receptors are shown in Table 14-2.

In the lungs, β-2 receptors are found in the smaller airways, alveolar walls, and submucosal glands. The primary goal of beta-2 adrenergic drugs is to combine with these receptors to initiate bronchodilation.

Adrenergic bronchodilators are classified as catecholamines or catecholamine derivatives.

Catecholamines. Catecholamines such as norepinephrine, epinephrine, isoproterenol, and isoetharine share the following characteristics: (1) rapid onset, (2) rapid degradation by catechol-O-methyltransferase (COMT) in the liver, kidney, and throughout the body and the intraneuronal enzyme monoamine oxidase (MAO), (3) ineffective when taken enterally, and (4) nonspecific receptor binding.

inotropic: affecting the contraction.

Catecholamine derivatives. Catecholamine derivatives such as metaproterenol, terbutaline, albuterol, and pirbuterol have a more complex chemical structure than catecholamines. The modification in the chemical structure results in more specific beta-2 receptor binding and delayed degradation by COMT and MAO. As a result, catecholamine derivatives (noncatecholamines) offer less cardiac adverse effects and prolonged bronchodilation than the catecholamines.

chronotropic: affecting the rate.

TABLE 14-2 Major Effects of Alpha and Beta Receptors

RECEPTOR	MAJOR EFFECTS
Alpha-1 (α-1)	Vasoconstriction Constriction of pupils
Alpha-2 (a-2)	Decreased gastrointestinal activity
Beta-1 (β-1)	Positive **inotropic** effect (↑ muscular contractility) Positive **chronotropic** effect (↑ heart rate)
Beta-2 (β-2)	Bronchodilation Peripheral vasodilation Decreased gastrointestinal activity

Additionally, resistance to COMT degradation makes these agents suitable for enteral administration—although, beta-2 specificity may be lost via this route (Rau, 2002).

Table 14-3 shows the relative receptor actions, dosage, and frequency of use of some common sympathomimetics.

Adverse Effects. The adverse effects of adrenergic bronchodilators include tachycardia, palpitations, skeletal muscle tremors, and nervousness. The degree of adverse effects depends on the mode of administration, dosage, frequency of administration, presence of

TABLE 14-3 Adrenergic Bronchodilators

CATECHOLAMINES	ACTION RECEPTOR	INHALATION	DOSAGE	FREQUENCY
Epinephrine (adrenaline)	a > β-1 > β-2	Neb (1%)	0.25 to 0.5 mL	QID
Racemic Epinephrine (MicroNefrin, Vaponefrin, Asmanefrin)	a > β-1 > β-2	Neb (2.25%)	0.25 to 0.5 mL	QID
Isoetharine (Bronkosol, Bronkometer)	β-1 = β-2	Neb (1%) MDI	0.25 to 0.5 mL 1 to 2 puffs	QID QID
Isoproterenol (Isuprel)	β-1 < β-2	Neb (0.5%)	0.25 to 0.5 mL	QID
CATECHOLAMINE DERIVATIVES				
Bitolterol (prodrug) (Tornalate)	β-1 < β-2	MDI	2 puffs	Q 4 to 6°
Metaproterenol (Alupent, Metaprel)	β-1 < β-2	Neb MDI	(5%) 0.3 mL 2 to 3 puffs	TID/QID Q 4°
Albuterol (Proventil, Ventolin)	β-1 < β-2	Neb (0.5%) MDI, DPI	0.5 mL 2 puffs	TID/QID TID/QID
Levalbuterol (Xopenex)	β-1 < β-2	Neb	0.63 to 1.25 mg	TID/QID
Terbutaline (Brethaire, Brethine, Bricanyl)	β-1 < β-2 DPI	MDI 1 puff	2 puffs QID	QID
Pirbuterol (Maxair)	β-1 < β-2	MDI	1 to 2 puffs	Q 4 to 6°
Salmeterol Xinafoate (Serevent)	β-1 < β-2	MDI, DPI	2 puffs	BID

preexisting cardiac disease, and the specific adrenergic agent used. In most cases the benefits of bronchodilation will outweigh the potential adverse effects.

Special Considerations. The primary purpose of beta agonists is bronchodilation. For patients with inflammatory airway disease (i.e., asthma and chronic bronchitis) intermittent use of beta agonists may not be sufficient. Deaths have been reported in asthmatics following regular and prolonged use of these agents. Uncontrolled inflammation and mucosal edema are likely the cause of this adverse outcome (Witek, 1994).

Desensitization of receptor sites has been documented with regular use of beta agonists. Two mechanisms appear to be responsible: (1) the loss of receptor from the surface of cells and (2) the failure of the cell to function (Cottrell et al., 1995). The practitioner may wish to combine beta agonists with other categories of drugs to achieve bronchodilation. For example, a combination of corticosteroid and beta agonist may potentiate their individual effects and produce bronchodilation.

However, paradoxical bronchospasm may occur with combined use of adrenergic agonist and corticosteroid. Its occurrence is rare, but the onset can be sudden. For this reason, practitioners should be aware of the hazard.

ANTICHOLINERGIC BRONCHODILATORS (PARASYMPATHOLYTICS)

Anticholinergic bronchodilators are agents that impede the impulses of the cholinergic, especially the parasympathetic nerve fibers of the autonomic nervous system.

Mechanism of Action. Parasympathetic receptors (muscarinic and nicotinic) are found throughout the body. They are classified according to whether they respond to muscarine or nicotine. In the lungs, muscarinic receptors are found in submucosal glands, mast cells, and smooth muscles of the larger airways.

The combination of **acetylcholine** with muscarinic receptors results in increased bronchial tone and increased secretion from mucosal glands. Anticholinergic agents (atropine and atropine derivatives) block these physiologic responses and may be useful for the reversal of vagally mediated bronchospasm. Table 14-4 shows the usage of three common anticholinergic bronchodilators.

Adverse Effects. When inhaled, atropine is readily distributed throughout the body and may cause systemic effects such as tachycardia, nervousness, headache, and dried secretions. Atropine easily penetrates the blood brain barrier and at higher levels may cause hallucination or mental confusion. Patients with atropine-induced

acetylcholine: An ester that plays a role in the transmission of nerve impulses at synapses and neuromuscular junctions. It is metabolized by an enzyme, cholinesterase. Too much or too little of acetylcholine at the motor endplates may lead to muscle blockade.

☑ Atropine is an anticholinergic agent used as a secondary bronchodilator. It is also used for symptomatic bradycardia and prophylactic drying of secretions before surgery.

Table 14-4 Anticholinergic Bronchodilators

DRUG	INHALATION DOSAGE		FREQUENCY
Tiotropium (Spiriva)	DPI (HandiHaler)	18 mcg	Once daily
Atropine	Neb	0.3 to 0.5 mL	Up to 4 times/day
Ipratropium bromide (Atrovent)	MDI Neb (0.025%)	1 to 2 puffs 1 to 2 mL	QID Q 4 to 6°
Glycopyrrolate (Robinul)	Neb (0.02%)	5.0 mL	Q 4 to 6°

hallucinations have been erroneously diagnosed with psychiatric disorders.

Other anticholinergic agents such as ipratropium bromide (Atrovent) and glycopyrrolate (Robinul, an atropine derivative) are not well absorbed systemically and when inhaled, produce fewer adverse effects than those produced by atropine. Drying of secretions is an adverse effect of Atrovent, but it can be prevented by proper humidification or systemic hydration.

Clinical Considerations. Ipratropium bromide is not indicated for the initial treatment of acute episodes of bronchospasm where immediate response is required. These agents are commonly used in addition to the rapid-acting beta agonists. For example, ipratropium bromide is premixed with albuterol sulfate for MDI use (Combivent). The normal dosage is 2 puffs of this mixture QID.

XANTHINE BRONCHODILATORS

The third class of bronchodilators, the **xanthines,** include the drugs theophylline and its salt form aminophylline. Theophylline is a stimulant found in tea leaves and is chemically related to other stimulants found in coffee and colas. To the consumers of caffeine, the effects of tachycardia, central nervous stimulation (wakefulness), and diuresis may be well known.

Xanthines are used for their relaxing effects on smooth muscles and ability to inhibit inflammation. Clinically, the xanthines are considered to be less effective in acute bronchospasm than the beta agonists and are more useful in the management of inflammation associated with asthma and COPD. For individuals with carbon dioxide retention, xanthines improve ventilation by heightening carbon dioxide sensitivity in the central nervous system and enhancing diaphragmatic contractility. Water-soluble aminophylline is suitable for intravenous administration and is indicated for acute bronchospasm or periods of apnea associated with narcotic overdose, head trauma,

xanthine broncho-dilators: Drugs that produce bronchodilation by inhibiting phosphodiesterase, an enzyme that inactivates cyclic 3′ 5-AMP (a substance that promotes bronchodilation). Examples are oral theophylline (Theo-Dur, Slo-bid), and aminophylline, a water-soluble theophylline (Aminophyllin, Somophyllin).

TABLE 14-5   Xanthine Bronchodilators

GENERIC NAME	TRADE NAMES	ADMINISTRATION
Theophylline (100% anhydrous)	(Aerolate, Constant-T, Respbid, Slo-bid, Theo-Dur, Uniphyl)	Oral
Aminophylline (78–86% theophylline, water soluble)	(Aminophyllin, Somophyllin)	Intravenous

and congestive heart failure (Cottrell et al., 1995). Table 14-5 lists the oral and intravenous xanthine bronchodilators.

Mechanism of Action.   Multiple theories on the mechanism of theophylline have been described. Although one generally accepted mechanism is that theophylline produces bronchodilation by inhibiting phosphodiesterase (PDE). Recall that PDE rapidly inactivates cyclic 3'5' AMP, the substance that relaxes the airway smooth muscles and inhibits mast cell histamine release. By inhibiting PDE, xanthine indirectly increases cyclic 3'5' AMP levels. A second theory describes theophylline as an adenosine antagonist. Normally, the stimulation of adenosine receptors results in histamine release, thus a blocking effect provides anti-inflammatory benefits. And finally, theophylline has been shown to increase catecholamine release in some studies. The enhanced sympathomimeticlike adverse effects experienced with a nonautonomic drug such as theophylline seems to support this finding (Rau, 2002).

☑ Inhibition of phosphodi-esterase, acting as an adenosine antagonist, and increased catecholamine release are three proposed mechanisms of action of theophylline.

Adverse Effects.   Unlike the adrenergic and anticholinergic bronchodilators, xanthines are not useful via inhalation due to their lack of ability to penetrate the mucosal lining of the airways. Xanthines are available for systemic administration via the intravenous and oral routes and, thus, produce widespread effects.

Some of the adverse effects (tachycardia and skeletal muscle and CNS stimulation) can occur even at therapeutic serum theophylline ranges of 5 to 15 mcg/mL. Routine monitoring of serum theophylline levels is one way to prevent these effects from intensifying to the degree of toxicity. However, the practitioner should be able to recognize the early warning signs of theophylline toxicity since a narrow margin between therapeutic and toxic levels exists. Patients with mild to moderate toxicity (20 to 30 mcg/mL) may experience tachypnea, palpitations, nausea, vomiting, headache, and agitation. Severe toxicity (>40 mcg/mL) is marked by gastric bleeding, arrhythmias, and seizures (Wilkins et al., 2003; Witek, 1994).

☑ Nausea, vomiting, abdominal pain, diarrhea, and nervousness are some initial signs of theophylline toxicity.

Clinical Considerations.   Nausea, vomiting, abdominal pain, diarrhea, and nervousness are some initial signs of theophylline toxicity. These signs may not be apparent in or communicated by

☑ Theophylline toxicity may be avoided by keeping its serum level within therapeutic range (5 to 15 mcg/mL).

the sedated or paralyzed patient. If xanthines are used in a paralyzed patient, the serum theophylline level should be monitored closely to prevent inadvertent overdose. Toxic adverse effects can be minimized when the serum theophylline level is within its therapeutic range (5 to 15 mcg/mL) (NIH Publication, 1997).

Most of the theophylline is metabolized by the liver and excreted in the urine. Patients at risk for theophylline toxicity are those with heart failure or liver disease. Diminished liver perfusion (due to heart failure) or impaired liver function can reduce the metabolism and clearance rate of theophylline. The end result is excessive theophylline accumulation and toxicity.

On the other hand, patients at risk for inadequate theophylline are those who smoke. Smoking increases the level of hepatic enzyme and theophylline clearance. The end result for these individuals is higher maintenance theophylline dosages to maintain bronchodilation (Cottrell et al., 1995).

corticosteroids: *Hormones that are released from the cortex of the adrenal gland. Their potent anti-inflammatory effects make corticosteroids useful in the treatment of asthma and chronic bronchitis. Corticosteroids are available for intravenous administration as well as inhalation. Examples of inhaled steroids are dexamethasone (Decadron, Respihaler), beclomethasone (Beclovent, Vanceril), flunisolide (AeroBid), and triamcinolone (Azmacort).*

ANTI-INFLAMMATORY AGENTS (CORTICOSTEROIDS)

Corticosteroids are powerful, naturally occurring hormones that are released from the adrenal cortex. Their anti-inflammatory effects make them first-line drugs in the management of chronic asthma and other long-term airway inflammatory conditions. In the intensive care setting, they have been used with favorable results in status asthmaticus, acute exacerbation of COPD, inhalation airway injury, drug-induced pneumonitis, septic shock, ARDS, and spinal cord injury.

Corticosteroids have no bronchodilator effect and should not be given alone during an acute asthma attack. The effects of corticosteroids require an onset time of about 2 to 24 hours, further demonstrating their inappropriateness in acute situations.

Mechanism of Action. The general functions of corticosteroids include (1) carbohydrate metabolism, (2) immunosuppression, and (3) reduced inflammation. Their specific mechanism in reducing inflammation is complex, involving genetic changes to target cells of inflammation. The combination of the steroid with its receptor site (nucleus of target cell) results in altered cellular function.

Normally, an inflammatory response results in the release of histamine and bradykinin (among other mediators) from the mast cell causing bronchoconstriction and increased capillary permeability. This leads to early-phase bronchoconstriction and late-phase submucosal edema and hyperactivity (Rau, 2002). With altered cellular function, these and other mediators are blocked and inflammation is reduced.

☑ Corticosteroids may be used when other traditional bronchodilators have failed to relieve bronchospasm.

Adverse Effects. Corticosteroids are available for oral, intravenous, and inhalation administration (Tables 14-6 and 14-7), and as with

TABLE 14-6   Corticosteroids for Metered-Dose Inhaler (MDI) Use

DRUG	MDI DOSAGE	FREQUENCY
Dexamethasone (Decadron, Respihaler)	2 to 3 puffs	3 to 4 times/day
Beclomethasone (Beclovent, Vanceril)	2 puffs	3 to 4 times/day
Flunisolide (AeroBid)	2 puffs	2 times/day
Triamcinolone (Azmacort)	2 puffs	3 to 4 times/day
Fluticasone propionate (Flovent)	2 puffs	2 times/day

✓ Corticosteroids return constricted airways to normal by blocking the inflammatory mediators.

most agents, the inhalation route is favored for its convenience, smaller dosage, and fewer adverse effects.

The most frequent adverse effects reported with metered-dose inhaler (MDI) use are hoarseness and oral fungal infections (e.g., candidiasis). To prevent fungal superinfections, patients should be instructed to rinse and gargle the mouth after each treatment. MDI corticosteroids are rarely used in the ventilator patient.

There are many serious adverse effects associated with systemic corticosteroid therapy. Abrupt withdrawal following long-term systemic therapy may cause serious complications from adrenal insufficiency. Recovery time varies depending on the dosage and duration of therapy. Another serious effect is an increased susceptibility to opportunistic infections.

Clinical Considerations.   Corticosteroids are not bronchodilators. Their use in the treatment of bronchospasm is limited to situations where patients have lost beta agonist responsiveness or when other bronchodilators have failed. Their primary role is in the management of long-term airway inflammation. Systemic corticosteroids should be used cautiously with patients receiving steroidal based neuromuscular blocking agents (vecuronium bromide and pancuronium bromide) because of the potential of prolonged blockade (Kupfer et al., 1987).

TABLE 14-7   Corticosteroids for Systemic Use

DRUG	ROUTE OF ADMINISTRATION
Hydrocortisone	Oral
Cortisone	Parenteral (intravenous, intramuscular, subcutaneous, or mucosal)
Prednisolone	
Dexamethasone	
Prednisone	Oral

MDI

Ventilator
Inspiratory
Tubing

Spacer

Figure 14-1 An MDI with spacer on a ventilator circuit.

DELIVERY OF MDI MEDICATIONS

Many bronchodilators and steroids come in a metered-dose inhaler (MDI). With proper adapter or fittings, MDI medications may be administered via the ventilator circuit without interruption to mechanical ventilation or airway pressure. MDI may be given with a right-angle adapter or with a spacer. Studies have shown that an MDI with spacer is a more efficient method for delivering inhaled medications to the lungs than the right-angle MDI port (Marik, Hogan & Krikorian, 1999; Mouloudi, Katsanoulas & Anastasaki et al., 1998). In addition, the efficacy of MDI medications does not improve with end-inspiratory pause during delivery (Mouloudi et al., 1998). Figure 14-1 shows a typical setup of an MDI on the ventilator circuit.

NEUROMUSCULAR BLOCKING AGENTS

Neuromuscular blocking agents are administered when temporary paralysis of skeletal muscles is desired. Pharmacological paralysis is most commonly induced to (1) ease endotracheal intubation, (2) relieve laryngeal spasm, (3) provide muscle relaxation during surgery, or (4) maintain mechanical ventilation.

TABLE 14-8   Benefits of Paralysis during Controlled Ventilation

1. Reduced combativeness and agitation
2. Relaxation of respiratory muscles
3. Increased chest wall compliance
4. Synchronization during unnatural modes of ventilation (e.g., inverse I:E)
5. Prevention of hypoxemia associated with increased work of breathing
6. Decreased intracranial pressures caused by excessive movement

Paralyzing agents are used on ventilator patients in difficult situations due to underlying pathology, unnatural modes of ventilation, or psychologic unacceptance. If any of these conditions prevent adequate ventilation, oxygenation or patient comfort, a paralyzing agent should be considered. The benefits of paralysis during controlled ventilation are given in Table 14-8.

Since serious adverse effects can occur with the use of these agents, they should not be given routinely or before alternative management is considered. If paralysis is indicated, a sedative drug, such as the benzodiazepines along with a narcotic analgesic should be provided for patient comfort. This is necessary because perception and pain threshold of a patient still exist with use of neuromuscular blocking drugs.

The following testimonies affirm the need for adequate sedation and analgesia during paralysis. One patient who was pharmacologically paralyzed and not sedated described his experience as "a feeling of being buried alive." Another patient thought that she had died (Halloran, 1991). A trauma survivor recalls the sensation of endotracheal tube suctioning being like that of a red-hot burning iron passed into the trachea (Hansen-Flaschen et al., 1993).

MECHANISM OF ACTION

During normal neuromuscular transmission, the nerve axon reaches the muscle fibers and it branches out to form many fine nerve terminals. These nerve terminals are rich in mitochondria, cytoplasmic enzymes, and vesicles. Acetylcholine (ACh), the major chemical in the transmission of nerve impulses, is stored in these vesicles.

When the nerve terminal is stimulated by nerve impulses, acetylcholine is released into the synaptic cleft. From there, some of the acetylcholine is broken down by acetylcholinesterase (ACHe) and other ACh diffuses to the muscle end plate producing depolarization and muscle contraction. Figure 14-2 is the functional illustration of neuromuscular transmission.

The sequence of events at the neuromuscular junction is as follows. A repeating sequence of depolarization and repolarization is required for continued and coordinated muscular movement. Interruption at

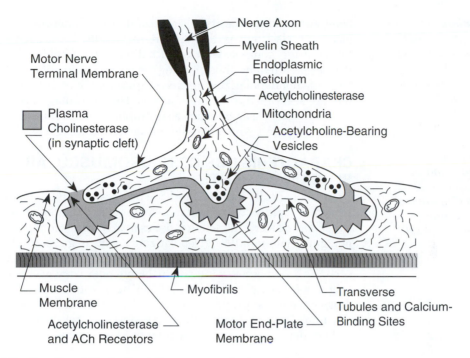

Figure 14-2   Functional illustration of neuromuscular transmission.

any point of the sequence causes muscle relaxation or paralysis, depending on the effective dosage.

Neuromuscular blocking drugs are typically divided into two groups depending on the modes of action at the neuromuscular junction.

Depolarizing Agents.   The first group of neuromuscular blockers is classified as **depolarizing agents.** This type of agent (e.g., succinylcholine) binds with the receptor site, producing quick onset and sustaining depolarization. Uncoordinated muscle contraction called fasciculation marks the onset. Subsequent neuromuscular transmission is inhibited during the time that adequate concentration of succinylcholine is bound to the receptor site (Ebadi, 1993).

There is no antidote for depolarizing agents. Succinylcholine is, however, rapidly hydrolyzed by plasma pseudocholinesterase (PCHE). A small percentage of the population has an abnormal plasma cholinesterase that does not hydrolyze succinylcholine within minutes, as expected. Plasma PCHE level may also be decreased in patients with insecticide poisoning, liver disorders (hepatitis, cirrhosis, obstructive jaundice), malnutrition, acute infections, and anemias (Kee, 2001). These individuals may require ventilatory support for hours because of insufficient plasma PCHE.

depolarizing agents: Drugs that prolong the depolarization phase of muscle contraction, thus rendering the repolarization/depolarization sequence (normal mechanism for muscle movement) impossible and causing muscle blockade. An example is succinylcholine (Anectine, Quelicin).

nondepolarizing agents: Drugs that compete with acetylcholine for the receptor sites at the motor endplates, thus blocking the normal action of acetylcholine and causing muscle blockade. Examples are tubocurarine chloride (Tubarine), and pancuronium bromide (Pavulon).

Nondepolarizing Agents. The second group of neuromuscular blockers is classified as **nondepolarizing agents.** These agents (e.g., tubocurarine) compete with acetylcholine for the receptor sites at the motor endplates, thus blocking the normal action of acetylcholine. Since the nondepolarizing agents compete for the receptor sites, they are also called competitive agents. They are antagonized by anticholinesterase agents such as endrophonium, pyridostigmine, and neostigmine. Anticholinesterase agents allow ACh levels to rise.

CHARACTERISTICS OF NEUROMUSCULAR BLOCKING AGENTS

Pharmacologically induced blockade progresses in the following sequence: rapidly contracting muscles (eyes and digits) followed by larger and slower contracting muscles (extremities, trunk, and diaphragm) (Halloran, 1991). Depolarizing agents (e.g., succinylcholine) have a quick onset but are short-lasting, making them the drugs of choice for emergency intubation. Nondepolarizing agents have longer onsets ranging from 3 to 10 min, but are longer lasting. These drugs are more appropriate for controlled ventilation in the intensive care unit. Table 14-9 shows the characteristics of selected depolarizing and nondepolarizing neuromuscular blocking agents.

FACTORS AFFECTING NEUROMUSCULAR BLOCKADE

Several factors can alter neuromuscular transmission and blockade. They include organ failure, drug interaction, electrolyte imbalance, and acid-base status.

☑ Organ failure may decrease drug clearance, increase drug accumulation and prolonged neuromuscular blockade.

Organ Failure. Patients with altered renal or hepatic function have an increased risk of prolonged blockade. These patients can remain profoundly weak long after the drug is discontinued. Both pancuronium bromide and vecuronium bromide have been implicated in drug accumulation in patients with renal insufficiency. Vecuronium is also poorly eliminated in patients with hepatic failure. Atracurium is preferred in the presence of organ failure because it is self-destroying and does not rely on organ metabolism and excretion (Halloran, 1991).

Drug Interaction. Some cardiovascular and antiarrhythmic agents may interact and potentiate the effects of nondepolarizing agents. They include beta blockers, procainamide, quinidine, calcium channel blockers, and nitroglycerine. High concentrations of antibiotics may also potentiate the effects of competitive agents by decreasing the release of ACh. These antibiotics include the aminoglycosides and polymyxins as well as tetracycline, erythromycin, and vancomycin (Halloran, 1991).

☑ Beta blockers, procainamide, quinidine, calcium channel blockers, and nitroglycerine may potentiate the effects of nondepolarizing agents.

Steroidal based vecuronium bromide and pancuronium bromide may be particularly dangerous if administered along with systemic

TABLE 14-9   Depolarizing and Nondepolarizing Agents

AGENTS	INITIAL DOSE (mg/kg)	ONSET (min)	DURATION	DRUG CLEARANCE
Depolarizing				
Succinylcholine (Anectine, Quelicin, Sux-Cert, Sucostrin)	0.3 to 1.1	1	Short	Metabolized by plasma cholinesterase
Nondepolarizing				
Tubocurarine chloride (Tubarine)	0.5	5	Long	Excreted unchanged in urine
Pancuronium bromide (Pavulon)	0.07	5 to 7	Long	Metabolized by liver, excreted in urine
Metocurine iodide (Metubine)	0.2 to 0.4	4	Long	Excreted unchanged in urine
Atracurium (Tracrium)	0.4 to 0.5	4 to 5	Intermediate	Self-destroying
Vecuronium bromide (Norcuron)	0.05	4 to 6	Intermediate	Metabolized by liver, excreted in urine
Pipecuronium bromide (Arduan)	0.05 to 0.06	4 to 6	Long	Renal
Doxacurium chloride (Neuromax)	0.03	8 to 12	Long	Renal
Mivacurium chloride (Mivacron)	0.01	3 to 6	Short	Metabolized by plasma cholinesterase
Rocuronium (Zemuron)	0.3	3 to 4	Short	Metabolized by liver

☑ ↑ Ca^{++} may lead to ↑ release of Ach and ↑ muscular contraction.

corticosteroids (Watling et al., 1994). A significant number of asthmatics receiving these neuromuscular blocking agents in combination with steroid therapy have experienced prolonged blockade for several days following discontinuation of the paralyzing agent (Kupfer et al., 1987). This prolonged blockade is possibly related to the comparable chemical structure of steroid and steroidal based agents. Figure 14-3 shows the basic steroid structure and pipecuronium, a steroidal based paralyzing agent. Until studies become conclusive, use of corticosteroids should be avoided during prolonged muscle blockade with

Figure 14-3 (A) Basic steroid structure; (B) A steroidal based neuromuscular blocking agent, pipecuronium.

steroidal based blocking agents (pancuronium bromide and vecuronium bromide) (Hansen-Flaschen et al., 1993).

Electrolyte Imbalance. The normal physiology of muscle contraction depends on the regulation of electrolytes. Abnormal levels of calcium and magnesium affect the quality of contraction, while imbalances in potassium and sodium levels alter the excitability at the motor endplate. For example, the release of ACh depends on extracellular calcium and magnesium concentrations. Calcium functions to release ACh from the vesicles and expose myosin-binding sites on actin. Myosin-binding site exposure is a structural change that is necessary for the sliding of thin myofilaments past thick myofilaments. The sliding of these filaments results in muscular contraction (Tortora et al., 2002). Magnesium works in opposition to calcium. It decreases the release of ACh as well as the membrane's sensitivity, thus inhibiting muscle contraction (Ebadi, 1993).

   Consequently, low calcium and high magnesium levels can enhance the effects of nondepolarizing agents. Increased magnesium levels can magnify the effects of depolarizing agents.

   Sodium and potassium function in the process of depolarization. When a muscle cell is at rest, or not depolarized, there is a considerable difference between the concentration of sodium and potassium outside and inside the plasma membrane. At rest, there is an increased concentration of sodium extracellularly and an increased concentration of

☑ ↑ Mg^{++} may lead to ↓ release of Ach and ↓ muscular contraction.

☑ ↓ Ca^{++} or ↑ Mg^{++} enhances neuromuscular blockade with *nondepolarizing* agents.

☑ ↑ Mg^{++} enhances neuromuscular blockade with *depolarizing* agents.

✓ Diuretic-induced hypokalemia causes ↑ blockade with nondepolarizing agents and ↓ blockade with depolarizing agents.

potassium intracellularly. The difference in charge on either side of the membrane of the resting cell is known as the resting potential and is said to be polarized or charged (Tortora et al., 2002).

An acute decrease in extracellular potassium will result in hyperpolarization and an increased resistance to depolarization. Hence, hypokalemia augments nondepolarizing agents and antagonizes depolarizing agents (Ebadi, 1993). Diuretic-induced hypokalemia should be corrected to prevent altered effects (potentiation of blockade with nondepolarizing agents; hinderance of blockade with depolarizing agents) (Halloran, 1991).

Acid-Base Status.   Acidemia intensifies neuromuscular blockade requiring a lower dosage of paralyzing agent or a higher dosage of reversal agent such as neostigmine (Kupfer et al., 1987). On the other hand, alkalemia necessitates a higher dosage of paralyzing agent to maintain neuromuscular blockade. These alterations are likely the result of potassium shift (extracellularly) associated with acidemia. H^+ moves into cells to be buffered, and K^+ moves out to maintain ionic neutrality. One might find these effects to be significant when intracranial pressure is being reduced via hyperventilation (respiratory alkalosis).

✓ Acidemia intensifies the effects of neuromuscular blockade.

✓ Alkalemia diminishes the effects of neuromuscular blockade.

Although the preceding factors can alter the action of neuromuscular blocking agents, the net effects following the initial dosage can be titrated based on the results of patient monitoring. Since there is no standard level of paralysis to be achieved, the desired depth of blockade will depend on the clinical objectives of the physician.

ADVERSE EFFECTS

Apnea is the most immediate and life-threatening adverse effect associated with both depolarizing and nondepolarizing agents. For this reason, practitioners experienced in airway management must be present when these drugs are administered. For a patient who is already intubated and committed to a mechanical ventilator, the following alarms should be employed.

- Apnea alarm
- Low pressure/disconnect
- Low exhaled tidal volume
- Low exhaled minute volume
- Low SaO_2 or SpO_2 (pulse oximetry)

Deaths due to apnea have been reported in cases where alarms were inappropriately set or inactivated. It is possible that the incidence of fatal outcome is underreported (Halloran, 1991).

Other undesirable effects of neuromuscular blocking agents include loss of cough mechanism, blunted neurologic assessment, emotional trauma due to inadequate sedation, disuse muscle atrophy, pressure sores, and increased iatrogenic morbidity and mortality associated with extended ICU exposure.

✓ Succinylcholine, tubocurarine, metocurine, and atracurium may provoke bronchospasm and hypotension due to histamine release.

Histamine release is a property shared by most nondepolarizing agents. The presence of histamine may be manifested clinically as vasodilation, flushing, and bronchospasm. The degree of histamine release differs among the drugs. Succinylcholine, tubocurarine, metocurine, and atracurium have been known to provoke bronchospasm and hypotension related to moderate histamine release, whereas pancuronium elicits only minimal release. Histamine release is not likely with the use of vecuronium (Ebadi, 1993).

Cardiovascular effects range from minimal to moderate, including bradycardia, tachycardia, arrhythmias, and circulatory collapse.

TABLE 14-10   Adverse Effects of Neuromuscular Blocking Agents

AGENTS	HISTAMINE RELEASE	CARDIOVASCULAR IMPAIRMENT	CLINICAL CONSIDERATIONS
Depolarizing			
Succinylcholine (Anectine, Quelicin, Sux-Cert, Sucostrin)	Moderate	Moderate	Caution with plasma cholinesterase disorder
Nondepolarizing			
Tubocurarine chloride (Tubarine)	Moderate	Moderate	
Pancuronium bromide (Pavulon)	Minimal	Moderate	Steroidal based Use corticosteroids with caution
Metocurine iodide (Metubine)	Moderate	Moderate	Appropriate dosage highly variable About 3 times as potent as tubocurarine, but shorter acting
Atracurium (Tracrium)	Moderate	Minimal	Not affected by organ dysfunction
Vecuronium bromide (Norcuron)	Not likely	Minimal	Steroidal based Use corticosteroids with caution
Pipecuronium bromide (Arduan)	Minimal	Minimal	
Doxacurium chloride (Neuromax)	Minimal	Minimal	Caution with plasma cholinesterase disorder
Mivacurium chloride (Mivacron)	Moderate	Minimal	Steroidal based
Rocuronium (Zemuron)	Minimal	Minimal	Use corticosteroids with caution

Sudden changes in drug levels associated with intermittent administration (versus continuous infusion) seem to be responsible for these adverse effects (Watling et al., 1994). Table 14-10 summarizes the bronchopulmonary and cardiovascular adverse effects of neuromuscular blocking agents.

EVALUATION OF NEUROMUSCULAR BLOCKADE

To prevent unintentional overdosing, clinicians must establish an objective method of monitoring the depth of paralysis. This is especially meaningful in the management of patients with potential for drug accumulation secondary to renal or hepatic dysfunction.

The Train-of-Four (ToF), a peripheral nerve stimulator, is a valuable tool used in the evaluation of patients who are pharmacologically paralyzed. It determines the degree of blockade by measuring the muscle twitches in response to a controlled stimulus. Two electrodes are placed along a nerve path where electrical stimuli delivered at 2 Hz are four times in 0.5 sec intervals. As the degree of blockade increases, the number of elicited responses (muscle twitches) decreases. The ulnar, facial, and posterior tibial nerves are commonly used because they are superficial and easy to locate. Figure 14-4 shows the electrode placement along the ulnar nerve.

Figure 14-4 Placement of the Train-of-Four electrodes along the ulnar nerve.

TABLE 14-11   Assessment of Neuromuscular Blockade Reversal

1. Head lift 5 sec
2. Tongue protrusion 5 sec
3. Hand grip
4. Arterial blood gases with PaO_2 >80 mm Hg and $PaCO_2$ <45 mm Hg*
5. Maximal inspiratory pressure (MIP) at least -25 cm H_2O
6. Vital capacity greater than 900 mL

Slightly higher $PaCO_2$ is acceptable for patients with chronic CO_2 retention.

☑ The ability to open eyes widely, sustain head lift, and protrude the tongue for more than 5 sec confirms adequate reversal of neuromuscular blockade.

☑ Return of diaphragm function is assessed by acceptable blood gases, MIP >-25 cm H_2O, VC >900 mL.

Most recommendations for ToF monitoring suggest titration of neuromuscular blocker to one or two twitches (>80% to 90% muscular blockade) in 2 sec, which is the current practice in using ToF monitoring. However, ToF of three twitches generally corresponds closely to 80% muscular blockade. This lighter level of muscular blockade may be adequate to assure patient-ventilator synchrony and lower airway pressures and to optimize oxygen delivery in most patients (Strange et al., 1997).

A clinically useful but less objective method of measuring the depth of blockade is by assessing the patient's spontaneous muscle effort. Recovery of muscle blockade occurs in a reverse sequence. The ability to open one's eyes widely, sustain head lift, and protrude the tongue for more than 5 sec confirms adequate reversal. Ventilator support, however, should not be discontinued until the diaphragm is able to provide adequate ventilation. Arterial blood gases and spontaneous maneuvers [e.g., maximal inspiratory pressure [MIP] and vital capacity [VC]) can provide evidence of partial or full diaphragm recovery (Halloran, 1991). Table 14-11 outlines the method for assessment of neuromuscular blockade reversal.

SEDATIVES AND ANTIANXIETY AGENTS (BENZODIAZEPINES)

benzodiazepines: A group of drugs with strong hypnotic and sedative actions; used mainly to reduce anxiety and to induce sleep.

Benzodiazepines are given to patients to reduce anxiety, provide amnesia, and improve tolerance of mechanical ventilation. In addition, they facilitate invasive procedures (e.g., bronchoscopy, intravenous access, suctioning), decrease oxygen consumption, and protect the patient from self-injury.

MECHANISM OF ACTION

Binding receptors for benzodiazepines have been identified in the limbic, thalamic, and hypothalamic levels of the central nervous system (Mohler et al., 1977). These receptor sites appear to be

Figure 14-5 Gamma-aminobutyric acid (GABA) receptor complex. GABA is the most common inhibitory neurotransmitter in the central nervous system (CNS). Activation of the postsynaptic GABA receptor increases chloride conductance through the ion channel thus hyperpolarizing it and inhibiting the postsynaptic neuron. Once the postsynaptic neurons are inhibited, depression of the CNS and neuromuscular blockade results.

gamma-aminobu-tyric acid (GABA): *A major central nervous system inhibitory transmitter that regulates the chloride ion channel and hyperpolarizes the neurons. Once the neurons are hyperpolarized and become resistant to repeated depolariza-tion, sedation results.*

anxiolysis: *Dimin-ishing anxiety.*

☑ With benzodi-azepines, the intravenous route of administration is preferred.

involved in a large molecular complex that includes **gamma-aminobutyric acid (GABA)** receptors and GABA-regulated chloride ion channels (Figure 14-5).

GABA Mechanism. GABA is a major central nervous system inhibitory transmitter that opens chloride ion channels. Once hyper-polarized by the GABA action, the neurons become more resistant to repeated depolarization and sedation results (Mohler et al., 1988). Benzodiazepines facilitate the action of GABA, thus producing clinical sedation, **anxiolysis,** anticonvulsant effects, amnesia, slowing of reaction time, visual accommodation difficulties, and ataxia.

Absorption. Benzodiazepines are normally well absorbed in the gastrointestinal (GI) tract. In unstable patients, GI tract absorption may be unreliable and parenteral administration is preferred. Lorazepam and midazolam are rapidly and completely absorbed intramuscularly, whereas the absorption of chlordiazepoxide and diazepam is slow and erratic (McEvoy, 1995). Because of the slower onset of action and pain associated with intramuscular administration, the intravenous route is preferred in the critically ill. The lipid solubil-ity of the drugs allows rapid distribution across the blood-brain bar-rier with midazolam being the most lipophilic, followed by diazepam and chlordiazepoxide, and then lorazepam (McEvoy, 1995).

Excretion. Benzodiazepines are metabolized in the liver to active and inactive metabolites that are excreted mainly in the urine. Although the pharmacokinetics of drugs are often used to explain correlations between plasma concentrations and effect, benzodiazepines do not exhibit this relationship. Furthermore, carefully controlled clinical trials have not shown the superiority of one agent over another for various ICU indications (Dasta et al., 1994). Therefore, the choice of benzodiazepine is often based on cost.

ADVERSE EFFECTS

☑ Dose-dependent adverse CNS effects include confusion, weakness, dizziness, drowsiness, ataxia, syncope, vertigo, and amnesia.

Dose-dependent adverse central nervous system effects are very common with benzodiazepines. They are an extension of the pharmacologic actions of the drugs and include confusion, weakness, dizziness, drowsiness, ataxia, syncope, vertigo, and amnesia (McEvoy, 1995). Central nervous system stimulation occurs occasionally in patients with underlying psychiatric disorders. These patients present with restlessness, mania, euphoria, acute rage reactions, and sleep disorders (McCartney et al., 1993). A withdrawal syndrome may occur if these drugs are abruptly discontinued in patients on prolonged therapy or high doses. This may be manifested by severe anxiety, tachycardia, diaphoresis, hypertension, and, occasionally, seizures (McCartney et al., 1994).

☑ Withdrawal syndrome (anxiety, tachycardia, diaphoresis, hypertension, and, occasionally, seizures) may occur if benzodiazepines are abruptly discontinued.

Parenteral administration of benzodiazepines may result in a dose-dependent respiratory depression (Forster et al., 1980) which is additive to that produced by narcotics. Elderly and COPD patients are at the greatest risk (Levine, 1994). Although depression of the respiratory drive is not usually as great with benzodiazepines as with other sedative agents, apnea may occur. Careful dosing of these agents is also necessary to avoid prolonged mechanical ventilation.

☑ Benzodiazepines may decrease the mean arterial pressure, stroke volume, cardiac output, and systemic vascular resistance.

Benzodiazepines may also have direct effects on cardiovascular hemodynamics. They have been shown to decrease mean arterial pressure, stroke volume, cardiac output, and systemic vascular resistance (Reves et al., 1990). Additive decreases in blood pressure may occur when narcotics are administered concurrently. Table 14-12 outlines the cardiovascular effects of benzodiazepines.

ASSESSMENT OF SEDATION

☑ Ramsay Scale is used to assess a patient's sedation state.

The indication for benzodiazepines and the estimated duration of therapy may be helpful in deciding whether to administer these drugs intermittently or continuously. If a short period of sedation is needed, intermittent intravenous bolus dosing may prevent oversedation.

TABLE 14-12 Cardiovascular Effects of Benzodiazepines

1. ↓ Mean arterial pressure
2. ↓ Stroke volume
3. ↓ Cardiac output
4. ↓ Systemic vascular resistance
5. ↓ Blood pressure

TABLE 14-13   Ramsay Scale for Assessment of Sedation

LEVEL/SCORE	CLINICAL DESCRIPTION
I	Anxious and agitated
II	Cooperative, oriented, tranquil
III	Responds only to verbal commands
IV	Asleep with brisk response to light stimulation
V	Asleep with sluggish response to stimulation
VI	Asleep without response to stimulation

☑ Ramsay Scale is not suitable for paralyzed patients since they cannot perform those required commands.

Ramsay Scale: The scoring system with a scale ranging from level I to level VI; used to assess the degree of sedation.

☑ Autonomic signs (tachycardia, diaphoresis, hypertension, and lacrimation) may suggest inadequate sedation or pain control.

If prolonged periods of sedation are required, a bolus followed by a continuous infusion may provide optimal patient comfort. If the indication is to facilitate an uncomfortable procedure, an intravenous bolus dose should be given.

Since individual patient response to benzodiazepines is highly variable, monitoring is essential to ensure correct dosing and reduce costs. Assessment of a patient's sedation state may be done with the **Ramsay Scale** for Assessment of Sedation as outlined in Table 14-13 (Ramsay et al., 1974). Using the Ramsay Scale and the appropriate types and dosages of benzodiazepines (Table 14-14), a desired level of sedation may be determined.

It is important to note that the Ramsay Scale is not suitable for paralyzed patients. Since they cannot perform those required commands for the Ramsay Scale, autonomic signs such as tachycardia, diaphoresis, hypertension, and lacrimation may suggest inadequate sedation or pain control (Shelly et al., 1986).

NARCOTIC ANALGESICS

Patients on mechanical ventilation may have a variety of medical or surgical problems that necessitate attention to pain control. In these patients, however, pain is difficult to assess because of their inability to speak.

TABLE 14-14   Common Benzodiazepines Used in Mechanical Ventilation

DRUG	INITIAL DOSE	ONSET	DURATION
Diazepam (Valium)	2.5 to 10 mg IV	Fast	Short initially; multiple doses result in prolonged effect
Lorazepam (Ativan)	0.5 to 2 mg IV	Intermediate	Intermediate
Midazolam (Versed)	1 to 5 mg IV	Fast	Short, but may be prolonged if not carefully dosed

TABLE 14-15   Adverse Patient Outcomes Associated with Pain

REACTION INDUCED BY PAIN	ADVERSE OUTCOMES
Tissue initiated stress hormone response	Breakdown of body tissue Increased blood clotting Increased metabolic rate Increased water retention Decreased immune function
Activation of autonomic functions	Increased blood pressure Increased heart rate
Muscle splinting	Decreased tidal volume Decreased respiratory rate Decreased minute ventilation
Immobility	Formation of deep vein thrombosis and pulmonary embolism
Diminished gastrointestinal function	Delay of bowel and gastric function

Hemodynamic and respiratory instability, and immediate life-threatening concerns also overshadow the presence of pain. Subsequently, pain control for these patients is often inadequate (Wheeler, 1993).

Pain can cause anxiety, discomfort, and delirium in patients on mechanical ventilation. Interference with sleep also compounds the level of anxiety thus further elevating the perception of pain. Pain is also associated with many adverse outcomes in the intensive care unit (Table 14-15). **Narcotic analgesics** are commonly used to control pain to allow earlier patient mobilization and to decrease hospital stay.

narcotic analgesics:
Drugs that are used to control pain via the central nervous system. Examples are morphine, codeine, and meperidine (Demerol, a synthetic compound).

MECHANISM OF ACTION

Narcotic analgesics produce analgesia by binding to opioid receptors in and outside the central nervous system. Several subtypes of opiate receptors have been identified. The mu, kappa, and sigma receptors are known to have important nociceptive (neural receptors for painful stimulus) properties in humans. Binding and activating these receptors also helps to explain the adverse pharmacologic profile of these drugs (Table 14-16) (Teeple, 1990).

Opiates may be further classified depending on whether they are agonists, agonist-antagonists, or pure antagonists at these receptors (Table 14-17). Full agonists produce a maximal response within cells to which they bind; agonist-antagonists activate one type of opiate receptor while blocking another; and antagonists only block opiate receptors (Teeple, 1990).

☑ Full agonists produce a maximal response within cells to which they bind.

Table 14-17 contains only representative samples from each class. It is not a complete listing of all opioids.

TABLE 14-16   Narcotic Receptor Classifications

PHYSICAL PARAMETER	mu	kappa	sigma
Pain sensation	−	−	0
Body temperature	−	0	+
Pulse rate	−	0	+
Pupils	−	−	+
Respiratory rate	−	−	+
CNS effect	Sedation	Hypnosis	Delirium

+ *increased effect*
− *reduced effect*
0 *no effect*

☑ Agonist-
antagonists acti-
vate one type of
opiate receptor while
blocking another.

☑ Antagonists
block opiate
receptors.

☑ Sedation, respi-
ratory depres-
sion, and shallow
breathing are the pri-
mary adverse effects
of narcotic anal-
gesics on the CNS.

Most agonist-antagonist drugs are agonists at the sigma receptor. As the dose of these drugs is increased for deeper analgesia, the more likely they may cause significant psychological effects such as delirium. This class of drugs is not routinely used in ventilator patients and will not be discussed further.

Antagonist drugs such as naloxone (Narcan) are primarily used to reverse overdose of narcotics. Special care must be exercised with the use of naloxone in a patient being treated for severe pain. It may reverse an untoward adverse effect such as respiratory depression while causing the return of severe pain (Levine, 1994).

ADVERSE EFFECTS

Narcotic analgesics produce many adverse effects. Table 14-18 outlines the adverse effects that may occur to various systems or body locations of the patient.

Central Nervous System.   Opiates cause sedation, respiratory depression, and myoclonus (twitching or spasm of muscles) and their effects are dose dependent (Levine, 1994). Clinically significant respiratory depression is more likely to occur with a large initial dose or in

TABLE 14-17   Opioid Drug Classifications

DRUGS [SELECTED EXAMPLES]	mu	kappa	sigma
1. Agonist [morphine, meperidine (Demerol), fentanyl (Sublimaze)]	+	+	0
2. Agonist-antagonist [pentazocine, butorphanol]	−	+	+
3. Antagonist [naloxone (Narcan)]	−	−	−

+ *agonist*
− *antagonist*
0 *no effect*

TABLE 14-18   Adverse Effects of Narcotic Analgesics

LOCATION	ADVERSE EFFECTS
Central nervous system	Sedation Respiratory depression Shallow breathing (and atelectasis)
Muscle groups	Myoclonus (twitching or spasm of muscles) Convulsions Chest wall rigidity
Cardiovascular	Direct vasodilation Vagally mediated bradycardia Hypotension
Gastrointestinal	Delayed gastric emptying Constipation Nausea
Others	Miosis (contraction of pupils) Altered levels of stress hormones Uncommon allergic reactions

patients with underlying pulmonary disease. Respiratory depression (decreased tidal volume and respiratory rate) is mediated by opioid agonist activity at the mu receptors of the brain stem (Teeple, 1990). Since opiates suppress deep breathing, they may induce atelectasis, which can be prevented by activating the automatic sigh mode on the ventilator.

☑ Myoclonus (twitching or spasm of muscles), convulsions, and chest wall rigidity are the primary adverse effects of narcotic analgesics on the muscle group.

Muscle Groups.   Myoclonus (twitching or spasm of muscles) and other neuroexcitatory phenomena have been reported with opioid analgesics. Myoclonus may be prevented by switching to another opioid, lowering the dosage, or using a benzodiazepine (Valium), an antianxiety and hypnotic agent. Convulsions have been reported with high doses of any opioid in an intolerant patient, but are most common with normeperidine—a liver metabolite of meperidine (Demerol) (Brucera et al., 1992). Naloxone (Narcan) may be used to reverse convulsions caused by opiates with the exception of those caused by use of meperidine.

Chest wall rigidity is a complication that may develop after administration of any opiate, but it is most commonly reported with fentanyl (Sublimaze). This adverse effect is most often seen at the time of anesthesia induction or after surgery. It may be so severe that the patient may require intubation, mechanical ventilation, and chemical paralysis. Patients at risk for this untoward effect appear to be the elderly, patients with renal failure, and those receiving large doses of opioids (Wheeler, 1993).

☑ Direct vasodila-
tion, vagally
mediated bradycar-
dia, and hypotension
are the primary
adverse effects of
narcotic analgesics
on the cardiovascular
system.

Cardiovascular Effects.   Opioids can affect a patient's hemodynamic status. Hypotension may develop as a result of direct vasodilation, histamine release, and vagally mediated bradycardia (Levine,
1994). These complications may be prevented by using the lowest
effective dose, providing an adequate intravascular volume, or
decreasing the rate of administration. [Note: Meperidine's (Demerol's)
structure resembles that of atropine; thus it may cause tachycardia
rather than bradycardia.]

Although opioids may produce a dose-dependent clinical spectrum ranging from pain relief to sedation, deep coma, and anesthesia,
low-dose opiates are often combined with low-dose sedatives (benzodiazepines) to minimize the adverse effects of these two agents.

☑ Delayed gastric
emptying, con-
stipation, and nausea
are the primary
adverse effects of
narcotic analgesics
on the GI system.

cathartic agents:
Active purgatives
used to produce
bowel movements.

Gastrointestinal Effects.   The gastrointestinal effects of opioids
include delayed gastric emptying, constipation, and nausea (Levine,
1994). Since tolerance to constipation does not occur, or occurs very
slowly during opiate administration, **cathartic agents** should be given
on a regular basis to activate bowel movements.

Nausea and vomiting during opiate administration may be due to
three different mechanisms. Opiates may reduce gastric motility that
results in nausea after eating. Secondly, opioids seem to cause nausea
that is due to sensitization of the vestibular apparatus. This type of
nausea is brought on by changes in position or head movement. Third,
these drugs may directly stimulate the medullary chemoreceptor trigger zone. Nausea from this mechanism is usually present continuously (Jacox et al., 1994).

Other adverse effects related to opioid use include miosis (contraction of pupils), altered levels of stress hormones, and uncommon
allergic reactions.

CLINICAL CONSIDERATIONS

Opioid tolerance, physical dependence, and psychological dependence are important concepts to understand when considering analgesic therapy. Misuse of these terms has led to ineffective practices
in prescribing, administering, and treatment of patients in pain.

Tolerance.   Tolerance is defined as the need to increase dosage
requirements to maintain effective pain relief. In addition, tolerance
may occur to some adverse opioid effects such as respiratory depression, miosis, sedation, and nausea (Foley, 1993).

Physical Dependence.   Physical dependence is defined as the pre-
cipitation of a withdrawal syndrome upon abrupt termination of the
drug or after administration of a narcotic antagonist (naloxone). Clinically, the withdrawal symptoms include irritability, joint pain, chills
and hot flashes, anxiety, nausea, vomiting, lacrimation, rhinorrhea,
diaphoresis, abdominal cramps, and diarrhea. Withdrawal symptoms

TABLE 14-19   Clinical Signs of Inadequate Pain Control

Tachycardia in the absence of hypoxemia

Blood pressure changes

Dilated pupils

Diaphoresis

Grimacing

Restlessness

Guarding

✓ Since ventilator patients cannot communicate effectively, these clinical signs may be used to reflect inadequate pain control.

barbiturates: A group of drugs that depresses the central nervous system. Adverse effects are many, including alteration of the respiration, heart rate, blood pressure, and temperature. It is used in seizure disorders, control of elevated intracranial pressure.

✓ Barbiturates may be preferred in seizure disorders, control of elevated intracranial pressure.

may be avoided in physically dependent patients by gradual dosage reduction of the opiate (Hammack et al., 1994).

Psychological Dependence.   Psychological dependence is an additive behavior characterized by drug seeking, preoccupation with obtaining and using the drug, and drug use for other than analgesic purposes (euphoria).

ASSESSMENT OF ADEQUATE PAIN CONTROL

Pain assessment is important in ensuring adequate pain relief and enhancing patient recovery. Cooperative, awake, and alert patients may be assessed with pain intensity and pain distress scales. Unfortunately, ventilator patients are frequently unable to participate in their pain management plan. In this case, clinical signs such as tachycardia, blood pressure changes, dilated pupils, diaphoresis, grimacing, restlessness, and guarding may be signs that indicate inadequate analgesia (Table 14-19).

AGENTS FOR SEIZURES AND ELEVATED INTRACRANIAL PRESSURE (BARBITURATES)

Barbiturates, once widely used in critically ill patients for sedation and anxiolysis, have limited applications in patients on mechanical ventilation because of respiratory and cardiovascular depression. For sedative action, they have been replaced by safer drugs such as benzodiazepines. Barbiturates may be preferred in certain situations, such as seizure disorders, control of elevated intracranial pressure (normal ICP 8 to 12 mm Hg, <20 mm Hg in clinical practice).

Table 14-20 lists the selected barbiturates that are used in different situations because of the wide range of duration of action, ranging from ultrashort-acting (0.2 hour) to long-lasting (4 to 12 hours).

TABLE 14-20   Selected Barbiturates

NAMES	DURATION OF ACTION	DURATION OF HYPNOTIC* EFFECT
Thiopental Methohexital	Ultra short-acting	0.2 hour
Pentobarbital	Short-acting	1 to 4 hours
Amobarbital	Intermediate-acting	2 to 8 hours
Phenobarbital	Long-acting	4 to 12 hours

*The anesthetic dose is about three times the hypnotic dose; the lethal dose is about six times the hypnotic dose (Cottrell et al., 1995; Ziment, 1978).

MECHANISM OF ACTION

Barbiturates are capable of producing all levels of CNS depression, ranging from mild sedation to hypnosis to deep coma to death. As previously discussed in the benzodiazepine section, GABA is the most common CNS inhibitory neurotransmitter. The GABA receptor exists as a complex involving the benzodiazepine receptor, the barbiturate receptor, and the GABA receptor and its associated chloride ion channel (Figure 14-5) (Olson, 1988). Drug binding to this receptor complex facilitates GABA-mediated hyperpolarization of the neuron via an increase in chloride ion entry into the cell. This hyperpolarization makes the neuron more resistant to depolarization causing depression of CNS function. The importance of this cellular mechanism in producing the clinical effects of barbiturates is unclear.

☑ GABA-mediated hyperpolarization of the neuron makes the neuron more resistant to depolarization causing depression of CNS function.

Higher doses of barbiturates may directly activate the chloride ion channel independent of the barbiturate-GABA receptor complex (Levine, 1994). This results in a progressive depression of central nervous system function ranging from deep sedation to coma. When coma is induced, these agents are capable of decreasing cerebral metabolic oxygen consumption. Through autoregulation, the brain decreases cerebral blood flow thereby lowering intracranial pressure.

ADVERSE EFFECTS

These once widely used agents now have limited applications in critically ill patients because of dose-dependent cardiovascular and respiratory depression (Price-Roberts, 1984). Venodilation with peripheral pooling of blood, tachycardia, and depressed myocardial contractility may result in hypotension especially in elderly patients with poor cardiac function.

☑ Venodilation with peripheral pooling of blood, tachycardia, and depressed myocardial contractility may result in hypotension in patients with poor cardiac function.

Respiratory adverse effects to barbiturates include blunted ventilatory response to hypoxia and hypercapnia, reduced tidal volume and respiratory rate. Other adverse effects attributed to barbiturates include rashes and gastrointestinal upset.

DRUG INTERACTIONS

✔ Barbiturates increase the clearance of those drugs that are metabolized by the liver.

Barbiturates may induce tolerance as well as physical and psychologic dependence. These concepts have been discussed at length in the section on narcotic therapy. Another problem complicating barbiturate therapy is the potential for numerous drug interactions. When barbiturates are in use, liver metabolism of other drugs may be enhanced thus decreasing their effects. Caution should be exercised when adding to or deleting a drug from a therapeutic regimen containing a barbiturate, giving consideration to the possible need for dosage adjustment.

✔ Barbiturates do not relieve pain and may paradoxically heighten the sensation of pain.

Barbiturates do not relieve pain and may paradoxically heighten pain intensity (Dundee et al., 1988). Therefore it is necessary to reassess analgesic efficacy when these drugs are used in patients requiring analgesia.

OTHER AGENTS USED IN MECHANICAL VENTILATION

Other agents used in mechanical ventilation include propofol (for sedation and maintenance of anesthesia), haloperidol (for sedation and reduction of anxiety), and nitric oxide (for dilation of pulmonary vessels).

PROPOFOL

✔ Depending on the dosage, propofol provides a spectrum of CNS depression ranging from light sedation to deep general anesthesia.

Propofol (Diprivan) is an intravenous (IV) drug administered together with other anesthetics to produce and maintain anesthesia. A hypnotic effect is produced within 40 sec after a rapid IV bolus administration (1 to 2.5 mg/kg). The maintenance dose is 0.05 to 0.2 mg/kg/min by IV infusion (Reiss et al., 2001). Propofol is used to provide sedation in ventilator patients and induction and maintenance of anesthesia.

Mechanism of Action.   Propofol appears to enhance GABA-activated chloride ion channel function [for a complete discussion, see Sedatives and Antianxiety Agents (Benzodiazepines) in this chapter] (Fragen et al., 1992). The mechanism of action may involve a separate receptor recognition site or may involve a different mechanism from that previously discussed for barbiturates and benzodiazepines.

✔ Propofol is formulated in an oil-in-water vehicle and it could contribute a significant amount of calories from fat.

Adverse Effects.   Adverse reactions reported with propofol use include apnea, bradycardia, laryngospasm, bronchospasm, coughing, dyspnea, hypotension, and burning or pain at the site of infusion. Discoloration of the urine to green or red-brown may occur due to liver metabolites of propofol (Mirenda et al., 1995; Reiss et al., 2001).

Propofol is highly fat soluble and is formulated in an oil-in-water vehicle. The soybean oil in this vehicle could contribute a significant amount of calories from fat. Therefore, other sources of dietary intake

☑ Since fat emul-
sion provides an
excellent medium
for microbial growth,
strict aseptic tech-
niques are essential.

☑ Propofol has no
analgesic prop-
erties. Additional
analgesics are
needed for pain
control.

must be adjusted to compensate for the amount of fat infused. In addition, patients receiving propofol should be monitored for elevations
in serum triglycerides. Because fat emulsion provides an excellent
medium for microbial growth, and propofol contains no preservatives,
strict aseptic administration techniques are important to prevent
iatrogenic sepsis.

Clinical Considerations.   Propofol has no analgesic properties,
therefore attention must be paid to providing adequate analgesia in
patients requiring pain relief. When opioid analgesics are used in combination with a propofol additive, hypotension may occur.

Since propofol does not promote salivation or vomiting, its use can
be an advantage for intubated patients (Reiss et al., 2001). The rapid
onset and offset of sedation may be a disadvantage if patients are
allowed to awaken abruptly in pain or to great environmental disorientation (Levine, 1994). This problem can be avoided by decreasing
the infusion rate so the patient awakens slowly.

As discussed previously in the benzodiazepine section, monitoring
the level of sedation is important to avoid over- or undersedation.
The Ramsay Scale [refer to Sedatives and Antianxiety Agents
(Benzodiazepines) in this chapter for a discussion] or computer-
assisted cerebral function monitoring can be used to determine the
patient's level of sedation. The latter notes changes in brain function
on a real-time basis and with adequate training, the changes may be
interpreted by caregivers.

HALOPERIDOL

☑ Haloperidol
(Haldol) may be
effective in sedating
patients who have
concurrent agitation
and delirium caused
by use of sedatives.

Pharmacotherapy for sedation and anxiolysis may in some patients
paradoxically cause agitation and delirium. Haloperidol (Haldol)
may be effective in these situations. Delirium may be defined as a
reversible global impairment of cognitive processes manifested chiefly
by disorientation, impaired short-term memory, arousal, attention,
illusions, and hallucinations (McCartney et al., 1993). The initial
approach to a ventilator patient presenting with delirium should be a
search for reversible causes. See Table 14-21 for examples of reversible
causes of delirium.

Nonpharmacologic approaches such as repeated reorientation and
explanation (explain treatment plans to the patient), minimize environmental stress and enhance communication (written or hand signals
in intubated patients may also be helpful). Drug therapy should be
added to nonpharmacologic approaches if the latter are ineffective
and a reversible cause is not found.

Indications.   Haloperidol is primarily used in the critically ill ventilator patient for the control of agitation and delirium. The intravenous
route of administration is preferred in the intensive care setting
although the drug may be given intramuscularly or orally.

TABLE 14-21   Reversible Causes of Delirium

WITHDRAWAL OF MEDICATIONS	IMPROVEMENT OF CLINICAL CONDITIONS
Alcohol	Fever
Analgesics	Head injury
Anticholinergics	Hepatic failure
Anticonvulsants	Hyperparathyroidism and hypoparathyroidism
Antihistamines	Hyperthyroidism and hypothyroidism
Antihypertensives	Renal failure
Antiparkinsonian agents	
Cardiac drugs	
Corticosteroids	
Psychiatric agents	

Mechanism of Action.   An increase in dopamine release and metabolism have been postulated as one of the central nervous system derangements manifesting as agitation and delirium. Haloperidol blocks dopamine receptors in the central nervous system (limbic, basal ganglia, and brain stem) producing a calming effect (McEvoy, 1995). In addition, haloperidol blocks dopamine receptors in the chemoreceptor trigger zone that may be responsible for its **antiemetic** activity.

antiemetic: Preventing nausea and vomiting.

Adverse Effects.   Blockade of dopamine receptors in the central nervous system may interfere with normal motor function. These adverse effects are called extrapyramidal reactions (EPS) and may include unilateral cervical muscle contraction with neck twisting (torticollis), swollen tongue (laryngeal dystonia), jaw muscle spasm (trismus), and flexion of head and feet backward (opisthotonus) (McEvoy, 1995). EPS occurs much less frequently with IV haloperidol than that observed with intramuscular or oral therapy. The reason for this is currently unknown (Fish, 1991).

☑ Neck twisting, swollen tongue, jaw muscle spasm, and flexion of head and feet backward are some adverse effects of haloperidol.

Neuroleptic malignant syndrome is a rare, idiosyncratic, life-threatening reaction that may occur after a single dose of haloperidol. Hyperthermia, altered consciousness, labile blood pressure, diaphoresis, and tachyarrhythmias are suggestive of this condition (Simon, 1993).

Haloperidol may also prolong the electrocardiographic QT interval that on rare occasions can produce a polymorphic form of ventricular tachycardia known as torsade de pointes (Fish, 1991).

☑ Combined use of benzodiazepine, opioid, and haloperidol is often necessary for control of extremely agitated, delirious patients.

Clinical Considerations.   Combination therapy including a benzodiazepine, opioid, and haloperidol is often necessary for control of extremely agitated, delirious patients requiring critical care. The critical care team must be diligent in the search for reversible causes of agitation and delirium and if found, correct them whenever possible.

NITRIC OXIDE

Nitric oxide is endogenously synthesized in vascular endothelium from the amino acid L-arginine (Palmer et al., 1987). After being released from the endothelium, nitric oxide diffuses into vascular smooth muscle cells where it stimulates production of 3' 5'-cyclic guanosine monophosphate (cGMP). cGMP decreases the concentration of calcium in the muscle resulting in vasodilatation. Because nitric oxide is extremely labile (rapidly inactivated by hemoglobin) it causes only local regulation of endothelial tone without systemic hypotensive effects.

Indications. Inhaled nitric oxide (iNO) therapy has been used as a treatment or supportive modality for a variety of clinical conditions. Some of these conditions include persistent pulmonary hypertension and hypoxemic respiratory failure of the newborn (Abman & Kinsella, 1999), respiratory distress syndrome and hypoxemic respiratory failure of older infants and children (Dobyns et al., 1999), and adult respiratory distress syndrome (Burke-Martindale, 1998). In addition, iNO therapy has been effective in increasing pulmonary blood flow and oxygenation and improving systemic cardiopulmonary hemodynamics in infants (Ochikubo et al., 1997).

☑ Inhaled nitric oxide produces local vasodilation of vascular smooth muscles.

Mechanism of Action. Inhaled nitric oxide produces local vasodilation of vascular smooth muscles. Because the gas is delivered to alveolar units still presumably participating in gas exchange, these alveolar capillary units are preferentially vasodilated, diverting blood from hypoxic capillary beds with high vascular resistance (Stamler et al., 1992). The net physiologic results are reduction of pulmonary vascular resistance, reversal of hypoxic pulmonary vasoconstriction in unobstructed airway (improvement of V/Q matching), and improvement of oxygenation (Figure 14-6).

☑ Pulmonary vasodilation may reduce pulmonary vascular resistance, correct V/Q mismatch, and improve oxygenation.

Adverse Effects. Adverse effects of iNO therapy are dependent on the dosage and concentration of inhaled NO. When combined with oxygen, NO is converted to nitrogen dioxide (NO_2). NO_2 levels of higher than 10 ppm can cause cell damage, hemorrhage, pulmonary edema, and death. However, at therapeutic dosages (less than 2 ppm), adverse effects and toxicity caused by inhalation of NO are rare (Linberg & Rydgren, 1999; Wilkins et al., 2003).

☑ Nitric and nitrous acid are lung inflammatory by-products of nitric oxide therapy.

NO and NO_2 may be converted to nitric acid (HNO_3) and nitrous acid (HNO_2), respectively, both of which may cause lung inflammation (interstitial pneumonitis). Toxicology information on these compounds is primarily available from administration of various concentrations of NO and NO_2 to healthy animals or volunteers with normal lungs (Lunn, 1995). Further research is necessary to determine the adverse

Figure 14-6 (A) Ventilation/perfusion (V/Q) relationship of an obstructed airway and a normal airway. The perfusion to both is decreased because of hypoxic vasoconstriction. In the obstructed airway, V/Q is absent. In the unobstructed airway, a high V/Q (deadspace ventilation) is seen. (B) Inhalation of nitric oxide (NO) selectively dilates the pulmonary vessels of the ventilated alveoli, thus improving perfusion and restoring normal V/Q in unobstructed airway.

effects of prolonged exposure of NO and NO_2 in patients with lung diseases.

NO is inactivated by combining with hemoglobin to form methemoglobin (hemoglobin in blood oxidized to ferric form that is incapable of transporting oxygen). The amount formed during therapy depends on the amount of NO administered and the amount of methemoglobin eliminated by an enzyme (methemoglobin reductase). Partial or complete deficiencies of this enzyme may exist in some patients, predisposing them to methemoglobinemia. The signs and symptoms of methemoglobinemia are listed in Table 14-22 (Dabney, 1990).

TABLE 14-22   Signs and Symptoms of Methemoglobinemia

METHEMOGLOBIN CONCENTRATION	CLINICAL SIGNS AND SYMPTOMS
10% to 20%	Central cyanosis of trunk and limbs, usually asymptomatic
20% to 45%	CNS depression (headache, dizziness, fatigue, lethargy, syncope)
45% to 55%	Coma, arrhythmia, shock, convulsion
>70%	High risk of death

Other potential adverse effects of NO are inhibition of platelet aggregation and possible negative inotropic effect.

Clinical Considerations.   Most of the patients who receive iNO therapy are on mechanical ventilation. Two components are necessary for the delivery of NO to these patients: in-line monitoring of NO and NO_2, and a delivery source of NO gas (Wessel et al., 1994).

At this time, NO is regulated by the Food and Drug Administration and is available as an investigational agent. It is supplied as cylinders containing either 800 parts per million (ppm) or 2,200 ppm with nitrogen as the inert balance gas.

Delivery System and Dosage.   INOvent (INO Therapeutics, Inc. for North America and Europe; Datex-Ohmeda for elsewhere) is a U.S. FDA-approved delivery system for inhaled nitric oxide therapy. It works with a ventilator or anesthesia machine to deliver a constant percent of nitric oxide, regardless of the ventilator setting or mode. Alarms are built-in to ensure safe and reliable therapy with continuous monitoring of NO, NO_2, and O_2. The INOvent design also integrates with a system for delivering nitric oxide via a manual resuscitator. For current NO therapy and dosage information, see the Suggested Reading section at the end of the chapter.

SUMMARY

In mechanical ventilation, different drugs are used to (1) provide bronchodilation, (2) facilitate intubation, (3) relieve pain and anxiety, and (4) treat seizures or elevated intracranial pressure. These drugs can be very useful when they are used as directed. At the same time, they must be used with care, since adverse effects can be dangerous or even life-threatening. For this reason, practitioners are expected to have a thorough knowledge of the indications, contraindications, and adverse effects of the drugs that are administered to patients on mechanical ventilation.

Self-Assessment Questions

1. Bronchodilation may be induced by all of the following mechanisms *except*:

   A. stimulating the sympathetic branch of the autonomic nervous system.
   B. stimulating the parasympathetic branch of the autonomic nervous system.

   C. inhibiting the enzyme phosphodiesterase.
   D. inhibiting the parasympathetic branch of the autonomic nervous system.

2. A patient who has been using Theo-Dur at home states that she experiences palpitations, nausea, vomiting, headache, and agitation each time after taking the medication.

The proper management technique for this patient includes monitoring of the _____ level and titrating the dosage to a therapeutic range of _____.

A. serum theophylline, 5 to 15 mcg/mL   C. serum theophylline, 40 to 60 mcg/mL
B. corticosteroid, 5 to 15 mcg/mL   D. corticosteroid, 40 to 60 mcg/mL

3. An asthmatic patient who has been using Ventolin for several months complains of shortness of breath and states that "the Ventolin is not working any more." The physician asks for your suggestion. You would recommend a trial use of:

A. Proventil.   C. Brethine.
B. Alupent.   D. Vanceril.

4. Which of the following is *not* an indication for using a neuromuscular blocking agent?

A. relieve laryngeal spasm   C. facilitate endotracheal suctioning
B. maintain mechanical ventilation   D. enhance endotracheal intubation

5. Succinylcholine (Anectine, Quelicin) is a _____ neuromuscular blocking agent. It induces muscle blockade by _____.

A. depolarizing, binding to the receptor   C. depolarizing, competing for the
   sites and causing sustained   receptor sites and blocking the
   depolarization   action of acetylcholine
B. nondepolarizing, binding to the   D. nondepolarizing, competing for
   receptor sites and causing sustained   the receptor sites and blocking the
   depolarization   action of acetylcholine

6. All of the following are potential complications of a neuromuscular blocking agent *except*:

A. oversedation.   C. apnea.
B. prolonged muscle blockade.   D. bronchospasm.

7. A patient who has been given Norcuron 1 hour ago is recovering in the surgical intensive care unit. The physician wants to know whether neuromuscular blockade reversal has occurred. You would check all of the following *except*:

A. tongue protusion.   C. hand grip.
B. serum Anectine level.   D. head lift.

8. A ventilator patient has been receiving diazepam (Valium) for better tolerance of mechanical ventilation and related procedures. The cardiovascular adverse effects for his patient may include:

A. decreased cardiac output.   C. increased mean arterial pressure.
B. increased stroke volume.   D. increased systemic vascular
                                              resistance.

9. The Ramsay Scale is commonly used to assess the degree of:

   A. ventilation.   C. bronchodilation.
   B. pain.   D. sedation.

10. Inadequate pain control may lead to all of the following complications *except*:

   A. increased blood pressure.   C. decrease of lung function.
   B. increased immune function.   D. decrease of patient mobility.

11. A patient is given naloxone upon returning from surgery. You may conclude that the patient has received too much _____ during surgery.

   A. narcotic analgesic   C. benzodiazepine
   B. neuromuscular blocking agent   D. nitric oxide

12. For seizure disorders and control of elevated intracranial pressure, _____ may be useful.

   A. neuromuscular blocking agent   C. barbiturate
   B. nitric oxide   D. corticosteroid

13. Haloperidol (Haldol) should be considered for controlling agitation and delirium:

   A. as soon as a patient is placed on   C. when a patient experiences pain.
      mechanical ventilator.
   B. when narcotic analgesic is given   D. after reversible causes of delirium
      to a patient.   have been ruled out.

14. Among other applications, inhaled nitric oxide (iNO) is used to treat _____. When iNO is combined with oxygen, _____ is formed.

   A. pulmonary hypotension, nitrogen   C. pulmonary hypertension, nitrogen
      dioxide   dioxide
   B. pulmonary hypotension, nitrogen   D. pulmonary hypertension, nitrogen
      trioxide   trioxide

Answers to Self Assessment Questions

1. B. stimulating the parasympathetic branch of the autonomic nervous system.

2. A. serum theophylline, 5 to 15 mcg/mL

3. D. Vanceril.

4. C. facilitate endotracheal suctioning

5. A. depolarizing, binding to the receptor sites and causing sustained depolarization

6. A. oversedation.

7. B. serum Anectine level.

8. A. decreased cardiac output.

9. D. sedation.

10. B. Increased immune function.

11. A. narcotic analgesic

12. C. barbiturate

13. D. after reversible causes of delirium have been ruled out.

14. C. pulmonary hypertension, nitrogen dioxide.

References

Abman, S. H., & Kinsella, J. P. (1998). Inhaled nitric oxide therapy for pulmonary disease in pediatrics. *Curr Opin Pediatr, 10*(3), 236–242.

Brucera, E., et al. (1992). Organic hallucinosis in patients receiving high doses of opiates for cancer pain. *Pain, 48,* 397–399.

Burke-Martindale, C. H. (1998). Inhaled nitric oxide therapy for adult respiratory distress syndrome. *Crit Care Nurse, 18*(6), 21–27.

Cottrell, G., et al. (1995). *Pharmacology for respiratory care practitioners*. Philadelphia: F.A. Davis.

Dabney, B. J., et al. (1990). Evaluation and treatment of patients exposed to systemic asphyxiants. *Emerg Care Q, 6*(3), 65–80.

Dasta, J. F., et al. (1994). Pattern of prescribing and administering drugs for agitation and pain in patients in surgical intensive care unit. *Crit Care Med, 22,* 974–980.

Dobyns, E. L., Cornfield, D. N., Anas, N. G., et al. (1999). Multicenter randomized controlled trial of the effects of inhaled nitric oxide therapy on gas exchange in children with acute hypoxemic respiratory failure. *J Pediatr, 134*(4), 406– 412.

Dundee, J. W., et al. (1988). *Intravenous anaesthesia* (2nd ed.). New York: Churchill Livingstone.

Ebadi, M. (1993). *Pharmacology* (2nd ed.). Boston: Little, Brown and Co.

Fish, D. N. (1991). Treatment of delirium in the critically ill patient. *Clin Pharmacy, 10,* 456–466.

Foley, K. M. (1993). Changing concepts of tolerance to opioids: What the cancer patient has taught us. In C. R. Chapman & K. M. Foley (Eds.), *Current and emerging issues in cancer pain: Research and practice* (pp. 331–350). New York: Raven Press.

Forster, A., et al. (1980). Respiratory depression by midazolam and diazepam. *Anesthesiology, 53,* 494–497.

Fragen, R. J., et al. (1992). Nonopioid intravenous anesthetics. In P. G. Barash, B. F. Cullen, & R. K. Stoetling (Eds.), *Clinical Anesthesia* (pp. 385–412). Philadelphia: J.B. Lippincott.

Halloran, T. (1991). Use of sedation and neuromuscular paralysis during mechanical ventilation. *Crit Care Nur Clin of North Am, 3*(4), 651–657.

Hammack, J. E., et al. (1994). Use of orally administered opioids for cancer-related pain. *Mayo Clinic Proc, 69,* 384–390.

Hansen-Flaschen, J., et al. (1993). Neuromuscular blockade in the intensive care unit: More than we bargain for. *Am Rev of Respir Dis, 147*(1), 234–236.

Jacox, A., et al. (1994, March). Management of cancer pain. *Clinical Practice Guideline No. 9* AHCPR Publication No. 94-0592. Rockville, MD. Agency for Health Care Policy and Research, U. S. Department of Health and Human Services, Public Health Service.

Kee, J. L. (2001). *Laboratory and diagnostic tests with nursing implications* (6th ed.). Englewood Cliffs, NJ: Prentice-Hall.

Kinsella, J. P., & Abman, S. H. (1999). Recent developments in inhaled nitric oxide therapy of the newborn. *Curr Opin Pediatr, 11*(2), 121–125.

Kupfer, Y., et al. (1987). Disuse atrophy in a ventilated patient with status asthmaticus receiving neuromuscular blockade. *Crit Care Med, 15*(8), 795–799.

Levine, R. L. (1994). Pharmacology of intravenous sedatives and opioids in critically ill patients. *Crit Care Clin, 10,* 709–731.

Lindberg, L., & Rydgren, G. (1999). Production of nitrogen dioxide during nitric oxide therapy using the Servo Ventilator 300 during volume-controlled ventilation. *Acta Anaesthesiol Scand, 43*(3), 289–294.

Lunn, R. J. (1995). Inhaled nitric oxide therapy. *Mayo Clin Proc, 70*(3), 247–255.

Marik, P., Hogan, J., & Krikorian, J. (1999). A comparison of bronchodilator therapy delivered by nebulization and meter-dose inhaler in mechanically ventilated patients. *Chest, 115*(6), 1653–1657.

McCartney, J. R., et al. (1993). Understanding and managing behavioral disturbances in the ICU. *J Crit Illness,* 87–97.

McCartney, J. R., et al. (1994). Anxiety and delirium in the intensive care unit. *Crit Care Clin, 10,* 673–680.

McEvoy, G. K. (Ed.). (1995). *AHFS drug information.* Bethesda, MD: American Society of Health System Pharmacists.

Mirenda, J., et al. (1995). Propofol as used for sedation in the ICU. *Chest, 108,* 539–548.

Mohler, H., et al. (1977). Demonstration of benzodiazepine receptors in the central nervous system. *Science, 198,* 849–851.

Mohler, H., et al. (1988). The benzodiazepine receptor: A pharmacological control element of brain function. *Eur J Anaesthesiology,* (Suppl. 2), 15–24.

Mouloudi, E., Katsanoulas, K., Anastasaki, M., et al. (1998). Bronchodilator delivery by metered-dose inhaler in mechanically ventilated COPD patients: Influence of end-inspiratory pause. *Eur Respir J, 12*(1), 165–169.

NIH Publication No. 97-4051 (1997). U.S. Department of Health and Human Services, National Asthma Education and Prevention Program. *Expert panel report 2: Guidelines for the diagnosis and management of asthma.*

Ochikubo, C. G., Waffarn, F., & Turbow, R., et al. (1997). Echocardiographic evidence of improved hemodynamics during inhaled nitric oxide therapy for persistent pulmonary hypertension of the newborn. *Pediatr Cardiol, 18*(4), 282–287.

Olson, R. W. (1988). Barbiturates. *Int Anesthesiol Clin, 26,* 254.

Palmer, R. M., et al. (1987). Nitric oxide release accounts for the biological activity of endothelium-derived relaxing factor. *Nature, 327,* 425–526.

Price-Roberts, C. (1984). Cardiovascular and ventilatory effects of intrevenous anaesthetics. *Clin Anaesth 2,* 203.

Ramsay, M. A. E., et al. (1974). Controlled sedation with alphaloxone-alphadone. *Br Med J, 2,* 656–659.

Rau, J. L. (2002). *Respiratory care pharmacology* (6th ed.). St. Louis, MO: Mosby.

Reiss, B. S., et al. (2001). *Pharmacological aspects of nursing care* (6th ed.). Clifton Park, New York: Thomson Delmar Learning.

Reves, J. G., et al. (1990). Nonbarbiturate intravenous anesthetics. Chapter 9. In R. D. Miller (Ed.), *Anesthesia* (3rd ed.). New York: Churchill Livingstone.

Shelly, M. P., et al. (1986). Assessing sedation. *Crit Care Clin, 3,* 170–178.

Simon, H. B. (1993). Hyperthermia. *New Eng Journal of Medicine, 329,* 483–486.

Stamler, J. S., et al. (1992). Biochemistry of nitric oxide and its redox-activated forms. *Science, 258*, 1899–1902.

Strange, C., et al. (1997). Comparison of train-of-four and best clinical assessment during continuous paralysis. *Am J Respir Crit Care Med, 156*(5), 1556–1561.

Teeple, J. R. E. (1990). Pharmacology and physiology of narcotics. *Crit Care Clin, 6,* 255–282.

Tortora, G., et al. (2002). *Principles of anatomy and physiology* (10th ed.). New York: Wiley Textbooks.

Watling, S. M., et al. (1994). Prolonged paralysis in an intensive care unit patient after the use of a neuromuscular blockade. *Crit Care Nur, 22*(5), 884–891.

Wessel, D. L., et al. (1994). Delivery and monitoring of inhaled nitric oxide in patients with pulmonary hypertension. *Crit Care Med, 22,* 930–938.

Wheeler, A. P. (1993). Sedation, analgesia and paralysis in the intensive care unit. *Chest, 104,* 566–576.

Wilkins, R. L., et al. (2003). *Egan's fundamentals of respiratory care* (8th ed.). St. Louis, MO: Mosby.

Witek, T. J. (1994). *Pharmacology and therapeutics in respiratory care.* Philadelphia: W.B. Saunders.

Ziment, I. (1978). *Respiratory pharmacology and therapeutics.* Philadelphia: W.B. Saunders.

Suggested Reading

Acute Pain Management Guideline Panel. (1992, February). Acute pain management: Operative or medical procedures and trauma. *Clinical Practice Guideline.* AHCPR Pub. No. 92-0032. Rockville, MD: Agency for Health Care Policy and Research, U.S. Department of Health and Human Services, Public Health Service.

Johnson, J. (1990). Delirium in the elderly. *Emerg Med Clin N Amer, 8,* 255–265.

Kehlet, H. (1989). Surgical stress: The role of pain and analgesia. *Br J Anaesth, 63,* 189–195.

Klein, J. M. (2005). Present guidelines for nitric oxide (NO) therapy. Retrieved from http://www.vh.org/pediatric/provider/pediatrics/iowaneonatologyhandbook/pulmonary/presentnoguidelines.html

Murray, M. J. (1990). Pain problems in the ICU. *Crit Care Clin, 6,* 235–253.

Reves, J. G., et al. (1990). Nonbarbiturate intravenous anesthetics. Chapter 9. In R. D. Miller (Ed.), *Anesthesia* (3rd ed.). New York: Churchill Livingstone.

Simon, H. B. (1993). Hyperthermia. *New Eng J Med, 329,* 483–486.

Wattwil, M. (1989). Postoperative pain relief and gastrointestinal motility. *Acta Chir Scand, 550* (Suppl.), 140–145.

Westreich, L., et al. (1992). Delirium and acute psychosis. *Postgrad Med, 92,* 319–332.

CHAPTER FIFTEEN

WEANING FROM MECHANICAL VENTILATION

David W. Chang
James H. Hiers

OUTLINE

KEY TERMS

- compliance rate oxygenation and pressure (CROP) index
- pressure support ventilation (PSV)
- respiratory frequency to tidal volume (f/V$_T$) ratio

- simplified weaning index (SWI)
- SIMV (synchronized intermittent mandatory ventilation)
- T-tube weaning
- weaning procedure

INTRODUCTION

Weaning is the process of withdrawing mechanical ventilatory support and transferring the work of breathing from the ventilator to the patient. Weaning may be accomplished abruptly with the patient being directly transitioned from full ventilatory support to unassisted spontaneous breathing. This weaning approach is sometimes referred to as "taking the patient off the ventilator" or simply "discontinuing the ventilator."

Some patients can tolerate an abrupt termination of ventilatory support; this would include those who have been on the ventilator for a relatively short time (usually no more than 1 to 2 days) and who have also regained normal cardiopulmonary function. Examples include patients recovering from postanesthesia, drug overdose, and status asthmaticus.

For other patients, successful weaning requires a more gradual withdrawal of mechanical ventilatory support. Generally, the longer the patient has been on mechanical ventilation, the more gradual the weaning process should be. The process of gradually reducing mechanical ventilatory support must be individualized for each patient and the weaning process may take from days to weeks or even months. Indeed, some patients become ventilator dependent and may not be able to maintain adequate ventilation without mechanical assistance. Examples of these patients include high cervical spine (C-2) injury and some neuromuscular diseases.

DEFINITION OF WEANING SUCCESS AND FAILURE

☑ The process of gradually reducing mechanical ventilatory support must be individualized for each patient.

The ability to breathe spontaneously is the criterion to gauge the success or failure of weaning attempts. Weaning success means that a patient is able to maintain spontaneous breathing for a prescribed period of time. This usually leads to termination of mechanical ventilation. Weaning failure generally means that a patient is returned to mechanical ventilation after a period of unsustained spontaneous breathing.

WEANING SUCCESS

☑ Weaning suc-
cess is defined
as effective sponta-
neous breathing
without any mechan-
ical assistance for
24 hours or more.

Weaning success is defined as effective spontaneous breathing without any mechanical assistance for 24 hours or more (Fiastro et al., 1988; Morganroth et al., 1984). While the spontaneous breaths are unassisted by mechanical means, supplemental oxygen, bronchodilators, pressure support, or continuous positive airway pressure are often used to support and maintain adequate spontaneous ventilation and oxygenation.

Success Rate. Not all patients can be weaned from mechanical ventilation successfully on first attempt. In one study, the first weaning trial was successful in only 52% of 110 patients requiring mechanical ventilation (Pardee et al., 1984). The duration needed to wean a patient from mechanical ventilation may also vary greatly. Nett et al. (1984) reported that 15% of ventilator patients required more than 7 days to be weaned successfully.

☑ Since medical
patients often
have coexisting
problems, they usu-
ally take more time
to complete the
weaning process
than surgical
patients.

The success rate of weaning attempts is partly dependent on the patient population. It is generally more difficult to predict the weaning outcome of medical patients. Since medical patients often have coexisting problems, they usually take more time to complete the weaning process than surgical patients (Yang et al., 1991).

WEANING FAILURE

Weaning failure is harder to define than weaning success. This is because whenever a patient is placed back on the ventilator, weaning attempt has failed in one form or another. However, most studies have defined weaning failure on the basis of abnormal blood gases at the end of weaning trial or clinical deterioration to an unacceptable critical threshold (Sahn et al, 1973; Tobin et al., 1986). Signs of worsening clinical condition include diaphoresis, evidence of increasing respiratory effort, tachycardia, arrhythmias, and hypotension (Yang et al., 1991).

☑ Signs of wean-
ing failure
include abnormal
blood gases,
diaphoresis, increas-
ing respiratory
effort, tachycardia,
arrhythmias, and
hypotension.

Determining the threshold of abnormal blood gases and clinical condition can be a rather subjective process, depending on the background and experience of the physician. Also, the aggressiveness of one's weaning approach may also differ as to at what point the weaning trial has failed.

Since there are no simple objective measures for the assessment of weaning failure, it is defined here that weaning failure has occurred when the patient is returned to mechanical ventilation after any length of weaning trial.

Impact of Weaning Failure. It is obvious that patients who require prolonged ventilator support have a severe impact on the use of health care resources, including financial, physical, and human resources. In addition, the longer a patient stays on the ventilator, emotional and psychological pains also take a toll. For these reasons, different strategies have been devised to enhance the weaning process. These strategies are

TABLE 15-1   Conditions That May Hinder a Successful Weaning Outcome

CONDITIONS	EXAMPLES
Patient/pathophysiologic	Fever
	Infection
	Renal failure
	Sepsis
	Sleep deprivation
Cardiac/circulatory	Arrhythmias
	Blood pressure (high or low)
	Cardiac output (high or low)
	Fluid imbalance
Dietary/acid-base/electrolytes	Acid-base imbalance
	Electrolytes disturbance
	Anemia/dysfunctional hemoglobins

designed to minimize the use of our limited resources, and to keep the patients from the uncomfortable and sometimes painful diagnostic and therapeutic procedures associated with mechanical ventilation.

PATIENT CONDITION PRIOR TO WEANING

☑ Before weaning is attempted, the patient should be fully recovered and be able to assume spontaneous breathing.

Perhaps the first criterion to consider before any weaning attempt is to assess the patient's overall clinical condition. Two important questions pertaining to the patient's clinical condition are (1) Has the patient significantly recovered from the disease or injury that prompted the need for mechanical ventilation? and (2) Are there other clinical conditions that may interfere with the patient's ability to maintain the work of spontaneous breathing?

Assessment of the patient's overall clinical condition should include an evaluation of the clinical conditions in Table 15-1. Depending on the severity of these clinical conditions, they should be corrected or normalized prior to a weaning attempt.

WEANING CRITERIA

Weaning criteria are used to evaluate the readiness of a patient for weaning trial and the likelihood of weaning success. Weaning is more likely to succeed if a patient meets most of the criteria. On the other

TABLE 15-2   Common Weaning Criteria

CATEGORY	EXAMPLES	VALUES
Ventilatory criteria	Spontaneous breathing trial	Tolerates 30 to 120 min
	$PaCO_2$	<50 mm Hg with normal pH
	Vital capacity	>10 to 15 mL/kg
	Spontaneous V_T	>5 to 8 mL/kg
	Spontaneous RR (f)	<30/min
	Minute ventilation	<10 L
Oxygenation criteria	PaO_2 without PEEP	>60 mm Hg at F_IO_2 up to 0.4
	PaO_2 with PEEP	>100 mm Hg at F_IO_2 up to 0.4
	SaO_2	>90% at F_IO_2 up to 0.4
	Q_S/Q_T	<20%
	$P(A-a)O_2$	<350 mm Hg at F_IO_2 of 1.0
	PaO_2/F_IO_2	>200 mm Hg
Pulmonary reserve	Max. voluntary vent.	$2\times$ min vent at F_IO_2 up to 0.4
	Max. insp. pressure	>-20 to -30 cm H_2O in 20 sec
Pulmonary measurements	Static compliance	>30 mL/cm H_2O
	Airway Resistance	Observe trend
	V_D/V_T	<60%

(Data from Burton et al., 1997; Caruso et al., 1999; Girault et al., 1994; MacIntyre, 2004; Tobin et al., 1990; Yang et al., 1991.)

hand, if a patient can only meet one or two of the weaning criteria, the success rate is likely to be low.

Both subjective and objective measurements have been developed to determine a patient's readiness for weaning. The common weaning criteria are summarized in Table 15-2.

VENTILATORY CRITERIA

The ventilatory status of a patient may be used to evaluate the readiness and outcome of weaning attempts. Weaning success will be more likely if the patient can sustain an adequate ventilation. The generally accepted ventilatory weaning criteria include a $PaCO_2$ of less than 50 mm Hg with normal pH, a vital capacity of greater than 10 to 15 mL/kg, a spontaneous V_T of greater than 5 to 8 mL/kg, a spontaneous respiratory rate of less than 30/min, and a minute ventilation of less than 10 L with satisfactory blood gases.

☑ The $PaCO_2$ should be between 35 and 45 mm Hg and the pH between 7.35 and 7.45 (for COPD patients, the $PaCO_2$ may be around 50 mm Hg with a pH near 7.35).

$PaCO_2$.   The partial pressure of carbon dioxide in the arterial blood ($PaCO_2$) is the most reliable indicator of the patient's ventilatory status. Weaning from mechanical ventilation should be attempted only when the $PaCO_2$ is less than 50 mm Hg with a compensated pH (in the non-COPD patient).

In patients with normal lung functions, the $PaCO_2$ should be within the normal range of 35 to 45 mm Hg and the pH should be between 7.35 to 7.45. However, in COPD patients, the acceptable $PaCO_2$ may be slightly higher and the pH slightly lower, depending on the patient's normal values prior to mechanical ventilation (Millbern et al., 1978).

Vital Capacity and Spontaneous Tidal Volume. The mechanical condition of the lungs may be evaluated by measuring the vital capacity and spontaneous tidal volume. It is generally accepted that the minimal vital capacity and spontaneous tidal volume consistent with successful weaning are 10 to 15 mL/kg and 5 to 8 mL/kg, respectively (Pierson, 1982, 1983; Tahvanainen et al., 1983). The results of 11 studies indicate that spontaneous tidal volume averaged 368 mL in weaned patients but only averaged 277 mL in nonweaned patients (Jabour et al., 1991).

If the patient has been receiving full ventilatory support, it is advisable to allow the patient to breathe spontaneously for 3 min under close observation prior to measuring the vital capacity and spontaneous tidal volume. An equilibration period is needed to obtain the spontaneous effort based on the patient's actual respiratory requirement.

Unlike spontaneous tidal volume, vital capacity requires active patient effort and cooperation. Vital capacity measures the maximal amount of volume that the patient can expire following a maximal inspiration. For this reason, its validity is effort-dependent, and proper teaching and coaching are required for accurate measurements. Poor effort or inability to follow commands may result in lower than actual vital capacity measurement.

Spontaneous Respiratory Rate. For a successful weaning outcome, the spontaneous respiratory rate should be less than 30 to 35 breaths per minute while the corresponding $PaCO_2$ should be less than 50 mm Hg (Pierson, 1983; Tahvanainen et al., 1983). A rate of greater than 35 breaths per minute is associated with an increased work of breathing that probably cannot be sustained by the patient. Increases in spontaneous respiratory rate after discontinuation of mechanical ventilation are strongly associated with weaning failure (Jabour et al., 1991).

As with the spontaneous tidal volume measurement, if the patient has been receiving full ventilatory support, the patient should be allowed to breathe spontaneously for 3 min off the ventilator prior to measuring the spontaneous respiratory rate. This method allows the patient ample time to normalize the breathing pattern, thus more reflective of the patient's response to the respiratory requirements.

Minute Ventilation. The patient's minute volume (either spontaneous or assisted) should be *less* than 10 L/min for a successful weaning outcome (assuming the corresponding $PaCO_2$ is normal). A high minute ventilation requirement (>10 L) needed to normalize the $PaCO_2$ implies that the work of spontaneous breathing will be

---

☑ The minimal vital capacity and spontaneous tidal volume consistent with successful weaning are 10 to 15 mL/kg and 5 to 8 mL/kg, respectively.

☑ The vital capacity maneuver is effort dependent. Proper teaching and coaching are required for accurate and valid measurements.

☑ For a successful weaning outcome, the spontaneous respiratory rate should be less than 30 to 35 breaths per minute, while the corresponding $PaCO_2$ should be less than 50 mm Hg.

☑ The patient's minute volume should be *less* than 10 L/min for a successful weaning outcome.

excessive. The patient is unlikely to be able to sustain the increased work of breathing once the ventilator rate begins to reduce.

An excessive minute volume requirement may result from increased carbon dioxide production secondary to an increased metabolic rate, an increase in alveolar deadspace, or metabolic acidosis. Causes for increased carbon dioxide production include extensive burn injuries, an elevated body temperature, and sometimes overfeeding, especially with carbohydrate supplements. Alveolar deadspace will be increased if the alveolar ventilation exceeds the alveolar perfusion (V/Q > 0.8). This condition may occur when (1) the alveoli are overventilated as in hyperinflation of the lungs (e.g., emphysema) and (2) the pulmonary circulation is underperfused (e.g., pulmonary embolism, decreased cardiac output).

OXYGENATION CRITERIA

The oxygenation status of a patient may be used to evaluate the readiness and outcome of weaning attempts. Weaning success will be more likely if the patient is adequately oxygenated. The generally accepted oxygenation weaning criteria include a PaO_2 of greater than 60 mm Hg (or $SaO_2 > 90\%$) on an F_IO_2 of 0.40 or less (Barnes, 1994), an intrapulmonary shunt of less than 20%, an alveolar-arterial oxygen tension gradient [$P(A-a)O_2$] less than 350 mm Hg, and a PaO_2/F_IO_2 ratio greater than 200 mm Hg (Feeley et al., 1975; Girault et al., 1994).

 For a successful weaning outcome, the PaO_2 should be >60 mm Hg on $F_IO_2 \leqslant 40\%$.

PaO_2 and SaO_2. A PaO_2 of 60 mm Hg corresponds to an SaO_2 of about 90%. It is essential to note that in patients with anemia or increased level of dysfunctional hemoglobins (carboxyhemoglobin), the PaO_2 and SaO_2 do not reflect the true oxygenation status of the patient. In those instances, the arterial oxygen content (CaO_2) should be measured and used.

If pulse oximetry is used to monitor a patient's oxygenation status, the pulse oximetry O_2 saturation (SpO_2) should be kept in the mid-90s for allowance of machine inaccuracies because SpO_2 readings in critical care are accurate to within 2% to 4% of the SaO_2 (Malley, 1990).

Q_S/Q_T. The physiologic shunt to total perfusion (Q_S/Q_T) ratio is used to estimate how much pulmonary perfusion is wasted. Shunted pulmonary perfusion cannot take part in gas exchange due to lack of ventilation (e.g., atelectasis). The Q_S/Q_T ratio can be calculated as follows using the classic physiologic shunt equation:

See Appendix 1 for example.

$$\frac{Q_S}{Q_T} = \frac{(CcO_2 - CaO_2)}{(CcO_2 - CvO_2)}$$

Q_S/Q_T: Shunt percent in %
CcO_2: End-capillary oxygen content in vol%
CaO_2: Arterial oxygen content in vol%
CvO_2: Mixed venous oxygen content in vol%

✔️ For a successful weaning outcome, the Q_S/Q_T should be <20%.

In clinical settings, a calculated physiologic shunt of 10% or less is considered normal. Shunt of 10% to 20% indicates mild physiologic shunt, and shunt of 20% to 30% shows significant physiologic shunt. Greater than 30% shunt reflects critical and severe shunt (Malley, 1990; Shapiro et al., 1994).

Since physiologic shunt in mechanical ventilation is usually intrapulmonary in origin (inadequate ventilation in relation to pulmonary perfusion), weaning failure becomes very likely when spontaneous ventilation cannot keep up with the pulmonary perfusion. For this reason, significant and severe intrapulmonary shunt ($Q_S/Q_T > 20\%$) should be corrected in order to enhance the weaning process and secure a successful weaning outcome.

$P(A\text{-}a)O_2$. The alveolar-arterial oxygen tension gradient [$P(A\text{-}a)O_2$] is used to estimate the degree of hypoxemia and the degree of physiologic shunt. The $P(A\text{-}a)O_2$ gradient may be obtained by subtracting the measured PaO_2 from the calculated P_AO_2 value. This gradient is directly related to the degree of hypoxemia or shunt (a larger gradient reflects more severe hypoxemia or shunt).

✔️ See Appendix 1 for example of $P(A\text{-}a)O_2$.

The alveolar-arterial oxygen tension gradient [$P(A\text{-}a)O_2$] can be calculated as follows:

$$P(A\text{-}a)O_2 = P_AO_2 - PaO_2$$

$P(A\text{-}a)O_2$: Alveolar-arterial oxygen tension gradient in mm Hg
P_AO_2: Alveolar oxygen tension in mm Hg
PaO_2: Arterial oxygen tension in mm Hg

✔️ On 100% oxygen, every 50 mm Hg difference in $P(A\text{-}a)O_2$ approximates 2% physiologic shunt.

On room air, the $P(A\text{-}a)O_2$ should be less than 4 mm Hg for every 10 years in age. For example, the $P(A\text{-}a)O_2$ should be less than 24 for a 60-year-old patient. On 100% oxygen, every 50 mm Hg difference in $P(A\text{-}a)O_2$ approximates 2% physiologic shunt (Barnes, 1994; Burton et al., 1997; Shapiro et al., 1994).

✔️ For a successful weaning outcome, the $P(A\text{-}a)O_2$ should be <350 mm Hg while on 100% O_2.

In mechanical ventilation, $P(A\text{-}a)O_2$ of less than 350 mm Hg while on 100% oxygen suggests a strong likelihood of weaning success. $P(A\text{-}a)O_2$ of 350 mm Hg while on 100% oxygen approximates 14% shunt and values of greater than 350 mm Hg may hinder the weaning process. Any large $P(A\text{-}a)O_2$ gradient (>350 mm Hg) should be corrected prior to the weaning trial.

✔️ For a successful weaning outcome, the PaO_2/F_IO_2 index should be 150 mm Hg to 200 mm Hg or higher.

PaO_2/F_IO_2. The arterial oxygen tension to inspired oxygen concentration (PaO_2/F_IO_2) index is a simplified method for estimating the degree of intrapulmonary shunt. A PaO_2/F_IO_2 index of 150 mm Hg to 200 mm Hg or higher is indicative of normal physiologic shunt and compatible to successful weaning trial (Girault et al., 1994; Grap et al., 2003; MacIntyre et al., 2001).

✔️ See Appendix 1 for example of PaO_2/F_IO_2.

PULMONARY RESERVE

A patient's pulmonary reserve may be assessed by measuring the vital capacity (VC) and maximum inspiratory pressure (MIP). The VC and MIP maneuvers require active patient cooperation and therefore these two measurements are effort dependent. Proper explanation, vigorous coaching, and allowance of an equilibration period to stimulate active respiratory drive are the prerequisites for valid and meaningful measurements.

☑ For a successful weaning outcome, the patient should have a VC >10 to 15 mL/Kg.

Vital Capacity. The vital capacity (VC) reflects a patient's pulmonary reserve as it includes three lung volumes: inspiratory reserve volume, tidal volume, and expiratory reserve volume. VC measures the maximum amount of lung volume that the patient can exhale following maximal inspiration. Typically the patient is instructed to breathe in as deep as possible and exhale all the air into a spirometer. Unlike the forced vital capacity obtained in the pulmonary function lab, this VC maneuver does not require forceful exhalation. For successful weaning, the patient should have a VC of greater than 10 to 15 mL/kg (Pierson, 1982, 1983; Tahvanainen et al., 1983).

☑ For a successful weaning outcome, the patient should be able to generate an MIP of >−30 cm H_2O.

Maximum Inspiratory Pressure. The maximum inspiratory pressure (also called negative inspiratory force) is the amount of negative pressure that the patient can generate in 20 sec when inspiring against an occluded measuring device (negative pressure manometer) (Marini et al., 1986). If the patient is alert, explain the procedure and encourage the patient to attempt to inspire as forcibly as possible. The MIP is considered a measure of ventilatory muscle strength and weaning will likely be successful if the patient can generate an MIP of at least −30 cm H_2O. The results of 11 studies indicate that the MIP averaged −37 cm H_2O for weaned patients versus only −30 cm H_2O for nonweaned patients (Jabour et al., 1991).

PULMONARY MEASUREMENTS

Static compliance, airway resistance, and deadspace to tidal volume (V_D/V_T) ratio are three measurements that are not dependent on a patient's cooperation or effort. They are used to indicate the amount of pulmonary workload that is needed to support spontaneous ventilation. In general, low compliance, high airway resistance, and high V_D/V_T ratio all contribute to an increased workload. When these undesirable conditions reach the patient's threshold, they may hinder the weaning process and outcome.

☑ For a successful weaning outcome, the compliance should be ≥30 mL/cm H_2O.

Static Compliance. The static lung compliance is measured by dividing the patient's tidal volume (measured at the airway opening) by the difference in the plateau pressure and the PEEP. The lower the compliance, the greater the work of breathing will be. The minimal compliance value consistent with successful weaning is 30 mL/cm H_2O or greater (Hess et al., 1991).

See Appendix 1 for example.

pressure support ventilation (PSV): PSV is a mode in which the patient's spontaneous tidal volume is aug-mented by the appli-cation of a preset pressure plateau to the patient's airway for the duration of a spontaneous breath. It is used to reduce the work of breath-ing imposed by the endotracheal tube and ventilator circuit.

SIMV (synchronized intermittent manda-tory ventilation): A mode of ventilation that permits spon-taneous breaths between preset (mandatory) venti-lator breaths. The ventilator breaths are synchronized (mandatory breaths that may come slightly sooner or later) to coincide with the patient's next inspiratory effort.

For a successful weaning out-come, the V_D/V_T ratio should be ⩽60%.

See Appendix 1 for example.

The static lung compliance may be calculated as follows:

$$C_{ST} = \frac{\Delta V}{\Delta P}$$

C_{ST}: Static lung compliance in mL/cm H_2O
ΔV: Corrected tidal volume in mL
ΔP: Pressure change (Plateau–PEEP) in cm H_2O

Airway Resistance. The airway resistance can be calculated by dividing the difference in the peak inspiratory pressure and the plateau pressure by *constant* inspiratory flow rate. The normal range for airway resistance is 0.6 to 2.4 cm H_2O/L/sec (Burton et al., 1991) and higher for ventilator patients because of the associated pathologi-cal conditions (e.g., bronchospasm) and tubing resistance (e.g., endo-tracheal tube, ventilator circuit).

Although no critical weaning value for airway resistance has been established in the literature, the higher the airway resistance, the greater the work of breathing will be. The endotracheal (ET) tube contributes significantly to the airway resistance. The effect of resis-tance through the tube can be minimized by ensuring that the ET tube is not kinked or the suction catheter of a continuous suction system (Ballard suction system) is not protruding into the tube. Since retained secretions and bronchospasm contribute to the airway resistance, the patient's airways and lungs should be suctioned as needed. Use of bronchodilators also may be helpful to reduce or reverse bronchospasm.

Pressure support ventilation (PSV) has been used successfully in reducing the circuit and airway resistance during spontaneous breath-ing. This strategy may be used in conjunction with the **SIMV** mode or other modes that include spontaneous ventilation.

Deadspace/Tidal Volume (V_D/V_T) Ratio. The deadspace to tidal volume (V_D/V_T) ratio indicates the amount of each breath that is "wasted" or not being perfused by pulmonary circulation. The higher the V_D/V_T ratio, the greater the minute volume demand will be. The V_D/V_T ratio can be calculated as the partial pressure of arterial carbon dioxide minus the mean partial pressure of the carbon dioxide in the exhaled air divided by the arterial blood carbon dioxide tension. For a successful weaning outcome, the V_D/V_T ratio should be 60% or less (Fitzgerald et al., 1976).

The deadspace to tidal volume (V_D/V_T) ratio can be calculated as follows:

$$\frac{V_D}{V_T} = \frac{(PaCO_2 - P\bar{E}CO_2)}{PaCO_2}$$

V_D/V_T: Deadspace to tidal volume ratio in %
$PaCO_2$: Arterial carbon dioxide tension in mm Hg
$P\bar{E}CO_2$: Mixed expired carbon dioxide tension in mm Hg

TABLE 15-3   Combined Weaning Indices

TERM	NORMAL THRESHOLD FOR SUCCESSFUL WEANING
Respiratory frequency to tidal volume ratio (f/V_T)	<100 breaths/min/L
Simplified weaning index (SWI)	<9/min
Compliance rate oxygenation and pressure (CROP) index	≥13 mL/breaths/min

☑ For a successful weaning outcome, the f/V_T ratio should be <100 cycles/L.

respiratory frequency to tidal volume (f/V_T) ratio: The f/V_T ratio quantifies rapid shallow spontaneous breathing as the f (rate of spontaneous breathing) is divided by the V_T (depth of spontaneous breathing) in liters. Absence of rapid shallow breathing, as defined by an f/V_T ratio of less than 100 cycles/L, is a very accurate predictor of weaning success.

☑ Rapid shallow breathing induces inefficient, deadspace ventilation.

COMBINED WEANING INDICES

In the early 1990s, some of the independent weaning criteria were combined to make up a cumulative index of weaning. Among the indices developed, three are simple to use and highly accurate in predicting weaning success. They are (1) respiratory frequency to tidal volume (f/V_T) ratio, (2) simplified weaning index (SWI), and (3) compliance rate oxygenation and pressure (CROP) Index. These combined weaning indices and the threshold values for successful weaning are listed in Table 15-3.

RESPIRATORY FREQUENCY TO TIDAL VOLUME (f/V_T) RATIO

Failure of weaning may be related to the development of a spontaneous breathing pattern that is rapid (high respiratory rate) and shallow (low tidal volume). The ratio of spontaneous respiratory rate divided by the spontaneous tidal volume (in liters) has been used to evaluate the presence and severity of this breathing pattern (Jacob et al., 1997; Tobin et al., 1986; Vassilakopoulos et al., 1998; Yang et al., 1991).

Rapid shallow breathing is quantified as the f (number of breaths per minute) divided by the V_T in liters and this breathing pattern induces inefficient, deadspace ventilation. When the f/V_T ratio becomes greater than 100 cycles per liter, it suggests potential weaning failure. On the other hand, absence of rapid shallow breathing, as defined by an f/V_T ratio of less than 100 cycles per liter, is a very accurate predictor of weaning success (Yang et al., 1991).

To measure the f/V_T ratio, the patient is taken off the ventilator and allowed to breathe spontaneously for 3 min or until a stable breathing pattern has been established. The minute expired volume (V_E) and respiratory frequency (f) are measured. The V_T is calculated by dividing the V_E by f. The procedure for measuring and calculating the f/V_T is outlined in Table 15-4.

TABLE 15-4   Procedures to Obtain the f/V$_T$ Ratio

PROCEDURE

1. Allow the patient to stabilize spontaneous breathing pattern

2. Measure expired volume and respiratory frequency for 1 min

3. Divide minute volume by frequency (f) to obtain an average tidal volume (V$_T$) in liter

4. Divide f by V$_T$ to obtain f/V$_T$ ratio

NOTE: See Appendix 1 for example.

SIMPLIFIED WEANING INDEX (SWI)

Calculation of the simplified weaning index (SWI) is based on the following parameters: ventilator respiratory rate (f_{mv}), peak inspiratory pressure (PIP), PEEP, spontaneous maximum inspiratory pressure (MIP), and PaCO$_2$ while receiving full ventilatory support (PaCO$_{2\ mv}$). The SWI can be calculated as follows:

☑ See Appendix 1 for example.

$$SWI = \frac{f_{mv}\,(PIP - PEEP)}{MIP} \times \frac{PaCO_{2\ mv}}{40}$$

simplified weaning index (SWI): SWI evaluates a patient's ventilatory endurance and the efficiency of gas exchange. An SWI of less than 9/min is highly predictive (93%) of weaning success.

SWI: Simplified weaning index/min
f_{mv}: Ventilator frequency
PIP: Peak inspiratory pressure
PEEP: Positive end-expiratory pressure
MIP: Maximal inspiratory pressure
PaCO$_{2\ mv}$: Arterial CO$_2$ tension while on ventilator

When the SWI is less than 9/min, it is highly predictive (93%) of weaning success and when the SWI is greater than 11/min, there is a 95% probability of weaning failure (Jabour et al., 1991). SWI evaluates a patient's ventilatory endurance and the efficiency of gas exchange. Even though SWI is a simplified version of the original weaning index, its simplicity and exclusive use of common parameters make this index a practical method of assessment during routine ventilator care.

☑ When the SWI is less than 9/min, it is highly predictive (93%) of weaning success.

COMPLIANCE RATE OXYGENATION AND PRESSURE (CROP) INDEX

The Compliance Rate Oxygenation and Pressure (CROP) Index evaluates a patient's pulmonary gas exchange and the balance between respiratory demands and respiratory neuromuscular reserve. A CROP index of 13 mL/breaths/min or higher is predictive of weaning success (Yang et al., 1991). The CROP index is calculated as follows:

$$CROP = \frac{\left[C_{DYN} \times MIP \times \dfrac{PaO_2}{P_AO_2} \right]}{f}$$

compliance rate oxy-
genation and pres-
sure (CROP) index:
*The CROP index
evaluates a patient's
pulmonary gas
exchange and the
balance between res-
piratory demands
and respiratory neu-
romuscular reserve.
A CROP index of
13 mL/breaths/min or
higher is predictive
of weaning success.*

weaning procedure:
*A systemic approach
to wean a patient off
mechanical ventila-
tion by using a set
of clinical measure-
ments as a guide.*

spontaneous breath-
ing trial: *A technique
of weaning by alter-
nating the patient
between sponta-
neous breathing
(5 min) and full venti-
latory support
(30 to 180 min). The
duration of sponta-
neous breathing trial
is gradually
increased as toler-
ated by the patient.*

CROP: Compliance rate oxygenation and pressure index
C_{DYN} (dynamic compliance): Volume delivered/(Peak Inspiratory Pressure − PEEP)
MIP (maximum inspiratory pressure): Most negative pressure recorded during 20 sec of airway occlusion
PaO_2: Arterial oxygen tension
P_AO_2: Alveolar oxygen tension
f (frequency): Spontaneous respiratory rate per minute

WEANING PROCEDURE

The **weaning procedure** may be carried out by one or more of the following procedures: **Spontaneous breathing trial,** synchronized intermittent mandatory ventilation (SIMV), and pressure support ventilation (PSV) (Keenan, 2002). Selection of the weaning proce-dure is dependent on the patient's ability to breathe spontaneously and the level of muscular strength to overcome the airway resistance. The suggested steps for each procedure are outlined in Table 15-5.

SPONTANEOUS BREATHING TRIAL

Once a decision is made to proceed with weaning, the patient may be discontinued from full ventilator support and placed on a sponta-neous breathing mode via the ventilator or aerosol T-tube (Brigg's adapter) by progressively decreasing the level of ventilatory support (Dries, 1997; Vallverdu et al., 1998). The spontaneous breathing trial weaning method may be useful for patients with normal cardiopul-monary status who require only brief mechanical ventilation. Abrupt ter-mination of ventilatory support is usually reserved for patients who have been on the ventilator for a relatively short time (usually for no more than 2 to 3 days), and who appear to have substantially recovered from the need for mechanical ventilation. Generally speaking, the longer a patient has been on the ventilator, the longer the weaning process.

If a patient is to be weaned gradually, there are basically three approaches that may be used. Prior to the introduction of IMV/SIMV, the only available method of "gradually" weaning a patient was the technique of alternating the patient between spontaneous aerosol T-tube breathing and full ventilatory support (Nett et al., 1984). Initially, the patient is placed on a T-tube for 5 min and returned to full support for approximately 30 to 180 min. The process is repeated with progressively more time on the T-tube and less time on full sup-port until either the patient is weaned or it appears that the patient is not ready to be weaned.

Spontaneous breathing via the ventilator circuit is possible without an aerosol setup. The patient receives the humidity via the humidifica-tion system of the ventilator. With SIMV or PSV, the mandatory rate

TABLE 15-5   Common Weaning Procedures

PROCEDURE	STEPS
Spontaneous breathing	(1) May use new aerosol setup or existing ventilator circuit; (2) Let patient breathe spontaneously for up to 5 min every 30 to 180 min; (3) Return patient to mechanical ventilation to rest; (4) Increase duration of spontaneous breathing gradually for up to 2 hours each time; (5) If patient tolerates step (4), consider extubation when blood gases and vital signs are satisfactory.
SIMV	(1) Reduce SIMV (ventilator) rate by 1 to 3 breaths per min; (2) Monitor SpO_2, obtain ABG as needed; (3) Reduce SIMV rate further until a rate of close to zero is reached. This may take only hours for patients with normal cardiopulmonary functions but days for those with abnormal functions; (4) If patient tolerates step (3), consider extubation when blood gases and vital signs are satisfactory.
PSV	(1) PSV may be used in conjunction with spontaneous breathing or SIMV mode; (2) Start PSV at a level of 5 to 15 cm H_2O (up to 40 cm H_2O) to augment spontaneous V_T until a desired (high) V_T or (low) spontaneous RR is obtained; (3) Decrease pressure support (PS) level by 3 to 6 cm H_2O intervals until a level of close to zero is reached; (4) If patient tolerates step (3), consider extubation when blood gases and vital signs are satisfactory.

(Data from Downs et al., 1974; Girault et al., 1999; MacIntyre, 1986; Milbern et al., 1978; Nett et al., 1984; Tobin et al., 1990.)

or pressure support level is gradually reduced and the patient is compelled to assume a higher level of spontaneous breathing.

SIMV

SIMV weaning alleviates the need to alternate the patient on T-tube and ventilatory support. Since most current generation ventilators have an SIMV mode, weaning with the SIMV mode is probably the most simple and common weaning approach. Weaning with SIMV is accomplished by progressive decreases in the mandatory SIMV respiratory rate (usually 1 to 3 breaths per minute at each step). Arterial blood gases are measured after 30 min or more at that setting (Tobin et al., 1990). If the pH remains above 7.30 or 7.35 (Downs et al., 1974; Milbern et al., 1978), the SIMV rate is further reduced in further steps until a rate of close to zero is reached. The pace of SIMV weaning is dictated by the patient's tolerance. Some patients may be weaned using SIMV in a few hours while other patients may take much longer.

☑ The pace of SIMV weaning is dictated by the patient's tolerance.

PRESSURE SUPPORT VENTILATION

Pressure support ventilation (PSV) or its adjuncts (e.g., proportional pressure support, volume-assured pressure support) may be applied during weaning. PSV helps to reduce the airway resistance imposed on the patient by the endotracheal tube and ventilator circuit. Some clinicians advocate weaning with pressure support as a stand-alone mode. Regardless of the weaning approach used, it is advisable to provide full ventilatory support at night to allow the patient to rest (Barnes, 1994).

✔ **Weaning with PSV is done by starting the pressure support level at 5 to 15 cm H_2O and adjusting it gradually (up to 40 cm H_2O) until a desired spontaneous V_T or spontaneous rate (<25/min) is obtained.**

Weaning with PSV is done by starting the pressure support level at 5 to 15 cm H_2O and adjusting it gradually (up to 40 cm H_2O) until a desired V_T is obtained (MacIntyre, 1986). Some practitioners titrate the pressure support level until a desired spontaneous rate is reached, typically 25/min or less. This approach is clinically relevant since an increased spontaneous tidal volume corresponds with a decreased spontaneous rate. If the patient tolerates the weaning process well, the pressure support level is gradually decreased by 3 to 6 cm H_2O increments until a level of close to 0 cm H_2O is reached. Extubation may be considered when the patient's blood gases and vital signs remain satisfactory (Tobin et al., 1990).

Automatic Tube Compensation. Automatic tube compensation (ATC) is a mode in the Evita 4 ventilator (Dräger Medical) that reduces the airflow resistance imposed by the artificial airway (endotracheal or tracheostomy tube). It allows the patient to have a breathing pattern as if breathing spontaneously without an artificial airway. This type of compensation may facilitate breathing efficacy and reduce the work of breathing throughout the weaning process.

OTHER MODES OF PARTIAL VENTILATORY SUPPORT

Sometimes SIMV and PSV are used together in patients who have failed the spontaneous breathing trial or have done poorly with SIMV or PSV alone. Under these circumstances, there are other modes of ventilation that provide partial ventilatory support (MacIntyre et al., 2001). These modes are volume support, volume-assured pressure support, mandatory minute ventilation, and airway pressure-release ventilation. For a more detailed discussion on these modes, refer to Chapter 4, Operating Modes of Mechanical Ventilation.

Volume support (VS) and volume-assured pressure support (VAPS) are a form of PSV that "guarantees" a preset tidal volume. In VS, the pressure support level is adjusted automatically to achieve the target tidal volume. In VAPS, it guarantees a preset tidal volume by incorporating inspiratory pressure support ventilation (PSV) with conventional volume-assisted cycles (VAV). Unlike typical PSV, VAPS assures stable tidal volume in patients with irregular breathing patterns. By decreasing the rate, the work of breathing is shifted to the patient.

Mandatory minute ventilation (MMV) is a form of SIMV in which the minute ventilation is guaranteed. The ventilator adjusts the rate automatically to achieve the target minute ventilation. By decreasing the MMV level, the patient assumes more spontaneous breathing.

Airway pressure-release ventilation (APRV) has two pressure levels: the higher airway pressure (e.g., 10 cm H_2O) and the lower release pressure (usually 0 cm H_2O). The *tidal volume* is determined by the pressure gradient between the airway pressure and the release pressure. In APRV, exhalation occurs during pressure release and inhalation occurs when the pressure returns to the airway pressure.

TABLE 15-6 Weaning Protocol for Mechanical Ventilation

STEP	CRITERIA	RESULTS
1	Does the patient show: • Evidence of some reversal of underlying cause for ventilatory failure? • Presence of inspiratory effort? • Hemodynamic stability? (absence of myocardial ischemia, hypotension, use of vasopressor) • Adequate oxygenation and acid-base status? (PaO$_2$ / F$_I$O$_2$ >150 mm Hg, PEEP <8 cm H_2O and pH $\geqslant$7.25) • Light sedation or better? (brief eye contact to voice command)	If YES to *all five* questions, proceed to STEP 2. If NO to *any one* question, postpone weaning till next day.
2	Perform and measure rapid shallow breathing index (RSBI or f/V$_T$) with mandatory rate and pressure support at 0, PEEP $\leqslant$5cm H_2O, measurements taken $\geqslant$3 min of spontaneous breathing. • RSBI or f/V$_T$ <100 cycles/min/L?	If YES, proceed to STEP 3. If NO, postpone weaning till next day.
3	Can patient tolerate: • Spontaneous breathing trial for up to 120 minutes without termination*? (See termination criteria below)	If YES, proceed to ventilator discontinuance or evaluate for extubation. If NO, repeat weaning till next day.

(Adapted from Grap et al., 2003 with additional data from Ely et al., 2001; MacIntyre et al., 2001).
*Termination criteria: Spontaneous rate >35/min for 5 min; SpO2 <90%, Heart rate >140/min or 120% of baseline; Systolic pressure >180 mm Hg or <90 mm Hg; Signs of anxiety or use of accessory muscles.

Weaning may be done by decreasing the frequency of pressure release. When the frequency of pressure release is zero, the patient is essentially on a CPAP mode.

WEANING PROTOCOL

Weaning protocol and clinical practice guideline for weaning are primarily used to outline the standard of care for the purpose of weaning from mechanical ventilation. In general, they often include three elements: the patient condition in which weaning may be attempted, the detailed process of weaning, and the evaluation of weaning outcomes.

There are many weaning protocols published in the literatures or developed by individual hospitals or departments. Each of them can be useful when the elements of weaning are incorporated with sound clinical judgment and implementation. The criteria in the protocol should be used as guidelines only and must not be carried out using a "cookbook" approach. Individual patient differences must also be considered since disease processes and patient characteristics are just two of many variables that may affect the outcomes of a weaning protocol (Keenan, 2002). Weaning protocols range from simple to complex and Table 15-6 provides a simple weaning protocol for mechanical ventilation (Grap et al., 2003).

SIGNS OF WEANING FAILURE

Once the weaning process has been started, the previously described weaning criteria should be monitored closely to insure that the patient is tolerating the weaning attempt. When the mechanical ventilatory support is decreased, part of the work of breathing is shifted to the patient. The goal for the patient is to maintain the work of spontaneous breathing and adequate oxygenation. If the patient tolerates the increased work of breathing and the weaning criteria remain within acceptable limits, then the amount of ventilatory support (e.g., SIMV rate, pressure support level) should again be decreased. This process is repeated if the patient tolerates the decrease of ventilatory support. The weaning process should be stopped if the patient shows signs of muscle fatigue or ventilatory failure.

☑ Early signs of weaning failure include: tachypnea, use of accessory muscles and paradoxical abdominal movements, dyspnea, chest pain, chest-abdomen asynchrony, and diaphoresis.

Early signs of weaning failure include tachypnea, use of accessory muscles, and paradoxical abdominal movements (Cohen et al., 1982). Other indications that the patient cannot maintain the work of breathing may include dyspnea, chest pain, chest-abdomen asynchrony, diaphoresis, and delirium (Ely et al., 2004; Jabour et al., 1991). Some specific indicators of weaning failure are listed in Table 15-7.

TABLE 15-7 Indicators of Weaning Failure

INDICATORS	EXAMPLES
Blood Gases	Increasing $PaCO_2$ (>50 mm Hg) Decreasing pH (<7.30) Decreasing PaO_2 (<60 mm Hg) Decreasing SpO_2 (<90%) Decreasing PaO_2/F_IO_2 (<150 mm Hg)
Vital Signs	Changing blood pressures (20 mm Hg systolic or 10 mm Hg diastolic) Increasing heart rate (by 20/min, or >110/min) Abnormal ECG (presence of arrhythmias)
Respiratory Parameters	Decreasing V_T (< 250 mL) Increasing f (>30/min) Increasing f/V_T ratio (>100 cycles/L) Decreasing MIP (<−20 cm H_2O) Decreasing static compliance (<30 mL/cm H_2O) Increasing V_D/V_T (>60%)

(Data from Burton et al., 1997; Girault et al., 1994; Jabour et al., 1991; Jubran & Tobin, 1997; MacIntyre, et al., 2001; Tobin et al., 1990; Yang et al., 1991.)

If the patient does not tolerate the weaning procedure, the patient should be returned to full ventilatory support and be allowed to rest. The patient should then be reassessed in order to determine the cause of weaning failure. Appropriate therapies may then be applied before attempting the weaning process again.

CAUSES OF WEANING FAILURE

☑ Weaning failure is generally related to (1) increase of air flow resistance, (2) decrease of compliance, or (3) respiratory muscle fatigue.

Aside from the pathological conditions that lead to the need for mechanical ventilation, weaning failure may occur when the work of spontaneous breathing becomes too great for the patient to sustain. Weaning failure is generally related to (1) increase of air flow resistance, (2) decrease of compliance, or (3) respiratory muscle fatigue.

INCREASE OF AIR FLOW RESISTANCE

☑ ET tubes of size 8 or larger should be used to reduce the air flow resistance.

Normal subjects using an endotracheal (ET) tube have an increase of 54% to 240% in the work of breathing depending on the size of the ET tube and ventilator flow rate (Fiastro et al., 1988). An 8-mm ET tube has a cross-sectional area of 50 mm², which is slightly smaller than the average cross-sectional area of the adult glottis (66 mm²), the narrowest part of the airway (Kaplan et al., 1991). To minimize the effects of artificial airway on air flow resistance, ET tubes of size 8 or larger should be used when it is appropriate to the patient's size. In addition, the ET tube may be cut to about an inch from the patient's lips so as to minimize the air flow resistance contributed by the length of the ET tube. The cut section of the ET tube should be displayed prominently so others would not presume that the ET tube had been moved deep into the brochus.

Other strategies for decreasing airway resistance can easily be done by periodic monitoring of the ET tube for kinking or obstructions by secretions, or other devices attached to the ET tube such as a continuous suction catheter, heat and moisture exchanger (HME, "artificial nose") or end-tidal CO_2 monitor probe. Frequent suctioning to remove retained secretions and use of bronchodilators to relieve bronchospasm have also been used successfully to reduce the air flow resistance.

Other causes for an increased work of breathing include abdominal distention or an increased carbon dioxide production. Abdominal distention may contribute to an increased work of breathing if it interferes with diaphragmatic movement. An increased metabolic rate will result in an increased carbon dioxide production which in turn will require an increased minute volume to "blow off" the CO_2. An increased metabolic rate may be due to disease or injury or it may result from excessive nutritional support, especially if carbohydrate substrates are being administered.

Tracheal obstruction may cause weaning failure in patients requiring long-term mechanical ventilation (Rumbak et al., 1999). The ventilator may also contribute to an increased work of breathing. A low demand valve sensitivity, a relatively long demand valve response time, or an inadequate inspiratory flow delivered by the ventilator are conditions that increase the patient's work of breathing.

DECREASE OF COMPLIANCE

Abnormally low lung or thoracic compliance impairs the patient's ability to maintain efficient gas exchange. Low compliance makes lung expansion difficult and it is a major contributing factor to respiratory muscle fatigue and weaning failure.

In situations where the compliance gradually decreases (ARDS), the resultant refractory hypoxemia and increased work of breathing may lead to muscle fatigue and ventilatory failure. When this occurs to a patient undergoing a weaning trial, return to the mechanical ventilator is almost inevitable. Table 15-8 shows some examples that lead to a decreased compliance measurement.

RESPIRATORY MUSCLE FATIGUE

Respiratory work is a product of transpulmonary pressure and tidal volume. Studies have been done to evaluate the relationship between the work of breathing and a patient's ability to sustain adequate spontaneous ventilation.

☑ Low lung or thoracic compliance makes lung expansion difficult and it is a major contributing factor to respiratory muscle fatigue and weaning failure.

TABLE 15-8 Clinical Conditions That Decrease the Compliance

TYPE OF COMPLIANCE	CLINICAL CONDITIONS
Static compliance	Atelectasis
	ARDS
	Tension pneumothorax
	Obesity
	Retained secretions
Dynamic compliance	Bronchospasm
	Kinking of ET tube
	Airway obstruction

$$\text{Work of Breathing} = P_{TP} \text{ (Transpulmonary Pressure)} \times V_T \text{ (Tidal Volume)}$$

The transpulmonary pressure is increased in conditions of low compliance or high airway resistance. Normally a threshold work value of 1.6 kg.m/min or less is needed before ventilator-dependent patients can be weaned and assume adequate spontaneous breathing. Conditions leading to an increased work load such as low compliance and high air flow resistance may lead to respiratory muscle fatigue and eventual ventilatory failure. A threshold work value of 1.7 kg.m/min or higher is associated with failure to wean from mechanical ventilation (Tobin et al., 1990; Vassilakopoulos et al., 1996).

Another condition that may cause respiratory muscle dysfunction is due to muscular atrophy secondary to prolonged full ventilatory support and muscle disuse. Other factors that may contribute to muscle weakness include a low oxygen delivery (low O_2 content or cardiac output), insufficient nutrition or electrolyte imbalance, especially hypokalemia, hypophosphatemia, hypocalcemia, and hypomagnesemia (Knochel, 1982).

Retraining of atrophied muscles may be accomplished by short T-tube trials that improve strength. Pressure support ventilation may also be tried as it increases diaphragmatic endurance (Hess et al., 1991).

TERMINAL WEANING

☑ Terminal weaning is defined as withdrawal of mechanical ventilation that results in the death of a patient.

Terminal weaning is defined as withdrawal of mechanical ventilation that results in the death of a patient. This differs from withholding of mechanical ventilation in which the patient is not placed on any mechanical ventilatory support.

Decisions to withdraw life-support measures (e.g., mechanical ventilation, nutritional support) have become more common. This trend is partly due to the public's awareness of the quality of life issue, and their knowledge that death is an inevitable process in spite of medical advances, state-of-the-art medical equipment, and pulmonary rehabilitation strategies (Jacavone & Young, 1998). It is also partly due to the availability of living wills, and the choices available to the patient and family members.

When terminal weaning is considered, three concerns must be evaluated and discussed: (1) patient's informed request, (2) medical futility, and (3) reduction of pain and suffering (Campbell et al., 1992).

☑ **Discussions on a patient's informed consent should be done over a period of time so that emotion, pain, and other intangible factors do not interfere with an informed and valid decision.**

Patients' informed consent means that patients agree to have the life-sustaining devices removed, and that they understand the potential consequences (including death). No matter who initiates the discussion, the talk with patients must be open and honest. These discussions should also be done over a period of time so that emotion, pain, and other intangible factors do not interfere with an informed and valid decision.

☑ **Terminal weaning may be justified if medical intervention is futile or hopeless.**

Terminal weaning may be justified if medical intervention is futile or hopeless. The interpretation of futility (hopelessness) is based on the past experience of the primary physician or specialist. Schneiderman et al. (1990) suggested that medical treatments may be futile if physicians have concluded that in the last 100 similar cases the treatments were useless. This type of objective assessment may be helpful to the patients or family members who have reservations about terminal weaning and uncertainties about the chances of recovery.

☑ **Another reason for terminal weaning is to stop pain and suffering.**

Another reason for terminal weaning is to stop pain and suffering associated with the disease process (e.g., cancer), medical treatments (e.g., radiation therapy), medical procedures (e.g., arterial puncture, incisional wounds), and psychologic trauma (e.g., being totally dependent on others in an unfamiliar surrounding, unable to care for self, to eat, or talk).

Terminal weaning carries many ethical and legal implications. Each health care facility should have resource persons and standard protocol on terminal weaning available to the patients and family members, preferably before the needs arise. It is beyond the scope of this section to cover the ethical implications of terminal weaning in detail. The readers are encouraged to seek other available medical ethics books to learn more about this topic.

PRIOR TO WITHDRAWAL

Prior to withdrawal of mechanical ventilation, all immediate caregivers who are uncomfortable with the process should be offered an opportunity to withdraw from the case. The patient's pastor or hospital-based chaplain should be notified. The room should provide a quiet atmosphere and unlimited visitations. All invasive monitoring devices/alarms and unnecessary lines and tubes should be removed. The equipment and supplies that remain should include only the basic vital sign monitoring devices and intravenous access for administration of analgesics and sedatives.

WITHDRAWAL

During the withdrawal process, the family members should be offered an opportunity to stay with the patient. The attending physician and chaplain are encouraged to be present. Analgesics and sedatives should be provided in sufficient quantity for patient comfort and relief of anxiety. The ventilator settings may be adjusted to provide minimal support (e.g., oxygen and humidity only) while the patient is still intubated. If the ventilator is turned off at this point, the patient is extubated and put on an oxygen mask to minimize prolonged hypoxia (Seton Healthcare Network, 2005). The airway is suctioned to ease patient's breathing efforts. Document the events following completion of terminal weaning per physician's pronouncement.

SUMMARY

Weaning from mechanical ventilation is not always easy because there are no absolute criteria that can guarantee successful weaning every time. The criteria for weaning provided in this chapter are based on results of research studies and experience of clinical trials from many sources. While these criteria cannot be expected to be accurate at all times, they are nevertheless very useful as a guide and a starting point for weaning trials.

From the review of available literature, it is reasonable to conclude that the more weaning criteria that are met by a patient, the more likely the weaning process will be successful. In addition to using as many clinical parameters as feasible, the patient's progress should also be monitored on a continuing basis. From these data and trends, changes and adjustments on the ventilator and treatment plan may then be made to enhance the weaning outcome.

Self-Assessment Questions

1. Which of the following patient conditions is the *least important* consideration prior to weaning a patient off mechanical ventilation?

   A. frequent arrhythmias
   B. ventilatory failure

   C. severe acidosis
   D. use of positive end-expiratory pressure (PEEP)

2. The physician asks you to evaluate the following ventilatory parameters for possible weaning attempt on a 40-year-old patient. You would report to the physician that the only parameter that suggests successful weaning is:

   A. spontaneous RR (f) = 40/min.
   B. spontaneous V_T = 7 mL/kg.

   C. minute ventilation = 12 L.
   D. $PaCO_2$ = 55 mm Hg.

3. The oxygenation status of a 30-year-old postoperative patient shows: PaO_2 = 65 mm Hg, SaO_2 = 85%, Q_S/Q_T = 25%, PaO_2/F_IO_2 = 118 mm Hg, F_IO_2 = 55%. Based on these measurements, you would recommend to the physician that weaning _____ begin because _____ of the measurements presented above are within the normal limits for a weaning attempt.

   A. should, 50%   C. should not, none
   B. should, all   D. should not, 50%

4. All of the following pulmonary measurements suggest readiness for weaning attempt *except*:

   A. maximal inspiratory pressure =   C. static compliance = 32 mL/cm H_2O.
      −18 cm H_2O.
   B. V_D/V_T = 50%.   D. maximum voluntary ventilation =
                                                three times the minute ventilation.

5. A ventilator patient has the following oxygen content measurements: CcO_2 = 21.1 vol%, CaO_2 = 18.8 vol %. CvO_2 = 14.4 vol %. The calculated shunt is about _____ and it can be interpreted as _____ shunt.

   A. 3.4%, mild   C. 34%, severe
   B. 17%, significant   D. 66%, severe

6. The PaO_2 of a ventilator patient is 250 mm Hg on 100% oxygen. If the P_AO_2 is 680 mm Hg, what is the alveolar-arterial oxygen tension gradient? What is the estimated shunt if every 50% mm Hg difference approximates 2% shunt?

   A. 430 mm Hg, 8%   C. 940 mm Hg, 17%
   B. 430 mm Hg, 17%   D. 940 mm Hg, 34%

7. Ms. Warren, a ventilator patient recovering from drug overdose, has a PaO_2 of 76 mm Hg on 30% (0.30) oxygen. What is the PaO_2/F_IO_2 ratio? Is it normal based on the oxygenation criteria for weaning?

   A. 25.3, normal   C. 253, normal
   B. 25.3, abnormal   D. 253, abnormal

8. A patient has the following measurements while receiving mechanical ventilation: corrected tidal volume = 480 mL, peak airway pressure = 45 cm H_2O, plateau pressure = 30 cm H_2O, PEEP = 8 cm H_2O. What is the calculated static compliance? Is it normal based on the pulmonary measurement criteria for weaning?

   A. 11 mL/cm H_2O, normal   C. 22 mL/cm H_2O, normal
   B. 11 mL/cm H_2O, abnormal   D. 22 mL/cm H_2O, abnormal

9 to 11. Match the combined weaning indices with the normal threshold for a successful weaning attempt.

COMBINED WEANING INDEX	NORMAL THRESHOLD
9. Respiratory frequency to tidal volume ratio (f/V_T)	A. <9/min
10. Simplified weaning index (SWI)	B. ≥13 mL/cycles/min
11. Compliance rate oxygenation and pressure (CROP) index	C. <100 breaths/min/L

12. _____ weaning is done by reducing the ventilator respiratory rate gradually.

A. T-tube
B. Synchronized intermittent mandatory ventilation (SIMV)
C. Spontaneous breathing trial
D. Pressure support ventilation (PSV)

13. According to the weaning protocol for mechanical ventilation (Table 15-6), the spontaneous breathing trial should be up to _____ unless terminated earlier.

A. 5 min
B. 30 min
C. 2 hours
D. 8 hours

14. All of the following trends may be used as indicators of weaning failure with the *exception* of:

A. decreasing PaO_2.
B. increasing $PaCO_2$.
C. increasing V_T.
D. decreasing static compliance.

15. Terminal weaning is defined as _____ of mechanical ventilation that results in the _____ of a patient.

A. withholding, vegetative state
B. withholding, death
C. withdrawal, vegetative state
D. withdrawal, death

Answers to Self-Assessment Questions

1. D. use of positive end-expiratory pressure (PEEP)

2. B. spontaneous $V_T = 7$ mL/kg

3. C. should not, none

4. A. maximal inspiratory pressure $= -18$ cm H_2O

5. C. 34%, severe

6. B. 430 mm Hg, 17%

7. C. 253, normal

8. D. 22 mL/cm H_2O, abnormal

9. C. <100breaths/min/L

10. A. <9/min

11. B. >13 mL/cycles/min

12. B. Synchronized intermittent mandatory ventilation (SIMV)

13. C. 2 hours

14. C. increasing V_T

15. D. withdrawal, death

References

Barnes, T. A. (1994). *Core textbook of respiratory care practice* (2nd ed.). St. Louis, MO: Mosby.

Baumeister, B. L., et al. (1997). Evaluation of predictors of weaning from mechanical ventilation in pediatric patients. *Pediatr Pulmonol, 24*(5), 344–352.

Burton, G. G., et al. (1997). *Respiratory care: A guide to clinical practice* (4th ed.). Baltimore: Lippincott Williams & Wilkins.

Campbell, M. L., et al. (1992). Terminal weaning from mechanical ventilation: Ethical and practical considerations for patient management. *Am J Crit Care, 3,* 52–56.

Caruso, P., et al. (1999). The unidirectional valve is the best method to determine maximal inspiratory pressure during weaning. *Chest, 115*(4), 1096–1101.

Cohen, C. A., et al. (1982). Clinical manifestations of inspiratory muscle fatigue. *Am J Med, 73,* 308–316.

Downs, J. B., et al. (1974). Intermittent mandatory ventilation: An evaluation. *Arch Surg, 109,* 519–523.

Dries, D. J. (1997). Weaning from mechanical ventilation. *J Trauma, 43*(2), 372–384.

Ely, E. W., et al. (2001). Mechanical ventilator weaning protocols driven by nonphysician health-care professionals. *Chest, 120*, 454S–463S.

Ely, E. W., et al. (2004). Delirium as a predictor of mortality in mechanically ventilated patients in the intensive care unit. *JAMA, 291*(14),1753–1762.

Feeley, T. W., et al. (1975). Weaning from controlled ventilation and supplemental oxygen weaning from intermittent positive pressure ventilation. *N Engl J Med, 292,* 903–906.

Fiastro, J. F., et al. (1988). Comparison of standard parameters and the mechanical work of breathing in mechanically ventilated patients. *Chest, 94,* 232–238.

Fiastro, J. F., et al. (1988). Pressure support compensation for inspiratory work due to endotracheal tubes and demand continuous positive airway pressure. *Chest, 93,* 499–505.

Fitzgerald, L. M., et al. (1976). Weaning the patient from mechanical ventilation. *Heart Lung, 5,* 228–234.

Girault, C., et al. (1994). Weaning criteria from mechanical ventilation. *Monaldi Arch Chest Dis, 49*(2), 118–124.

Girault, C., et al. (1999). Noninvasive ventilation as a systematic extubation and weaning in acute-on-chronic respiratory failure: A prospective, randomized controlled study. *Am J Respir Crit Care Med, 160*(10), 86–92.

Grap, M. J., et al. (2003). Collaborative practice: Development, implementation, and evaluation of a weaning protocol for patients receiving mechanical ventilation. *J Crit* Care, *12,* 454–460.

Hess, D., et al. (1991). Mechanical ventilation: Initiation, management and weaning. In G. G. Burton, J. E. Hodgkin, J. J. Ward (Eds.), *Respiratory care: A guide to clinical practice* (3rd ed.). Philadelphia: J.B. Lippincott.

Jabour, E. R., et al. (1991). Evaluation of a new weaning index based on ventilatory endurance and the efficiency of gas exchange. *Am Rev Respir Dis, 144,* 531–537.

Jacavone, J., & Young, J. (1998). Use of pulmonary rehabilitation strategies to wean a difficult-to-wean patient: Case study. *Crit Care Nurse, 18*(6), 29–37.

Jacob, B., et al. (1997). The unassisted respiratory rate/tidal volume ratio accurately predicts weaning outcome in postoperative patients. *Crit Care Med, 25*(2), 253–257.

Jubran, A., & Tobin, M. J. (1997). Pathophysiologic basis of acute respiratory distress in patients who fail a trial of weaning from mechanical ventilation. *Am J Respir Crit Care Med, 155*(3), 906–915.

Kaplan, J. D., et al. (1991). Physiologic consequence of tracheal intubation. *Clin Chest Med, 12,* 425–432.

Keenan, S. P. (2002). Weaning protocols: Here to stay. *Lancet, 359,* 186–187.

Knochel, J. P. (1982). Neuromuscular manifestations of electrolyte disorders. *Am J Med, 72,* 521–533.

Lynn, J., et al. (2000). *Improving Care for the End of Life: A Sourcebook for Health Care Managers and Clinicians.* New York: Oxford University Press.

MacIntyre, N. R. (1986). Respiratory function during pressure support ventilation. *Chest, 89,* 677–683.

MacIntyre, N. R., et al. (2001). Evidence-based guidelines for weaning and discontinuing ventilatory support: A collective task force facilitated by the American College of Chest Physicians; the American Association for Respiratory Care; and the American College of Critical Care Medicine. *Chest, 120* (6 Suppl.), 375S–395S.

MacIntyre, N. R. (2004). Evidence-based ventilator weaning and discontinuation. *Respir Care, 49*(7), 830–836.

Malley, W. J. (1990). *Clinical blood gases—Application and noninvasive alternatives.* Philadelphia: W.B. Saunders.

Marini, J. J., et al. (1986). Estimation of inspiratory muscle strength in mechanically ventilated patients: The measurement of maximal inspiratory pressure. *J Crit Care, 1,* 32–38.

Millbern, S. M., et al. (1978). Evaluation of criteria for discontinuing mechanical ventilatory support. *Arch Surg, 113,* 1441–1443.

Morganroth, M. L., et al. (1984). Criteria for weaning from prolonged mechanical ventilation. *Arch Intern Med, 144,* 1012–1016.

Nett, L. M., et al. (1984). Weaning from mechanical ventilation: A prospective and review of techniques. In R. C. Bone (Ed.), *Critical care: A comprehensive approach.* Park Ridge, IL: American College of Chest Physicians.

Pardee, N. E., et al. (1984). Bedside evaluation of respiratory distress. *Chest, 85,* 203–206.

Pierson, D. J. (1982). Acute respiratory failure. In S. A. Sahn (Ed.), *Pulmonary emergencies.* New York: Churchill Livingstone.

Pierson, D. J. (1983). Weaning from mechanical ventilation in acute respiratory failure: Concepts, indications and techniques. *Respir Care, 28,* 646–662.

Rumbak, M. J., et al. (1999). Significant tracheal obstruction causing failure to wean in patients requiring prolonged mechanical ventilation: A forgotten complication of long-term mechanical ventilation. *Chest, 115*(4), 1092–1095.

Sahn, S. A., et al. (1973). Bedside criteria for discontinuation of mechanical ventilation. *Chest, 63,* 1002–1005.

Scheinhorn, D. J., et al. (2001). Outcomes in post-ICU mechanical ventilation—a therapist-implemented wearing protocol. *Chest, 119,* 236–242.

Schneiderman, L. J., et al. (1990). Medical futility: Its meaning and ethical implications. *Ann Intern Med, 112,* 949–954.

Seton Healthcare Network. (2005). Sourcebook: Improving care for the end of life: 4.4 ventilator withdrawal guidelines. Retrieved May 20, 2005, from http://www.mywhatever.com/cifwriter/content/66/4214.html.

Shapiro, B. A., et al. (1994). *Clinical application of blood gases* (5th ed.). St. Louis, MO: Mosby.

Tahvanainen, J., et al. (1983). Extubation criteria after weaning from intermittent mandatory ventilation and continuous positive airway pressure. *Crit Care Med, 11,* 702–707.

Tobin, M. J., et al. (1986). The pattern of breathing during successful and unsuccessful trials of weaning from mechanical ventilation. *Am Rev Respir Dis, 134,* 1111–1118.

Tobin, M. J., et al. (1990). Weaning from mechanical ventilation. *Crit Care Med, 6*(3), 725–747.

Vallverdú, I., et al. (1998). Clinical characteristics, respiratory functional parameters, and outcome of a two-hour T-piece trial in patients weaning from mechanical ventilation. *Am J Respir Crit Care Med, 158*(6), 1855–1862.

Vassilakopoulos, T., et al. (1996). Respiratory muscles and weaning failure. *Eur Respir J, 9*(11), 2383–2400.

Vassilakopoulos, T., et al. (1998). The tension-time index and the frequency/tidal volume ratio are the major pathophysiologic determinants of weaning failure and success. *Am J Respir Crit Care Med, 158*(2), 378–385.

Walsh, T. S., et al. (2004). Evaluation of simple criteria to predict successful weaning from mechanical ventilation in intensive care patients. *Br J Anaesth, 92*(6), 793–799.

Yang, K. L., et al. (1991). A prospective study of indexes predicting the outcome of trials of weaning from mechanical ventilation. *N Engl J Med, 324,* 1445–1450.

Suggested Reading

Terminal Weaning
American Thoracic Society Medical Section of the American Lung Association. (1991). Withholding and withdrawal of life-sustaining therapy. *Am Rev Respir Dis. 144,* 726–731.

Ankrom, M., et al. (2001). Elective discontinuation of life-sustaining mechanical ventilation on a chronic ventilator unit. *J Am Geriatr, 49*(11),1549–1554.

Bone, R. C., et al. (1990). ACCP/SCCM consensus panel: Ethical and moral guidelines for the initiation, continuation and withdrawal of intensive care. *Chest, 97,* 949–958.

Campbell, M. L., et al. (1999). Patient responses during rapid terminal weaning from mechanical ventilation: A prospective study. *Crit Care Med, 27*(1), 73–77.

Fair allocation of intensive care unit resources. (1997). Official Statement of the American Thoracic Society. *Am J Respir Crit Care Med 156,* 1282–1301.

Gilligan, T., & Raffin, T. A. (1996). Withdrawing life support: Extubation and prolonged terminal weans are inappropriate. *Crit Care Med, 24*(2), 352–353.

Robb, Y. A. (1997). Ethical considerations relating to terminal weaning in intensive care. *Intensive Crit Care Nurs, 13*(3), 156–162.

Tasota, F. J., & Hoffman, L. A. (1996). Terminal weaning from mechanical ventilation: Planning and process. *Crit Care Nurs Q, 19*(3), 36–51.

Therapist-driven Protocol

Ely, E. W., et al. (1999). Large scale implementation of a respiratory therapist-driven protocol for ventilator weaning. *Am J Respir Crit Care Med, 159*(2), 439–446.

Weaning Protocol

Scheinhorn, D. J., et al. (2001). Outcomes in post-ICU mechanical ventilation—a therapist-implemented weaning protocol. *Chest, 119,* 236–242.

Weaning

Chao, D. C., & Scheinhorn, D. J. (1998). Weaning from mechanical ventilation. *Crit Care Clin, 14*(4), 799–817, viii.

Cohen, J. D., et al. (2002). Automatic tube compensation-assisted respiratory rate to tidal volume ratio improves the prediction of weaning outcome. *Chest, 122,* 980–984.

Leitch, E. A., et al. (1996). Weaning and extubation in the intensive care unit. Clinical or index-driven approach? *Intensive Care Med, 22*(8), 752–759.

Martin, A. D., et al. (2002). Use of inspiratory muscle strength training to facilitate ventilator weaning*—a series of 10 consecutive patients. *Chest, 122,* 192–196.

Twibell, R., et al. (2003). Subjective perceptions and physiological variables during weaning from mechanical ventilation. *Am J Crit Care,* 12, 101–112.

Vassilakopoulos, T., et al. (1999). Weaning from mechanical ventilation. *J Crit Care, 14*(1), 39–62.

Weaning of Infant/Pediatric Patients
Baumeister, B. L., et al. (1997). Evaluation of predictors of weaning from mechanical ventilation in pediatric patients. *Pediatr Pulmonol 24*(5), 344–352.

Khan, N., et al. (1996). Predictors of extubation success and failure in mechanically ventilated infants and children. *Crit Care Med 24*(9), 1568–1579.

CHAPTER SIXTEEN

NEONATAL MECHANICAL VENTILATION

Kent B. Whitaker

OUTLINE

───── **KEY TERMS** ─────

- **compression factor**
- **extracorporeal membrane oxygenation (ECMO)**
- **high frequency ventilation (HFV)**
- **high frequency jet ventilation (HFJV)**
- **high frequency oscillatory ventilation (HFOV or HFO)**
- **mean airway pressure (mPaw)**

- **nasal CPAP (N-CPAP)**
- **peak inspiratory pressure**
- **power**
- **pressure-limited ventilation**
- **surfactant**
- **surfactant replacement**
- **volume-limited ventilation**

───── **INTRODUCTION** ─────

Neonatal mechanical ventilation provides a different kind of challenge to many respiratory care practitioners because neonates have different requirements (normal and abnormal physiologic and laboratory values) from those of adults. Also, caring for neonates often requires very different respiratory care equipment, supplies, and techniques. Above all, keen senses and the ability to observe and evaluate a neonate in distress is the most critical element because they cannot talk.

This chapter provides a working outline of respiratory care procedures in caring for a neonate in distress. These procedures focus on neonatal care and range from intubation and surfactant instillation immediately after birth to different types of neonatal mechanical ventilation.

✔ Intubation is indicated in (1) inadequate bag mask ventilation; (2) low heart rate during chest compressions; (3) endotracheal administration of epinephrine or surfactant;(4) the presence of meconium, slow heart rate (<100/min), poor respirations, or poor muscle tone; and (5) extreme prematurity.

INTUBATION

In most instances, intubation of the trachea is a necessary part of mechanical ventilation of the neonate. An exception is the use of external negative thoracic pressure. It is beyond the scope of this chapter to cover in detail the procedure for neonatal intubation. Those interested in studying the procedure are referred to any of the several excellent neonatal/pediatric respiratory texts for that information. Here, the indications, equipment, and general considerations of neonatal mechanical ventilation are covered.

INDICATIONS

Endotracheal intubation of a neonate is indicated when (1) prolonged or inadequate bag mask ventilation is present; (2) chest compressions are needed and heart rate remains low; (3) endotracheal administration of epinephrine or surfactant is indicated; (4) meconium

TABLE 16-1   Apgar Score

	0	1	2
Heart rate	None	Slow (<100) Irregular	Over 100
Respiratory effort	Apnea	Irregular, shallow Gasping	Good, crying
Muscle tone	Flaccid	Some flexion of extremities	Well flexed
Reflex	No response to stimulus	Grimace	Cough or sneeze
Color	Pale blue	Blue extremities, pink body	Pink all over

is present on delivery and the neonate has slow heart rate (<100/min), poor respirations, or poor muscle tone. Intubation needs to be done as quickly as possible to remove meconium from the airway before manual ventilation and (5) the neonate is extremely premature and mechanical ventilation is inevitable.

Other less common indications may include presence of obstructive lesions such as trachealmalacia, tracheal web, tracheal stenosis, laryngeal paralysis, and extrinsic masses. Diaphragmatic hernia, removal of pulmonary secretions, maintaining the airway during surgery, and obtaining tracheal aspirates also require intubation.

Table 16-1 shows the method of assessing a neonate using the Apgar score. Parameters listed are assigned points based on findings shown in the table. Resuscitation of a neonate should continue while scoring the Apgar. The scores range from 0 to 10 and they are given at 1 and 5 min. Scoring stops if the score is 7 or higher at 5 min. However, scoring should continue every 5 min up to 20 min if the score is less than 7.

EQUIPMENT

☑ Use laryngo-scope blade size 0 for most newborns and all preemies; size 1 for larger infants (>5 kg).

The basic equipment and supplies for intubation include a laryngoscope, an appropriately sized laryngoscope blade with light, and an endotracheal tube (ETT). Miller blade sizes of 00, 0, and 1 are used to intubate extremely premature infants to term infants. Selection of an ETT is based on the birth weight or gestational age of the neonate. Table 16-2 shows the guidelines for selecting an ETT for neonates as

TABLE 16-2   Selection of Neonatal Endotracheal Tubes

TUBE SIZE (ID MM)	WEIGHT	GESTATIONAL AGE
2.5	Below 1,000 g	Below 28 weeks
3.0	1,000 to 2,000 g	28 to 34 weeks
3.5	2,000 to 3,000 g	34 to 38 weeks
4.0	Above 3,000 g	Above 38 weeks

published in the Neonatal Resuscitation Program (NRP) by The American Academy of Pediatrics. These guidelines are commonly used by hospitals with labor and delivery rooms.

Other essential equipment may include airway suctioning devices, adhesive tape or other ETT stabilizers, flow inflating bag with 500- to 750-mL capacity and a flow restricting valve, airway manometer, and masks of different sizes (i.e., preemie, neonate, and infant) to fit over the tip of chin, mouth, and nose. An oxygen blender should be able to deliver a wide range of F_IO_2 (up to 100% oxygen) so that weaning from oxygen may be guided by SpO_2 readings and clinical signs. The SpO_2 for premature infants less than 32 weeks gestation should be maintained between 85% and 92% to minimize the incidence of retinopathy of prematurity (ROP).

Intubation.   Intubation should be done by two persons. The person performing the intubation should take care of the bag-mask ventilation, intubation, and stabilization of the ETT. Another person may help by passing the intubation equipment, monitoring the patient and vital signs, and timing of the procedure. Each intubation attempt should be limited to 20 sec and bag-mask ventilation with oxygen between attempts must be done to maintain acceptable SpO_2 and vital signs.

The infant should be put in a sniffing position and the blade should sweep the tongue from right to left as you place the blade into the infant's mouth. Gently slide the blade into the vallecula (if curve blade is used) and view the glottis area and vocal cords. Apply cricoid pressure as needed and advance the ETT through the vocal cords under direct vision.

If the tube has a vocal cord marking, it should be at or slightly beyond the vocal cords. If the tube does not have a vocal cord marking, a rule to estimate the depth of intubation is to add 6 to the body weight in kilograms (kg). For example, the depth of ETT for a 2-kg infant should be 8 cm (6 + 2) at the lips.

Listen for breath sounds and place a CO_2 detector on the ETT and verify change in color. However, a CO_2 detector should not be used when intubating for meconium removal. After confirming endotracheal placement, the tube is taped securely. A chest radiograph is done to confirm the depth of ETT placement.

> ✓ Each intubation attempt should be limited to 20 sec. Bag-mask ventilation with oxygen must be done between attempts.

> ✓ The vocal cord marking on the ETT should stop at or slightly beyond the vocal cords.

> ✓ A rule to estimate the depth of intubation is to add six to the body weight in kilograms.

> ✓ The primary cause of RDS is surfactant deficiency.

surfactant: *A natural phospholipid that lowers the surface tension of the lungs. Deficiency of surfactant causes high surface tension in the lungs and increases the work of breathing.*

SURFACTANT REPLACEMENT THERAPY

It has long been understood that the primary dysfunction in respiratory distress syndrome (RDS) is abnormally high alveolar surface tension resulting from a lack of pulmonary **surfactant.** Thus it became an item of major interest in the scientific community to develop a surfactant that can be administered to an infant to replace that which is lacking (Robertson & Halliday, 1998).

Naturally occurring surfactant is composed of several phospholipids and lipids, and four or more specific apoproteins. Each component appears to have its own distinct characteristics with regard to production, secretion, and removal (Jobe & Ilkegami, 1993). These factors have made it difficult to produce an ideal replacement surfactant.

Approximately 90% of surfactant is phospholipid, with phosphatidylcholine (PC) comprising 85% of the total amount. Roughly 60% of the PC is dipalmitoyl phosphatidylcholine (DPPC). It is the DPPC that allows surfactant to lower the surface tension of alveoli (Holm & Waring, 1993). The remaining phospholipids are phosphatidylglycerol (PG) and phosphatidylinositol (PI). Cholesterol is the predominant neutral lipid in surfactant. The four proteins found in surfactant, given the names of surfactant proteins A, B, C, and D (SP-A, etc.), make up 5% to 10% of the total. While small in quantity, their presence is essential for proper activity of pulmonary surfactant (Holm & Waring, 1993).

HISTORY

Early studies were discouraging as researchers could not find the right combination of components that formed an effective surfactant. Effective dosages and ideal method of delivery were two other questions that hindered the development of **surfactant replacement** therapy.

Early surfactants were made with DPPC and were nebulized into the trachea. This type of surfactant alone and *method* of delivery did not produce the desired results. Continued research and later studies of surfactant and its biochemical and biophysical properties illustrated the important role of the other proteins and lipids. New surfactants were developed that included the additional lipids and proteins. Delivery was changed from nebulization to direct instillation of surfactant into the trachea at higher dosages than had previously been used. These discoveries had dramatic effects on the surfactant-deficient premature lung, with rapid weaning of pressures and F_IO_2 levels.

INDICATIONS

There are two protocols for the administration of surfactant. Prophylactic use of surfactant is indicated for infants who are at high risk of developing RDS because of the short gestation and low body weight. However, routine treatment of infants at risk based on these two criteria may unnecessarily commit some infants to the complications of intubation, mechanical ventilation, and surfactant administration. At one medical institution, infants born at or less than 26 weeks gestation and with PaO_2/P_AO_2 <0.22 are treated prophylactically on a routine basis (British Columbia). Birth weight of less than 1,250 g is also an indication for prophylactic use of surfactant (Survanta drug insert). Since protocols vary greatly among institutions, infants with gestational age or birth weight outside these criteria must be monitored and evaluated for possible inclusion.

surfactant replacement: *Direct instillation of bovine-prepared surfactant (Survanta®) or synthetic surfactant (Exosurf Neonatal®) into the trachea.*

☑ Surfactant is given by direct instillation into the trachea.

☑ Prophylactic use of surfactant is indicated for infants who are at high risk of RDS, <26-week gestation, PaO_2/P_AO_2 <0.22, birth weight <1,250 g.

Prophylactic use of surfactant is also given to "micropreemies" in many neonatal intensive care units (NICUs). These infants are usually <30 weeks and typically weigh between 500 g and 1 kg. They are intubated in the delivery room within the first few minutes of birth and given surfactant through the ETT. Pulse oximeter, oxygen blender, and the use of Neopuff, a device that allows delivery of set PIP and PEEP, should be considered because of the rapid changes in oxygenation and compliance. In many cases, rapid weaning of F_IO_2 to 21% and minimal pressures for ventilation is possible due to the improvement in compliance. Many of these premature infants are extubated to CPAP or high flow devices such as Vapotherm.

☑ Therapeutic ("rescue") use of surfactant is indicated in RDS (grunting, nasal flaring, retraction), increasing oxygen or ventilatory requirement, positive chest radiograph.

Therapeutic ("rescue") use of surfactant is indicated for infants with established RDS (hyaline membrane disease or HMD). Eligible infants should fulfill the usual clinical and radiographic criteria for a diagnosis of RDS. The clinical signs may include grunting, nasal flaring, retraction, cyanosis along with an increasing oxygen or ventilatory requirement (i.e., from CPAP to mechanical ventilation). The bilateral ground glass appearance on the chest radiograph supports the diagnosis of RDS. Infants who exhibit these clinical and radiographic signs are usually born <34 weeks gestation and with an arterial/alveolar (PaO_2/P_AO_2) ratio of <0.22 (British Columbia). The indications for prophylactic and therapeutic use of surfactant are summarized in Table 16-3.

☑ Survanta® is produced by mincing cow lung tissue. Exosurf Neonatal® is a synthetic preparation.

TYPES OF SURFACTANT AND DOSAGES

Currently used surfactants fall into one of two categories: those obtained from mammalian lungs and those that are synthetically produced. Typically, the mammalian preparations contain all surfactant proteins, whereas the synthetics may be protein free (Exosurf®) or with proteins (KL4®, Venticute®). In addition to the group of synthetic

Table 16-3   Indications for Surfactant Administration

APPLICATION	CRITERIA
Prophylactic use	1. Gestational age ≤26 weeks 2. PaO_2/P_AO_2 <0.22 3. Birth weight of <1,250 g
Therapeutic (rescue) use	1. Signs of RDS (grunting, nasal flaring, retraction, cyanosis) 2. Positive chest radiograph for RDS (bilateral ground glass appearance) 3. Increasing oxygen requirement PaO_2/P_AO_2 <0.22 4. Increasing ventilatory requirement (from CPAP to mechanical ventilation) 5. Gestational age generally <34 weeks

✓ Exosurf® is a synthetic surfactant. Survanta®, Infasurf®, and Alveofact® are naturally produced from cow lung tissue. Curosurf® is produced from pig lung tissue.

surfactants that are FDA approved, there are two groups of natural surfactants that are extracted from cows and pigs. From the cow (bovine), lung tissues include Survanta®, Infasurf®, and Alveofact®. From the pig (porcine), lung tissue is Curosurf®. A randomized trial comparing the two surfactants failed to find any advantage in using synthetic or natural surfactant (Horbar et al., 1993). Both surfactants have been found to be effective for the treatment of RDS (Modanlou et al., 1997).

In prophylactic therapy Exosurf Neonatal® (colfosceril palmitate) is administered as soon as possible after birth in a dosage of 5 mL/kg birth weight. (Each milliliter of Exosurf contains 13.5 mg of active ingredient.) If necessary, second and third doses may be given 12 and 24 hours following the initial dose. For rescue therapy, 5 mL/kg is given, and it is followed by another dose 12 hours later (Witek & Schachter, 1994).

The recommended dosage for prophylactic or rescue use of Survanta (beractant) is 4 mL/kg birth weight. (Each milliliter of Survanta contains 25 mg of active ingredient.) Up to three additional doses of the same amount may be given at least 6 hours following the preceding dose (Witek & Schachter, 1994; Robertson & Halliday, 1998).

Table 16-4 summarizes the recommended dosages of some commonly used surfactants. The reader should refer to the current inserts from the manufacturers of each respective surfactant.

Table 16-4   Recommended Dosages of Common Surfactants

TYPE OF SURFACTANT	DOSAGE
Synthetic	
(A) Without proteins (Exosurf®)	Prophylactic dose = 5 mL/kg every 12 hours up to 3 total doses. (For prophylactic use, give first dose within 15 to 30 min of birth) Rescue dose = 5 mL/kg every 12 hours up to 2 total doses.
(B) With proteins (KL4®, Venticute®)	Not yet available in the United States
Natural	
(A) Bovine (Survanta®, Infasurf®, Alveofact®)	Survanta® = 4 mL/kg every 6 hours up to 4 total doses in the first 48 hours. Infasurf®: 3 mL/kg every 12 hours up to 3 doses.
(B) Porcine (Curosurf®)	Initial dose = 2.5 mL/kg. Up to 2 additional doses at 1.25 mL/kg at 12-hour intervals. (Divide each dose into two halves and give these halves doses 30 sec apart)

OUTCOMES

☑ Surfactant replacement therapy reduces the severity of RDS and the incidence of some related cardiopulmonary complications.

On the positive side, surfactant replacement therapy appears to reduce the severity of RDS, pulmonary interstitial emphysema (PIE), and epithelial necrosis (Pinar et al., 1994), reduces pulmonary vascular resistance (Kaapa et al., 1993), improves lung function (Yuksel et al., 1993), and has beneficial long-term effects on airway resistance (Abbasi et al., 1993). Additionally, synthetic surfactants may reduce the incidence of bronchopulmonary dysplasia (BPD) and intraventricular hemorrhage (IVH) (Long, 1993).

Another study found that surfactant replacement therapy may actually predispose an infant to intraventricular hemorrhage (IVH) (Gunkel & Banks, 1993). Surfactant replacement does not work on all patients. It is not known why some patients have a transient response and others have no response. Perhaps as knowledge and understanding continue to advance in this area, we will discover those unknown factors that prevent successful use of surfactant replacement therapy in all neonates.

Since coming of age, surfactant replacement therapy has dramatically decreased the mortality rate from RDS in neonates. It should now be considered the standard of care for those neonates with RDS who require mechanical ventilation (Parmigiani et al., 1997; Wiswell & Mendiola, 1993).

NASAL CPAP

Some infants may be able to ventilate satisfactorily but unable to maintain sufficient oxygenation in spite of traditional oxygen therapy. If the hypoxemia is due to mild to moderate intrapulmonary shunting, it may be corrected without mechanical ventilation. Use of nasal continuous positive airway pressure can be an effective strategy in the management of these infants.

USE OF NASAL CPAP

Continuous positive airway pressure (CPAP) was introduced in 1971. It reduces V/Q mismatch by improving the functional residual capacity and reducing intrapulmonary shunting. CPAP was originally administered via an endotracheal tube. Over the years, nasal CPAP (N-CPAP) was developed and has become a less risky procedure to reduce the F_IO_2 requirement and the need for mechanical ventilation. Recent publications have reported that N-CPAP is both feasible and effective in most very-low-birth-weight infants and those with acute respiratory failure. Early rescue treatment with surfactant replacement with a brief intubation has further increased the effectiveness of N-CPAP (Jeena et al., 2002; Malik et al., 2003).

A bubble CPAP device creates CPAP by an underwater seal with vigorous bubbling. Infants receiving CPAP by an underwater seal were observed to have chest vibration at frequencies similar to high-frequency ventilation (HFV). In one study, lower minute ventilation, respiratory rate, and better gas exchange were observed when compared with ventilator derived CPAP device. It suggests that the chest vibrations produced with bubble CPAP may have contributed to these findings (Lee et al., 1998).

Unlike the CPAP provided by a ventilator, the flow-generating CPAP device uses flow to maintain CPAP and has no exhalation valve. Since this CPAP device does not have an exhalation valve, it may offer a lower resistance than the ventilator CPAP. There are different size prongs and masks for better fitting on the patient. Different size hats are also available for stabilization of the flow-generating attachment. The expiratory limbs of the circuit hang loose and the flow is driven out the tube opening to room air. These devices can be noisy but the manufactures have produced a baffle device to reduce the noise level.

All CPAP devices should be humidified. One humidification manufacturer recommends setting temperature to 39°C because of cooling effects distal to the humidification system.

✔ The initial N-CPAP settings for most infants range from 4 to 7 cm H_2O with flow rates from 5 to 10 L/min.

The initial N-CPAP settings for most infants range from 4 to 7 cm H_2O with flow rates from 5 to 10 L/min. For infants with RDS, the CPAP level should start at 6 cm H_2O. If the infant with RDS is having recurrent apnea, persistent respiratory acidosis (pH less than 7.20), or unsatisfactory PaO_2 on >50% of oxygen with N-CPAP, intubation and surfactant therapy should be considered.

BASIC PRINCIPLES OF NEONATAL VENTILATION

Many mechanical ventilators used in the neonatal population are classified as pressure-limited ventilators. They generate a sufficient flow and deliver variable tidal volumes by a preset pressure limit. Recently, mechanical ventilation by monitoring and adjusting the volume setting (volume-limited ventilation) has gained popularity.

PRESSURE-LIMITED VENTILATION

pressure-limited ventilation: A preset PIP is used to deliver tidal volumes; the delivered volumes are variable.

In **pressure-limited ventilation,** a preset peak inspiratory pressure (PIP) is used to deliver the volume. The volume is variable depending on the changing compliance and airflow resistance characteristics of the infant. A decreasing compliance or an increasing airflow resistance requires a higher pressure to maintain the same tidal volume. As the patient's condition improves (increased compliance or decreased air-flow resistance), the pressure must be decreased to avoid excessive volume and possible barotrauma. An example of this observation is the successful use and response to surfactant replacement. The lung compliance of the infant increases dramatically and rapidly soon after surfactant administration. The PIP must be reduced accordingly to avoid overexpansion of the lungs.

VOLUME-LIMITED VENTILATION

volume-limited ventilation: A desired tidal volume is preset; the PIP needed to deliver each tidal volume is variable.

Volume-limited ventilation has gained popularity because the volume is preset using variable pressures. This strategy reduces the incidence of overexpansion of the lungs. For extremely low-birth-weight infants, some ventilators (e.g., Drager Babylog) can provide a tidal volume as low as 2 mL. This is an important feature when trying to maintain a range of 3 to 7mL/kg for extremely low-birth-weight infants (e.g., as low as 500 g birth weight). Typically, an initial tidal volume of 5 mL/kg is used to ventilate these infants and the volume may be titrated up or down to meet the infant's needs.

VENTILATOR CIRCUITS AND HUMIDIFIERS

During mechanical ventilation, some of the ventilator volume is "lost" within the circuit and humidifier and is not delivered to the patient. This wasted volume is called the compressible volume, and it is partly caused by the positive pressure applied to these devices. Higher inspiratory pressures would cause the circuit and humidifier to expand more than those under low pressures. This compressible volume is also dependent on the characteristics of the circuit and humidifier. More compliant circuits and humidifiers would expand more under positive pressure than those with low compliance.

compression factor: The amount of expansion of the ventilator circuit or humidifier during the inspiratory phase measured in mL/cm H_2O. This volume is considered "lost" and unavailable to the patient.

Circuit Compression Factor. Neonatal ventilator circuits should have a very low **compression factor**, that is, they should have minimal expansion when pressure is applied. A highly compliant circuit would expand under pressure and absorb a large portion of the volume of gas that should be delivered to the patient.

✔ To minimize volume loss the circuit and humidifier used in a neonatal ventilator should have small compressible volume.

Humidifiers. Humidifiers that are used in a neonatal circuit should possess a small compressible volume. The larger the compressible volume, the more expansion occurs under pressure. A humidifier with a large compressible volume may hold more volume than the patient's lungs and thus greatly reduce patient ventilation.

The ideal humidifiers for neonatal ventilation are types that incorporate a wick-type system, as they provide excellent warming and humidifying properties and maintain a low compressible volume.

Ideally, the temperature of the gas at the trachea should be 32°C to 34°C (Chatburn, 1991). When inspired gas temperature is measured at the patient connection, the humidifier must heat the gas 3 or 4 degrees above the desired temperature to overcome the loss of heat after the gas exits the humidifier. One problem that occurs in this type of ventilator circuit is condensation or "rain-out" inside the tubing.

Rain-out occurs when the warmed and humidified gas exits the humidifier and makes contact with the cooler walls of the tubing. This causes the gas temperature to decrease and condensation to occur on the tubing wall. The water accumulated in the ventilator tubing may result in increased airway resistance, a higher risk of contamination, and the potential of accidentally draining the water into the patient's lungs. A water trap placed in-line with the ventilator circuit helps to prevent these hazards.

☑ Heated wire inside the inspiratory tubing reduces condensation.

Heated Wire Circuits.   To counter this problem, many ventilator circuits have a heated wire inside the inspiratory tubing that runs from the humidifier to the patient connection, shown in Figure 16-1. The heated wire is attached to a servo-controller before its entry into the circuit. The temperature of the gas is measured as it exits the canister and is controlled by the humidifier. The temperature is again measured at the patient connection by the servo-controller.

Figure 16-1   Heated wire circuit inside the inspiratory tubing that runs from the humidifier to the patient connection. The heated wire is attached to a servo-controller for temperature regulation.

The servo heats the gas flow in the inspiratory tubing by heating the wire, which then heats the inspired gas. Both the humidifier and servo work from a negative feedback mechanism. The desired temperature becomes the set point and as the actual temperature drops below the set point, power is increased until the temperature returns to the desired level. Newer circuits heat the expiratory gas in addition to the inspiratory flow, thus minimizing condensation in the expiratory line.

One potential problem with this system is found when the distal temperature probe is placed at the patient connection inside a heated incubator that is set at a higher temperature than the humidifier. As the inspiratory tubing enters the incubator, the gas is heated to the set temperature of the incubator environment. This causes the temperature probe to sense the higher temperature and shut down the heater wires. The result is a buildup of condensation in the inspiratory tubing.

The solution to this problem is to place the distal temperature probe just outside the inlet to the incubator. This allows the probe to measure the actual gas temperature and properly regulate the heater wires (Chatburn, 1991).

✔ To prevent premature shutdown (power off) of the heated wire, the temperature probe should be placed just outside the inlet to the incubator.

INITIATION OF NEONATAL VENTILATOR SUPPORT

Indications for neonatal ventilatory support are based on three general guidelines: apnea, hypercapnia, and hypoxemia. These guidelines are similar to those used for adult patients. Unlike adult ventilators that use a tidal volume control to adjust the tidal volume, neonatal ventilators use a peak inspiratory pressure control to deliver an approximate tidal volume. Another unique feature of most neonatal ventilators includes the use of the flow rate and inspiratory time (I time) to fine tune the tidal volume. The suggested initial ventilatory parameters for neonatal mechanical ventilation are discussed below.

INDICATIONS FOR MECHANICAL VENTILATION

Mechanical ventilation provides two important physiologic functions. First, it maintains elastic properties and lung volumes by preventing or correcting atelectasis. By maintaining an appropriate FRC, lung compliance is maintained at an optimal level. Mechanical ventilation supplies the work of breathing when the patient is unable to maintain these properties. Second, mechanical ventilation provides the appropriate removal of CO_2 and the addition of inspired oxygen to meet the needs of the patient who cannot maintain arterial PO_2 or PCO_2 at normal levels.

Table 16-5   General Indications for Initiating Neonatal Mechanical Ventilation

1. Apnea
   a. due to prematurity
   b. secondary to intraventricular hemorrhage
   c. due to drug depression

2. $PaCO_2$ acutely rising with concurrent decrease in pH

3. PaO_2 acutely below 50 mm Hg with supplemental oxygen

☑ Mechanical ventilation is indicated when the patient is unable to maintain adequate blood gas values through sponta- neous breathing.

Mechanical ventilation is therefore indicated when any condition causes a decrease in lung function and an increase in work of breathing that the patient is unable to overcome and when the patient is unable to maintain normal blood gas values through spontaneous breathing. The exact criteria used to determine the need for mechanical ventilation are difficult to define. Each institution establishes its own criteria for initiation of mechanical ventilation. Table 16-5 lists general guidelines used to indicate the need for mechanical ventilation.

INITIAL VENTILATOR PARAMETERS

The initial ventilator parameters depend on several factors, including the gestational age and weight of the neonate, the disease state present, and the type of ventilator being used. In general, the smaller the neo- nate, the higher the incidence of barotrauma. Therefore, it is desirable to initiate these patients at lower pressures when possible. Disease states in which lung compliance is reduced will require higher initial pressures than normal or high compliance states. The presence of air leaks requires low pressures and high rates. Finally, some ventilators may require a tidal volume to be set by the operator.

☑ The initial pres- sure setting is higher for neonates with low compliance; lower for air leaks.

Initial Settings Based on Compliance.   With respect to the above factors, Table 16-6 lists suggested starting ventilation based on compliance.

Since the tidal volume (V_T) control is not available on a pressure-limited ventilator, an estimated V_T can be calculated by multiplying the inspiratory time (I time) and flow rate, as follows:

Example: On a pressure-limited ventilator, the I time and flow rate are set at 0.5 sec and 6 L/m, respectively. What is the calculated V_T?

V_T = I Time (second) × Flow Rate (liters per minute)
    = 0.5 sec × 6 L/m
    = 0.5 sec × 6000 mL/60 sec
    = 0.5 sec × 100 mL/sec
    = 50 mL

TABLE 16-6   Initial Settings for Neonatal Mechanical Ventilation Based on Compliance

PARAMETER	NORMAL COMPLIANCE	LOW COMPLIANCE
PIP	15 to 20 cm H_2O	20 to 40 cm H_2O
PEEP	3 to 5 cm H_2O	Up to 8 cm H_2O
V_T*	6 to 10 mL/kg	6 to 10 mL/kg
Rate	40/min	Up to 150/min (esp. with air leak)
Flow Rate	6 to 8 L/min	6 to 8 L/min
I Time	0.5 sec	Change according to rate to maintain an I:E ratio of 1:1
I:E Ratio	1:1.5 to 1:2	At least 1:1
F_IO_2	Set to keep patient pink using SpO_2 or transcutaneous pO_2 readings	Set to keep patient pink using SpO_2 or transcutaneous pO_2 readings. Use with appropriate PEEP level

On ventilators that are capable of providing a preset tidal volume (volume-controlled ventilation).
(Data from Bandy et al., 1992; Goldsmith et al., 1993; Deakins et al., 2001.)

Initial Settings Based on Birth Weight.   In addition to the previous settings for neonatal mechanical ventilation, alternatives are possible by using the birth weight as a guide to determine the initial settings. Four primary parameters are discussed here for volume-limited ventilation: rate, inspiratory time, volume, and PEEP.

The rate on many neonatal ventilators is controlled by adjusting the expiratory time after setting the flow and inspiratory time. Typically the rate is adjusted to 30 to 60/min for premature infants and 20 to 50/min for term infants, depending on the ventilatory requirement and disease process. The inspiratory time is usually set at 0.4 to 0.5 sec with a shorter inspiratory time when the rate is high or presence of air trapping. The PEEP is set between 4 to 7 cm H_2O depending on the oxygenation status of the infant. A higher PEEP is used initially if the infant's F_IO_2 requirement is high or evidence of severe intrapulmonary shunting. Table 16-7 provides the primary settings for volume-limited ventilation using birth weight as a guide.

TABLE 16-7   Initial Settings for Neonatal Mechanical Ventilation Based on Weight

PARAMETER	VERY LOW BIRTH WEIGHT	LOW BIRTH WEIGHT	TERM
Rate	30 to 60/min	30 to 60/min	20 to 50/min
Inspiratory time	Match gestational age >0.25 sec	Match gestational age, may add 10%	Match gestational age, may add 10%
Volume	3 to 7mL/kg starting at 5mL/kg	3 to 7mL/kg starting at 5mL/kg	3 to 7mL/kg starting at 5mL/kg
PEEP	4 to 7 cm H_2O	4 to 7 cm H_2O	4 to 7 cm H_2O

☑ The normal arterial blood gases for neonates are PO$_2$ >50 mm Hg, a PaCO$_2$ 35 to 45 mm Hg, and a pH between 7.3 to 7.45. For capillary samples, a lower PO$_2$ is acceptable.

Once mechanical ventilation is initiated, the ventilator settings are fine tuned until appropriate arterial blood gases are achieved. Blood gas measurement can be achieved by obtaining arterial blood from a peripheral or umbilical artery catheter (UAC), peripheral artery puncture, or capillary blood from a finger or heel stick. Under most circumstances, a PaO$_2$ >50 mm Hg, a PaCO$_2$ 35 to 45 mm Hg, and a pH between 7.3 to 7.45 are acceptable for a UAC sample. An appropriately done capillary sample will roughly correlate with arterial PCO$_2$, pH and HCO$_3^-$, and thus share the same acceptable values. A capillary PO$_2$ is usually not acceptable as a determinant of oxygenation status and requires the use of a pulse oximeter or transcutaneous PO$_2$ monitor. Common exceptions to these values are in the case of chronic lung disease patients such as pulmonary interstitial emphysema in which higher PaCO$_2$ are acceptable, and patients treated for pulmonary hypertension, where high PO$_2$ low PCO$_2$ and high pH are used.

high frequency ventilation (HFV): A type of ventilation that uses very high frequencies. It is subdivided into three categories: high frequency positive pressure ventilation (60 to 150 cycles per minute); high frequency jet ventilation (240 to 660 cycles per minute); and high frequency oscillatory ventilation (480 to 1,800 cycles per minute).

HIGH FREQUENCY VENTILATION (HFV)

Since the explosion of research in neonatal medicine started some 20 years ago, there is an ongoing search for a better method of ventilation to maintain adequate blood gas levels without inflicting damage on the premature lung. Several exciting methods have evolved to address these concerns.

The normally held understanding of ventilation is that the tidal volume must exceed the amount of physiologic deadspace for alveolar ventilation to occur. Conventional ventilation utilizes this principle by inflating the patient's lungs with a tidal volume that exceeds deadspace and inflates the alveoli. Expiration then occurs by the passive recoil of the thorax and lung.

High frequency ventilation (HFV) is a ventilation technique that delivers small tidal volumes at very high frequencies. Early studies involving HFV showed that adequate ventilation occurred even when tidal volumes far below deadspace were used (Carlo & Chatburn, 1988).

☑ HFV is a technique of ventilation that delivers small tidal volumes at very high frequencies.

The major advantage of delivering small tidal volumes is that it can be done at relatively low pressures, greatly reducing the risk of barotrauma. Despite the fact that HFV offers the advantage of oxygenation and ventilation at a lower risk of barotrauma, it has not been shown to be superior to conventional ventilation and its use is often limited to those situations in which conventional ventilation has failed. It appears to be most useful in treating RDS and pneumonia (Clark, 1994).

☑ HFV uses low pressures to deliver small tidal volumes. This reduces the risk of barotrauma.

HFV is delivered at rates between 150 and 3,000 cycles per minute (breaths per minute). The major types of HFV are categorized by the frequency of ventilation and the method with which the tidal volume is delivered. The three categories examined here are high frequency positive pressure ventilation, high frequency jet ventilation, and high frequency oscillation (Table 16-8).

TABLE 16-8   Classification of High Frequency Ventilation

TYPE OF HIGH FREQUENCY VENTILATOR	FREQUENCY (HERTZ)*	FREQUENCY (CYCLES PER MIN)
High frequency positive pressure ventilation (HFPPV)	1 to 2.5 Hz	60 to 150
High frequency jet ventilation (HFJV)	4 to 11 Hz	240 to 660
High frequency oscillatory ventilation (HFOV or HFO)	8 to 30 Hz	480 to 1800

1 Hertz (Hz) = 1 cycle per sec or 60 cycles per min

HIGH FREQUENCY POSITIVE PRESSURE VENTILATION (HFPPV)

High frequency positive pressure ventilation (HFPPV) is simply conventional ventilatory breaths delivered at rates between 60 and 150 breaths per minute (1 to 2.5 Hz). The delivery of tidal volume during HFPPV appears to occur via convective air movement, in which tidal volume exceeds deadspace (Boynton, 1986). Modern neonatal ventilators can deliver HFPPV at rates up to 150/minute.

Indications.   HFPPV is indicated on those patients who are hypoxemic or hypercapnic despite adequate and appropriate conventional ventilation. Studies have shown a reduction in $PaCO_2$ and in F_IO_2 when HFPPV was used on these patients. These studies additionally showed a lower incidence of pneumothoraces in the neonates ventilated with HFPPV when compared to those receiving conventional ventilation (Boynton, 1986). There are also studies that have shown that fighting the ventilator by the neonate may be eliminated at ventilatory rates of 100 to 120 breaths per minute (Milner & Hoskins, 1989).

Clinical Use.   In the presence of severely noncompliant lungs, increases in peak inspiratory pressure may reach dangerous levels before an adequate tidal volume is achieved. In these cases, the rate is increased to increase minute ventilation, allowing the peak pressure to remain lower. As rates increase, the inspiratory time is decreased to allow adequate exhalation of the tidal volume. This requires that time constants be low to allow exhalation and prevent air trapping. Continuous monitoring of $PaCO_2$ and PaO_2 will help the practitioner achieve the rate needed to attain the desired minute ventilation.

Hazards.   As the rate of positive pressure breaths increases, the **mean airway pressure (mPaw)** increases concurrently. The increasing mPaw greatly heightens the risk for barotrauma and cardiac compromise.

☑ HFPPV is indicated on those patients who are hypoxemic or hypercapnic despite adequate and appropriate conventional ventilation.

mean airway pressure (mPaw): The average airway pressure during a complete respiratory cycle. It is directly affected by the respiratory rate, inspiratory time, peak inspiratory pressure, and positive end-expiratory pressure.

☑ HFPPV increases the risk of barotrauma and cardiac compromise.

The neonate is also at a higher risk of developing intracranial bleeding with increasing mPaw. The ability to suction the airway is diminished, as even short-term removal from the ventilator may result in severe hypoxemia and hypercapnia.

 See Appendix 1 for example.

$$mPaw = \left[\left(\frac{RR \times I\ time}{60} \right) \times (PIP - PEEP) \right] + PEEP$$

mPaw: Mean airway pressure
RR: Respiratory rate
I time: Inspiratory time
PIP: Peak inspiratory pressure
PEEP: Positive end-expiratory pressure

high frequency jet ventilation (HFJV): Ventilation through a specially designed endotracheal tube, generally at a rate between 240 and 660/min (4 to 11 Hz).

HIGH FREQUENCY JET VENTILATION (HFJV)

High frequency jet ventilators generally operate at rates between 240 and 660/min (4 to 11 Hz). The high frequency jet ventilator delivers a high pressure pulse of gas to the patient's airway. This is done through a special adaptor attached to the endotracheal tube, or through a specially designed endotracheal tube that allows the pulsed gas to exit inside the endotracheal tube, depicted in Figure 16-2.

 The indications for using HFJV include severe pulmonary disease that is complicated by air leaks and other pulmonary problems.

Indications.   The indications for using HFJV include severe pulmonary disease that is complicated by air leaks, pulmonary hypoplasia, restrictive lung disease, and persistent pulmonary hypertension (Gordin, 1989).

Clinical Use.   HFJV is used in tandem with conventional ventilators. The purpose of the conventional ventilator is threefold. First, it provides

Figure 16-2   The high frequency jet ventilator (HFJV) delivers a high pressure pulse of gas to the patient's airway through a specially designed endotracheal tube that allows the pulsed gas to exit inside the endotracheal tube.

occasional sighs that help stimulate the production of surfactant and prevent microatelectasis. Second, the conventional ventilator provides PEEP to the patient's airway. Third, it makes a continuous flow of gas available at the endotracheal tube for entrainment by the jet ventilator (Gordin, 1989).

Hazards. The principle hazard of HFJV is damage to the trachea and large airways leading to necrotizing tracheobronchitis. Originally thought to be caused by poor humidification, it is now believed to be caused by the impact of the high pressure gas "bullets" on the wall of these airways (Milner & Hoskins, 1989).

To offset damage, HFJV should only be delivered through a special catheter that exits internally to the endotracheal tube or via a special triple-lumen endotracheal tube, previously mentioned. The triple-lumen tube incorporates the jet injector and a pressure monitoring port in the lumen of standard-sized endotracheal tubes.

Other hazards include gas trapping, hyperinflation, obstruction of the airway with secretions, hypotension, and inflammatory injury to the trachea (Gordin, 1989; Richardson, 1988).

Of concern with the use of HFJV is the difficulty encountered in assessing the patient. Auscultation of breath sounds and heart sounds is difficult due to the constant vibration and noise produced by the ventilator. Assessment of these patients is based on the observation of other clinical signs. Decreased lung compliance and pneumothoraces are observed by a decrease in chest wall vibration, increased $PaCO_2$, and a decreased PaO_2. A decrease in chest wall vibration and an increase in $PaCO_2$, without a drop in PaO_2, indicate an obstruction or malposition of the endotracheal tube. Microatelectasis and hyperinflation may be seen clinically as a decrease in the PaO_2. Neonates on HFJV should also be closely monitored for fluid, electrolyte, and neurological status (Gordin, 1989).

HIGH FREQUENCY OSCILLATORY VENTILATION (HFOV)

High frequency oscillatory ventilation (HFOV) utilizes the highest of rates, usually in the range of 480 to 1,800/min (8 to 30 Hz). The oscillatory waves that deliver the gas to the lungs are produced by either a piston pump or by the use of a loudspeaker.

Concept of Operation. A unique feature of HFOV is that it produces a positive as well as a negative stroke, which assists both inspiration and expiration (Figure 16-3). The HFOV device is placed in-line with the endotracheal tube and a gas source is passed perpendicularly into the tube, as illustrated in Figure 16-4 .

As the fresh gas enters the endotracheal tube, it is driven to the patient by the waves coming from the oscillator. Expiration occurs opposite to where the gas enters the endotracheal tube through an

The principle hazard of HFJV is damage to the trachea and large airways leading to necrotizing tracheobronchitis.

To minimize tracheal damage, the high pressure pulse of gas exits inside the endotracheal tube via a special tube.

Transillumination of the infant chest can be used to detect tension pneumothorax.

high frequency oscillatory ventilation (HFOV): Ventilation produced by a piston pump or loudspeaker, usually at a rate between 480 and 1,800/min

Figure 16-3 In high frequency oscillatory ventilation (HFOV), positive and negative strokes are provided to assist both inspiration and expiration.

expiratory limb that has a high impedance to oscillations, but low impedance when there is a steady flow of gas. Modern HFOV devices use traditional endotracheal tubes and are not used in tandem with conventional ventilators (Meredith, 1995).

Theories of Gas Exchange. As with all theories of gas exchange during HFV, it may be easiest to just say "We don't know why, it just

Figure 16-4 The oscillator or high frequency oscillatory ventilation (HFOV) device is placed in-line with the endotracheal tube and a gas source is passed perpendicularly into the tube.

works." Even those who experiment, compute, and mathematically examine these theories, conclude that what happens in simulations may not be what is happening in real lungs (Pedley et al., 1994).

☑ HFOV should be considered when conventional ventilation fails to provide adequate ventilation or oxygenation to neonates of all birth weights and gestational ages.

Indications. HFOV should be considered when conventional ventilation fails to provide adequate ventilation or oxygenation to neonates of all birth weights and gestational ages (Clark et al., 1994; Grenier & Thompson 1996). Since hyaline membrane disease is the most common condition in the neonatal ICU, premature infants are most likely to be considered for HFOV (Vierzig et al., 1994). The indications for HFOV are highly variable and dependent on the diagnosis and progression of the patient condition. Infants with congenital diaphragmatic hernia (Miguet et al., 1994), diffuse alveolar disease, non-homogeneous lung disease, air leak, and pulmonary hypoplasia are potential candidates for HFOV. The major clinical conditions for HFOV are summarized in Table 16-9.

While HFOV can be useful to treat a variety of conditions, it is of interest to note that the presence of airleaks and lack of early improvement indicate a poor prognosis (Chan et al., 1994).

Benefits. Three benefits of HFOV have been demonstrated. First it appears as though HFOV prevents the release of inflammatory chemical mediators in the lung, resulting in less lung injury than is seen with conventional ventilation (Imai et al., 1994). When used in conjunction with surfactant replacement therapy during the first hours of life, the incidence and severity of BPD may be reduced (Jackson et al., 1994). The third benefit of HFOV is that when applied early to maintain ventilation with optimal lung volume, oxygenation is increased in acute

TABLE 16-9   Clinical Conditions for HFOV

CLINICAL CONDITION	NOTES
Failing conventional ventilation	Unable to maintain acceptable blood gases Deteriorating clinical condition
Increasing ventilation requirement	F_IO_2 >50%, rate >30/min, and PIP >20 cm H_2O for infants <1,000 g (PIP in high 20 for infants >1,500 g)
Rapidly increasing F_IO_2 requirement (without pneumothorax)	Oxygen index >10 e.g., patent ductus arteriosus
Chest radiograph consistent with diffuse, homogeneous lung disease (without air trapping)	e.g., hyaline membrane disease (HMD)
Pulmonary hypertension	Nitric oxide candidates, oxygen index ≥15

stage of RDS. This improvement in oxygenation reduces the need for surfactant administration (Plavka et al., 1999).

Complications.   The ability of HFOV to oxygenate the blood is not as good as with other methods. This often requires the use of high levels of PEEP, often in excess of 15 cm H_2O (Milner & Hoskins, 1989). Combined with evidence that HFOV causes hyperinflation of the alveoli, high levels of PEEP may compromise cardiac output and lead to a higher risk of developing barotrauma (Milner & Hoskins, 1989).

There are several technical problems encountered in the use of HFOV. One problem is in the measurement of pressure at the distal end of the endotracheal tube. It is likely that alveolar pressures are quite different from those measured at the carina. An additional problem is a general lack of HFOV devices and training for its use in level I and level II nurseries.

As with HFJV, cardiopulmonary assessment of the patient is difficult when HFOV is being used. The infant must be frequently assessed for signs of pallor, cyanosis, bradycardia, hypotension, and increased respiratory effort, all of which indicate a worsening of status.

INITIAL HFOV SETTINGS
Once an infant is committed to HFOV, the following sequence may be used to set up the ventilator: mean airway pressure (mPaw), flow, power, frequency, inspiratory time%, F_IO_2. Each of these parameters and settings is discussed below. Table 16-10 provides the initial HFOV settings. A summary of the HFOV guidelines for specific clinical conditions is provided in Table 16-11.

Mean Airway Pressure (mPaw).   The mPaw affects mostly the oxygenation of the patient. The initial setting of mPaw on HFOV should be based on the mPaw during conventional ventilation. Generally a higher initial mPaw is used for HMD and a lower initial mPaw is used for nonhomogenous lung disease. Changes should be made in increments of 1 to 2 cm H_2O unless the PO_2 demands require dynamic changes for increasing or decreasing the mPaw. When lung compliance and oxygenation improve, a subtle drop in the mPaw may be observed.

During weaning, changes in the mPaw should be done every 6 hours, sooner if rib expansion of greater than nine ribs posterior continues.

Flow.   The initial flow settings are 20 L/min for infants weighing more than 2,000 g. For infants less than 2,000 g, 10 to 15 L/min should be adequate.

Power.   The power setting determines the amplitude of oscillation (ΔP) and thus the tidal volume and degree of ventilation. In HFOV, the tidal volume produced by the power setting is less than the deadspace volume. The CO_2 is drawn out actively during oscillation.

☑ During HFJV and HFOV, cardiopulmonary assessment of the patient is difficult. Signs of pallor, cyanosis, bradycardia, hypotension, and increased respiratory effort indicate a worsening of status.

☑ In addition to the F_IO_2, the mPaw affects mostly the oxygenation of the patient.

power: *A setting during HFOV that determines the amplitude of oscillation, tidal volume, and degree of ventilation.*

TABLE 16-10   Initial HFOV Settings

PARAMETER	INITIAL SETTINGS
mPaw (dependent on power setting)	Maintain mPaw 3 to 4 cm H_2O > during conventional ventilation for diffuse alveolar disease (e.g., HMD)
	Maintain mPaw ≤ less than during conventional ventilation for non-homogeneous lung disease or air leak (permissive hypercapnia should be considered for these infants).
Bias flow	20 L/M (>2000 g) 10 to 15 L/M (<2000 g)
Power [amplitude of oscillation (ΔP) − increasing the power increase delivered tidal volume]	Adjust power in increments of 2 to 4 cm H_2O until adequate chest wiggle
Frequency (Hz)—*decreasing* the frequency or Hz increase delivered tidal volume	12.5 to 15 Hz (<1,000 g) 10 to 12.5 Hz (1,000 to 1,500 g) 10 Hz (>1,500 to 2,000 g) 8 to 10 Hz (>2,000 g)
Inspiratory Time%	33% for an I:E ratio of 1:2
F_IO_2	Initially 100%; titrate following stabilization of the patient to maintain adequate SpO_2

(Data from Deakins et al., 2001)

✓ The power setting determines the amplitude of oscillation and thus the tidal volume and degree of ventilation.

✓ When the power (amplitude) setting is changed, the mPaw requires adjustment and the piston should be centered.

Initially, the power setting should be increased in increments of 2 to 4 cm H_2O unless the PCO_2 demands require dynamic changes for increasing or decreasing the amplitude.

Changes in the power setting will affect the mPaw, thus requiring readjustment of the mPaw. The piston should be centered continuously when changes are made.

Frequency.   The initial frequency setting is 8 to 15 Hz depending on the size of the infant and the diagnosis. The frequency may need adjustment when changes are made to amplitude or mPaw. The piston should be centered continuously when changes are made. Increasing the power (amplitude of oscillation or ΔP) or *decreasing* the frequency (Hz) increase delivered tidal volume and decrease $PaCO_2$.

Inspiratory Time %.   The inspiratory time % determines the I:E ratio and is usually set at 33%. This setting provides an I:E ratio of 1:2. This parameter is not routinely changed.

F_IO_2.   The initial F_IO_2 may be set at 100%. After stabilization of the patient, the F_IO_2 is titrated to keep SpO_2 between 90% and 95%.

TABLE 16-11   HFOV Guidelines for Specific Clinical Conditions*

CLINICAL CONDITION		POWER (ΔP OR AMPLITUDE)	MEAN AIRWAY PRESSURE (mPaw) CV: mPaw DURING CONVENTIONAL VENTILATION	FREQUENCY (Hz)
Diffuse alveolar disease	Premature infant	Adequate chest wiggle**	1 to 2 cm H_2O >CV	10 to 15 Hz
	Term or near term	Adequate chest wiggle	2 to 4 cm H_2O >CV	8 to 10 Hz
Nonhomogeneous lung disease	Meconium aspiration syndrome (with air trapping)	Good to adequate chest wiggle	=CV if tolerated	6 to 10 Hz
	Meconium aspiration syndrome (diffuse)	Good to adequate chest wiggle	2 to 4 cm H_2O >CV if tolerated	6 to 10 Hz
	Focal pneumonia	Adequate chest wiggle	=or 1 cm H_2O <CV if tolerated	8 to 10 Hz
Air leak	Premature (PIE)	Minimal chest wiggle	1 cm H_2O <CV if tolerated	10 to 15 Hz
	Premature (gross air leak)	Adequate chest wiggle	=or 1 cm H_2O >CV if tolerated	10 to 15 Hz
	Term/Near Term (gross air leak)	Adequate chest wiggle	=or 2 cm H_2O >CV if tolerated	8 to 10 Hz
Pulmonary hypoplasia	Uniform disease	Minimal chest wiggle (may need to increase to maintain PCO_2)	=CV (may need to ↑ to improve SaO_2)	10 to 15 Hz (may need to ↓ to maintain PCO_2)
	Nonuniform disease	Minimal chest wiggle (may need to increase to maintain PCO_2)	=to 2 cm H_2O>CV (use good lung to guide)	10 Hz (may need to ↓ to maintain PCO_2)

*These guidelines should be used as initial settings only and they must be adjusted for changing clinical conditions. Appropriate patient assessment and monitoring must be provided at all times before and during HFOV.

**Chest wiggle is determined by observable chest movement down to the eight ribs or umbilicus during HFOV.

OTHER METHODS OF VENTILATION

In addition to research into new ventilatory techniques, several advances have been made in the use of conventional ventilation. Much of the focus is on synchronizing the ventilator with the neonate's own spontaneous breathing to lessen the effect of fighting the ventilator and to improve flow dynamics into the airways. One new mode is flow-synchronization, in which the patient triggers the ventilator, with flow changing to meet the patient's inspiratory needs. This method of ventilation has been shown to allow weaning and extubation more rapidly when compared to conventional ventilation (Donn, 1990).

Other approaches include synchronized assisted ventilation (Blocker et al., 1994; Visveshwara et al., 1991), negative pressure ventilation, pressure support ventilation, and pressure-controlled inverse ratio ventilation. Some of these methods of mechanical ventilation are discussed elsewhere in this book.

LIQUID VENTILATION

An exciting technology in the area of neonatal ventilation is liquid ventilation. Although not a new concept, the ability to successfully utilize this technology has only recently been developed. The concept behind liquid ventilation is to obliterate the air/liquid interface in the alveoli with resultant lowering of surface tension. Mechanical inflation could then occur at pressures low enough to prevent damage to lung tissues.

Perfluorocarbon (PFC) liquids are the first substances that have been shown to support respiration while remaining relatively nontoxic to the lungs.

Liquid ventilation has potential applications for use in several diseases that traditionally have been difficult to treat. Included are RDS, aspiration syndromes, persistent pulmonary hypertension of the newborn, and pneumonia (Greenspan, 1993). While the potential of a favorable impact on the treatment of neonates is nearer, much research is still necessary before liquid ventilation takes its place among current treatment modalities.

EXTRACORPOREAL MEMBRANE OXYGENATION (ECMO)

extracorporeal membrane oxygenation (ECMO): Oxygenation of blood outside the body through a membrane oxygenator.

With patients for whom it is difficult or near impossible to maintain adequate oxygenation by conventional means (oxygen therapy, CPAP, PEEP), it may become necessary to oxygenate the blood outside the body. One method used with moderate success is the procedure of **extracorporeal membrane oxygenation (ECMO)**.

HISTORY

Oxygenation of blood outside the body, through a membrane oxygenator, was first developed for use in open heart surgery in the 1950s. The technology continued to improve and modifications allowed long-term use of the technique in the 1960s (Carlo & Chatburn, 1988).

The first use of the extracorporeal membrane oxygenator on an infant was done and described in 1971 (Zwischenberger et al., 1986). This paved the way for perfection and refinement of the technique. Today ECMO is used in many institutions across the country.

PATIENT SELECTION

Because of the potential risks associated with ECMO, the clinical criteria used selects only those infants who are at an 80% or greater risk of mortality if conventional methods are used.

Several limitations have been established that help to define the ECMO population. Those infants at a gestational age less than 34 weeks or weighing less than 2,000 g are excluded from consideration. This is due to the significant mortality associated with intracranial hemorrhage (ICH) (Revenis et al., 1992). Any patient with an existing ICH is not a candidate for ECMO. This is because of the need for systemic heparinization during the procedure, which could worsen an intracranial bleed. This also requires that any coagulopathy be corrected before initiating ECMO.

ECMO is contraindicated when mechanical ventilation has been used for more than 2 weeks prior to the initiation of ECMO. This is because of the likelihood of the development of chronic lung disease, which ECMO cannot reverse (Short, 1994). Additionally, candidates must have a reversible lung disease and should be free of significant cardiac disease.

ECMO CRITERIA

Since ECMO therapy is reserved for candidates with an extremely high mortality rate (80% or greater) under conventional ventilator care strategies, there are three ways to predict the occurrence of this mortality rate: (1) alveolar-arterial oxygen pressure gradient [P(A-a)O$_2$ or A-aDO$_2$], (2) oxygen index, and (3) PaO$_2$ or pH measurements.

Using the P(A-a)O$_2$. The P(A-a)O$_2$ is measured and calculated with the patient on 100% oxygen:

$$P(A\text{-}a)O_2 = \text{barometric pressure} - 47 - PaCO_2 - PaO_2$$

P(A-a)O2 of 605 to 620 mm Hg (at 100% FIO2) for 4 to 12 hours indicates a need for ECMO therapy.

Using the Oxygen Index. The OI is determined as follows:

$$OI = \frac{(mPaw \times F_IO_2)}{PaO_2}$$

☑ ECMO is not recommended for infants of less than 34 weeks gestational age, weighing less than 2,000 g, having evidence of intracranial hemorrhage (ICH).

☑ ECMO candidates should have less than 2 weeks of ventilator assistance, and have reversible lung disease.

☑ The mortality rate of infants under conventional ventilator care strategies can be predicted by three methods: P(A-a)O$_2$, oxygen index, PaO$_2$ or pH measurements.

☑ See Appendix 1 for example.

TABLE 16-12   Criteria for ECMO Therapy

PARAMETER	CRITICAL VALUE
Alveolar-arterial oxygen tension gradient (A-aDO$_2$) on 100% F$_I$O$_2$	605 to 620 mm Hg for 4 to 12 hours
Oxygen index (OI)	0.35 to 0.6 for 0.5 to 6 hours
PaO$_2$	35 to 50 mm Hg for 2 to 12 hours
pH	<7.25 for 2 hours with hypotension

An oxygen index of 0.35 to 0.6 for 0.5 to 6 hours is inclusive for ECMO therapy.

A study by Durand and associates (1990) described the use of the OI in addition to mPaw to identify a select group of meconium aspiration patients for ECMO. Their conclusions were that an OI greater than 0.4 in association with a mPaw of 20 cm H$_2$O or greater, may be helpful in identifying those patients who could benefit from ECMO.

Using the PaO$_2$ or pH.   A third criteria used is the presence of a PaO$_2$ of 35 to 50 mm Hg for 2 to 12 hours or a pH of <7.25 for 2 hours with hypotension (Short, 1994). Table 16-12 summarizes the parameters and critical values that may be used to determine the need for ECMO therapy.

MECHANISMS OF BYPASS

Two types of ECMO can be done: venoarterial and venovenous.

Venoarterial.   In the venoarterial route, blood is drawn from the right atrium via the internal jugular vein. The oxygenated blood is returned to the aortic arch via the right common carotid artery, as shown in Figure 16-5. Venoarterial ECMO not only oxygenates the blood, but also supports the cardiac function of the patient, because the blood return to the aortic arch is supported by the ECMO machine. For this reason, the venoarterial route is most commonly used for the ECMO procedure (Donn, 1990).

Venovenous.   In the venovenous route, blood is removed from the right atrium via a catheter inserted in the right internal jugular vein. The oxygenated blood is returned to the right atrium through a catheter inserted via the femoral vein. This method oxygenates the blood and does not support cardiac output.

In the venovenous method, blood flow from right to left heart remains the sole function of the heart.

ECMO Circuit.   The ECMO circuit uses a modified heart-lung bypass machine consisting of a venous-blood drainage reservoir, a blood pump, the membrane oxygenator where the exchange of O$_2$

☑ In the venoarterial route, blood goes from the right atrium (via the internal jugular vein) to the aortic arch (via the right common carotid artery). This route oxygenates the blood and supports the patient's cardiac function.

☑ In the venovenous route, blood goes from the right atrium (via the right internal jugular vein) and returns to the right atrium (via the femoral vein). This route oxygenates the blood only and does not support the patient's cardiac function.

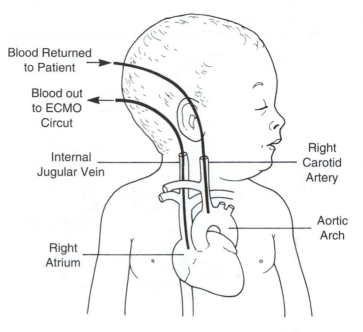

Blood Returned to Patient

Blood out to ECMO Circut

Internal Jugular Vein

Right Carotid Artery

Aortic Arch

Right Atrium

Figure 16-5 Venoarterial route of ECMO setup. Blood is drawn from the right atrium via the internal jugular vein. The oxygenated blood is returned to the aortic arch via the right carotid artery.

and CO_2 takes place, and a heat exchanger to maintain temperature. Figure 16-6 depicts a typical ECMO circuit.

COMPLICATIONS

Complications of ECMO are both mechanical and physiologic. Common physiologic complications of ECMO are those related to bleeding, secondary to the high level of heparin required for anticoagulation. Intracranial hemorrhage (ICH) has been reported to affect 14% of ECMO patients in one study (Donn, 1990). The incidence of ICH may be decreased if cephalic jugular venous drainage is used in conjunction with ECMO (O'Connor, 1993).

There is also a high incidence of seizures in ECMO patients. It is unknown whether the seizures are caused by the therapy, the disease, or both (Donn, 1990). Pulmonary edema, the release of vasoactive substances secondary to platelet-membrane interaction, and pulmonary hemorrhage are potential pulmonary complications.

Cardiovascular complications arise from hypo- and hypervolemia leading to hypo- and hypertension in the infant. Hypertension is seen in about 7% of ECMO patients (Donn, 1990). Alteration of the renin-angiotensin-aldosterone cycle, secondary to the nonpulsatile perfusion, may lead to renal complications.

☑ Bleeding, ICH, pulmonary edema, and hemorrage are some potential complications of ECMO therapy.

Desired Gas Mixture

Heat Exchanger

Patient Bridge

Membrane Oxygenator

Infusion Sites

Reservoir Bladder

Roller Pump

Figure 16-6   A typical ECMO circuit.

Anemia, leukopenia, and thrombocytopenia are all possible hematologic complications caused by the consumption of blood components by the membrane oxygenator (Carlo & Chatburn, 1988). Due to the invasive nature of ECMO, there is an increased risk of infection. Roughly 6% of patients on ECMO have positive blood cultures (Donn, 1990).

Mechanical complications arise in approximately 10% of ECMO cases and include failure of the pump, rupture of the tubing, failure of the membrane, and difficulties with the cannulas (Donn, 1990).

Implications.   The initial hope that ECMO could provide a safe means of ventilating the sick neonate has not been realized. It became apparent early on that there are many hazards and complications that make the procedure suitable in only a few selected clinical conditions. The long-term complications of ECMO are still unknown. It is necessary to permanently ligate the carotid artery used to cannulate the patient, and the effects of having a single carotid artery as the patient grows older have yet to be determined.

The ECMO procedure is expensive and requires around-the-clock monitoring by specially trained personnel, which increases the cost tremendously. The high cost is often offset, however, by a decreased number of days spent in the hospital. Patients receiving ECMO averaged 25 days in the hospital, compared to 76 days for those treated conventionally (Wagner, 1989).

SUMMARY

Neonatal mechanical ventilation is an area that requires additional training and clinical experience beyond the basics of respiratory care. Neonates are not just smaller adults because the ventilator settings, normal values, and treatment plans are all unique and sometimes wearisome to manage. This is particularly true for respiratory care practitioners who "wear more than one hat" and work in both the adult and neonatal intensive care units.

Since the materials presented in this chapter are relevant to actual clinical practice, they should be very useful to respiratory care students as they get ready to practice in the neonatal intensive care units. For seasoned practitioners, the reference sources should provide additional information on the topics presented in this chapter.

Self-Assessment Questions

1. Intubation of neonates following delivery is indicated under all of the following conditions *except*:

    A. meconium staining of amniotic fluid.
    B. difficulty ventilating by bag and mask.
    C. Apgar score greater than 8.
    D. presence of diaphragmatic hernia.

2. For neonates below 1,000 g body weight, the proper size of laryngoscope blade should be size _____ and endotracheal tube size _____ (internal diameter, mm):

    A. 0, 1.5
    B. 0, 2.5
    C. 1, 1.5
    D. 1, 2.5

3. The most common cause of respiratory distress syndrome in newborns is:

    A. surfactant deficiency.
    B. oxygen toxicity.
    C. congenital heart disease.
    D. low body weight.

4. A preterm infant has a diagnosis of respiratory distress syndrome. You would expect to read in the chart that, immediately after delivery, the neonate showed all of the following signs *except*:

    A. expiratory grunting.
    B. nasal flaring.
    C. apnea.
    D. chest retraction.

5. Which of the following statements is *true* regarding surfactant replacement therapy?

    A. Survanta® is a synthetic preparation.
    B. Exosurf Neonatal® is a preparation from cow lung tissue.
    C. Surfactant replacement works on all preterm infants.
    D. Surfactant replacement reduces the severity of RDS.

6. The major difference between adult and neonatal ventilators is that neonatal ventilators are mostly _____-limited and they deliver a variable _____ depending on a patient's lung compliance or airway resistance.

    A. pressure, volume   C. volume, pressure
    B. pressure, pressure   D. volume, volume

7. Keeping the same preset pressure on a pressure-limited ventilator, a lower tidal volume would result when the patient's compliance is _____ or airway resistance is _____.

    A. increased, increased   C. decreased, increased
    B. increased, decreased   D. decreased, decreased

8. A blood gas report done on a neonate shows a $PaCO_2$ of 58 mm Hg. The physician asks you to increase the tidal volume to be delivered by the pressure-limited ventilator. You would increase the _____ setting on the ventilator.

    A. tidal volume   C. expiratory time
    B. inspiratory pressure   D. positive end-expiratory pressure

9. During mechanical ventilation, the volume loss in the circuit and humidifier may be minimized by using a circuit and humidifier with:

    A. large mechanical deadspace volume.   C. low compression factor.
    B. heated wire.   D. high compression factor.

10. A heated wire is sometimes placed on the inspiratory side of the circuit to reduce _____ in the ventilator circuit.

    A. airway resistance   C. contamination
    B. condensation   D. circuit temperature

11. The general indications for mechanical ventilation include all of the following *except*:

    A. acute alveolar hyperventilation.   C. acute respiratory acidosis.
    B. apnea.   D. acute hypoxemia (PaO_2 <50 mm Hg with supplemental oxygen).

12. When using a pressure-limited ventilator, the tidal volume delivered by the ventilator may be estimated by:

    A. I time + Flow rate.   C. I time + E time.
    B. I time $\times$ Flow rate.   D. Flow rate / I time.

13. The normal blood gas values of an umbilical artery sample include all of the following *except*:

    A. pH from 7.3 to 7.45.   C. PO_2 greater than 50 mm Hg.
    B. PCO_2 from 35 to 45 mm Hg.   D. SaO_2 from 60% to 90%.

14. High frequency ventilation has the advantages of delivering _____ and reducing the incidence of _____.

    A. small tidal volume, barotrauma

    B. large tidal volume, barotrauma

    C. large mean airway pressure, necrotizing trachbronchitis

    D. low peak inspiratory pressure, air trapping

15 to 17. Match the type of high frequency ventilator with the respective frequency (cycles/minute). Use each answer once.

Type of High Frequency Ventilator	Frequency (Cycles Per Minute)
15. High frequency jet ventilation (HFJV)	A. 60 to 150
16. High frequency oscillatory ventilation (HFOV or HFO)	B. 240 to 660
17. High frequency positive pressure ventilation (HFPPV)	C. 480 to 1800

18. To minimize tracheal damage caused by high pressure gas jets in high frequency jet ventilation (HFJV), a specially-designed tube allows pulsed gas to exit _____ the endotracheal tube.

    A. at the distal end of

    B. at the proximal end of

    C. at the middle and inside of

    D. at the middle and outside of

19. During high frequency jet ventilation (HFJV) or high frequency oscillatory ventilation (HFOV), assessment of a patient's cardiopulmonary status is difficult. Signs of deterioration may include all of the following *except*:

    A. respiratory distress.

    B. tachycardia.

    C. hypotension.

    D. pallor.

20. Candidates for HFOV may exhibit all of the following clinical conditions with the *exception* of:

    A. difficult to wean from conventional ventilation.

    B. increasing ventilation requirement.

    C. rapidly increasing F_IO_2 requirement.

    D. chest radiograph consistent with diffuse, homogeneous lung disease.

21. A neonate is being ventilated by a high frequency oscillator. Her physician would like to lower the patient's $PaCO_2$. You would increase the level of ventilation by increasing the _____ or decreasing the _____.

    A. increasing the power (amplitude), increasing the frequency (Hz)

    B. increasing the power (amplitude), decreasing the frequency (Hz)

    C. decreasing the power (amplitude), increasing the frequency (Hz)

    D. decreasing the power (amplitude), decreasing the frequency (Hz)

22. In addition to the F_IO_2 control on a high frequency oscillator, a patient's oxygenation status can be improved by increasing the:

    A. power.
    B. frequency.
    C. mean airway pressure.
    D. amplitude.

23. A neonate who is diagnosed with severe RDS has been deteriorating over the past 12 hours. The physician asks you to evaluate this neonate for possible extracorporeal membrane oxygenation (ECMO) therapy. You would *recommend* the neonate for ECMO therapy if she:

    A. has a gestational age of more than 34 weeks.
    B. weighs less than 2,000 g.
    C. has evidence of intracranial hemorrhage (ICH).
    D. has been mechanically ventilated for more than 2 weeks.

24. Extracorporeal membrane oxygenation (ECMO) therapy should be considered only when the patient has a(n) _____ percent mortality rate using the conventional ventilator management strategies.

    A. 20
    B. 40
    C. 60
    D. 80

25. All of the following may be used to predict an 80% mortality rate under conventional ventilator management strategies *except*:

    A. A-a gradient of 605 to 620 mm Hg for 4 to 12 hours.
    B. oxygen index of 0.35 to 0.6 for 30 min to 6 hours.
    C. PaO_2 of 35 to 50 for 2 to 12 hours.
    D. pH of less than 7.25 for 2 hours with hypertension.

26. Which of the following statements is *true* concerning the *venoarterial* route in ECMO therapy?

    A. Blood is removed from the right common carotid artery.
    B. Blood is removed from the brachial or femoral artery.
    C. Blood is returned to the aortic arch via the right common carotid artery.
    D. Blood is returned to the aortic arch via the internal jugular vein.

27. Which of the following statements is *true* concerning the *venovenous* route in ECMO therapy?

    A. Blood is removed from the right atrium via the right carotid artery.
    B. Blood is removed from the right atrium via the femoral vein.
    C. Blood is returned to the right atrium via the femoral vein.
    D. Blood is returned to the aortic arch via the internal jugular vein.

28. The _____ route in ECMO therapy supports cardiac function because the blood is returned to the _____.

    A. venoarterial, aortic arch via the common carotid artery

    B. venoarterial, right atrium via the femoral vein

    C. venovenous, aortic arch via the common carotid artery

    D. venovenous, right atrium via the femoral vein

Answers to Self-Assessment Questions

1. C. Apgar score greater than 8.

2. B. 0, 2.5

3. A. surfactant deficiency.

4. C. apnea.

5. D. Surfactant replacement reduces the severity of RDS.

6. A. pressure, volume

7. C. decreased, increased

8. B. inspiratory pressure

9. C. low compression factor.

10. B. condensation

11. A. acute alveolar hyperventilation.

12. B. I time × Flow rate

13. D. SaO_2 from 60% to 90%

14. A. small tidal volume, barotrauma

15. B. 240 to 660 cycles per min

16. C. 480 to 1800 cycles per min

17. A. 60 to 150 cycles per min

18. C. at the middle and inside of

19. B. tachycardia.

20. A. difficult to wean from conventional ventilation.

21. B. increasing the power (amplitude), decreasing the frequency (Hz)

22. C. mean airway pressure.

23. A. has a gestational age of more than 34 weeks

24. D. 80

25. D. pH of less than 7.25 for 2 hours with hypertension.

26. C. Blood is returned to the aortic arch via the right common carotid artery.

27. C. Blood is returned to the right atrium via the femoral vein.

28. A. venoarterial, aortic arch via the common carotid artery

References

Abbasi, S., et al. (1993). Long-term pulmonary consequences of respiratory distress syndrome in preterm infants treated with exogenous surfactant. *J Pediatr, 122*(3).

Bandy, K. P., et al. (1992, May/June). Volume-controlled ventilation for severe neonatal respiratory failure. *Neonatal Intensive Care, 5*(3), 70–73.

Blocker, D., et al. (1994, November/December). Synchronized assisted ventilation of infants (SAVI) examined as part of a quality improvement study: West Paces Medical Center, Atlanta, Georgia. *Neonatal Intensive Care,* 32–35.

Boynton, B. R. (1986). High frequency ventilation in newborn infants. *Respir Care, 31*(6), 480–490.

Carlo, W. A., & Chatburn, R. L. (1988). *Neonatal respiratory care* (2nd ed.). Chicago: Year Book Medical Publishers.

Chan, V., et al. (1994). High frequency oscillation for preterm infants with severe respiratory failure. *Arch Dis Child Fetal Neonatal Ed,* 70, F44-46.

Chatburn, R. L. (1991). Principles and practice of neonatal and pediatric mechanical ventilation. *Resp Care, 36*(6), 569–593.

Clark, R. H. (1994). High frequency ventilation in acute pediatric respiratory failure. (Editorial). *Chest, 105*(3), 652–653.

Clark, R. H. et al. (1994). Prospective, randomized comparison of high frequency oscillation and conventional ventilation in candidates for extracorporeal membrane oxygenation. *J Pediatr, 124*(3), 447–454.

Deakins, K., et al. (2001). Selecting appropriate ventilator parameters. Retrieved September 7, 2004, from http://www.rtmagazine.com/issues.ASP?issueid=0409

Donn, S. M. (1990). ECMO indications and complications. *Hosp Pract, 25*(6), 143–146, 149–150, 153–157.

Durand, M., et al. (1990). Oxygenation index in patients with meconium aspiration: Conventional and extracorporeal membrane oxygenation therapy. *Crit Care Med, 18*(4), 373–377.

Goldsmith, J. P., et al. (1993). Ventilatory management casebook. *J Perinatology, 13,* 72–75.

Gordin, P. (1989). High frequency jet ventilation for severe respiratory failure. *Pediatr Nurs, 15*(6), 625–629.

Greenspan, J. S. (1993). Liquid ventilation: A developing technology. *Neonatal Netw, 12*(4), 23–32.

Grenier, B., & Thompson, J. (1996). High-frequency oscillatory ventilation in pediatric patients. *Respir Care Clin N Am, 2*(4), 545–575.

Gunkel, J. H., & Banks, P. L. (1993). Surfactant therapy and intracranial hemorrhage: Review of the literature and results of new analyses. *Pediatrics, 92*(6), 775–786.

Holm, B. A., & Waring, A. J. (1993). Designer surfactants: The next generation in surfactant replacement. *Clin Perinatol, 20*(4), 813–829.

Horbar, J. D., et al. (1993). A multicenter randomized trial comparing two surfactants for the treatment of neonatal respiratory distress syndrome. *J Pediatr, 123*(5), 757–766.

Imai, Y., et al. (1994). Inflammatory chemical mediators during conventional ventilation and during high frequency oscillatory ventilation. *Am J Resp Crit Care Med, 150*(6, Pt. 1), 1550–1554.

Jackson, J. C., et al. (1994). Reduction in lung injury after combined surfactant and high frequency ventilation. *Am J Resp Crit Care Med, 150*(2), 534–539.

Jeena, P., et al. (2002). Nasal CPAP in newborns with acute respiratory failure. *Ann Trop Paediatr, 22,* 201–207.

Jobe, A. H., & Ikegami, M. (1993). Surfactant metabolism. *Clin Perinatol, 20*(4), 683–696.

Kaapa, P., et al. (1993). Pulmonary hemodynamics after synthetic surfactant replacement in neonatal respiratory distress syndrome. *J Pediatr, 123*(1), 115–119.

Lee, K. S., et al. (1998). A comparison of underwater bubble continuous positive airway pressure with ventilator-derived continuous positive airway pressure in premature neonates ready for extubation. *Biol Neonate, 73,* 69–75.

Long, W. (1993). Synthetic surfactant. *Semin Perinatol, 17*(4), 275–284.

Malik, R. K., et al. (2003). A two year experience in continuous positive airway pressure ventilation using nasal prongs and pulse oximetry. *Med J Armed Forces Ind, 59,* 36–39.

Meredith, K. S. (1995). High frequency ventilation. In S. L. Barnhart, & M. P. Czervinske, *Perinatal and pediatric respiratory care.* Philadelphia: W.B. Saunders.

Miguet, D., et al. (1994). Preoperative stabilization using high frequency oscillatory ventilation in the management of congenital diaphragmatic hernia. *Crit Care Med, 22*(Suppl. 9), 77–82.

Milner, A. D., & Hoskins, E. W. (1989). High frequency positive pressure ventilation in neonates. *Arch Dis Child, 64*(1), [Fetal Neonatal ed.], 1–3.

Modanlou, H. D., et al. (1997). Comparative efficacy of Exosurf® and Survanta® surfactants on early clinical course of respiratory distress syndrome and complications of prematurity. *J Perinatol, 17*(6), 455–460.

O'Connor, T. A. (1993). Decreased incidence of intracranial hemorrhage using cephalic jugular venous drainage during neonatal extracorporeal membrane oxygenation. *J Pediatr Surg, 28*(10), 1332–1335.

Parmigiani, S. et al. (1997). Evolution of respiratory mechanics in preterm babies after surfactant administration in the neonatal period. *Acta Biomed Ateneo Parmense, 68*(Suppl. 1), 65–73.

Pedley, T. J., et al. (1994). Gas flow and mixing in the airways. *Crit Care Med, 22*(Suppl. 9), 24–36.

Pinar, H., et al. (1994). Pathology of the lung in surfactant-treated neonates. *Pediatr Pathol, 14*(4), 627–636.

Plavka, R., et al. (1999). A prospective randomized comparison of conventional mechanical ventilation and very early high frequency oscillatory ventilation in extremely premature newborns with respiratory distress syndrome. *Intensive Care Med, 25*(1), 68–75.

Revenis, M. E., et al. (1992). Mortality and morbidity among lower birth weight (2000 to 2500 grams) infants treated with extracorporeal membrane oxygenation (ECMO). *J Pediatr, 121*(3), 452–458.

Richardson, C. (1988). Hyaline membrane disease: Future treatment modalities. *J Perinat Neonat Nurs, 2*(1), 78–88.

Robertson, B. & Halliday, H. L. (1998). Principles of surfactant replacement. *Biochim Biophys Acta, 1408*(2–3), 346–361.

Short, B. L. (1994). Extracorporeal membrane oxygenation. In G. B. Avery et al. (Eds.), *Neonatology: pathophysiology and management of the newborn* (4th ed.). Philadelphia: J.B. Lippincott.

Vierzig, A., et al. (1994). Clinical experiences with high frequency oscillatory ventilation in newborns with severe respiratory distress syndrome. *Crit Care Med, 22*(Suppl. 9), S583–S587.

Visveshwara, N., et al. (1991). Patient-triggered synchronized assisted ventilation of newborns. Report of a preliminary study and three years' experience. *J Perinatol, 11*(4), 347–354.

Wagner, M. (1989). New technology for critically ill newborns needs solid planning. *Mod Healthc, 19*(29), 48.

Wiswell, T. E., & Mendiola, J. (1993). Respiratory distress syndrome in the newborn: Innovative therapies. *Am Fam Phys, 47*(2), 407.

Witek, T. J., & E. N. Schachter. (1994). *Pharmacology and therapeutics in respiratory care.* Philadelphia: W. B. Saunders.

Yuksel, B., et al. (1993). Respiratory function at follow-up after neonatal surfactant replacement therapy. *Respir Med, 87*(3), 217–221.

Zwischenberger, J. B., et al. (1986). The role of extracorporeal membrane oxygenation in the management of respiratory failure in the newborn. *Resp Care, 31*(6), 491–497.

Suggested Reading

Invasive and Noninvasive Mechanical Ventilation
Donn, S. M., et al. (2003). Invasive and noninvasive neonatal mechanical ventilation. *Respir Care, 48(4), 426–439.*

Mechanical Ventilation and Monitoring

Bignall, S., et al. (1997). Monitoring interactions between spontaneous respiration and mechanical inflations in preterm neonates. *Crit Care Med, 25*(3), 545–553.

Despotova-Toleva, L., & Petrov, A. (1997). Feasibility for evaluation of the efficacy of conventional ventilatory support in very low birth weight infants. *Folia Med* (Plovdiv), *39*(4), 55–64.

Mammel, M. C., & Bing, D. R. (1996). Mechanical ventilation of the newborn. An overview. *Clin Chest Med, 17*(3), 603–613.

Sinha, S. K., et al. (1997). Randomized trial of volume controlled versus time cycled, pressure limited ventilation in preterm infants with respiratory distress syndrome. *Arch Dis Child Fetal Neonatal Ed, 77*(3), F202–205.

High-Frequency Ventilation

Hoehn, T., et al. (1998). High-frequency ventilation augments the effect of inhaled nitric oxide in persistent pulmonary hypertension of the newborn. *Eur Respir J, 11*(1), 234–238.

Jouvet, P., et al. (1997). Assessment of high-frequency neonatal ventilator performances. *Intensive Care Med, 23*(2), 208–213.

Kalenga, M., et al. (1998). High-frequency oscillatory ventilation in neonatal RDS: Initial volume optimization and respiratory mechanics. *J Appl Physiol, 84*(4), 1174–1177.

Extracorporeal Gas Exchange

Alpard, S. K., & Zwischenberger, J. B. (1998). Extracorporeal gas exchange. *Respir Care Clin N Am, 4*(4), 711–738, ix.

CHAPTER SEVENTEEN

HOME MECHANICAL VENTILATION

David W. Chang

OUTLINE

--------------------------------- **KEY TERMS** ---------------------------------

- acute care
- acute exacerbation
- desaturation
- home care

- learning objectives
- quality of life
- team approach

--------------------------------- **INTRODUCTION** ---------------------------------

Home mechanical ventilation made its first major appearance in the United States during the poliomyelitis epidemics of the mid-twentieth century. At that time, negative pressure ventilators (iron lungs) were used to sustain the lives of those who lost the ability to breathe. Today, health care reform and cost containment strategies are limiting the resources available for acute care in the hospitals. Since there are few nursing homes or extended care facilities that will accept the increasing number of ventilator patients, home care becomes an important and viable option for ventilator-dependent patients.

GOALS OF HOME MECHANICAL VENTILATION

acute care: Patient care provided in facilities where life-sustaining equipment and qualified personnel are always available.

quality of life: The most important, positive features of daily living for a patient based on his/her current physical and mental conditions. The quality varies among different individuals and its definition may change over time.

Mechanical ventilation provided in the home is drastically different from that delivered in an **acute care** setting. In an acute care setting such as the hospital, the patient is surrounded by an array of medical equipment and supplies. Specialized health care practitioners are available at all times to provide diagnostic and therapeutic procedures. In addition, the patient in an acute care setting gets little rest because of frequent vital sign assessments and routine laboratory tests. For patients who require long-term mechanical ventilation, it may not be logical or financially feasible to provide mechanical ventilation in an acute care setting.

An alternative to the acute care setting is to provide mechanical ventilation in a nonacute environment such as the patient's home. Three unique and beneficial goals of home ventilator care have been identified and they are (1) extension of the patient's life and enhancement of the **quality of life,** (2) creation of an environment that will develop and strengthen the patient's physical and physiological functions, and (3) reduction of the cost for ventilator care (O'Donohue et al., 1986).

Extension of the patient's life is a primary goal of medical and health care procedures. Quality of life is an important issue since a life that has poor quality or little meaning may cause the patient a great deal of anxiety and unnecessary suffering. For this reason, the patient must be involved and be part of the decision-making process before changing the ventilator care plan from an acute care setting to the patient's home.

> ☑ To spend much of the day in a familiar home environment is one benefit that cannot be provided by the hospital.

To be able to spend much of the day in a familiar home environment is one benefit that cannot be provided by the hospital. At home, the patient is likely to become more active in the rehabilitation process. There is an incentive for the patient to try to get well and be weaned off the ventilator. Furthermore, interactions with family members and friends will enhance the patient's psychologic well-being and quality of life.

> ☑ The cost savings of providing mechanical ventilation at home can be drastic but it should not be the *primary* consideration.

Reduction of the cost for patient care is another goal of home mechanical ventilation. The cost savings of providing mechanical ventilation at home can be drastic but should not be the primary consideration. It is vital to ensure that quality care is provided to the patient at or below the cost of patient care in an acute care setting.

As we see later in this chapter, the success of home ventilator care requires a team that consists of medical professionals (physicians, nurses, respiratory therapists, social workers) and nonmedical lay-persons (relatives, friends, support group members). No matter what their background or training, a **team approach** dedicated and committed to quality care is vital to any successful home ventilator care program (Gower et al., 1985).

> *team approach:* A unified and supportive way of taking care of a patient by medical and non-medical individuals who share a common goal.

> ☑ A team approach dedicated and committed to quality care is vital to any successful home ventilator care program.

INDICATIONS

Before a decision is made to provide home ventilator care for a patient, four questions may help to assess the need for home ventilator care: (1) Does the patient have a disease state (high cervical spine injury, severe respiratory muscle paralysis) which may result in ventilatory failure and the need for long-term ventilator care? (2) Does the patient exhibit clinical characteristics (impending ventilatory failure, cerebral hypoxia) that require mechanical ventilation? (3) Is the patient clinically stable enough to be managed outside an acute care setting? and (4) Are there other noninvasive alternatives besides artificial airway and mechanical ventilation (diaphragm pacing, pneumo-belt) suitable for the patient (O'Donohue et al., 1986)?

DISEASES THAT MAY JUSTIFY HOME MECHANICAL VENTILATION

Lung diseases that may justify ventilator care provided outside an acute care setting may be grouped into four categories. They are (1) chronic obstructive lung diseases (COPD), (2) restrictive lung diseases, (3) ventilatory muscle dysfunction, and (4) central hypoventilation syndromes (Ferns, 1994; Goldstein et al., 1995; O'Donohue et al.,

TABLE 17-1   Diseases That May Justify Home Mechanical Ventilation

PULMONARY PROBLEM	CLINICAL COURSE
COPD	Air flow obstruction Excessively high compliance Air trapping Acute exacerbation (pneumonia)
Restrictive lung disease	Reduction of lung volumes and capacities Deadspace ventilation Muscle fatigue
Ventilatory muscle dysfunction	Inefficient ventilatory muscle Atelectasis and pneumonia
Central hypoventilation syndrome	Apnea Chronic hypoventilation Atelectasis and pneumonia

1986). Since the severity and coexisting conditions of a disease vary greatly among patients with the same diagnosis, a thorough patient evaluation is a prerequisite for home ventilator care. The diseases that may benefit from home mechanical ventilation are summarized in Table 17-1.

COPD.   COPD is a group of lung impairments that includes chronic asthma, chronic bronchitis, emphysema, and bronchiectasis. Air flow obstruction is the primary clinical feature of these patients. Typically, stable COPD patients require only minimal care such as bronchodilators, flu vaccines, and bronchopulmonary hygiene. Only on rare occasions do they require ventilatory assistance.

acute exacerbation: A sudden aggravation of symptoms or increase in the severity of a disease. This condition is often caused by a secondary medical problem such as a severe infection.

COPD patients who require mechanical ventilation are those who develop ventilatory failure or oxygenation failure, or both. On occasion, these patients may deteriorate to a point requiring mechanical ventilation as a result of pneumonia or major surgical procedure. When this occurs, blood gases usually reveal acute ventilatory failure (acute respiratory acidosis) superimposed on chronic ventilatory failure (compensated respiratory acidosis). This condition of acute hypercapnia in COPD is also called **acute exacerbation** of COPD (Malley, 1990). Table 17-2 shows the changes in blood gas reports when a stable COPD patient goes into ventilatory failure requiring mechanical ventilation.

☑ COPD patients are difficult to wean because of insufficient alveolar ventilation caused by air flow obstruction, loss of elastic recoil, and air trapping.

Once placed on a ventilator, COPD patients may be difficult to wean off mechanical ventilation because of insufficient alveolar ventilation. This problem is primarily due to air flow obstruction, loss of elastic recoil, and air trapping. In addition, COPD patients usually have coexisting medical problems that are related to the primary lung disease. Some examples of these related medical problems are ventilation/perfusion mismatch, pulmonary hypertension, and cor pulmonale.

TABLE 17-2   Blood Gas Characteristics of Acute Exacerbation of COPD

CONDITION	TYPICAL BLOOD GASES
Chronic ventilatory failure in a stable COPD patient	pH = 7.36, $PaCO_2$ = 55 mm Hg, PaO_2 = 50 mm Hg, HCO_3^- = 30 mEq/L
Acute ventilatory failure in a normal patient due to pneumonia or major surgical procedure	pH = 7.30, $PaCO_2$ = 55 mm Hg, PaO_2 = 75 mm Hg, HCO_3^- = 26 mEq/L
Acute ventilatory failure superimposed on chronic ventilatory failure (e.g., COPD patient with pneumonia)	pH = 7.27, $PaCO_2$ = 74 mm Hg, PaO_2 = 43 mm Hg, HCO_3^- = 33 mEq/L

desaturation: A significant decrease in arterial oxygen saturation (SaO_2) or pulse oximetry saturation (SpO_2) from the normal baseline value.

COPD patients also require a high level of care in maintaining the airway. Because of copious amounts of pulmonary secretions and inability to clear secretions effectively, they often require suctioning of the airways and bronchopulmonary drainage. The oxygenation levels also fluctuate widely depending on unanticipated events such as bronchospasm and mucus plugging. Since the weaning process for COPD patients may take days or weeks, home ventilator care becomes a viable option once they are clinically stable and without significant oxygen **desaturation.** When significant oxygen desaturation (SaO_2 or SpO_2 < 90%) occurs, its cause must be identified and corrected before transferring the patient from hospital to home.

Restrictive Lung Diseases.   Restrictive lung diseases such as pulmonary fibrosis and atelectasis limit the patient's ability to expand the lungs. As a result, lung volumes and capacities are reduced. Since minute ventilation requires an adequate tidal volume and respiratory rate, patients with restrictive lung disease assume a rapid breathing pattern because of the reduction of tidal volume.

✓ The amount of deadspace ventilation is increased in rapid shallow breathing.

The amount of deadspace ventilation is increased in rapid shallow breathing. Furthermore, the work of breathing in restrictive lung diseases is increased because of low lung compliance. High inflation pressures and respiratory rates are usually required to maintain adequate ventilation in these patients. Over time, these patients develop ventilatory failure secondary to excessive work of breathing and muscle fatigue. Home ventilator care should be considered for patients who have chronic restrictive lung disease and are clinically stable.

Ventilatory Muscle Dysfunction.   Patients with ventilatory muscle dysfunction include those afflicted with spinal cord injury or polyneuropathy. Since the primary problem of ventilation is with the ventilatory muscles, they usually have healthy lungs and a good prognosis. Home ventilator care is usually carried out without any complications. Unless there is an infection, these patients generally maintain healthy lungs and normal lung functions. When lung infection occurs, it often leads to pneumonia and atelectasis.

Long-term mechanical ventilation is often necessary for these patients because of the chronic nature of the diseases affecting the respiratory system. These patients often recover and do not require prolonged mechanical ventilation except in cases of high spinal (cervical 1 and 2) injuries. Aggressive airway care and broncho-pulmonary hygiene should be done to avoid complications resulting from the use of mechanical ventilation and artificial airway.

Central Hypoventilation Syndrome.   Patients with central hypoventilation syndrome often exhibit apnea or variable periods of hypoventilation due to failure or dysfunction of the autonomic control of breathing. Because of the range of severity and complications in central hypoventilation syndrome, some patients may require mechanical ventilation only during sleep while others may need it continuously. In patients who have persistent hypoventilation, poor lung expansion may lead to lung infection, atelectasis, and pneumonia. Careful evaluation of these patients in the hospital can help to formulate a care plan for mechanical ventilation in the home.

PATIENT SELECTION

Not all patients receiving mechanical ventilation in an acute care setting are suitable candidates for home ventilator care. Typically, a patient who requires a good deal of monitoring and laboratory tests or one who is clinically unstable is ruled out for home ventilator care. Aside from the evaluations based on the medical perspective, four nonmedical factors are crucial in the patient selection process. They are (1) desires of the patient, (2) desires of the family, (3) cost, and (4) available resources (Eigen et al., 1990; O'Donohue et al., 1986; Smith, 1994).

DESIRES OF THE PATIENT

✔ Discussions concerning home ventilator care should not take place when the patient is hypoxic, confused, or under emotional distress.

Likely candidates for home ventilator care should be told about the potential advantages and disadvantages of leaving the hospital. The advantage of being at home is the opportunity for the patient to stay closer to family members and to live in a familiar environment. The disadvantage of leaving the hospital is the feeling of isolation from professional help and the assumption of medical care by self and family members. The discussion on the topic of home ventilator care should be done when the patient can comprehend the meaning and implications of leaving the acute care setting. It should not take place when the patient is hypoxic, confused, or under emotional distress.

home care: Patient care provided in the home or other nonacute care settings (nursing homes, extended care facilities) where minimal medical equipment and personnel are available.

✔ Adaptation of home ventilator care depends on the level of communication within the family and the degree of commitment between all family members.

✔ The cost of home ventilator care varies greatly and depends primarily on the type of equipment and the extent of professional care required.

Finally, the decision to implement home ventilator care should not be rushed. Ample time should be provided to the patient so that the decision may reflect the patient's true desire. Hasty discussions and decisions often lead to inaccurate perceptions and poor transition from the hospital to the **home care** setting.

DESIRES OF THE FAMILY

The desires of family members must be considered because they will be the key persons taking care of the patient and ventilator at home. Depending on the level of ventilator care required by the patient, personal sacrifices must be made. These sacrifices may range from giving up some free time and leisure activities to terminating one's job or career (Smith, 1994). Successful home ventilator care requires a total commitment from family members. They must also be able and willing to assume this unfamiliar task of home ventilator care for the duration of time that the patient remains on the ventilator. In one study, the most important factor associated with adaptation of home ventilator care was the level of communication within the family and the degree of commitment between all family members (Glass, 1993).

COST

The cost of home ventilator care varies greatly and depends primarily on the type of equipment and the extent of professional care required. Ventilator, a backup ventilator, and oxygen supplies are some major equipment expenditures, either obtained by purchase or through a rental agreement. Use of home care professionals can also be costly. Depending on the patient's needs, nurses and respiratory therapists may be a costly expenditure (Murray, 1989; O'Donohue et al., 1986).

The complexity and available features of a ventilator can affect the equipment cost. As a rule, more complex equipment and supplies cost more. For patients who cannot breathe spontaneously and require continuous ventilatory support, a backup ventilator may also be necessary. Those patients who require around-the-clock care may also need medical professionals to make frequent home visits. Family members may also need to hire a home care aide to provide periodic relief for leisure time and other family or work obligations.

A study on the financial aspects of pediatric home ventilator care, it shows a significant reduction in the total cost (Hazlett, 1989). Of course, home ventilator care cannot be justified from a financial standpoint if its total cost is higher than the cost of comparable hospital care. Careful cost analysis should be done based on the patient's requirements. The resultant cost for the entire home ventilator care program may be part of the patient selection process.

AVAILABLE RESOURCES

The primary resources that are vital to the success of home ventilator care include physical environment, technical support, and emotional support. The physical environment for home ventilator care must provide adequate space for the ventilator, special bed, wheelchair, oxygen units, and supplies. Suitable and sufficient electrical outlets are also needed for the ventilator, alarms, and other related equipment. Technical support should include one or more home health agencies that have ample equipment and supplies, qualified medical professionals, and around-the-clock coverage. Emotional support may include psychosocial assistance provided to the patient and family members by community agencies, support groups, and friends.

EQUIPMENT SELECTION

Although positive pressure ventilation with an artifical airway is the most common modality in home ventilator care, there are several factors to consider before prescribing the equipment for the patient. The primary factor of equipment selection should result in a ventilator or device that suits the patient's immediate and long-term needs. The secondary factor should deal with the use and maintenance of the equipment.

TYPES OF VENTILATORY SUPPORT

If the patient does not have adequate spontaneous ventilation for an extended time, positive pressure or negative pressure ventilators are the equipment of choice. Positive pressure ventilation requires an artificial airway whereas negative pressure ventilation can be provided without an artificial airway. One exception to this practice is the presence of significant airway obstruction.

> ✔ A backup ventilator may be necessary if the patient is totally dependent on mechanical ventilation.

A backup ventilator may be necessary if the patient is totally dependent on mechanical ventilation. For patients who are using mechanical ventilation on a part-time basis (e.g., during sleep), a backup system may not be needed or financially justifiable.

Other modes of ventilatory support include the chest cuirass, raincoat or wrap, pneumobelt, rocking bed, and diaphragmatic pacing. A chest cuirass ventilator is a shell that fits over the patient's chest wall (Figure 17-1). The raincoat or wrap is an airtight jacket that seals at the arms, hips, and neck (Figure 17-2). It covers a larger area than the chest cuirass and does not impinge on the chest and abdomen. For this reason, it offers a larger inspiratory volume to the user. The raincoat or wrap is more difficult to get into and usually requires help from another person in the home. The pneumobelt is a corsetlike belt attached to a positive pressure generator. The positive pressure inflates the belt, squeezes the abdomen, and pushes the diaphragm upward. An alternating sequence of positive pressure and ambient pressure provided to the pneumobelt produces active ventilation. The rocking bed relies on motion to displace the abdominal contents

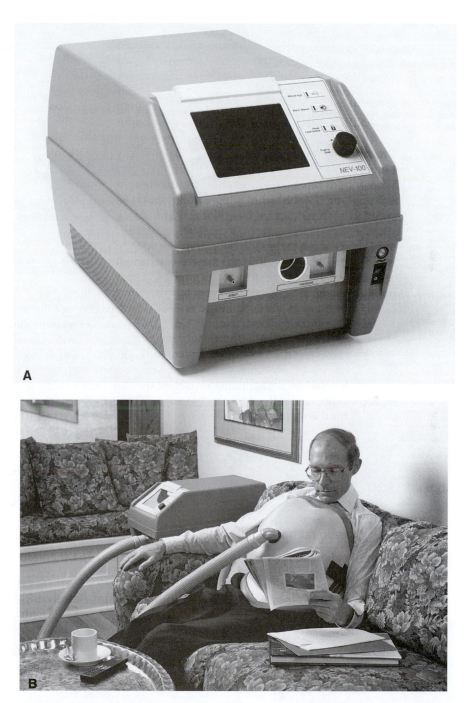

Figure 17-1 (A) LIFECARE's noninvasive extrathoracic ventilator NEV-100; (B) NEV-100 in use with a chest shell (cuirass);

(continued)

Figure 17-1 *(continued)* (C) LIFECARE Soft Seal Chest Shell. (Courtesy of LIFECARE.)

to facilitate diaphragmatic motion and ventilation (Hill, 1994; Votroubek, 1995).

Diaphragmatic Pacing. Diaphragmatic pacing or bilateral pacing of the phrenic nerves does not actually provide mechanical ventilation. Rather, it is used to augment spontaneous ventilation. Diaphragmatic pacing has been used in infants and children for more than a decade (Ilbawi et al., 1985). The pacing system includes an external transmitter and antenna placed on the skin over a receiver implanted subcutaneously. At a predetermined interval, the receiver sends electrical energy to an electrode placed near the thoracic phrenic nerves.

Figure 17-2 (A) LIFECARE's Nu-Mo suit; (B) pulmo wrap. (Courtesy of LIFECARE.)

When the phrenic nerves are stimulated by electrical energy, the diaphragm contracts (Votroubek, 1995).

RELIABILITY AND SAFETY

☑ A home care ventilator and its safety features must not be too complicated for those working with the patient and ventilator.

The ventilator used at home should be highly dependable and require little or no maintenance by nonmedical personnel such as the patient, family members, and home care aides. Each ventilator should have safety features such as high pressure, low pressure, and ventilator failure alarms. These features must not be too complicated for those working with the patient and ventilator.

SIMPLICITY AND PORTABILITY

☑ Ventilators with built-in rechargable battery packs are versatile in the event of brief power failure. The patient may also take advantage of this feature to make physician office visits or brief shopping trips.

The operation and maintenance of home care ventilators should be direct and simple. Dials and alarms on the ventilator that are illogical and hard to understand are likely to confuse the users. The ventilator circuits should be easy to clean if they are reusable.

Ventilators that are small, compact, and portable will provide the most flexibility when the patient wants to move around the home. Ventilators with built-in rechargeable battery packs are also very versatile in the event of brief power failure. The patient may also take advantage of this feature to make physician office visits or brief shopping trips.

RESOURCES FOR HOME MECHANICAL VENTILATION

Learning Objectives for Positive Pressure Ventilation in the Home is published by The National Center for Home Mechanical Ventilation. This publication lists the detailed educational objectives to aid respiratory care professionals in customizing an educational program for caregivers of ventilator-dependent patients. For further information, contact National Center for Home Mechanical Ventilation, 1400 Jackson Street, Room J105a, Denver, CO 80206.

Tracheostomy Tube Adult Home Care Guide is a booklet published by Shiley Tracheostomy Tubes to help home health care providers to teach home tracheostomy care. This guide is available from Mallinckrodt Medical TPI, Inc., P.O. Box 19614, Irvine, CA 92713-9614. 800/854-4071.

SUMMARY

Mechanical ventilation has been used effectively to support patients suffering from ventilatory or oxygenation failure. Many of these patients require continuing ventilatory support due to irreversible problems such as high cervical or head injuries. As a result, they are required to stay in an acute care setting longer than other patients. Since acute care settings are traditionally more costly, home mechanical ventilation has gained popularity in caring for patients requiring prolonged ventilatory assistance.

The successful management of a patient on a home mechanical ventilator demands proper patient selection, careful planning, detailed home instruction, and a programmatic follow-up by the health care team. The team approach is probably the most critical element of successful ventilator care in the home. The health care professionals and especially the family members must be able and willing to make a long-term commitment in caring for the patient in the home.

Self-Assessment Questions

1. Which of the following is *not* a goal of mechanical ventilation provided in the home?

   A. extension of the patient's life and quality of life
   B. development and improvement of the patient's body functions
   C. elimination of staff positions in an acute care setting
   D. reduction of the cost for acute ventilator care

2. Providing or receiving mechanical ventilation in the home:

   A. needs careful evaluation in selecting a suitable patient.
   B. gives the patient less time to interact with family members and friends.
   C. requires little or no commitment from family members.
   D. is more costly than one provided in an acute care setting.

3. Some essential team members for a successful home ventilator program should include all of the following *except*:

   A. physician.
   B. insurance clerk.
   C. respiratory therapist.
   D. nurse.

4. Dr. Kingston asks you to evaluate Mr. Lange, a patient who has been on the ventilator for 3 weeks, for continuation of ventilator care in the home. You would evaluate all of the following *except*:

   A. age of patient.
   B. clinical stability of the patient.
   C. type of ventilator suitable for the patient.
   D. laboratory and clinical assessment of the patient.

5 to 8. Match the type of pulmonary problem with the respective clinical characteristics. Use each answer once.

Pulmonary Problem	Characteristics
5. COPD	A. Apnea and chronic hypoventilation
6. Restrictive lung disease	B. Inefficient ventilation, atelectasis, and pneumonia
7. Ventilatory muscle dysfunction	C. Air flow obstruction and air trapping
8. Central hypoventilation syndrome	D. Reduction of lung volumes/capacities and deadspace ventilation

9. A COPD patient has an admitting diagnosis of lobar pneumonia affecting three of five lobes. When this pulmonary problem triggers a rapid deterioration of the patient's clinical status, it is called:

    A. acute bronchitis and COPD.

    B. acute exacerbation of COPD.

    C. chronic ventilatory failure with metabolic acidosis.

    D. respiratory failure of COPD.

10. Which of the following blood gas reports illustrates the condition in Question #9?

Blood Gas Report
A. pH = 7.26, $PaCO_2$ = 78 mm Hg, PaO_2 = 44 mm Hg, HCO_3^- = 34 mEq/L
B. pH = 7.40, $PaCO_2$ = 45 mm Hg, PaO_2 = 81 mm Hg, HCO_3^- = 27 mEq/L
C. pH = 7.39, $PaCO_2$ = 52 mm Hg, PaO_2 = 56 mm Hg, HCO_3^- = 31 mEq/L
D. pH = 7.49, $PaCO_2$ = 30 mm Hg, PaO_2 = 43 mm Hg, HCO_3^- = 22 mEq/L

11. In addition to V/Q mismatch and pulmonary hypertension, COPD patients usually have:

    A. low lung compliance.

    B. high elastic recoil of lung tissues.

    C. air trapping.

    D. reduced lung volumes and capacities.

12. Mechanical ventilation may be necessary for patients with restrictive lung disease because they have:

    A. high lung compliance.

    B. increased lung volumes and capacities.

    C. low lung inflating pressure requirement.

    D. increased work of breathing.

13. Apnea, hypoventilation, infection, and atelectasis are some signs of patients diagnosed with:

    A. central hypoventilation syndrome.

    B. COPD.

    C. restrictive lung disease.

    D. spinal cord injury at the C-5 level.

14. Selection of patient for a home mechanical ventilation program should be based on all of the following considerations *except* the:

    A. desires of the patient.

    B. desires of the physician.

    C. available equipment and financial resources.

    D. cost for the home care program.

15. Ms. Lange has been receiving around-the-clock mechanical ventilation for two months due to a head injury sustained in an automobile accident. Prior to transfer to her home for ventilator care, which of the following is the most essential safety feature based on her condition?

    A. insurance coverage

    B. high and low pressure alarms

    C. live-in health care assistance

    D. backup ventilator

Answers to Self-Assessment Questions

1. C. elimination of staff positions in an acute care setting

2. A. needs careful evaluation in selecting a suitable patient.

3. B. insurance clerk.

4. A. age of patient.

5. C. Air flow obstruction and air trapping

6. D. Reduction of lung volumes/capacities and deadspace ventilation

7. B. Inefficient ventilation, atelectasis, and pneumonia

8. A. Apnea and chronic hypoventilation

9. B. acute exacerbation of COPD

10. A. pH = 7.26, $PaCO_2$ = 78 mm Hg, PaO_2 = 44 mm Hg, HCO_3^- = 34 mEq/L

11. C. air trapping.

12. D. increased work of breathing.

13. A. central hypoventilation syndrome.

14. B. desires of the physician.

15. D. backup ventilator

References

Eigen, H., et al. (1990). Home mechanical ventilation of pediatric patients. *Am Rev Respir Dis, 141*(1), 258–259.

Ferns, T. (1994). Home mechanical ventilation in a changing health service. *Nurs Times, 90*(40), 43–45.

Glass, C. A. (1993). The impact of home based ventilator dependence on family life. *Paraplegia, 31*(2), 93–101.

Goldstein, R. S., et al. (1995). Home mechanical ventilation: Demographics and user perspectives. *Chest, 108*(6), 1581–1586.

Gower, D. J., et al. (1985). Home ventilator dependence after high cervical cord injury. *South Med J, 78*(8), 1010–1011.

Hazlett, D. E. (1989). A study of pediatric home ventilator management: Medical, psychosocial, and financial aspects. *J Pediatr Nurs, 4*(4), 284–294.

Hill, N. S. (1994). Use of negative pressure ventilation, rocking beds, and pneumobelts. *Respir Care, 39,* 532–549.

Ilbawi, M. N., et al. (1985). Diaphragm pacing in infants: Techniques and results. *Ann Thorac Surg, 40,* 323–329.

Malley, W. J. (1990). *Clinical blood gases: Application and noninvasive alternatives.* Philadelphia: W. B. Saunders.

Murray, J. E. (1989, October). Payment mechanisms for pediatric home care. *Caring,* 33–35.

O'Donohue, W. J., et al. (1986). Long-term mechanical ventilation: Guidelines for management in the home and at alternate community sites (Report of the ad hoc committee, Respiratory Care Section, American College of Chest Physicians). *Chest,* (Suppl. 90, 1), 1S–37S.

Smith, C. E. (1994). Caregiver learning needs and reactions to managing home mechanical ventilation. *Heart Lung, 23*(2), 157–163.

Votroubek, W. L. (1995). Home mechanical ventilation: What are all the options? *J Home Health Care Prac, 7*(3), 21–26.

Suggested Reading

Banaszak, E. F., et al. (1981). Home ventilator care. *Respir Care, 26*(12), 1262–1268.

Carroll, P. F. (1987). Home care for the ventilator patient: A check list you can use. *Nursing, 17*(10), 82–83.

Feldman, J., et al. (1982, March/April). Mechanical ventilation: From hospital intensive care to home. *Heart Lung, 11,* 162.

Glenn, K. A., et al. (1993). *Learning objectives for positive pressure ventilation in the home.* Denver, CO: National Center for Home Mechanical Ventilation.

Goldberg, A . I. (1989). Home care for life-supported persons: The French system of quality control, technology assessment, and cost containment. *Public Health Rep, 104*(4), 329–335.

Hughes, S. L., et al. (1987). Impact of long-term home care on hospital and nursing home use and cost. *Health Serv Res, 22*(1), 19–47.

Hughes, S. L., et al. (1992). A randomized trial of the cost effectiveness of VA hospital-based home care for the terminally ill. *Health Serv Res, 26*(6), 801–817.

Sivak, E., et al. (1983, August). Home care ventilation. *Chest, 84,* 239.

Smith, J. E., & Shneerson, J. M. (1996). A laboratory comparison of four positive pressure ventilators used in the home. *Eur Respir J, 9*(11): 2410–2415.

White, K. D., et al. (1986). Your ventilator patient can go home again. *Nursing, 16*(12), 54–56.

CHAPTER EIGHTEEN

CASE STUDIES

CASE 1: COPD

INTRODUCTION

A 74-year-old Caucasian male with a diagnosis of pulmonary emphysema, made six years prior, was seen in the emergency department with a complaint of shortness of breath. He has had respiratory problems on and off since diagnosis, including two hospital admissions, each of several days duration. He stated he caught a cold the previous week that moved down into his chest, and since that time breathing has become increasingly more difficult. He related that in his usual state of health, he was able to move freely about his home and yard and enjoyed his hobby of gardening, but now was unable to do either. Sleeping in bed had become such a problem that for the previous two nights he slept sitting back in his easy chair. His normal sputum production of about a tablespoon per day had increased to about 1/4 cup a day and had turned from white to yellow in color. He gained 6 lb in the past 4 days and noticed that his ankles were swollen by the end of the day. When questioned about his smoking history, he stated that he had smoked two packs per day for 40 years, and had tried unsuccessfully to quit after his diagnosis of emphysema was made. He now smokes a half pack per day of a "lighter" brand. His home medications include an albuterol metered-dose inhaler (MDI), 1–2 puffs every 2 to 6 hours, as needed.

☑ The inability to breathe comfortably unless standing or sitting up is termed orthopnea and is a common clinical manifestation of pulmonary disease.

☑ Sudden weight gain with dependent edema in a COPD patient is a sign of cor pulmonale.

PHYSICAL EXAMINATION

General. The patient is a mildly obese male, weight 100 kg, height 72 in., in moderately severe respiratory distress, sitting on the edge of the bed leaning forward supporting his weight with his palms and breathing through pursed lips.

Vital Signs.   Heart rate 124/min, blood pressure 150/90 mm Hg, respiratory rate 28/min, and temperature 100.5°F.

HEENT.   Some cyanosis of the lips, otherwise unremarkable.

Neck.   Trachea in the midline, no masses, stridor, lymphadenopathy, or thyromegaly. Carotid pulses ++ without bruit. There is marked use of accessory muscles of the neck with mild jugular venous distention.

☑ Paradoxical motion of the abdomen during ventilation is an indication of diaphragmatic muscle fatigue.

Chest.   The anteroposterior diameter of the chest is increased with a deep suprasternal notch and some paradoxical motion of the abdomen. Decreased tactile fremitus and absent point of maximal impulse (PMI) are noted with hyperresonance to percussion bilaterally.

Heart.   Sounds are distant with no irregularity in rate or rhythm noted, no gallops or murmurs.

Lungs.   Bilaterally diminished with scattered expiratory wheezing, bibasilar rhonchi, and a prolonged expiratory phase.

Abdomen.   Mild hepatomegaly, paradoxical movement with breathing, otherwise unremarkable.

Extremities.   Slight digital cyanosis with +2 pitting edema in both ankles.

INITIAL ASSESSMENT AND TREATMENT

In the emergency room, a portable chest radiograph and arterial blood gas with co-oximetry were obtained, the patient was placed on a 2 L/min nasal cannula and given an aerosol treatment with 2.5 mg albuterol sulfate in NS. Room air blood gas results revealed:

pH	7.32
$PaCO_2$	70 mm Hg
PaO_2	44 mm Hg
HCO_3^-	35 mEq/L
BE	+6
SaO_2	85%
Hb	16 g/dL
HBCO	3%

☑ Acute on chronic ventilatory failure in the COPD patient is an indication for admission to the ICU.

The chest radiograph revealed evidence of hyperinflation, an increase in vascular markings, and an infiltrate in the RLL. Because of the patient's clinical condition, chest radiograph findings, and the acute imposed-on chronic ventilatory failure indicated by the blood gas, the patient was transferred immediately to the medical intensive care unit (ICU) for further evaluation and treatment.

☑️ Aminophylline
(theophylline)
improves diaphrag-
matic function in the
COPD patient.

☑️ Corticosteroids
are only useful
in the treatment of
COPD if the patient
has evidence of
reversible airway
disease.

The patient was then started on the following regimen: supplemental oxygen at 2 L/min by nasal cannula, nebulized albuterol sulfate,
2.5 mg in NS Q2H, 2.5 mg/kg loading dose of aminophylline over
30 min, followed by a maintenance dose of 0.5 mg/kg per hour IV
(titrated according to serum levels), furosemide, 40 mg, IV push,
and methylprednisolone, 120 mg IV, Q6H. Sputum for Gram stain
and culture was obtained and sent to the lab. The patient was also
started on a prophylactic broad-spectrum antibiotic. The report on
the Gram stain came back later and showed numerous gram-positive
diplococci.

INDICATIONS

Over the next hour, the patient's respiratory status continued to deteriorate despite intervention. Respiratory rate rose to 36/min and paradoxical abdominal motion became more pronounced. The rising
respiratory rate in conjunction with the abdominal paradox and the
increasing $PaCO_2$ from the first blood gas are indicative of increasing
ventilatory fatigue. Impending acute ventilatory failure must be
assumed.

INITIAL SETTINGS

☑️ In the alert and
cooperative
patient with intact
airway defenses,
noninvasive ventila-
tion can provide
ventilatory support
without the risks
associated with
intubation.

On the basis of clinical and laboratory data, a decision was made
to assist the patient's ventilation. In lieu of endotracheal intubation,
bilevel positive airway pressure (bilevel PAP) was initiated via nasal
mask at the settings below. The IPAP and EPAP levels were titrated
to 15/5 resulting in an SpO_2 endpoint of around 90%.

Mode	Spontaneous
IPAP	15 cm H_2O
EPAP	5 cm H_2O
Sup. O_2	2 L/min

The patient was poorly compliant with the therapy, removing the
mask at regular intervals, complaining of not being able to get enough
air. After 1 hour, an arterial blood gas was obtained and revealed the
following:

pH	7.25
$PaCO_2$	80 mm Hg
PaO_2	56 mm Hg
HCO_3^-	34 mEq/L
BE	+3
SaO_2	89%
Hb	16 g/dL
HBCO	2%

On the basis of the worsening ventilatory failure despite noninvasive ventilatory assistance, the patient was intubated with a size

8.5 endotracheal tube, and volume-targeted mechanical ventilation was initiated on the following settings:

Mode	CMV
V_T	750 mL
f	10/min
PIF	55 L/min, resulting in an I:E ratio = 1:4
F_IO_2	0.40
PEEP	5 cm H_2O
Flow Trigger	3 L/min

After 30 min, an arterial blood gas was obtained and revealed the following:

pH	7.36
$PaCO_2$	65 mm Hg
PaO_2	88 mm Hg
HCO_3^-	36 mEq/L
BE	+6
SaO_2	96%
Hb	16 g/dL
HBCO	1%

On the basis of the blood gas, an order was written to titrate the patient's F_IO_2 to maintain the $SpO_2 \geq 92\%$. No other changes were made to the ventilatory parameters. Albuterol orders were changed to MDI, 8 puffs in-line Q4H. The patient was suctioned prn for moderate amounts of thick pale yellow secretions.

PATIENT MONITORING

✓ In order to minimize theophylline toxicity, the therapeutic range for serum theophylline level should be kept from 5 to 15 mcg/mL.

Over the course of the next 72 hours the patient was rested on the ventilator and treated appropriately for his pneumonia and right heart failure. The patient remained alert and cooperative with his care. A chest radiograph done on day three of ICU admission demonstrated clearing of the pneumonic process in the RLL. Findings characteristic of emphysema were also present including hyperlucent lung fields, flattened diaphragm, widely spaced ribs, and a narrow heart shadow. Serum theophylline levels were monitored daily, averaging 9 mcg/mL.

The ventilator settings were adjusted appropriately and currently are:

Mode	SIMV
V_T	750 mL
f	6
PIF	55 L/min, resulting in an I:E ratio = 1:4
F_IO_2	0.35
PEEP	5 cm H_2O
PSV	7 cm H_2O
Flow Trigger	3 L/min

Spontaneous Parameters

Spont. f	12
Spont. V_T	550 mL
VC	2.21 L
MIP	-36 cm H_2O

The arterial blood gas drawn on the current ventilator settings shows:

pH	7.39
$PaCO_2$	57 mm Hg
PaO_2	74 mm Hg
HCO_3^-	34 mEq/L
BE	+7
SaO_2	94%
Hb	15.5 g/dL
HBCO	1%

PATIENT MANAGEMENT

The patient's vital signs have normalized and along with ventilator care, fluid status was normalized and bronchodilator therapy was continued to relieve bronchospasm and help promote mucociliary clearance. Antibiotic therapy was continued and adjusted on the basis of the culture and sensitivity report. Secretion volume and consistency have decreased and color has changed from yellow to white.

WEANING

As the patient's condition continued to improve, ventilatory support was gradually withdrawn over the next 3 days. He was placed on the spontaneous breathing mode (CPAP mode) at an F_IO_2 of 0.35 with a pressure support of 5 cm H_2O and CPAP of 5 cm H_2O. After 4 hours, spontaneous ventilatory parameters were measured and an arterial blood gas was obtained. The results are as follows:

☑ f/ V_T ratio <100/min/L is predictive of weaning success.

f	18
V_T	525 mL
VE	9.45 L
f/V_T	34/min/L
VC	2.85 L
MIP	-44 cm H_2O
pH	7.38
$PaCO_2$	59 mm Hg
PaO_2	68 mm Hg
HCO_3^-	34 mEq/L
BE	+7
SaO_2	92%
Hb	15.1 g/dL
HBCO	1%

☑ A comprehensive rehabilitation program teaches the patient about his or her disease, self-care, maintenance of an active lifestyle, and smoking cessation.

COMPLICATIONS

On the basis of the patient's clinical condition and diagnostic results, he was extubated and placed on 2 L/min O_2 via nasal cannula. He was moved to the medical floor later that day, and was subsequently discharged 2 days later after being enrolled in the hospital's comprehensive outpatient rehabilitation program. His home medications included albuterol via MDI, ipratropium via MDI, and oral theophylline.

CASE 2: STATUS ASTHMATICUS

INTRODUCTION

P.W., a 32-year-old, 48-kg female, was gravida 14, para 0-4-9-4, and about 21½ weeks pregnant at the time of her admission. She was evaluated for acute exacerbation of asthma with upper respiratory tract infection. The patient stated that she was "doing fine" until approximately midnight at which time she began having difficulty breathing. Her shortness of breath continued despite taking her bronchodilator inhalers.

☑ Aminophylline is commonly used to reverse severe bronchospasm in acute asthma that has not responded to epinephrine.

☑ Hypoxemia is severe since the PaO_2 is only 59 mm Hg with a nonrebreathing mask.

In the emergency room, she was tachypneic with inspiratory and expiratory wheezes, rhonchi, and dry crackles throughout all lung fields. She was placed on oxygen with a nonrebreathing mask at 10 L/min and given one Proventil nebulizer treatment. A stat blood gas was done and she was started on IV aminophylline. Her respiratory rate at that time was 28/min, with the following blood gas results:

pH	7.47
$PaCO_2$	34 mm Hg
PaO_2	59 mm Hg
HCO_3^-	24.2 mEq/L
Hb	12.8 g %
SpO_2	91%
Mode	Nonrebreathing mask
Oxygen	10 L/min
RR	Spontaneous 28/min

☑ $PaCO_2$ of 34 mm Hg indicates the work of breathing is excessive in order to maintain borderline oxygenation.

☑ Increase in respiratory rate from 28 to 36/min is an ominous sign in the progression of acute asthma.

Four hours later her respiratory rate had increased to 36/min and she had received medication nebulizer treatments every hour with Proventil. However, inspiratory and expiratory wheezes persisted. A follow-up blood gas revealed:

pH	7.42
$PaCO_2$	36 mm Hg
PaO_2	58 mm Hg
HCO_3^-	23.2 mEq/L
Hb	12.8 g %

☑ PaO$_2$ does not show much improvement in spite of increase in spontaneous respiratory rate.

SpO$_2$	91%
Mode	Nonrebreathing mask
Oxygen	10 L/min
RR	Spontaneous 36/min

INDICATIONS

Subsequent blood gases indicated that the patient's ventilatory status quickly deteriorated and she became unable to maintain hyperventilation. Her PaCO$_2$ began rising toward normal.

Rising PaCO$_2$ from a low level (hyperventilation) toward normal is indicative of muscle fatigue. Impending ventilatory failure is likely if not treated aggressively.

In asthma, the increased work of breathing is related to a combination of bronchospasm, airway inflammation, and mucus accumulation. This condition increases the airway resistance and work of breathing, which perpetuates the degranulation of mast cells. Asthmatic patients may not respond to bronchodilators and eventually may show signs of exhaustion and progressive somnolence with hypoxemia and hypercapnea. At that point, intubation and mechanical ventilation are indicated.

INITIAL SETTINGS

The patient was initially set on assist/control (AC) mode at rate of 10/min, V$_T$ of 600 mL, F$_I$O$_2$ of 90%, and PEEP of 5 cm H$_2$O. The peak flow was increased to match her inspiratory demand, approaching 110 L/min. Every effort was made to reduce the work of breathing and decrease her anxiety level from a ventilatory standpoint. Blood gases obtained revealed the following:

pH	7.42
PaCO$_2$	33 mm Hg
PaO$_2$	55 mm Hg
HCO$_3^-$	21.3 mEq/L
Hb	12.4 g %
SpO$_2$	90%
Mode	A/C
RR	10/min
V$_T$	600 mL
F$_I$O$_2$	90%
PEEP	5 cm H$_2$O

☑ PC-IRV may improve oxygenation and minimize occurrence of barotrauma.

Although pharmacologic sedation is generally not recommended for asthmatic patients, she was medicated and changed to inverse I:E ratio ventilation on pressure control (PC-IRV) mode at a 2:1 ratio to improve oxygenation and prevent barotrauma related to positive pressure ventilation. She was started at a rate of 20/min, an inspiratory pressure of 40 cm H$_2$O, T$_I$ of 0.5 sec, F$_I$O$_2$ of 60%, and PEEP of 10 cm H$_2$O. Blood gases were as follows:

pH	7.36
$PaCO_2$	44 mm Hg
PaO_2	64 mm Hg
HCO_3^-	24 mEq/L
Hb	11.8 g %
SpO_2	92%
Mode	PC-IRV
T_I	0.5 sec
I:E ratio	2:1
Rate	20/min
P_{INSP}	40 cm H_2O
F_IO_2	60%
PEEP	10 cm H_2O

No changes in her care or ventilator parameters were made at that time. Breath sounds revealed wheezes and coarse rhonchi throughout all lung fields. She continued with her bronchodilator therapy and was suctioned appropriately.

PATIENT MONITORING

The chest radiograph shows the characteristic hyperinflation of the lungs. The distance between the adjacent ribs is widened and the diaphragm is depressed. Infiltrates or areas of edema are also noted on the chest radiograph (Figure 18-1). Other than these signs, the chest radiograph is normal.

Over the next 3 days, the ventilator settings were changed accordingly and the latest settings were pressure control at 30 cm H_2O, T_I of 0.7 sec for a 2:1 ratio, F_IO_2 of 50%, and PEEP of 10 cm H_2O. She was beginning to show signs of reduced inflammation of her airway with only occasional inspiratory and expiratory wheezes. Small amounts of cloudy, clear secretions were suctioned from her endotracheal tube. Peak and trough levels of serum theophylline were drawn to monitor possible toxicity. Blood gas results were as follows:

✓ The therapeutic range of serum theophylline is between 5 to 15 mcg/mL.

pH	7.43
$PaCO_2$	36 mm Hg
PaO_2	78 mm Hg
HCO_3^-	23 mEq/L
Hb	12 g %
SpO_2	93%
Mode	IR-PCV
T_I	0.7 sec
I:E ratio	2:1
Rate	20/min
P_{INSP}	30 cm H_2O
F_IO_2	50%
PEEP	10 cm H_2O

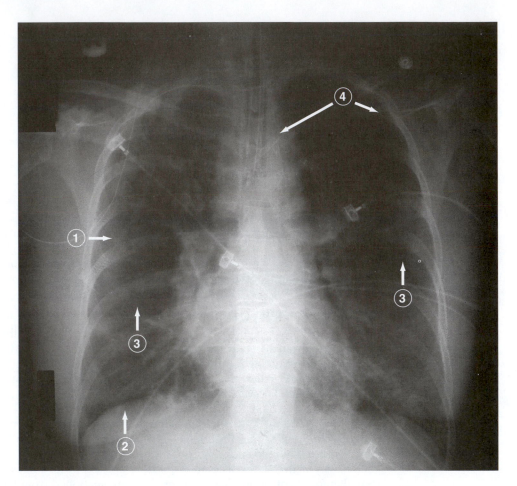

Figure 18-1 Status asthmaticus. Hyperinflation is evident on this chest radiograph since the distance between the adjacent ribs is widened (1) and the diaphragm is depressed (2). Infiltrates or areas of edema are noted (3). The central venous line (4) is also visible on this chest radiograph.

She was becoming more alert and subsequently changed to SIMV with pressure support to supplement her own efforts to breathe. She appeared calm at first but became increasingly restless and combative over the afternoon and evening. She frequently motioned for the endotracheal tube to be removed and was frustrated about her inability to talk.

PATIENT MANAGEMENT

In addition to the ventilator management strategies, adequate hydration was provided to promote mucociliary clearance and bronchopulmonary hygiene. Bronchodilators, glucocorticosteroids, and mast cell stabilizers were used to bring the bronchospasm under control.

☑ Intal is not given in acute asthma episodes but is used as a prophylactic measure to control airway hyperreactivity.

KEY MEDICATIONS

The patient was treated with aminophylline given intravenously, sympathomimetic beta adrenergics (Proventil and Serevent) via MDI and given in-line through the ventilator circuit every 3 to 4 hours. These served to control the symptoms associated with asthma while she was started on triacinolone acetonide (Azmacort), a corticosteroid inhaler to control the inflammation. She was also started on two puffs of cromolyn sodium (Intal) to help prevent the degranulation of mast cell mediators responsible for reactive airway disease.

WEANING

The weaning process was uneventful as the patient continued to improve. She was eventually placed on CPAP without pressure support or PEEP for assessment of possible extubation. Her spontaneous ventilatory parameters revealed the following results:

$$f = 15 \quad V_E = 8.1\ L \quad V_T = 0.54\ L \quad VC = 2.19\ L \quad MIP = -43$$
$$f/V_T = 28/min/L$$

She eventually extubated herself, while restrained, and was placed on a nasal cannula at 6 L/min, which maintained saturations above 90%.

COMPLICATIONS

Her oxygen demands decreased over several days where she continued on her bronchodilators, weaned to room air, and was discharged after 6 days. There were no apparent complications throughout her hospital stay and she was advised to seek and follow medical care through her primary care provider. She remained on an oral steroid (Prednisone) and an antibiotic (Erythromycin) for an additional 10 days after discharge from the hospital.

Note: This case study on status asthmaticus describes the evaluative, diagnostic, and ventilatory management techniques employed at the time it was first written. For additional information, please refer to the guidelines outlined by the National Institute of Health (1997, Oct). *Practical guide for the diagnosis and management of asthma. NIH Publication No. 97-4053.*

CASE 3: POSTABDOMINAL SURGERY

INTRODUCTION

C.T., a 78-year-old, 90-kg, 5'4" female, was admitted to the emergency room (ER) with complaints of the following ailments that had persisted for the past several days: abdominal pain, nausea, fatigue,

☑ An f/V_T ratio of less than 100/min/L is highly predictive of weaning success.

☑ Leukocytosis (↑WBC) is generally caused by infection and is usually transient. It may also occur after hemorrhage.

☑ Low hematocrit leads to tissue hypoxia and it may account for her symptoms of shortness of breath, fatigability, weakness, and decreased exercise tolerance.

☑ Thrombocytopenia (↓platelets) occurs in acute infections, anaphylactic shock, and some hemorrhagic diseases and anemias.

☑ Discharge $PaCO_2$ (50 mm Hg) will serve as the target value in subsequent weaning attempts.

☑ Blood transfusion is indicated because of ↓ hematocrit and ↓ platelets.

☑ Normal cuff pressure is between 27 and 40 cm H_2O, lower for patients with hypotension.

weakness, shortness of breath, decreased exercise tolerance, vomiting, and black tarry stools.

She had a history of steroid-dependent asthma, COPD, coronary artery disease, diabetes, and arthritis. Her medications at home included Lasix, Diabeta, nitroglycerin, aspirin, Prozac, potassium, Proventil, Intal, Azmacort, and oxygen at 2 to 3 L/min.

In the ER her abdominal exam revealed severe pain in all quadrants and her abdominal radiograph showed free air in all areas. Respiratory assessments showed severe peripheral cyanosis, respiratory rate 32/min, heart rate 120/min, decreased breath sounds in all lobes with fine inspiratory crackles in the lower lobes, and accessory muscle use during inspiration.

Laboratory studies were done upon admission with the following results: WBC 22.2×10^3 (*normal 3.2 to 9.8 $\times 10^3$*), hematocrit (Hct) 25% (*female average 42%*), platelets 34.2×10^3 (*normal 130 to 400 $\times 10^3$*). The electrocardiograph (ECG) showed sinus tachycardia with nonspecific ST and T wave changes.

Other medical history was not significant. The patient's last hospitalization was 3 years ago for asthma. Upon discharge from the hospital, her room air blood gases were pH 7.43, $PaCO_2$ 50 mm Hg, PaO_2 42 mm Hg, HCO_3^- 32 mEq/L, and SaO_2 77%. She was placed on supplemental O_2 at home at that time.

After her exam the patient received two units of packed red blood cells (RBCs) and one unit of plasma to treat her low hematocrit. Due to her acute and severe condition, she was taken to the operating room for abdominal exploratory surgery.

INDICATIONS

The patient was heavily sedated during her abdominal exploratory surgery and required large amounts of IV fluids, including blood products to maintain her blood pressure during surgery and to increase her low hematocrit level. A bleeding gastric ulcer and a perforated duodenal ulcer were found and repaired without complications. The patient was returned to the ICU, intubated, and placed on mechanical ventilation for postanesthesia recovery.

INITIAL SETTINGS

The patient was intubated with a size 8.0 cuffed endotracheal tube secured at the 23 cm mark at the lips. The cuff pressure was maintained at 35 cm H_2O to prevent air leak around the cuff. The settings on the Puritan-Bennett 7200 ventilator were: SIMV mode, rate 10/min, V_T 800 mL, F_IO_2 100%, no PEEP, peak flow 45 L/min, and sensitivity -2 cm H_2O. Her initial static compliance was 74 mL/cm H_2O. Breath sounds were equal bilaterally with fine inspiratory crackles in both lower lobes. Blood gases showed:

pH	7.44
$PaCO_2$	36 mm Hg

☑ The PaO₂ is too high and the F₁O₂ should be reduced.

PaO₂	102 mm Hg
SaO₂	97%
HCO₃⁻	24 mEq/L
Mode	SIMV
Rate	10/min
V_T	800 mL
F_IO_2	100%
PEEP	0 cm H_2O
Peak Flow	45 L/min
Sensitivity	−2 cm H_2O
C_{ST}	74 mL/cm H_2O

PATIENT MONITORING

The major monitoring tools used during her recovery were pulse oximetry, end-tidal CO_2 monitor, and central venous pressure (CVP). Her SpO₂ was 96%. The $P_{ET}CO_2$ was about 33 to 35 mm Hg (*normal 2 mm Hg below PaCO₂*), and her CVP was consistently between 10 and 12 mm Hg (*normal 1 to 7 mm Hg*).

☑ SpO₂ (96%) correlates well with the SaO₂ (97%).

☑ CVP is higher than normal. The systemic venous volume status should be monitored closely.

PATIENT MANAGEMENT

The patient was maintained for several hours on SIMV, rate 10, V_T 800 mL, F_IO_2 40%, peak flow 45 L/min. The patient had no spontaneous ventilation after 6 hours despite being fully alert and oriented. After the F_IO_2 was decreased to 40%, the blood gas results were:

☑ Since the patient was a chronic CO₂ retainer, the target PaCO₂ (50 mm Hg) should be used to manage this patient.

pH	7.40
PaCO₂	38 mm Hg
PaO₂	65 mm Hg
SaO₂	92%
HCO₃⁻	23 mEq/L
Mode	SIMV
Rate	10/min
V_T	800 mL
F_IO_2	40%
PEEP	0 cm H_2O
Peak Flow	45 L/min

Fluid intake was adjusted to maintain a CVP reading between 10 and 12 mm Hg. Other vital signs were within normal limits for her age. Proventil and Intal treatments were started for her asthma and her static compliance remained in the 70 sec.

The spontaneous respiratory parameters measured 8 hours post-surgery showed MIP −22 cm H_2O, vital capacity 700 mL. A trial of CPAP of 5 cmH_2O at an F_IO_2 of 40% was unsuccessful as she developed periods of apnea with intermittent tidal volumes of between 300 and 350 mL.

☑ The PaCO₂ can be increased (from the current 38 mm Hg to patient's target 50 mm Hg) by decreasing the SIMV rate or changing to CPAP mode.

☑ Preexisting asthma, postanesthesia, and tissue hypoxia are three major factors that lead to failure of CPAP trial.

☑ Since the rate (f) and V_T are 16/min and 0.476 L (476 mL), respectively, the f/V_T ratio is 34/min/L (16/0.476).

☑ An f/V_T ratio of less than 100/min/L is highly predictive of weaning success.

Over the next several hours, her cardiopulmonary status showed steady improvement from the anesthesia effects and the patient was again tried on CPAP. She tolerated the procedure very well this time, and her spontaneous respiratory parameters at the end of the CPAP trial were: MIP −40 cm H_2O, vital capacity 1,500 mL, spontaneous rate 16, and average V_T of 476 mL. She was successfully extubated and placed on a 50% Venturi mask and eventually weaned to nasal cannula at 3 L/min later that evening.

Some minor complications with the patient's oxygenation and perfusion status were adequately managed using oxygen, blood, and fluids. Her recovery from the abdominal exploratory surgery was gradual but uneventful, and she was discharged from the hospital a few days later.

COMPLICATIONS

The chest radiograph done 16 hours postextubation revealed increasing atelectasis and pneumonia in both bases with bilateral pleural effusions. Breath sounds showed increasing crackles with occasional rhonchi and wheezing. Aerosol treatments were started with Proventil TID and Intal BID. Her SpO_2 on 3 L/min of oxygen was consistently in the mid- to low-80s and she was placed back on a Venturi mask at 40% during the night. The F_IO_2 was increased to 50% at times during periods of desaturation on 40% oxygen.

Her hematocrit increased from 25% to 30% (*female average 42%*) after several transfusions of Hespan, plasma, and packed red blood cells. Her most recent vital signs before discharge were: SpO_2 90%, heart rate 95/min, blood pressure 140/90 mm Hg, and CVP 20 mm Hg (*normal 1 to 7 mm Hg*).

CASE 4: HEAD INJURY

INTRODUCTION

T.A., a 16-year-old, 52-kg female, was brought to the emergency department after sustaining multiple trauma from a moving vehicle accident. She was a passenger in a small car involved in a high-speed collision with a truck. It was unknown if she was restrained prior to the accident but paramedics required approximately 30 to 45 min to extract her from the vehicle. She was reportedly conscious at the scene but became combative and hysterical when she arrived at the hospital. Her blood pressure (BP) was 149/87 mm Hg, pulse 104/min, temperature 34.8°C, and she was able to move all of her extremities.

Due to the extent of her injuries, she was orally intubated and maintained by sedation. The routine trauma laboratory studies revealed

✓ Leukopenia (decrease in WBC) may be due to the trauma or adverse effects of drugs.

✓ Glasgow coma score of 3 reflects a severe coma state. See Appendix B. Glasgow Coma Score.

✓ Pupils that are reactive to light mean that cerebral circulation and oxygenation are adequate.

✓ CT scan of the head and radiographs of the spine and major organs are indicated for head trauma patients.

✓ In head injury, the lungs are not affected unless there are coexisting complications (e.g., aspiration).

✓ Drug-induced coma is done to reduce metabolic rate and minimize intracranial pressure (ICP).

✓ Hyperventilation (e.g., $PaCO_2$ 29 mm Hg) should be done to reduce intracranial pressure in the initial stage of management.

the following results: WBC count of 2.3×10^3 (*normal 3.2 to 9.8 $\times$ 10³*), hematocrit (Hct) 37% (*female average 42%*), platelets of 269×10^3 (*normal 130 to 400 $\times$ 10³*), prothrombin time (PT) of 13 sec (*normal 9 to 12 sec*), and partial thromboplastin time (PTT) of 27 sec (*normal 22 to 37 sec*). Radiographs of the abdomen and chest were unremarkable. However, due to the extent of her head injuries, she was flown by air transport and transferred to a nearby trauma center.

Throughout transport, she was reportedly in and out of consciousness, and upon her arrival to the trauma center her BP was 119/70 mm Hg, pulse 92/min, Glasgow coma score of 3 with no spontaneous eye opening, no movement of her arms or legs. During assessment, she was nonverbal and noted to have a cephalhematoma in the right frontal region with a large laceration in the occipital area. Pupils were equal, round, and reactive to light. She was in a normal sinus rhythm, had equal breath sounds, and her SpO_2 was 100% while being manually ventilated.

INDICATIONS

A computerized tomography (CT) scan of her head revealed an occipital condylar fracture on the right with a small intrahemispheric subdural hematoma that did not require surgical intervention. Radiographs of her spine were unremarkable and there was no evidence of spleen or liver injury. The chest radiograph was also normal (Figure 18-2). She was transported to the ICU in critical condition and placed on a mechanical ventilator due to her extensive head injuries and therapeutic drug-induced coma.

INITIAL SETTINGS

Since heavy sedation and sustained hyperventilation were desired, the initial ventilator settings on the Puritan-Bennett 7200 consisted of assist/control (A/C) mode at a rate of 14/min, V_T of 600 mL, F_IO_2 of 60%, and no PEEP.

PATIENT MONITORING

The initial blood gas analysis after 20 min of mechanical ventilation showed:

pH	7.30
$PaCO_2$	29 mm Hg
PaO_2	256 mm Hg
HCO_3^-	13.9 mEq/L
Hb	11 g %
Mode	A/C
Rate	14
V_T	600 mL
F_IO_2	60%
PEEP	0 cm H_2O

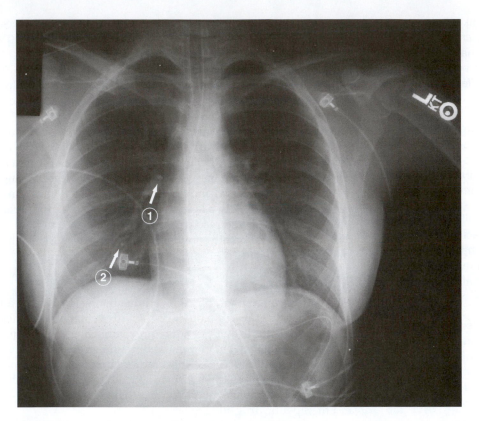

Figure 18-2 Head injury. The chest radiograph is normal. The small round markings (1 and 2) are the pulmonary blood vessels running parallel to the roentgen ray (X-ray).

☑ An ICP of less than 10 mmHg is the desirable target for this patient.

The patient was closely monitored using continuous intracranial pressure (ICP) measurements between 6 and 8 mm Hg, hemodynamics with indwelling pulmonary artery and arterial catheters revealed a heart rate of 118/min, BP of 116/84 mm Hg, and a pulmonary capillary wedge pressure (PCWP) of 11 mm Hg.

PATIENT MANAGEMENT

Carbon dioxide in the blood is a very potent vasodilator. This serves to promote swelling and edema following an acute injury to the brain. Blood flow to the area, and the subsequent swelling, may be reduced during the first 24 hours by maintaining the $PaCO_2$ between 25 and 35 mm Hg while monitoring the ensuing edema with an ICP monitor.

☑ Hyperventilation is used to maintain a $PaCO_2$ between 25 and 30 mm Hg.

Consequently, hyperventilation is used as a means to reduce the $PaCO_2$ level in the blood as well as to regulate the pressure resulting from swelling of the brain after the injury. Following the insertion

☑ Cerebrospinal fluid may also be drained to minimize the rise of intracranial pressure from subsequent swelling of the brain.

☑ PEEP is contraindicated in head injuries unless severe hypoxemia is present.

☑ Neurologic assessment should be done after recovery from drug-induced sedation.

of the ICP monitor, the level of hyperventilation can be assessed and titrated to maintain that pressure preferentially below 10 mm Hg to minimize further injury.

The PEEP level is usually maintained at or below 5 cm H_2O because the lungs are generally not affected by head injury, and that additional pressure is transmitted to the head by the use of positive pressure to ventilate the patient. This level is desirable unless the patient's oxygen requirements exceed 60% F_IO_2 when higher levels of PEEP may be indicated.

The ventilator settings were adjusted during the next several hours and the patient was weaned to a rate of 12/min resulting in a pH of 7.46 and $PaCO_2$ of 28 mm Hg.

KEY MEDICATIONS

The patient remained sedated with Phenytoin, Phenobarbital, Diazepam, and Midazolam during the acute phase (i.e., 24 to 48 hours following the accident) of her hospitalization to minimize the risk of further injury. She was then allowed to awaken for neurologic assessment.

Since the lungs were relatively unaffected, she was not given bronchodilator therapy, but was monitored for complications including atelectasis and consolidation resulting from inactivity, oral intubation, and subsequent ventilation. She was suctioned appropriately as necessary and was given periodic oral care to minimize the occurrence of infection.

WEANING

The patient was allowed to awaken fully and was changed to SIMV mode at 10/min with a pressure support level at 15 cm H_2O in an attempt to begin the weaning process. Blood gas analysis revealed the following:

pH	7.39
$PaCO_2$	40 mm Hg
PaO_2	83 mm Hg
HCO_3^-	23.3 mEq/L
Hb	13.8 g%
Mode	SIMV
Rate	10
V_T	600 mL
F_IO_2	60%
Pressure Support	15 cm H_2O

Weaning parameters done each morning included respiratory rate, minute volume, tidal volume, vital capacity, maximum inspiratory pressure, and frequency to tidal volume ratio. The weaning criteria done on the second day after admission showed that her ventilatory effort was adequate and she was weaned off the ventilator only with minor neurologic deficit.

She was alert and oriented to time and place but without memory of the accident. She appeared comfortable, cooperative, able to follow commands, and was not diaphoretic or febrile. She was not anxious and was spontaneously breathing on CPAP with 10 cm H_2O of pressure support at a RR of 14/min, HR of 88/min, BP of 112/78 mm Hg, SpO_2 of 96% on 35% F_IO_2 with satisfactory blood gases.

She was extubated and placed on a nasal cannula at 3 L/min of O_2. She was weaned off oxygen and discharged from the hospital 6 days after admission.

COMPLICATIONS

The patient had no apparent pulmonary complications; however, there were minor neuromotor obstacles to overcome including the loss of short-term memory and minimal motor sensory perception to the left. She will undergo physical and occupational therapy regimens after her release from the hospital to rehabilitate her injuries.

CASE 5: SMOKE INHALATION

INTRODUCTION

F.H. was a 64-year-old, 76-kg male admitted to the emergency department from his home where he was found in a smoke-filled room. He was unable to communicate with rescuers, appeared confused, and presented with first- and second-degree burns over 50% of his upper torso. His facial features contained dark smoke and soot about his nose and mouth, a singed mustache, and he had a strong odor of alcohol on his breath.

The initial blood pressure was 139/100 mm Hg, temperature was 35.8°C with a pulse of 102/min, and respirations of 24/min while breathing on a nonrebreathing mask at 15 L/min. He was immediately fluid resuscitated with 1,000 mL of D_5W, and treated empirically for cyanide toxicity, which interferes with oxidative metabolism at the cellular level by impairing the utilization of oxygen.

The clinical signs of cyanide poisoning may include the following:

Blood cyanide concentration 0.2 to 0.3 mg/L	↑ HR, ↑ RR, dizziness
Blood cyanide concentration 0.3 to 1 mg/L	↑ lethargy, arrhythmias, apnea
Blood cyanide concentration >1 mg/L	Death

✓ Patient history suggests potential complications of burn and smoke inhalation: infection, bronchospasm, carbon monoxide (CO), and cyanide poisoning.

✓ Cyanide is one of the by-products of combustion.

✓ With adequate spontaneous ventilation, the initial supportive measure for smoke inhalation is 100% O_2.

✓ Pulse oximetry should not be used in smoke inhalation because it cannot distinguish carboxyhemoglobin and provides false high SpO_2 readings.

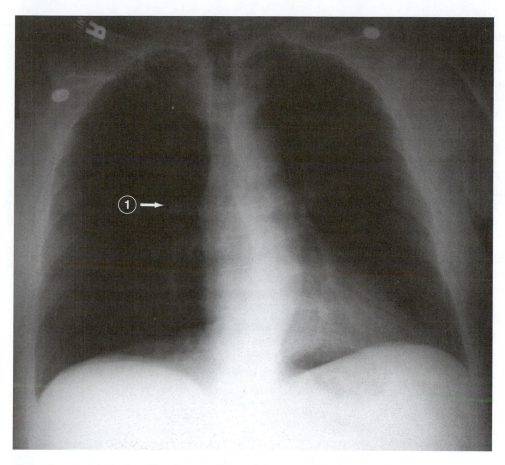

Figure 18-3 Smoke inhalation. The chest radiograph is normal. The lungs typically are not affected unless there is edema formation secondary to smoke inhalation. The small round marking (1) represents a pulmonary blood vessel running parallel to the roentgen ray (X-ray).

Upon admission into the hospital, the chest radiograph was normal (Figure 18-3). His breath sounds were mostly clear but dramatically changed following IV fluids to basilar crackles with expiratory wheezes throughout, and a prolonged expiratory phase. Although the patient maintained an SpO_2 of 99% per pulse oximetry, he did not appear short of breath. A stat blood gas was ordered in the emergency room followed immediately by a nebulizer treatment with 0.5 mL of 0.5% Proventil in 2.5 mL of normal saline. The results of the blood gases were as follows:

☑ Blood gases with carboxy-hemoglobin (HbCO) capability must be done in managing patients with smoke inhalation.

pH	7.29
$PaCO_2$	41 mm Hg
PaO_2	155 mm Hg
HCO_3^-	19.4 mEq/L

☑ In CO poisoning, the CaO_2 should be used to evaluate the patient's oxygenation status.

☑ In spite of normal Hb and satisfactory SaO_2, the measured CaO_2 is low (12.7 vol %) because of the high HbCO level (21.2 g %).

☑ Elective intubation is done to maintain a patent airway in anticipation of airway edema and obstruction.

HbCO	21.2 g %
Hb	14.4 g %
CaO_2	12.7 vol %
SaO_2	92%
Mode	Nonrebreathing mask
Flow	15 L/min

The patient was then transported to the intensive care unit for further evaluation and treatment.

INDICATIONS

Physical examination revealed that the patient had received a moderate thermal burn to the airway as well as to his torso and extremities. He was electively intubated to maintain an adequate airway and as expected, he became edematous to the point that his facial features were no longer recognizable.

INITIAL SETTINGS

He was lightly sedated and placed on CPAP with pressure support of 15 cm H_2O and the spontaneous rate was 16/min. He maintained a spontaneous V_T of 550 mL at an F_IO_2 of 100% and PEEP of 6 cm H_2O. After 30 min, blood gases revealed:

☑ The measured CaO_2 showed improvement (from 12.7 to 14.7 vol %) after initiation of CPAP, PS, and 100% O_2.

pH	7.42
$PaCO_2$	36 mm Hg
PaO_2	255 mm Hg
HCO_3^-	22.8 mEq/L
HbCO	19.2 g %
Hb	14.4 g %
CaO_2	14.7 vol %
SaO_2	94%
Mode	CPAP
PEEP	6 cm H_2O
Pressure Support	15 cm H_2O
RR (spontaneous)	16/min
V_T (spontaneous)	550 mL
F_IO_2	100%

The patient was maintained on the same ventilator settings as he had normal acid-base balance and was breathing spontaneously. A high F_IO_2 was maintained to reduce the half-life of HbCO.

The half-life of HbCO is as follows:

F_IO_2 of 100% and one atmospheric pressure	80 to 90 min
F_IO_2 of 21% (air) and one atmospheric pressure	280 to 320 min

PATIENT MONITORING

Careful observation should be carried out to assess any evidence of pulmonary complications such as thermal injuries to the airway or pulmonary edema. These injuries also increase the incidence and severity of ARDS. Impaired gas exchange or hypoxia caused by increased levels of CO may be treated by the use of PEEP. The patient's mental functions should be monitored to prevent CO-induced anoxic brain syndrome.

PATIENT MANAGEMENT

The patient was closely monitored for 2 days while on mechanical ventilation for evidence of further injuries (i.e., decreasing lung compliance, thermal airway injuries, and hypoxia).

KEY MEDICATIONS

The patient was given MDI treatments with 10 puffs of Proventil given in-line through the ventilator circuit and continued with medication nebulizer treatments with Proventil after extubation.

WEANING

The swelling to the airway was significantly reduced and the patient was extubated after the return of adequate ventilation. He was immediately given an aerosol treatment of 0.5 mL racemic epinephrine (Micronephrine) in distilled water to minimize stridor and edema to the upper airway. Blood gases after extubation revealed:

☑ Reduction of peak inspiratory pressure, improvement of breath sounds, and dynamic compliance are signs that the swelling to the airway has improved.

pH	7.42
$PaCO_2$	38 mm Hg
PaO_2	104 mm Hg
HCO_3^-	23.6 mEq/L
HbCO	2.8 g %
Hb	14.1 g %
CaO_2	18.8 vol %
SaO_2	96%
Mode	Cool aerosol mask
RR (spontaneous)	16/min
F_IO_2	28%

The patient remained in the hospital for three more days where he was weaned from the oxygen and required fewer medication nebulizer treatments to control intermittent wheezing.

COMPLICATIONS

The patient experienced no lasting complications from his injuries. He was weaned to room air and discharged from the hospital after a 6-day convalescence period.

CASE 6: DRUG OVERDOSE

INTRODUCTION

K.L. was a 78-year-old white male, 5 ft 8 in., medium build who weighed about 73 kg (160 lb). Upon admission to the 200-bed community hospital, his respiratory rate was 6/min and shallow. His skin color was pale but showed no cyanosis.

The paramedics stated that the patient was found by his neighbors in the bathroom on his back next to a pool of vomitus. The neighbors told the paramedics that the patient had a history of asthma and that he had been depressed since his girlfriend left him 2 weeks ago. An albuterol inhaler was found next to the patient and two empty bottles of tricyclic antidepressants were found on the kitchen table. Additional medical history revealed that the patient smoked about one pack of cigarettes each day.

The paramedics used a bag/mask resuscitator to ventilate the patient with O_2 at a rate of about 20/min. They suctioned and removed large amounts of vomitus from his airway en route to the hospital.

Upon arrival at the emergency room, the respiratory therapist provided bag/mask ventilation. A nasogastric tube was inserted to prevent gastric distention and aspiration.

Cardiopulmonary assessments provided the following information: heart rate 45/min, weak pulses, systolic blood pressure 90 mm Hg, SpO_2 90%, spontaneous respiratory rate 8/min, and shallow breath sounds with crackles and wheezes bilaterally.

Arterial blood gases on 100% O_2 revealed: pH 7.08, $PaCO_2$ 70 mm Hg, PaO_2 54 mm Hg, SaO_2 85%, and HCO_3^- 20 mEq/L.

☑ Blood gases show acute ventilatory failure with moderate hypoxemia.

INDICATIONS

The patient was intubated with a size 8.0 endotracheal (ET) tube. After checking for bilateral breath sounds, the ET tube was secured at the 24 cm mark at the lips. The end-tidal CO_2 reading was 20 mm Hg. During intubation, large amounts of watery brown secretions were suctioned from the airway and a sample was collected and sent to the laboratory for analysis.

☑ An end-tidal CO_2 reading of 20 mm Hg confirms placement of an ET tube in the airway.

After the ET tube cuff was properly inflated, activated charcoal was put into the stomach via the nasogastric tube in order to absorb the remaining tricycles.

While the activated charcoal was being administered, the airways and lungs were lavaged with normal saline and suctioned. This procedure was repeated until the return solution became clear.

☑ Repeat suctioning is indicated because watery brown secretions (stomach content) have been suctioned from the ET tube.

Chest radiograph done later showed that the ET tube was 4 cm above the carina. Hazy infiltrates were noted in both lungs indicating that the patient had aspirated.

Another blood gas was drawn with the patient intubated and being bagged at a rate of 20/min. The results were: pH 7.34, PCO_2 35 mm Hg, PO_2 350 mm Hg.

INITIAL SETTINGS
The patient was transferred to the adult ICU and placed on a Puritan-Bennett 7200 ventilator. The initial settings were CMV mode, RR 20/min, V_T 720 mL, F_IO_2 100%, PEEP 5 cm H_2O, peak flow 60 L/min, and square flow pattern. With these settings, the peak inspiratory pressure was 25 cm H_2O, plateau pressure was 20 cm H_2O, and corrected V_T was 710 mL. All alarms were set appropriately.

pH	7.32
$PaCO_2$	32 mm Hg
PaO_2	264 mm Hg
HCO_3^-	16 mEq/L
SpO_2	98%
Mode	CMV
Rate	20/min
V_T	720 mL
F_IO_2	100%
PEEP	5 cm H_2O
P_{PEAK}	25 cm H_2O
$P_{PLATEAU}$	20 cm H_2O

PATIENT MONITORING
A continuous SpO_2 monitor was placed on the patient with the low alarm set at 90%. A good waveform was noted, and the heart rate matched that on the cardiac monitor.

Respiratory monitoring of the patient consisted of Q 2° ventilator checks to include the peak and plateau pressures, returned volumes, minute volumes, F_IO_2 and compliance. Other clinical information and procedures included RR, breath sounds, suctioning, and ET tube cuff pressure.

Due to the potential complications of aspiration, of particular importance was the monitoring of high peak and plateau pressure, F_IO_2, and PaO_2. A Swan-Ganz catheter and an arterial line were used to monitor the patient's hemodynamic status (i.e., arterial blood pressure, central venous pressure, pulmonary artery pressure, pulmonary capillary wedge pressure, cardiac output, and mixed venous saturation). Laboratory studies included serum electrolytes.

PATIENT MANAGEMENT
Initially, the patient's respiratory status was stable but it began to deteriorate on the second day. The ventilator settings were changed to accommodate the patient's needs. The ventilator settings were: CMV

✔ Since aspiration is likely to have occurred, PEEP of 5 cm H_2O is used to prevent atelectasis.

✔ Alarms should include low minute volume, low tidal volume, PEEP, high pressure, low pressure, high respiratory rate and apnea alarms.

✔ Potential complications of aspiration may include aspirations pneumonia and ARDS.

✔ ARDS is usually preceded by increasing peak and plateau pressures (due to decreasing lung compliance), and increasing F_IO_2 requirement (due to intrapulmonary shunting).

mode, RR 35/min, V_T 720 mL, F_IO_2 100%, 20 cm H_2O PEEP. The peak inspiratory pressure was 80 cm H_2O and plateau pressure was 70 cm H_2O. The blood gas results were:

pH	7.27
$PaCO_2$	43 mm Hg
PaO_2	72 mm Hg
HCO_3^-	19 mEq/L
SpO_2	92%
Mode	CMV
Rate	35/min
V_T	720 mL
F_IO_2	100%
PEEP	20 cm H_2O
P_{PEAK}	80 cm H_2O
$P_{PLATEAU}$	70 cm H_2O

☑ In PCV, the initial pressure may be set at 10 cm H_2O below the peak inspiratory pressure on CMV.

Because of the increasing pressure requirement, pressure control ventilation (PCV) was started so as to minimize the occurrence of volume- or pressure-induced lung injuries. The pressure on PCV was initially set at 70 cm H_2O (10 cm H_2O below the peak inspiratory pressure on CMV). Other ventilator parameters for PCV were: inspiratory time 1 sec, RR 35/min, F_IO_2 100%, 20 cm H_2O PEEP. The blood gases were as follows:

pH	7.31
$PaCO_2$	41 mm Hg
PaO_2	56 mm Hg
HCO_3^-	20 mEq/L
SpO_2	88%
Mode	PCV
Pressure	70 cm H_2O
Rate	35/min
F_IO_2	100%
PEEP	20 cm H_2O

☑ In PCV, the minute volume is primarily determined by the pressure, inspiratory time, and lung compliance.

The inspiratory time was then increased to 2 sec to keep the PaO_2 in the 70s. The I:E ratio was changed to 4:1 to provide longer inspiratory time. Subsequently the minute volume was increased with these settings and the pressure was lowered to 50 cm H_2O. Blood gases on these settings were satisfactory. The minute volume of the patient was trended carefully during the use of PCV.

The patient was placed on a Roto-bed and was administered neuromuscular and sedative agents to minimize agitation and oxygen consumption. For proper airway management, a tracheostomy was performed because extended mechanical ventilation was anticipated.

☑ In ARDS, the lungs will heal faster with lower airway pressures.

To further minimize pressure-induced lung injuries, the pressure on PCV was further decreased until the tidal volume was about 450 mL.

The $PaCO_2$ was allowed to reach 80 mm Hg (permissive hypercapnia) while the pH was maintained near 7.35 by bicarbonate infusion and kidney compensation.

KEY MEDICATIONS

☑ Permissive hypercapnia is used to reduce the pressure and volume requirement for ventilation.

No medication was needed for intubation because the patient was unconscious at the time of intubation. Additional medications were withheld because of the uncertain drug interaction with other unknown drugs that the patient might have taken.

The patient was given neuromuscular blocking agents and sedatives while on mechanical ventilation. As the respiratory status improved, the patient was weaned from these drugs. Albuterol was given PRN for wheezing.

WEANING

Over the next 2 weeks, the patient continued to improve. Weaning was done by alternating CPAP with pressure support (during day) and SIMV (during night). Both modes of ventilation were supported with flow triggering. The SIMV mode allowed the patient to rest. He was also ambulated daily to strengthen his respiratory muscles and exercise endurance.

☑ An f/V_T ratio of less than 100/min/L is highly predictive of weaning success.

As he regained strength, the following spontaneous respiratory parameters were obtained: RR <35/min, minute volume around 9 L, vital capacity >1 L, MIF >−30 cm H_2O and f/V_T <100/min/L.

Eventually, the patient was weaned to CPAP of 5 cm H_2O, F_IO_2 35%, and pressure support of 5 cm H_2O. A spontaneous rate of 16 to 20/min yielded these ABG results:

pH	7.37
$PaCO_2$	43 mm Hg
PaO_2	80 mm Hg
HCO_3^-	24 mEq/L
SpO_2	95%
Mode	CPAP
PEEP	5 cm H_2O
F_IO_2	35%
Pressure Support	5 cm H_2O
Spontaneous Rate	16 to 20/min

After 2 days of CPAP, the patient continued to improve and he was placed on a nasal cannula at 4 L/min and his fenestrated tracheostomy tube was buttoned allowing the patient to breathe through his upper airway. He tolerated the closure of his tracheostomy very well, and it was left this way for 2 days. Two more days later, he was transferred to the rehabilitation floor.

✓ Tension pneumothorax was probably caused by excessive airway and pulmonary pressures.

✓ To prevent self-extubation, neuromuscular blocking agents and sedatives may be used to provide comfort. An alternative is to use active restraints.

✓ Chest tube is used to remove air, blood, or fluid accumulated in the pleural space.

✓ Hypotension and tachycardia are two common signs of inadequate blood volume.

✓ Tension pneumothorax or hemopneumothorax shifts the mediastinum to the unaffected (opposite) side.

✓ Colloids are used to enhance fluid balance in the early phase of volume replacement.

✓ Hemodynamic instability is mainly due to blood loss.

COMPLICATIONS

During the course of mechanical ventilation, a left-sided tension pneumothorax occurred and this led to decreased lung compliance, decreased O_2 saturation, and decreased breath sounds on the left side. Chest radiograph showed shift of the mediatinum to the right side. The tension pneumothorax gradually resolved with the placement of a chest tube.

At one point during weaning the patient became very combative and he self-extubated. He was reintubated without delay. Cloth restraints were then used to secure his extremities.

CASE 7: TENSION HEMOPNEUMOTHORAX

INTRODUCTION

P.S. was a 50-year-old, 96-kg male transferred from another hospital with a complicating right-sided pneumonia and hemothorax. At the onset, a small right pleural effusion was found that required drainage via a needle thoracentesis. This effusion again reaccumulated and a second thoracentesis was performed that was productive of over 400 mL of thin, cloudy fluid. A chest tube was placed following the procedure, which continued to drain thin, cloudy fluid followed by frank blood. This output continued throughout the day requiring massive transfusions to maintain his blood pressure, thus, he was transferred to a tertiary care facility for definitive therapy. Prior to air transport, the patient was volume resuscitated with both blood and fluid, nasally intubated, and noted to have inadequate drainage of the right hemothorax.

Upon arrival to the ICU, the patient developed further hemodynamic instability with a systolic pressure of 70 mm Hg (*normal 120 mm Hg*) and a heart rate of 120/min (*normal 60 to 100/min*). He had weak pulses bilaterally, dullness to percussion of the right hemithorax, expiratory wheezes, and coarse rhonchi with the left being greater than the right. The chest tube drained about 950 mL of bloody fluid. The patient was resuscitated with colloids followed by blood transfusions. A chest radiograph revealed a complete opacification on the right with concurrent mediastinal shift to the left side (Figure 18-4).

INDICATIONS

The patient was electively intubated prior to transport to establish and maintain an adequate airway. Mechanical ventilation was established because of hemodynamic instability, reduction of lung volumes, and increased work of breathing.

Figure 18-4   Tension hemopneumothorax. Right-sided hemopneumothorax shifts the mediastinum and trachea (1) to the left. The shift is not significant, possibly due to patient rotation when the radiograph was taken. The *white* area (2) on the radiograph is caused by the *blood* in the pleural space (Note: *air* in pleural space would appear *dark*). Compression of the left lung is noted (3). Chest tube (4) can be seen on the right side.

INITIAL SETTINGS

> ☑ Reduction of lung volumes is caused by compression of the lungs by blood and air in the pleural space.

The patient was lightly sedated and placed on a Puritan-Bennett 7200 ventilator in the assist/control mode at 16/min with V_T of 800 mL, F_IO_2 of 100%, and PEEP of 5 cm H_2O. There was no spontaneous respiratory effort.

The peak inspiratory pressures exceeded 70 cm H_2O with each breath and the tidal volume delivered was about 8 mL/kg of body weight. This low volume maintained adequate ventilation without excessive cardiovascular compromise induced by positive pressure ventilation.

✔ Increase in work of breathing is caused by reduction of lung compliance and/or increase of airway resistance.

✔ The peak inspiratory pressure was high (>70 cm H_2O) because of low lung compliance (due to compression of lung parenchyma by blood and air in the pleural space).

The patient was hemodynamically stabilized using stored blood and clinically evaluated with a chest radiograph and arterial blood gas analysis. The initial blood gas results were as follows:

pH	7.30
$PaCO_2$	40 mm Hg
PaO_2	83 mm Hg
HCO_3^-	18.9 mEq/L
B.E.	−6.8 mEq/L
Hb	15.8 g %
CaO_2	20.9 vol %
SaO_2	94%
SpO_2	89%
Mode	A/C
RR	16/min
V_T	800 mL
F_IO_2	100%
PEEP	5 cm H_2O

Twenty-five minutes later, the patient remained in critical but stable condition while continuing to bleed into the chest tube. The endotracheal tube position was noted and secured in the airway awaiting visualization on the chest radiograph. Blood gases were drawn to evaluate his acidosis and quantify the degree of blood loss from the tension hemothorax. These were outlined as follows:

✔ Change in the hemoglobin level (from 15.8 to 10.7 g %) greatly diminishes the patient's arterial oxygen content (from 20.9 to 15 vol %).

pH	7.40
$PaCO_2$	33 mm Hg
PaO_2	196 mm Hg
HCO_3^-	19.6 mEq/L
B.E.	−4.2 mEq/L
Hb	10.7 g %
CaO_2	15 vol %
SaO_2	96%
SpO_2	95%
Mode	A/C
RR	16/min
V_T	800 mL
F_IO_2	100%
PEEP	5 cm H_2O

✔ The F_IO_2 was reduced to 60% because the PaO_2 (196 mm Hg) was excessive.

The F_IO_2 was reduced to 60%. Chest radiograph confirmed proper placement of the endotracheal tube and noted a tension hemothorax on the right side. He was taken to the operating room for an emergency thoracotomy and relief of the tension hemothorax resulting from a spontaneous intercostal bleed.

By the end of thoracotomy and repair of the bleed, he received 11 units of blood prior to returning to the ICU. Later, he received nine more units of blood in the ICU.

PATIENT MONITORING

Upon return from the operating room (OR), the patient was placed back on mechanical ventilation at 1,000 mL tidal volume on assist/control with a rate of 12/min, F_IO_2 of 60%, and 5 cm H_2O of PEEP. Peak inspiratory pressures returned to 36 cm H_2O, he was hemodynamically stable, and allowed to awaken from the anesthesia. Blood gases 10 min after returning from surgery revealed the following:

pH	7.41
$PaCO_2$	39 mm Hg
PaO_2	55 mm Hg
HCO_3^-	24.1 mEq/L
B.E.	−2.7 mEq/L
Hb	11.4 g %
CaO_2	17.7 vol %
SaO_2	90.5%
SpO_2	87%
Mode	A/C
RR	12/min
V_T	1,000 mL
F_IO_2	60%
PEEP	5 cm H_2O

In an effort to minimize the effects of oxygen toxicity, the ventilator was adjusted by increasing the PEEP to 8 cm H_2O to increase the PaO_2 without raising the F_IO_2 past 60%.

PATIENT MANAGEMENT

☑ Cardiac output and pulmonary wedge pressures are used to monitor the adequacy of circulating blood volume.

This patient was recovered from surgery in the ICU on mechanical ventilation in an effort to minimize any postsurgical complications associated with continued blood loss and to guard against the development of respiratory distress.

Following rapid infusion of 20 units of blood to cover his losses, hemodynamic measurements including cardiac output and pulmonary wedge pressures help to assure adequate perfusion to the tissues. Oxygenation, under the conditions presented, may be complicated by the use of stored blood used for volume replacement. Of particular importance is the fact that stored blood contains limited amounts of 2,3 diphosphoglycerate (DPG), which effectively shifts the oxyhemoglobin dissociation curve to the left. Thus, stored blood reduces the unloading of oxygen at the tissues causing hypoxia, necrosis, and possibly sepsis if not managed properly. As a result, the patient's PaO_2 was closely monitored to maintain adequate oxygenation and saturation. He was also monitored for clinical signs of tissue hypoxia. At that time, follow-up blood gases revealed these results:

pH	7.46
$PaCO_2$	34 mm Hg

PaO_2	124 mm Hg
HCO_3^-	24.1 mEq/L
B.E.	−1.7 mEq/L
Hb	11.4 g %
CaO_2	15.5 vol %
SaO_2	95.7%
SpO_2	94%
Mode	A/C
RR	12/min
V_T	1,000 mL
F_IO_2	60%
PEEP	8 cm H_2O

☑ Reduce F_IO_2 when PaO_2 is too high.

The F_IO_2 was reduced to 50% and the patient was continuously monitored by the SpO_2 and SvO_2 measurements.

RESPIRATORY CARE PROCEDURES

Based on the preadmission diagnosis of complicating pneumonia, the patient was aggressively treated with frequent suctioning and a moderate amount of cloudy secretions was removed. Bronchopulmonary toilet was initiated and he was immediately started on bronchodilator therapy with 20 puffs of Proventil via a metered dose inhaler (MDI) given in-line through the ventilator circuit via Aerochamber®, and he was frequently turned from side-to-side to help prevent atelectasis.

WEANING

Two days following surgery, the patient began to breathe spontaneously and he was changed to SIMV in an attempt to wean him from the ventilator. Initially, his rate was decreased to 8/min, and all spontaneous breaths were supported by 10 cm H_2O of pressure support. He was able to initiate 20 breaths above the set rate and maintained a tidal volume of 400 to 600 mL at this level of support. His machine breaths were set at 1,000 mL tidal volume and over that time, his PEEP was reduced to 5 cm H_2O and his F_IO_2 was reduced to 40%. As his muscular effort improved, the tidal volume increased and his pressure support was quickly weaned to 6 cm H_2O while maintaining the same tidal volume. He remained at that level throughout the day without signs of fatigue, hypoxemia, tachypnea, hypertension, evidence of desaturation, or excessive tachycardia.

That night he was placed on assist/control in an effort to rest the muscles of inspiration. Weaning began at six o'clock the next morning on CPAP with pressure support of 12 cm H_2O, PEEP of 5 cm H_2O, and F_IO_2 of 40%. Spontaneous parameters obtained 2 hours later revealed:

☑ An f/V_T ratio of less than 100/min/L is highly predictive of weaning success.

$f = 26$ $V_E = 12.4$ L $V_T = 0.47$ L   VC = 1.09 L
MIP = −52 cm H_2O $f/V_T = 55$/min/L

Based on stable spontaneous parameters and clinical condition, he was removed from the ventilator and allowed to breathe on a "T-piece" at 40% F_IO_2 for 4 hours. Subsequent evaluations led to successful weaning and extubation. He was placed on a nasal cannula at 6 L/min and continued to improve.

COMPLICATIONS

Besides the tension hemopneumothorax, there were no apparent complications from either the right-sided pneumonia or throughout the postoperative period resulting from the mechanical ventilation. He was followed throughout his hospital stay with respiratory therapy and continued treatments with deep breathing regimens and with bronchodilator therapy for wheezing. His oxygen demands were monitored with daily pulse oximetry and the oxygen cannula was titrated to maintain the SpO_2s above 90%. He was discharged on the eighth postsurgical day from the tertiary care facility on room air and without further complications.

CASE 8: CHEST TRAUMA

INTRODUCTION

A.P. was a 24-year-old, 56-kg female involved in a moving vehicle accident. The patient was unrestrained and was struck on her side of the vehicle. She was thrown from the vehicle but her car was found to contain multiple prescription pain medication bottles. She was apparently comatose at the scene with no spontaneous breathing or pulse. However, her vital signs returned to normal en route to the hospital.

Upon arrival to the emergency department, her vital signs revealed a blood pressure (BP) of 122/80 mm Hg, pulse of 80/min, normal sinus rhythm, and temperature of 35.8°C. Her breathing was assisted by the respiratory care practitioner (RCP) with a manual resuscitator bag. Breath sounds revealed diffuse coarse rhonchi bilaterally without wheezing.

Laboratory and radiology results revealed a white blood cell (WBC) count of 17.5×10^3 (*normal 3.2 to 9.8 $\times 10^3$*), hemoglobin (Hb) of 12.7 g % (*normal 12 to 15 g %*), platelets of 195×10^3 (*normal 130 to 400 $\times 10^3$*), prothrombin time (PT) of 13 sec (*normal 9 to 12 sec*), and a partial thromboplastin time (PTT) of 30 sec (*normal 22 to 37 sec*). A portable chest radiograph (Figure 18-5) revealed rib fracture on the right and bilateral infiltrates in which the left were greater than the right. The left hemidiaphragm, heart border, and parenchymal changes were consistent with pulmonary contusion or possible aspiration pneumonitis.

☑ The white blood count is significantly elevated.

☑ Pulmonary contusion is an internal injury of the lung parenchyma in which the skin is not broken.

☑ Bilateral rib fractures and pneumothoraces with blood accumulation limit chest expansion and hinder ventilation and oxygenation.

Figure 18-5 Chest trauma. Rib fracture is noted on the right side (1) of this chest radiograph. Infiltrates on the left side (2) cause a greater density than the right side (3). The diaphragm shadow on the left is lost (4) likely due to pulmonary contusion or possible aspiration pneumonitis. Left-sided atelectasis pulls the mediastinum and trachea (5) to the left. The shift does not appear to be significant, possibly due to patient rotation when the radiograph was taken.

The patient underwent an extensive evaluation of her injuries including a computerized tomography (CT) of her head that was essentially normal. Scans of her chest and abdomen revealed bilateral rib fractures, pneumothoraces with blood accumulation, and rupture of her spleen with evidence of free peritoneal fluid. Also noted was an apparent transverse process fracture of the lumbar spine as well as possible posterior element fractures of the T1 vertebrae. She also had multiple contusions and lacerations including a large laceration to the right axilla and in the right wrist region.

☑ History of smok-
ing and chronic
bronchitis limit
the patient's lung
functions.

☑ Chest trauma,
unstable and
worsening cardio-
pulmonary and
hemodynamic status
are the primary indi-
cations for mechani-
cal ventilation.

☑ $PaCO_2$ of 25 mm
Hg shows alveo-
lar hyperventilation
and it indicates ven-
tilatory insufficiency
(i.e., hyperventilation
to maintain a PaO_2
of 83 mm Hg).

☑ When the patient
fatigues, it leads
to deteriorating ven-
tilation and oxygena-
tion status.

☑ Pressure
Control-Inverse
Ratio Ventilation
(PC-IRV) uses a pre-
determined inspira-
tory pressure to
minimize the occur-
rence of pressure-
induced barotrauma.

☑ PC-IRV increases
the mean airway
pressure, central
venous pressure,
and pulmonary
artery pressure.

Her previous history included smoking one pack of cigarettes per day and chronic bronchitis.

INDICATIONS

Due to the extent of her injuries, she was hemodynamically stabilized with a transfusion of four units of blood, paralyzed with a short-acting paralytic (Succinylcholine), and intubated with a 8.0 mm endotracheal tube. She was subsequently transferred to the intensive care unit (ICU) in critical but stable condition requiring mechanical ventilation.

INITIAL SETTINGS

She was immediately placed on a Puritan-Bennett 7200 ventilator on assist/control at 15/min control rate, V_T 600 mL, F_IO_2 60%, and PEEP 5 cm H_2O. Chest tubes were placed to evacuate the pleural space of blood and air. Her initial blood gases after 10 min on the ventilator were:

pH	7.45
$PaCO_2$	25 mm Hg
PaO_2	83 mm Hg
HCO_3^-	17.3 mEq/L
Hb	13.7 g %
Mode	A/C
Rate	15
V_T	600 mL
F_IO_2	60%
PEEP	5 cm H_2O

Over the next 24 hours, her condition quickly deteriorated requiring 100% F_IO_2 and increasing levels of PEEP to maintain adequate oxygenation.

PATIENT MONITORING

The increasing pressure required to ventilate her lungs began to compromise her cardiac output and, as such, limit perfusion to her tissues. As a result, she was heavily sedated and changed to *pressure control-inversed ratio ventilation* (PC-IRV) *mode* at a rate of 12/min and an inspiratory pressure of 30 cm H_2O. Her inspiratory time (T_I) was set at 1.0 sec resulting in a 3:1 I:E ratio. Her PEEP and F_IO_2 requirements were 8 cm H_2O and 100%, respectively. These settings provided hyperexpansion of the chest in order to stabilize the thorax and limit movement of the rib fractures. She was monitored by an end-tidal CO_2 monitor. Frequent blood gases were ordered to evaluate her ventilatory and oxygenation status. Blood gases drawn at this time revealed the following:

pH	7.36
$PaCO_2$	42 mm Hg

PaO_2	62 mm Hg
SaO_2	90%
HCO_3^-	22.9 mEq/L
Hb	11.2 g %
Mode	PC-IRV
T_I	1.0 sec
I:E ratio	3:1
Rate	12
P_{INSP}	30 cm H_2O
F_IO_2	100%
PEEP	8 cm H_2O

☑ Increase in central venous pressure lowers the systemic arterial and venous pressure gradient. Decreased venous return to the heart causes a lower cardiac output.

The patient appeared to tolerate these changes well. However, within 1 hour her hemodynamic values (including cardiac output) were reduced as a result of pressure ventilation. The T_I was decreased to 0.82 sec (2:1 ratio) and respiratory rate was increased to 24/min. The PEEP was increased to 15 cm H_2O. Arterial and mixed venous blood gases revealed the following:

Arterial
pH	7.38
$PaCO_2$	38 mm Hg
PaO_2	90 mm Hg
SaO_2	95%
HCO_3^-	21.8 mEq/L
B.E.	-2.4 mEq/L
Hb	11.1 g %
CaO_2	14.9 vol %

Mixed Venous
pH	7.36
PvO_2	47 mm Hg
SvO_2	78%
A-aDO_2	462 mm Hg
Qs/QT	42%

Ventilator Settings
Mode	PC-IRV
T_I	0.82 sec
I:E ratio	2:1
Rate	24
P_{INSP}	30 cm H_2O
F_IO_2	100%
PEEP	15 cm H_2O

☑ Ventilator settings should be adjusted based on the patient's ventilation and oxygenation requirement, as well as the patient's hemodynamic status.

The patient remained on a 2:1 I:E ratio and other ventilator settings were manipulated to normalize ventilation and oxygenation. To maintain a PaO_2 greater than 65 mm Hg, the required settings were: inspiratory pressure 30 cm H_2O, PEEP 18 cm H_2O, and F_IO_2 70%.

PATIENT MANAGEMENT

For the next 14 days, the patient was monitored closely for adverse signs while in a drug-induced coma. She was placed on a fentanyl citrate drip to manage her pain and was given narcotic medications to limit her movements while on pressure control ventilation. Vigorous pulmonary toilet was begun and she was suctioned with a closed directional tip catheter to the main-stem bronchi. This produced a large amount of thick, yellow secretions. She also received frequent acetylcystine (Mucomyst) lavage every 4 hours and was confined to a Rotorest® bed to help prevent pulmonary complications associated with atelectasis.

✔ Aggressive pulmonary hygiene is important in managing patients who are intubated and receiving prolonged mechanical ventilation.

KEY MEDICATIONS

She was given nebulizer treatments with 0.5 mL of 0.5% albuterol sulfate (Proventil) and 0.5 mg ipratropium bromide (Atrovent) every 4 hours for wheezing. Broad spectrum antibiotics including a fourth generation cephalosporin were used to treat pneumonia from long-term ventilation.

WEANING

Several days later, the patient's oxygen was weaned to 45% and respiratory rate of 22/min. Her condition continued to improve over time and the RCPs were also able to wean the PEEP to 15 cm H_2O. Blood gases on these settings revealed:

✔ For ventilator patients requiring high F_IO_2 and PEEP, wean F_IO_2 first to about 40% before weaning PEEP.

pH	7.58
$PaCO_2$	26 mm Hg
PaO_2	87 mm Hg
SaO_2	96%
HCO_3^-	23.5 mEq/L
B.E.	3.3 mEq/L
Hb	11.7 g %
CaO_2	15.8 vol %
Mode	IR-PCV
Rate	22
P_{INSP}	30 cm H_2O
F_IO_2	45%
PEEP	15 cm H_2O

At this point, she was removed from pressure control ventilation and allowed to awaken. As her spontaneous breathing resumed, she was quickly weaned to continuous positive airway pressure (CPAP) with 5 cm H_2O of PEEP and pressure support of 20 cm H_2O without difficulty. She maintained a respiratory rate of less than 24/min with tidal volumes of about 300 mL. As her muscular effort improved, tidal volume increased and her pressure support was titrated to maintain the same tidal volume and assure adequate alveolar ventilation and lung expansion.

✔ During weaning attempt, the pressure support level should be titrated based on the appropriate tidal volume and respiratory rate.

At night, she was rested on assist/control at a V_T of 600 mL, backup rate of 12/min. She maintained a spontaneous rate of 14/min. This regimen continued for the next 3 days where she was placed on CPAP with pressure support titrated to assist her spontaneous tidal volumes during the day, and rested during the night. Spontaneous parameters were obtained each morning to determine suitability to wean and monitor her effort to breathe on her own. Eventually, rather than returning to assist/control, she was able to tolerate synchronized intermittent mandatory ventilation (SIMV) mode with pressure support of 15 cm H_2O during the night. The following day, she remained on CPAP with 20 cm H_2O of pressure support throughout the next 36 hours without signs of respiratory insufficiency or distress.

She was evaluated for extubation, and her spontaneous respiratory parameters over the last 5 days were:

Day 1: $f = 50$ $V_E = 14.8$ L $V_T = 0.3$ L $VC = 0.80$ L
         $MIP = -46$ $f/V_T = 167$

Day 2: $f = 40$ $V_E = 10.6$ L $V_T = 0.27$ L $VC = 0.85$ L
         $MIP = -48$ $f/V_T = 148$

Day 3: $f = 37$ $V_E = 9.5$ L $V_T = 0.26$ L $VC = 0.87$ L
         $MIP = -56$ $f/V_T = 142$

Day 4: $f = 33$ $V_E = 8.2$ L $V_T = 0.3$ L $VC = 1.02$ L
         $MIP = -57$ $f/V_T = 110$

Day 5: $f = 32$ $V_E = 10.3$ L $V_T = 0.32$ L $VC = 1.14$ L
         $MIP = -42$ $f/V_T = 100$

☑ The weaning criteria on day 5 are satisfactory. See other weaning criteria in Chapter 14.

☑ An f/V_T ratio of less than 100 is highly predictive of weaning success.

Extubation decisions are frequently made in conjunction with spontaneous breathing parameters as well as other clinical indicators that may predict success. Ideally, every member of the patient care team may give input concerning this important decision. The frequency (f) should be below 30/min. The minute volume (V_E) should be around 10 L with a tidal volume of >5 to 8 mL/kg and a vital capacity >10 to 15 mL/kg. The maximum inspiratory pressure (MIP) should be greater than -20 to -30 cm H_2O where muscle strength is directly proportional to the volume generated for inspiration. The frequency to tidal volume ratio (f/V_T), sometimes called the rapid, shallow breathing test, measures the patient's volume as compared to the respiratory rate. Patients breathing rapidly with shallow volumes may only ventilate the anatomic deadspace (i.e., conducting zones within the lungs without effective alveolar ventilation). This ratio, then, should be below 100/min/L before effective weaning may take place.

Realize, however, that these indicators are only idealistic values and should not be taken individually as predictors of success. Other clinical signs such as level of consciousness, sensorium, ability to follow commands, character and volume of secretions, and hemo-dynamics may also help in predicting a successful postextubation course.

COMPLICATIONS

The patient followed a gradual resolution of her multiorgan dysfunction and severe refractory pulmonary difficulties after an 18-day ventilator course. She was recovered and discharged to a home health agency where she was advised to abstain from prescription narcotics, continued on Gentamicin 360 mg IV once per day, and Ciprofloxacin 750 mg twice daily for 10 days. Her SpO_2 at discharge was 90% on room air while walking.

CASE 9: ADULT RESPIRATORY DISTRESS SYNDROME

INTRODUCTION

M.I. was a 22-year-old, 54-kg female with a history of systemic lupus erythematosus, congenital mitral regurgitation, and syncopes. For the past several months, she complained of mild productive cough while lying down. One week prior to her admission she developed severe cough, progressive dyspnea without the use of accessory muscles, and associated pain throughout her chest wall and into her upper abdomen.

Her medical history also included chronic anemia (hemoglobin 8.7 g %, *normal 12 to 15 g %*) and was on iron supplement at the time. Her white blood cell (WBC) count was 21×10^3 (*normal 3.2 to 9.8 $\times 10^3$*), hematocrit (Hct) 27% (*female average 42%*) without evidence of blood loss. Blood pressure was 93/59 mm Hg (*normal 120/80 mm Hg*), pulse 114, respirations were shallow and guarded at 20 breaths per minute. Tenderness was noted across the upper abdomen and the lower ribs without organomegally or other masses present.

She was 4 months postpartum with gradual onset abdominal pain, progressive dyspnea with nonproductive coughs, and was admitted to the hospital for further evaluations.

The patient's nonspecific symptoms led to a wide range of diagnostic tests for her condition which included lupus, mitral regurgitation, and pulmonary insufficiency. Initial blood gases on room air were obtained in the emergency room, the patient was admitted to the medical floor, and a sputum culture was ordered to evaluate pathology concerning the respiratory tract.

✔ Iron supplement is used to increase the O_2^- carrying capacity of hemoglobin.

✔ Hemoglobin, WBC, Hct, and blood pressure are all outside normal limits.

☑ Alveolar
   hyperventilation
($PaCO_2$ 31 mm Hg)
with moderate
hypoxemia (PaO_2
67 mm Hg) could
lead to fatigue of
respiratory muscles
if causes of hypox-
emia are not identi-
fied and treated
promptly.

☑ Impending venti-
   latory failure
   typically shows
increasing $PaCO_2$
and decreasing PaO_2.

☑ Postural drain-
   age and chest
physiotherapy were
done to facilitate
loosening and
removal of
secretions.

☑ CPAP requires
   adequate spon-
taneous breathing.
Development of
respiratory muscle
fatigue is the pri-
mary concern for
prolonged CPAP
usage in critically ill
patients.

The initial blood gases were as follows:

pH	7.49
$PaCO_2$	31 mm Hg
PaO_2	67 mm Hg
HCO_3^-	22.7 mEq/L
Hb	8.4 g %
Mode	Spontaneous
F_IO_2	21%

Her breath sounds were unremarkable but she was moderately fatigued and continued to be short of breath. She was started on a nasal cannula at 2 L/min and was encouraged to deep breathe and cough. At this point, the patient was still able to adequately ventilate as evidenced by the $PaCO_2$. However, her condition deteriorated during the course of her evaluation and workup. Shortly thereafter, she developed intermittent wheezing for which albuterol nebulizer treatments were ordered.

INDICATIONS

Her blood gases continued to deteriorate, and 6 days later she required a nonrebreathing mask to maintain her SpO_2 above 90%. She showed signs of impending ventilatory failure evidenced by the rising $PaCO_2$s and acidotic pH on blood gases. A chest radiograph showed areas of bibasilar atelectasis and haziness with bilateral infiltrates. No pulmonary consolidation was noted. Postural drainage and chest physiotherapy were started but she was too weak to generate a productive cough.

Family members refused permission to obtain a diagnostic bronchoscopy or any attempts at percutaneous biopsies. Three days later, her oxygen requirements had increased to the point where she required a heated nebulizer analyzed at an F_IO_2 of 95% bled into her nonrebreathing mask at 15 L/min, and a nasal cannula at 6 L/min simply to maintain oxygen saturation of 86% to 92%. Practitioners were able to convince the family to utilize free standing CPAP at 12 cm H_2O and F_IO_2 of 50% to improve oxygenation, but the patient became fatigued to the extent that she was only able to tolerate the procedure 20 min every 2 hours. At that time she had a vital capacity of 0.9 L and MIP of -75 cm H_2O. This continued for 2 days as she became refractory to oxygen therapy and was unable to maintain adequate oxygen saturation.

INITIAL SETTINGS

Every attempt was made to forestall ventilatory failure and prevent intubation but the patient's condition continued to deteriorate, and she became progressively fatigued. Her age and previous health were positive factors in postponing ventilatory failure, but she eventually became overwhelmed by fatigue. She was moderately sedated, intubated with a

7.5 mm endotracheal tube, and placed on a Puritan-Bennett 7200 for mechanical ventilation. Initially, she was set on assist/control at 25/min, V_T of 800 mL, F_1O_2 of 100%, and PEEP of 8 cm H_2O. Arterial and mixed venous blood gases on these settings revealed the following:

Arterial
pH	7.55
$PaCO_2$	33 mm Hg
PaO_2	58 mm Hg
SaO_2	88%
HCO_3^-	29.5 mEq/L
Hb	10.1 g %

Mixed Venous
pH	7.38
PvO_2	33 mm Hg
SvO_2	58%
$C(a-v)O_2$	4.6 vol %
Qs/QT	37%

Ventilator Settings
Mode	A/C
Rate	25/min
V_T	800 mL
F_1O_2	100%
PEEP	8 cm H_2O

Her ventilator rate was reduced to 14/min, and her PEEP was increased to 10 cm H_2O.

PATIENT MONITORING

In addition to blood gases and vital signs, other cardiopulmonary monitoring included chest radiograph and hemodynamic measurements. Her chest radiograph at that time revealed initial findings consistent with adult respiratory distress syndrome (ARDS), including a uniform reticulogranular pattern or ground glass appearance throughout both lung fields. Arterial and pulmonary artery catheters were used to monitor the cardiac output and hemodynamic status. Cardiac output was stable at 4.2 L. The pulmonary capillary wedge pressure (PCWP) was around 11 mm Hg and thus ruled out cardiogenic edema.

For unknown reasons, the patient developed a parenchymal injury causing progressive inflammation, alveolar collapse, and hypoxemia.

Hypoxemia in ARDS may be summarized as follows:

Hypoxic vasoconstriction in ARDS increases the vascular resistance and diminishes the cardiac output. The lack of oxygen in the pulmonary circulation also causes necrosis of the tissue lining of the alveolar-capillary membrane that, in turn, induces capillary leak into

☑ The ventilator rate was decreased because of the low $PaCO_2$ (33 mm Hg).

☑ The PEEP was increased because of the low PaO_2 (58 mm Hg).

☑ With cardiogenic pulmonary edema, the PCWP is usually elevated (>18 mm Hg).

☑ Pulmonary edema with normal PCWP is likely caused by lung parenchymal changes (e.g., ARDS).

the interstitium (third spacing) and hence, impairs gas exchange. This eventually causes a severe V/Q mismatch and further hypoxemia. As a result of these factors, perfusion must be maintained and oxygenation restored for effective management of ARDS.

PATIENT MANAGEMENT

Management strategies for ARDS include correcting hypoxemia and acid-base disturbance, restoring cardiac function, and treating the underlying disease or other precipitating factors. This is generally accomplished with mechanical ventilation at 10 to 12 mL/kg of body weight and the application of PEEP or CPAP to correct refractory hypoxemia.

High level of positive pressure may be required to produce adequate ventilation and oxygenation, but its adverse effect on cardiac function must be monitored carefully. Some patients may benefit from pressure control (PC) ventilation to minimize the mean airway and parenchymal pressures. In PC mode the inspiratory time is increased and pressures are generally reduced, but the mean airway pressure may remain nearly the same or slightly increased. This ultimately shortens the expiratory time, inverts the I:E ratio, and potentially increases alveolar ventilation. As inspiratory time increases, and the elastic limit of the lung is reached, intrinsic PEEP increases air trapping and thus, may increase the $PaCO_2$ while also increasing the occurrence of pneumothorax in an already stiff lung. These important considerations must be kept in fine balance with each factor receiving equal attention.

In an attempt to decrease the pressures exerted within the thorax, the patient was placed on pressure control ventilation with an inverse ratio of 2:1 at pressure of 30 cm H_2O, T_I of 0.84 sec, F_IO_2 of 60%, and PEEP of 10 cm H_2O. Blood gases taken at the time revealed:

pH	7.42
$PaCO_2$	47 mm Hg
PaO_2	60 mm Hg
HCO_3^-	30 mEq/L
Hb	11.1 g %
SpO_2	90%
Mode	PC-IRV
T_I	0.84 sec
I:E ratio	2:1
Rate	14
P_{INSP}	30 cm H_2O
F_IO_2	60%
PEEP	10 cm H_2O

The pressures were then titrated in an effort to improve oxygenation and normalize her condition, but without success.

✓ Hypoxemia caused by intrapulmonary shunting may be supported by PEEP (with mechanical ventilation) or CPAP (with spontaneous breathing).

✓ Pressure control ventilation limits the inspiratory pressure during mechanical ventilation.

✓ As in IPPB, the tidal volume delivered by pressure control ventilation is directly related to the inspiratory pressure.

Mucomyst and
Pulmozyme
are used to mobilize
thick, retained
secretions.

KEY MEDICATIONS

The patient was placed in a Rotorest® bed to prevent development of atelectasis. She was also heavily sedated and maintained in a medicated coma for over 30 days but without significant improvement. She was given medication nebulizers with Proventil every 4 hours, lavaged with a combination of 2.0 mL normal saline (NS), 0.5 mL of 0.5% Proventil, and 4.0 mL of 10% Mucomyst solution, and suctioned every 4 hours with her treatment to improve bronchopulmonary hygiene. By this time she had a large amount of thick, yellow secretions and 0.5 mL of dornase alpha (Pulmozyme) in NS was used to loosen and remove her retained secretions.

WEANING

The deteriorating hemodynamic status prevented continuing use of inverse I:E ratio ventilation. She was returned to conventional methods throughout the remainder of her hospitalization. This included ventilation in the assist/control mode at a rate of 24/min. The patient initiated inspiratory effort to 28/min. She was set to a V_T of 500 mL, F_IO_2 of 80%, and PEEP of 8 cm H_2O. Arterial blood gases on these settings produced these results:

Low V_T is used
to minimize the
airway pressures.

pH	7.43
$PaCO_2$	48 mm Hg
PaO_2	64 mm Hg
HCO_3^-	31 mEq/L
Hb	11.1 g %
CaO_2	13.9 vol %
SpO_2	91%
Mode	A/C
RR	24/min
V_T	500 mL
F_IO_2	80%
PEEP	8 cm H_2O

The respiratory rate was increased to 30 breaths per minute to override her excessive and demanding respiratory efforts. PEEP was increased to 10 cm H_2O, and F_IO_2 was reduced to 70%.

Blood gases were drawn 30 min later with the following results:

pH	7.50
$PaCO_2$	47 mm Hg
PaO_2	59 mm Hg
HCO_3^-	36.4 mEq/L
B.E.	12.4 mEq/L
Hb	9.6 g %
CaO_2	12.4 vol %
SpO_2	91%

Mode	A/C
RR	30/min
V_T	500 mL
F_IO_2	70%
PEEP	10 cm H_2O

Several unsuccessful weaning attempts were made. Over several days she was weaned to a rate of 24/min on assist/control with a V_T of 380 mL, F_IO_2 of 50%, and PEEP of 8 cm H_2O and remained on those settings for nearly 1 week. Due to her deteriorating condition and persistent complications, it was decided to remove her from ventilatory support, and she died a short time later.

COMPLICATIONS

Through the course of her hospitalization the patient experienced many complicating injuries which contributed to her failure to recover. These included barotrauma to the lung parenchyma (pneumothorax was corrected with a chest tube), pneumomediastinum, and interstitial emphysema verified through serial chest radiographs, subcutaneous emphysema, and ultimately death. Many of these complications could have been expected as a result of her hospital course because ARDS, even without her related complicating factors, carries a 50% mortality rate.

✔ Complicating ARDS carries a 50% mortality rate.

Note: This case study on ARDS describes the evaluative, diagnostic, and ventilatory management techniques employed at the time it was first written. Recently, however, the National Heart, Lung, and Blood Institute of the National Institute of Health has released a statement concerning the ARDS Network Clinical Trial. This included research at a consortium of 10 clinical centers conducted at 24 hospitals across the United States. For further information, please refer to this statement outlined by the NIH (1999, Mar). *NHLBI Clinical Trial Stopped Early: Successful Ventilator Strategy Found for Intensive Care Patients on Life Support.* NIH Press Release at http://www.nih.gov/news/pr/mar99/nhlbi-15.htm (July 23, 2004)

Data from this clinical trial on the first 800 patients showed approximately 25% fewer deaths among patients receiving small, rather than large, tidal volumes from a mechanical ventilator. Patient tidal volume is based on an ideal body weight calculation. This is calculated from the following equation:

Male: 50 + 2.3 (Height in Inches − 60) × 6cc

Female: 45.5 + 2.3 (Height in Inches − 60) × 6 cc

Although the patient in this case study was not on this protocol, it seems worth mentioning that these new guidelines have proved to be useful in clinical practice. This is especially true with the ARDS protocol.

CASE 10: MYASTHENIA GRAVIS

INTRODUCTION

G.L. was a 72-year-old Caucasian male (6'1", 74 kg) with a history of myasthenia gravis for 25 years, but it had been in remission until about 6 months ago. His last hospitalization was 2 months ago because of ongoing shortness of breath, easy fatigability, inability to complete a sentence without taking a breath, chronic cough, malaise, yellow sputum production, and difficulty in swallowing. The diagnosis was pneumonia and he required mechanical ventilation for 17 days. He was eventually weaned off mechanical ventilation and discharged. During that hospitalization, he had repeated guaiac positive stool samples indicative of the presence of occult blood in the feces.

He had been home for 4 weeks and continued to have shortness of breath, fatigability, muscle weakness, orthopnea, and had to sleep sitting up in his recliner. He came to the outpatient radiology clinic for barium and chest radiograph studies. Upon arrival to the radiology department he was extremely short of breath and after his exams were completed he was referred to the emergency room. The patient declined to be seen and went home with his wife.

Within 5 min of arrival home the patient suffered a respiratory arrest. His wife reported that he just stopped breathing and turned blue. The paramedics arrived and attempted to intubate but were unsuccessful after three attempts. While being transported to the ER, the patient had some spontaneous respirations but poor diaphragmatic movement.

The initial blood gas analysis done upon arrival to the ER revealed the following results:

pH	6.95
$PaCO_2$	143 mm Hg
PaO_2	115 mm Hg
SaO_2	96%
HCO_3^-	30 mEq/L
Mode	Ambu bag and mask
F_IO_2	About 100%
Notes	Poor ventilation

INDICATIONS

The patient was intubated in the ER and bagged at a rate of 20/min and F_IO_2 of 100%. Vital signs included: blood pressure 138/40 mm Hg, heart rate 60/min, temperature 95.2°F, SpO_2 97%, and Glasgow coma score 15. Bilateral breath sounds were present. Chest radiograph (Figure 18-6) showed proper ET tube position, good thoracic expansion, but barium in the left lower lobe.

Sidebar notes

☑ Barium study is done to evaluate the cause of guaiac positive stools.

☑ Chest radiograph is done to evaluate the residual effects of pneumonia.

☑ Blood gas report indicates that the primary problem is acute ventilatory failure imposed on chronic ventilatory failure.

☑ $PaCO_2$ indicates that the bag/mask system in the ambulance was not ventilating the patient.

☑ HCO_3^- is elevated as a compensatory mechanism of the patient's pre-existing ventilatory failure.

Figure 18-6 Myasthenia gravis. Aspiration of barium on the left side (1) is seen. The right hemidiaphragm shadow is flat with a poorly defined costophrenic angle (2). This condition may be caused by pleural effusion.

✔ Glasgow coma score of ≤7 indicates coma. A score of 15 rules out coma.

✔ Chest radiograph shows aspiration of barium in the left lower lobe.

INITIAL SETTINGS

The patient was initially placed on a Puritan-Bennett 7200ae ventilator with the following settings: CMV 16/min, V_T 750 mL, F_IO_2 80%, PEEP 0 cmH$_2$O. The patient had the following arterial blood gas (ABG) results:

pH	7.48
PaCO$_2$	43 mm Hg
PaO$_2$	168 mm Hg
SaO$_2$	97%
HCO$_3^-$	30.5 mEq/L
Mode	CMV

☑ PaO$_2$ 168 mm Hg is too high and the F$_I$O$_2$ should be decreased.

Rate	16
V$_T$	750 mL
F$_I$O$_2$	80%
PEEP	0 cm H$_2$O

PATIENT MANAGEMENT

(Day 1) The patient was continued on mechanical ventilation and the F$_I$O$_2$ was weaned to 40% with the following results:

☑ PaCO$_2$ 21 mm Hg is too low and the rate should be decreased.

pH	7.58
PaCO$_2$	21 mm Hg
PaO$_2$	122 mm Hg
SaO$_2$	96%
HCO$_3^-$	19.1 mEq/L
Mode	CMV
Rate	16
V$_T$	750 mL
F$_I$O$_2$	40%
PEEP	0 cm H$_2$O

The patient's set respiratory rate was decreased to 12 and the blood gas results were:

☑ PaCO$_2$ 25 mm Hg is still too low and the rate should be decreased again.

pH	7.52
PaCO$_2$	25 mm Hg
PaO$_2$	128 mm Hg
SaO$_2$	97%
HCO$_3^-$	20 mEq/L
Mode	CMV
Rate	12
V$_T$	750 mL
F$_I$O$_2$	40%
PEEP	0 cm H$_2$O

The CMV rate was further decreased to 8/min for the rest of Day 1.

(Day 2) The next morning the patient was on CMV of 8/min, V$_T$ 750 mL, F$_I$O$_2$ 40%, and no PEEP. He had the following spontaneous parameters: V$_E$ 9.7 L, V$_T$ 660 mL, rate 15/min, MIP −24 cm H$_2$O, and a vital capacity of 2,080 mL. The patient was alert and responsive. A CPAP/pressure support (CPAP/PS) trial was done with PS of 5 cm H$_2$O, base flow of 2 L/min, PEEP of 5 cm H$_2$O, and an F$_I$O$_2$ of 40%. The patient tolerated this for 4 hours with spontaneous tidal volumes of 600 to 700 mL and a spontaneous rate of 16 to 21/min. Breath sounds showed fine inspiratory crackles throughout the anterior bases. All vital signs were within normal limits.

☑ The increased WBC may be due to aspiration of barium and subsequent aspiration pneumonitis.

(Day 3) The patient was rested on CMV overnight. Spontaneous parameters were: V$_E$ 7.8 L, V$_T$ 720 mL, rate 12/min, MIP −12 cm H$_2$O, and a vital capacity of 4,020 mL. Heart rate, blood pressure, and temperature were all within normal limits. The patient's WBC spiked at a high of 16.2×10^3 (*normal 3.2 to 9.8 $\times 10^3$*), chest radiograph showed the endotracheal tube was in proper position, and the bilateral opacities were consistent with barium aspiration.

He tolerated the previous CPAP/PS settings for 4 hours and was taken off CPAP/PS when he began to show extreme accessory muscle use. Blood gases during spontaneous breathing revealed:

☑ $PaCO_2$ 34 mm Hg indicates hyperventilation. It may lead to fatigue of respiratory muscles.

pH	7.38
$PaCO_2$	34 mm Hg
PaO_2	87 mm Hg
SaO_2	97%
Mode	Spontaneous breathing
F_IO_2	40%

(Day 4) The patient was rested overnight on CMV, spontaneous parameters were: V_E 9.9 L, V_T 550 mL, rate 18, MIP −26 cm H_2O, and a vital capacity of 3 L. Vital signs revealed: heart rate 76/min, temperature 38°C, blood pressure 120/74 mm Hg. The patient tolerated two trials of CPAP/PS at previous settings for 2 hours each time. Breath sounds were markedly decreased in both lower lobes. Patient was very anxious, restless, and had difficulty sleeping at night. He was started on Ativan for his anxiety. The patient had a feeding tube placed today for total nutrition.

(Day 5) He was rested overnight on CMV. Spontaneous parameters were: V_E 12.9 L, V_T 720 mL, rate 18/min, MIP −29 cm H_2O, and a vital capacity of 3.4 L. Patient had a repeat endoscopy and was heavily sedated. One CPAP/PS trial was done before the patient was sedated. The spontaneous respiratory rate was between 15 and 17/min and the spontaneous tidal volume was in the low 400 mL range. Patient's vital signs were: heart rate 73/min, temperature 36.8°C, and blood pressure 120/59 mm Hg. The patient's endoscopy biopsy was positive for cytomegalovirus and he was started on Ganciclovir and Prilosec.

(Day 6) The patient was again rested on CMV overnight. He was only able to tolerate partial spontaneous parameters and the results were: MIP −28 cm H_2O and a vital capacity of 1.1 L. The patient tolerated 90 min on CPAP/PS before he was extremely short of breath and exhibited an increased work of breathing with marked accessory muscle use. The patient's daily chest radiograph showed increasing bilateral infiltrates consistent with pneumonia/aspiration and the presence of barium in the left lower lobe. The patient had bilateral lower lobe rhonchi and was being suctioned for copious amounts of light yellow secretions. The patient also spiked a temperature to 39°C. Pulmonary consultation was obtained at this time.

PATIENT MONITORING

The patient's spontaneous breathing parameters from Day 2 through Day 6 are summarized as follows. On Day 6, the patient could perform only part of the breathing parameters.

☑ The overall breathing parameters are not satisfactory for a weaning attempt.

Day	V_E (L)	V_T (mL)	Rate (min)	MIP (cm H_2O)	VC (L)
2	9.7	660	15	−24	2.08
3	7.8	720	12	−12	4.02
4	9.9	550	18	−26	3.0
5	12.9	720	18	29	3.4
6	N/A	N/A	N/A	−28	1.1

WEANING

This patient was eventually weaned from mechanical ventilation after 25 days. He was weaned by using SIMV ventilation to build up his respiratory muscle strength before weaning to CPAP/PS again. The PS level was much higher than with previous attempts. The PS level was gradually weaned down each day as the patient's own spontaneous tidal volumes increased. He was then weaned to CPAP only and eventually extubated from CPAP to a face mask at 30%.

A vigorous program of physical therapy was started to assist the patient with overall strengthening of his weakened muscle. A dietary consult was obtained and a metabolic study performed in order to adjust his feedings to appropriate nutritional levels needed for successful weaning.

Notes: Adequate nutrition prior to and during weaning is necessary for a successful outcome. Appropriate nutrition helps to maintain and build respiratory muscle mass and strength, which enhances the likelihood of weaning.

The patient was also started on albuterol Q 4° with postural drainage and percussion. Antibiotics were used to treat the pneumonia. The patient was given neostigmine for his myasthenia gravis crisis.

☑ Neostigmine (Prostigmin) is a cholinergic drug used to treat myasthenia gravis.

COMPLICATIONS

Weaning attempts on this patient were complicated by three major factors: (1) myasthenia gravis, (2) aspiration pneumonia, (3) premature weaning attempts.

The history of myasthenia gravis (a neuromuscular disease) inhibits the transmission of nerve impulses at the myoneural junction. These patients typically have chronic fatigability and weak muscles in the face and throat. They can also suffer what is known as a

☑ Myasthenia gravis, aspiration pneumonia, and poor nutritional intake all contributed to the failure of earlier weaning attempts.

myasthenia gravis crisis—an acute exacerbation of muscle weakness that leads to respiratory distress and periods of apnea.

Aspiration pneumonia from the barium study increased the work of breathing and made it difficult for him to tolerate weaning procedures.

Premature and inconsistent weaning attempts during the first 3 days of his hospitalization made subsequent weaning attempts more difficult.

CASE 11: GUILLAIN-BARRÉ

INTRODUCTION

K.D. was a 14-year-old, 49-kg, right-handed male who sustained two minor head injuries at school over a period of 1 week. One injury occurred while playing basketball when a heavier student fell on him and the other occurred in an altercation during a break. Neither injury resulted in the loss of consciousness. He presented to the clinic complaining of headache and back pain but did not complain of slurred speech until being started on pain medication (Dolobid®) one day prior to admission. His medical history is noncontributory and consists of one hospitalization for a hernia repair in the distant past. He denied blurred vision but admitted to having transient nausea and had recently refused food. Since his slurred speech had become more pronounced he was admitted for further evaluation.

On examination, the patient was afebrile and had these vital signs: BP 110/70 mm Hg, pulse 78/min, respirations 14/min (up to 40/min on occasion). His facial muscles showed symmetry. He had trouble sitting up due to excessive pain in his lower extremities, especially on the left. Lung sounds revealed basilar crackles on the right with decreased aeration on the left. A chest radiograph showed left lower lobe atelectasis. The cranial nerves 2–12 appeared intact and motor strength showed marked weakness. The patient was able to lift his right heel 2 to 3 in with great difficulty but was unable to lift his left heel at all. His deep tendon reflexes were completely absent.

Laboratory results revealed WBCs of 14,000 with 84 segs. The electrolytes and urinalysis were normal. His FEV_1 and FVC were 1.4 L and 1.7 L, respectively. The FEV_1/FVC ratio was 82%. CT scan of the brain revealed a normal study. Chest radiograph at the time showed bilateral consolidation secondary to muscle weakness and left lower lobe atelectasis.

☑ Restrictive lung disease typically shows reduction in FEV_1 *and* FVC, resulting in a normal FEV_1/FVC%.

INDICATIONS

The patient had a 5-day history of progressive muscular weakness. For this reason, simple spirometry studies were done Q4 hours through the night. His predicted forced vital capacity (FVC) was 3.38 L

✔ Mechanical ventilation is indicated when the vital capacity falls below 1 L or twice the patient's predicted tidal volume.

✔ Bilateral breath sounds suggests proper endotracheal intubation. This sign should coincide with absence of respiratory distress, presence of adequate SpO_2, and stable vital signs.

✔ Chest radiograph is done to confirm proper placement of endotracheal tube and to rule out inadvertent mainstem intubation.

and his initial vital capacity was 1.7 L (50% of the predicted value), which he maintained through the early evening. His predicted FEV_1 was 3.12 L and his initial measurement revealed 1.4 L (48% of predicted) for an 82% FEV_1/FVC ratio. By 03:30 am, the patient's vital capacity had dropped to 1.2 L (35% of predicted) and an arterial blood gas (ABG) at that time, on room air, revealed the following:

pH	7.37
$PaCO_2$	45 mm Hg
PaO_2	46 mm Hg
SaO_2	76%
HCO_3^-	24.9 mEq/L
RR	24/min
F_IO_2	21%

Oxygen therapy was initiated at 2 L/min per nasal cannula. He rested well until 08:22 the next morning. The vital capacity at that time was slightly over 1 L (30% of predicted) and the ABGs revealed:

pH	7.38
$PaCO_2$	43 mm Hg
PaO_2	52 mm Hg
SaO_2	86%
HCO_3^-	25.2 mEq/L
RR	22/min

Every attempt was made to forestall clinical deterioration. Trends of spirometry and blood gases showed that the patient was going into ventilatory failure. By 10:30, the patient's vital capacity had dropped to 0.7 L (20% of predicted) and maintaining adequate oxygenation was becoming more difficult. Consequently, a decision was made to perform elective intubation. Preparation was made to notify family members of the impending ventilatory compromise, and the respiratory therapist gathered the necessary equipment for a controlled intubation. The patient was mildly sedated and intubated with a 7.5 mm endotracheal tube without difficulty. Bilateral breath sounds were heard and a portable chest radiograph was ordered.

INITIAL SETTINGS

Following intubation and confirmation of proper tube placement, the patient was placed on a Puritan-Bennett 7200a ventilator in A/C mode, backup rate of 12, tidal volume of 600 mL, and F_IO_2 of 40%. PEEP was not initiated at that time. ABGs revealed the following:

pH	7.37
$PaCO_2$	43 mm Hg
PaO_2	53 mm Hg
SaO_2	86%
HCO_3^-	23.7 mEq/L

Mode	A/C
Rate	12/min
Spont. Rate	17 min
V_T	600 mL
F_1O_2	40%

The ventilator settings were changed accordingly to a backup rate of 14/min, F_1O_2 of 50%, and PEEP of 5 cm H_2O. Follow-up ABGs showed:

pH	7.45
$PaCO_2$	42 mm Hg
PaO_2	73 mm Hg
SaO_2	94%
HCO_3^-	28 mEq/L
Mode	A/C
Rate	14/min
V_T	600 mL
F_1O_2	50%
PEEP	5 cm H_2O

The patient remained relatively stable and was monitored closely for signs of respiratory distress. The ventilator peak flow was adjusted to meet the patient's inspiratory demand without compromise to alveolar ventilation. By the third ventilator day, the F_1O_2 was increased to 60% and the PEEP was increased to 8 cm H_2O. These changes were made to prevent atelectasis and improve alveolar ventilation as evidenced by a declining PaO_2 on his morning blood gas. These revealed the following:

pH	7.44
$PaCO_2$	35 mm Hg
PaO_2	57 mm Hg
SaO_2	87%
HCO_3^-	22.5 mEq/L
Mode	A/C
Rate	14/min
V_T	600 mL
F_1O_2	60%
PEEP	8 cm H_2O

The patient's PEEP was subsequently increased to 10 cm H_2O without cardiac or hemodynamic compromise. F_1O_2 was decreased to 50% because of improving SpO_2 values. Follow-up ABGs revealed:

pH	7.46
$PaCO_2$	35 mm Hg
PaO_2	132 mm Hg
SaO_2	97%
HCO_3^-	23.5 mEq/L
Mode	A/C

Rate	14/min
V_T	600 mL
F_IO_2	50%
PEEP	10 cm H_2O

The F_IO_2 was again lowered to 40% and he remained stable for the next 2 days.

KEY MEDICATIONS

On day four of mechanical ventilation, a persistent low-grade fever and thick tenacious secretions necessitated initiation of vigorous pulmonary toilet. Albuterol with Mucomyst via small volume nebulizer was started Q4 hours in-line with the ventilator circuit as well as postural drainage and percussion to the bilateral lower lobes. Bronchoalveolar lavage with 4 mL of 10% Mucomyst, 0.5 mL of 0.5% albuterol, and 5 mL of normal saline facilitated suction of moderate to large amounts of thick secretions. Gradual clearing of retained secretions and atelectasis became evident by follow-up chest radiographs. These management strategies in pulmonary toilet were continued for the remainder of the ventilatory period.

Immobility was a major factor in the patient's clinical deterioration. Extensive physical therapy was begun with range of motion and activity as tolerated. However, extreme pain made these sessions almost unbearable to the patient.

☑ Each week of muscle immobility requires 4 weeks of rehabilitation of his diminished muscle mass.

PATIENT MONITORING

Respiratory parameters were obtained every morning in an effort to trend his ventilatory mechanics. The parameters listed in Table 18-1 were obtained on representative days and are not necessarily concurrent (please note on ventilator day 6 through 26 the patient was mainly unable to breathe on his own).

PATIENT MANAGEMENT

Management strategy for Guillain-Barre was mainly supportive as the ascending paralysis typically runs its course. Being predominantly idiopathic in nature, treatment included plasma phoresis in an attempt to reverse the pathology. However, by the sixth ventilator day it was apparent that long-term management strategies would be necessary. As such, a pediatric feeding tube was inserted and tracheostomy was performed in an effort to facilitate removal of secretions and to make oral care more accessible. A metabolic study was performed to ascertain the patient's nutritional status and feedings were adjusted in terms of optimizing the resulting V/Q ratio and total caloric intake. He was placed in a Rotorest bed and continuously turned from side to side and kept comfortable with antianxiolytics. The patient was closely monitored for signs of hypercapnea, hypoxia, and respiratory distress.

TABLE 18-1   Respiratory Parameters

VENT DAY	RR (f)	V$_T$ (mL)	FVC (L)	V$_E$ (L)	F/V$_T$	MIP (cm H$_2$O)	COMPLIANCE (mL/cm H$_2$O)
2	37	140	0.67	5.30	264	−20	28
3	50	60	0.32	5.30	833	−15	32
4	25	80	0.69	2.60	312	−13	38
5	23	80	0.10	5.40	287	−2	62
26	6	410	0.41	4.90	15	−15	45
28	10	440	0.45	5.00	23	−15	52
32	23	70	0.65	1.03	328	−10	34
36	30	135	0.55	4.00	222	−26	48
42	29	110	0.54	3.10	263	−11	41
46	32	85	0.25	2.73	376	−10	44
52	27	200	0.36	4.20	135	−14	51
54	23	210	0.57	4.83	1.09	−17	53
56	32	115	0.52	3.70	278	−17	55
58	21	240	0.68	4.60	88	−15	64
60	25	250	0.96	6.22	100	−23	70
62	29	175	1.02	5.09	165	−24	58
64	25	240	0.68	5.89	104	−26	55
66	19	210	1.15	4.91	90	−30	54
68	18	200	1.07	6.11	90	−37	54

It is important to note that the patient was not able to initiate any significant spontaneous tidal volume. The ventilator was thus completely responsible for his total alveolar ventilation. Blood gas analysis after tracheostomy by general anesthesia revealed the following:

pH	7.40
PaCO$_2$	52 mm Hg
PaO$_2$	122 mm Hg
SaO$_2$	96%
HCO$_3^-$	31 mEq/L
Mode	A/C
Rate	14/min
V$_T$	600 mL
F$_I$O$_2$	40%
PEEP	10 cm H$_2$O

In order to improve alveolar ventilation, the rate was increased to 16/min and the tidal volume was increased to 670 mL as he was still unable to initiate spontaneous ventilation. Due to his unstable ventilatory status, blood gas results from the following morning revealed:

pH	7.39
$PaCO_2$	48 mm Hg
PaO_2	90 mm Hg
SaO_2	94%
HCO_3^-	28 mEq/L
Mode	A/C
Rate	16/min
V_T	670 mL
F_IO_2	40%
PEEP	10 cm H_2O

In order to minimize airway pressures and risk of barotrauma, the $PaCO_2$ was allowed to stay in the mid to upper 40s. The patient appeared to rest comfortably. Blood gases obtained on the eighteenth ventilator day revealed:

pH	7.48
$PaCO_2$	47 mm Hg
PaO_2	114 mm Hg
SaO_2	97%
HCO_3^-	34 mEq/L
Mode	A/C
Rate	18/min
V_T	670 mL
F_IO_2	40%
PEEP	10 cm H_2O

These parameters were maintained until the 24 ventilator day when the patient appeared to improve clinically and began to breathe significantly on his own. Although he became increasingly uneasy about his breathlessness and, as a result, was changed to SIMV mode, rate of 18 breaths per minute, tidal volume of 750 mL, and F_IO_2 of 40%. PEEP was reduced to 5 cm H_2O and pressure support was initiated to augment his spontaneous volume. Blood gases taken after these changes indicated marked improvement in oxygenation and acid-base balance:

pH	7.47
$PaCO_2$	38 mm Hg
PaO_2	117 mm Hg
SaO_2	94%
HCO_3^-	27 mEq/L
Mode	SIMV
Rate	18/min
V_T	750 mL
F_IO_2	40%

PEEP	5 cm H_2O
Press. Support	15 cm H_2O

At this point, the F_IO_2 was reduced to 35% and remained relatively stable for the next 19 days. A bronchoscopy was performed on ventilator day 32 to clear an obstructed left lower lobe bronchus. This was achieved without difficulty and by ventilator day 39, the rate was decreased from 18 to 12/min. The following day, the rate was decreased to 10/min. His spontaneous rate ranged between 29 and 32/min.

WEANING

On ventilator day 40, the patient continued to show evidence of improved alveolar ventilation. Brief trials of ventilator discontinuance, as little as 10 to 15 min every 2 to 4 hours were initiated to encourage the use of respiratory muscles. Gradually, by the 54th ventilator day, he was able to tolerate short periods of ventilator discontinuance of 30 min to an hour twice a day on CPAP with minimal pressure support (10 to 15 cm H_2O). At this pressure support range, the patient was able to achieve an alveolar tidal volume of 300 to 400 mL. As muscle strength returned and gradually improved, less pressure support was necessary to maintain an adequate volume. The patient was allowed to rest completely at night on A/C mode and weaning was resumed each morning to CPAP with low level of pressure support.

> ✓ The pressure support level is titrated and subsequently adjusted until spontaneous tidal volume = 10 to 15 mL/kg or spontaneous respiratory rate <25/min.

By day 59, the patient progressed to 40 min to an hour of ventilator discontinuance every 2 hours during the day while resting at night. Each day brought the same monotonous routine but he continued to improve. On ventilator day 68 he was able to remain off the ventilator 24 hours per day. Real rehabilitation had just begun!

COMPLICATIONS

This patient encountered almost complete paralysis in the acute pathologic phase of his disease as he was only able to blink his eyes. He was under severe emotional and psychologic stress throughout his hospitalization. He developed GI bleeding from a duodenal ulcer for which he was treated with Zantac via his feeding tube. Otitis media developed and was treated with broad spectrum antibiotics, and a persistent left lower lobe pneumonitis requiring bronchoscopy. Rehabilitation was begun and he was transferred out of the intensive care unit with humidified O_2 at an F_IO_2 of 30%. The tracheostomy was gradually buttoned. He required only 2 L/min of oxygen via nasal cannula while recovering in rehab. The patient was discharged after 154 days of hospital stay (last 94 days in extensive rehabilitation) on room air requiring only 25 mg of prednisone and follow-up physical therapy. He continued to progress and, eventually, demonstrated no residual effects from this debilitating illness.

CASE 12: BOTULISM

INTRODUCTION

J.D. was a 66-year-old, 50-kg female in her usual state of health until she consumed a partial jar of home-canned salsa. The following day she developed abdominal cramping thought to be the flu. Her intermittent cramping continued for 48 hours postingestion, then she developed slurred speech and blurred vision. In addition to these symptoms, the patient experienced vertigo and diplopia at times and sought medical attention when diffuse upper motor weakness appeared. Her bulbar weakness and generalized fatigue necessitated admission for close observation in the ICU. *Clostridium botulism* was cultured from the salsa and also found to be present in the patient's stool. Community and state health officials were contacted for an antitoxin and subsequently this case was reported to the Centers for Disease Control and Prevention (CDCP) in Atlanta. Within 24 hours of admission the patient received trivalent botulism antitoxin but she encountered progressive deterioration with concomitant respiratory compromise.

INDICATIONS

On examination, the patient exhibited no evidence of distress. She did, however, manifest bilateral ptosis (drooping of eyelids) with decreased facial expression. Neck was supple, lungs were clear, and her mental status appeared normal. Pupillary light reflexes revealed sluggish reactions bilaterally. The tongue was midline with evidence of slurred speech. Motor examination revealed diffuse weakness of the upper extremities. Symmetrical fatigability of the biceps, deltoids, and grips were also noted. Gait revealed mild weakness, and electromyogram (EMG) studies showed decreased amplitude of repetitive nerve action potentials.

The patient was admitted for close observation. Vital capacities and maximum inspiratory pressure (MIP) were done Q2 hours. Her white blood cell count was 6,900 on admission and 12,500 (*normal 3.2 to 9.8 $\times$ 10^3*) 48 hours later. Vital signs revealed blood pressure of 168/56 mm Hg, heart rate of 88/min, temperature of 36.4°C, and respirations of 24/min. Her initial arterial blood gases on room air revealed:

pH	7.45
$PaCO_2$	36 mm Hg
PaO_2	72 mm Hg
SaO_2	95%
HCO_3^-	24.5 mEq/L
RR	24/min
F_IO_2	21%

Her vital capacity at 03:30 was 1.6 L (62% of predicted) with a MIP of −18 cm H_2O. By 08:00, the condition of the patient remained relatively unchanged except that her MIP had decreased to −12 cm H_2O. Due to progressive fatigue of respiratory muscles, she was nasally intubated at 10:00 with a 7.5 mm nasotracheal tube for mechanical ventilation.

In spite of normal $PaCO_2$, mechanical ventilation is indicated because of progressive muscle weakness (decreasing MIP) and anticipated outcome of botulism.

INITIAL SETTINGS

She was started on a Puritan-Bennett 7200a ventilator in assist/control (A/C) mode, backup rate of 12/min, tidal volume of 400 mL/PEEP of 5 cm H_2O, and F_IO_2 of 35%. ABGs drawn 30 min later revealed the following:

pH	7.54
$PaCO_2$	25 mm Hg
PaO_2	120 mm Hg
SaO_2	96%
HCO_3^-	21.1 mEq/L
Mode	A/C
Rate	12/min
Spont. Rate	22/min
V_T	400 mL
F_IO_2	35%
PEEP	5 cm H_2O

Based on these results, the rate was decreased to 8/min and the F_IO_2 was reduced to 30%. ABGs were ordered for the following morning. The results showed:

pH	7.42
$PaCO_2$	37 mm Hg
PaO_2	110 mm Hg
SaO_2	97%
HCO_3^-	23.6 mEq/L
Mode	A/C
Rate	8/min
Spont. Rate	12/min
V_T	400 mL
F_IO_2	30%
PEEP	5 cm H_2O

The patient remained febrile and weak as manifested by serial MIPs performed on the ventilator and on the fifth ventilator day, the patient underwent an elective tracheostomy for comfort and to prevent development of septic sinusitis from prolonged nasal intubation. She tolerated the procedure well.

TABLE 18-2   Serial Vital Capacities and Maximum Inspiratory Pressure

VENT DAY	RESPIRATORY RATE (f)	FORCED VITAL CAPACITY (VC) L	MAXIMUM INSPIRATORY FORCE (MIP) cm H$_2$O
1	18	1.03	−30
2	22	1.30	−30
3	28	1.11	−33
4	32	1.13	−36
5	34	1.06	−35
6	30	1.45	−39
7	28	1.42	−36
8	28	1.21	−50
9	24	1.40	−38
10	20	1.80	−34
11	24	1.70	−38
12	24	1.60	−40
13	18	1.65	−43
14	18	2.10	−46

PATIENT MONITORING

Her respiratory mechanics showed no signs of improvement initially but gradually improved over time. She was monitored for progressive muscle strength. Serial vital capacities and maximum inspiratory pressure (MIP) measurements while on CPAP every morning indicated gradual improvement. The serial measurements are are listed in Table 18-2. The patient continued to improve over the latter half of her hospitalization and after 14 days of mechanical ventilation, she exhibited evidence that she could support her own respiratory status without assistance.

PATIENT MANAGEMENT

☑ Management strategy for botulism consists mainly of supportive measures.

Management strategy for botulism consists mainly of supportive measures as she was mechanically ventilated for 14 days. Patient supportive measures included turning the patient from side to side, assisting the patient to an ortho chair at the bedside, and using medications for comfort. Her nutritional status was maintained through I.V. fluids alone. The patient continued to improve and on the seventh ventilator day she was transferred to a subacute unit for further recovery and monitoring.

KEY MEDICATIONS

The patient's lungs remained diminished but clear throughout. There were no abnormal secretions when she was suctioned. However, vigorous pulmonary toilet was done to prevent lung pathology while in the step-down ICU. She was treated, prophylactically, on small volume nebulizer therapy with 0.5 mL of 0.5% albuterol in 2.0 mL of saline Q 4 hours in-line with the ventilator circuit. These were discontinued after her removal from the ventilator.

WEANING

Beginning on the tenth day of mechanical ventilation, the patient began CPAP trials. She tolerated this procedure well for up to 8 to 10 hours at a time. She was then returned to SIMV mode with a backup rate of 6/min, tidal volume of 400 mL, PEEP of 5 cm H_2O, F_IO_2 of 30%, and pressure support of 10 cm H_2O to rest for the night. Her respiratory rate remained in the mid to high 20s and her return volume was consistently between 350 mL and 450 mL. She did not complain of shortness of breath, difficulty breathing, or discomfort, and appeared to rest comfortably. By the twelfth day of continuous mechanical ventilation, the patient was able to tolerate CPAP of 5 cm H_2O and F_IO_2 of 30% 24hours/day. Her ABGs revealed the following:

pH	7.42
$PaCO_2$	46 mm Hg
PaO_2	91 mm Hg
SaO_2	96%
HCO_3^-	29.9 mEq/L
Mode	CPAP
Spont. Rate	28/min
F_IO_2	30%
PEEP	5 cm H_2O

At that point, she was removed from the ventilator and placed on a humidified T-piece (Briggs "T" adapter) at an F_IO_2 of 30%. She was monitored via a continuous pulse oximeter that revealed SpO_2 between 92% and 94%. Her respiratory rate remained in the low 20s. She was closely observed for signs of respiratory distress or tachypnea (>30/min). Three days later, ABGs again were obtained while on the T-piece at an F_IO_2 of 30%. These revealed:

pH	7.46
$PaCO_2$	45 mm Hg
PaO_2	87 mm Hg
SaO_2	96%
HCO_3^-	30.9 mEq/L
RR	24/min

On the fourteenth day, her tracheostomy was buttoned and she was placed on a nasal cannula at 2 L/min without complications.

COMPLICATIONS

The patient showed no serious and lasting complications from this episode of botulism and was discharged from the hospital on room air 21 days following her admission. She did exhibit some generalized weakness and mild ptosis that continued to improve after discharge.

CASE 13: MECONIUM ASPIRATION/ PATENT DUCTUS ARTERIOSUS

☑ Long gestational age has a higher incidence of meconium aspiration syndrome.

☑ Visualization of the vocal cords helps to determine if meconium is present in the upper airway. If the vocal cords are stained green, suction should be done prior to the first breath so as to prevent or minimize meconium aspiration.

INTRODUCTION

L.F. was a 42-week (normal 40-week) gestation female Caucasian baby born to a 24-year-old gravida III mother. The birthweight was 3,054-gm (6.7 lb). All previous births were normal. The mother experienced spotting and early labor at 4 months, but the labor was halted at that time with terbutaline.

Shortly before delivery, the amniotic membrane ruptured and thick meconium was noted in the amniotic fluid. Upon delivery, the infant initiated her first breath and cried before visualization of the cords and suctioning could be performed. Immediately thereafter, the respiratory therapist visualized the cords and found meconium staining present at and below the vocal cords. Suctioning was performed immediately to remove as much meconium as possible.

The Apgar scores were 7 and 8 at 1 and 5 mins, respectively. They were scored as shown below.

	0	1	2	1 min	5 min
Heart rate	None	Slow Irregular	Over 100	2	2
Respiratory effort	Apnea	Irregular shallow Gasping	Yelling, crying	1	1
Muscle tone	Flaccid	Some flexion of extremities	Well flexed	2	2
Reflex	No response to stimulus	Grimace	Crying	2	2
Color	Pale blue	Blue extremities Body pink	Pink all over	0	1
Total				7	8

INDICATIONS

After stabilization at the delivery room, the infant female was admitted to the regular nursery with blow-by oxygen. Within a few hours of arrival, she became dusky and presented with moderate to severe intercostal and substernal retractions. As her condition continued to deteriorate, she was transferred to the NICU for further evaluation and treatment. Umbilical artery catheter (UAC) and orogastric (OG) tube were placed and mask CPAP on an F_1O_2 of 100% was initiated. Phenobarbital was begun to improve oxygenation. UAC blood gas results were:

> ☑ Phenobarbital is used to reduce seizure activity and facilitate ventilation and oxygenation.

pH	7.32
$PaCO_2$	40 mm Hg
PaO_2	43 mm Hg
HCO_3^-	20 mEq/L
B.E.	−6 mEq/L
Hct	41%
Mode	Mask CPAP
F_1O_2	100%

In spite of CPAP and 100% oxygen, the infant's oxygenation status continued to deteriorate. Her respiratory rate increased as she tried to compensate for the hypoxia. Capillary refill time was increased from 4 to 5 sec. Her extremities were cold and the mean arterial pressure was 35 mm Hg.

> ☑ Increased capillary refill indicates shunting of blood flow from the extremities or increased peripheral vascular resistance.

Based on the condition and prognosis of this infant, she was electively intubated with a 3.5 mm endotracheal (ET) tube and placed on a pressure-limited ventilator. During the initial hours of mechanical ventilation, large amounts of bright red secretions were suctioned from the ET tube.

INITIAL SETTINGS

The initial settings of the pressure-limited ventilator were: A/C, rate 60/min, PIP/PEEP 28/5 cm H_2O, T_{INSP} 0.5 sec, F_1O_2 100%. At these settings, the mean airway pressure was 14.5 cm H_2O and blood gases from a UAC sample showed:

pH	7.30
$PaCO_2$	44 mm Hg
PaO_2	39 mm Hg
HCO_3^-	21.2 mEq/L
B.E.	−5.9 mEq/L
Mode	A/C
PIP/PEEP	28/5 cm H_2O
Rate	60/min
T_{INSP}	0.5 sec
F_1O_2	100%
Mean Airway Pressure	14.5 cm H_2O

> ☑ PIP of 28 cmH_2O should be increased to enhance alveolar recruitment and oxygenation.

✓ Since the initial rate is 60/min (or 1/sec), the T_{EXP} is $1 - T_{INSP} = 1 - 0.5$ sec = 0.5 sec. The I:E ratio is 1:1.

✓ The rate should be reduced to allow more time for expiration.

✓ The increase in PIP and PEEP causes a higher mean airway pressure (from 14.5 to 16.5 cm H_2O). This may (1) lower the production of natural surfactant, (2) cause patent ductus arteriosus, and (3) increase the risk of barotrauma.

The PIP/PEEP were changed to 32/6 cm H_2O and the rate was changed to 50/min. At these settings, blood gases and transcutaneous gas tension showed:

pH	7.43
$PaCO_2$	32 mm Hg
PaO_2	43 mm Hg
HCO_3^-	21.1 mEq/L
B.E.	−2.7 mEq/L
SpO_2	86%
$P_{tc}O_2$	28 mm Hg
$P_{tc}CO_2$	30 mm Hg
Mode	A/C
PIP/PEEP	32/6 cm H_2O
Rate	50/min
T_{INSP}	0.5 sec
F_IO_2	100%
Mean Airway Pressure	16.5 cm H_2O

An echocardiogram was performed at this time that showed a patent ductus arteriosus (PDA) with a right-to-left shunt and evidence of persistent pulmonary hypertension of the newborn. The patient was started on dopamine and dobutamine.

Ninety minutes after dopamine and dobutamine administration, the blood gases showed:

pH	7.58
$PaCO_2$	27 mm Hg
PaO_2	66 mm Hg
HCO_3^-	24.9 mEq/L
B.E.	3.1 mEq/L
SpO_2	96%
$P_{tc}O_2$	53 mm Hg
$P_{tc}CO_2$	28 mm Hg
Mode	A/C
PIP/PEEP	38/6 cm H_2O
Rate	60/min
T_{INSP}	0.3 sec
F_IO_2	100%
Mean Airway Pressure	16.5 cm H_2O

Over the course of the next 12 hours, three doses of artificial surfactant were needed. The following results were obtained after the third dose:

pH	7.37
$PaCO_2$	42 mm Hg

✓ The PDA has partially closed allowing a decrease of the right to left shunt. This lowers the peak inspiratory pressure and improves gas exchange. The risk of barotrauma is therefore lowered.

✓ The administration of surfactant helps to increase the pulmonary compliance and to lower the peak inspiratory pressure, F_IO_2, and mean airway pressure requirements.

✓ An important aspect of weaning in this case is to maintain the PaO_2 at a safe level (50s mm Hg) so as to prevent increase of PVR and reopening of PDA.

PaO_2	56 mm Hg
HCO_3^-	24.2 mEq/L
B.E.	-0.9 mEq/L
SpO_2	90%
$P_{tc}O_2$	47 mm Hg
$P_{tc}CO_2$	66 mm Hg
Mode	A/C
PIP/PEEP	25/6 cm H_2O
Rate	36/min
T_{INSP}	0.4 sec
F_IO_2	51%
Mean Airway Pressure	12 cm H_2O

Over the next 2 days the ventilator was weaned by gradually decreasing the PIP, PEEP, rate, and F_IO_2. The patient continued to improve and was finally extubated to an oxyhood at 36% F_IO_2.

KEY MEDICATIONS

MEDICATION	MAIN PURPOSE
Decadron	Improves lung function in infants requiring prolonged ventilation. It also decreases tracheal edema to facilitate extubation
Dopamine	Improves cardiac output and blood pressure
Dobutamine	Decreases pulmonary vascular resistance
Phenobarbital	May have some value in preventing intraventricular hemorrhage (IVH). Aids in sedation to improve mechanical ventilation. Limits seizure activity
Albumin	Used for volume expansion when treating RDS. Shock may be seen after correction of acidosis or hypoxia (due to ↓ systemic vascular resistance and ↓ blood pressure)
Ampicillin	Broad spectrum antibiotic
Surfactant	Prevention and treatment of RDS by increasing the lung compliance and decreasing the alveolar surface tension

SPECIAL CONSIDERATIONS

Meconium aspiration is most likely to occur in term or postterm infants who have intrauterine distress or hypoxia. When meconium is seen in the amniotic fluid, vigorous suctioning of the oral cavity and upper airway should be done, preferably before the first breath. This is done to prevent aspiration of meconium and airway obstruction by these particles.

An infant diagnosed with meconium aspiration runs a high risk of barotrauma when mechanical ventilation is instituted. Ongoing assessment of the chest is of vital importance. Monitoring the mPaw is the best indicator of impending barotraumatic events. It is important to keep the mPaw as low as possible.

With the presence of PDA revealed by the echocardiogram, an adequate PaO_2 should be provided and maintained in an attempt to minimize an increase of the pulmonary vascular resistance (PVR). Surely we will try to reduce the F_IO_2 requirement, but this must be done slowly to prevent the PVR from increasing.

☑ Excessive PaO_2 may cause oxygen toxicity and related problems.

☑ Insufficient PaO_2 may cause hypoxemia and an increase of the PVR.

CASE 14: PERSISTENT PULMONARY HYPERTENSION OF THE NEWBORN

INTRODUCTION

B.G. was a 30-week gestation, 1,398-gm male infant born without prenatal care. The 1- and 3-min Apgar scores were 5 and 6, respectively.

Inspite of an Apgar score of 6 at 3 min, the cardiopulmonary status of the infant continued to deteriorate and cardiopulmonary resuscitation (CPR) became necessary. CPR was started using 100% oxygen via a resuscitation bag with pressure manometer attached. The infant was subsequently intubated with a 3.0 mm endotracheal tube and placed on a pressure-limited ventilator without complications.

An umbilical artery catheter (UAC) was inserted and secured. After a period of stabilization on the ventilator, the infant still appeared dusky. His capillary refill was slow indicating poor peripheral perfusion but the extremities were warm. The anterior fontanel was soft with slightly overlapping sutures. Breath sounds were diminished bilaterally.

Arterial blood was drawn from the UAC while using a resuscitation bag and 100% oxygen with pressures of 28/4 mm Hg at a rate of 40/min. The results were:

☑ The 3-min Apgar score should show significant improvement over the one-minute score.

☑ Peripheral perfusion status is a gross indicator of cardiac output or tissue perfusion.

☑ The blood gases show oxygenation failure because the PaO_2 is much lower than one that can be caused by a $PaCO_2$ of 48 mm Hg.

UAC Sample
pH   7.27
PaCO$_2$ 48 mm Hg
PaO$_2$ 22 mm Hg
HCO$_3^-$ 21.6 mEq/L
B.E.   −7.2 mEq/L
Mode   Bag/mask ventilation
F$_I$O$_2$ 100%
P$_{INSP}$ 28 mm Hg
PEEP   4 mm Hg
Rate   40/min

☑ If hyperventilation (to pH 7.5 and PaCO$_2$ between 20 and 25 mm Hg) provides significant improvement to the PaO$_2$, PPHN is likely the cause of hypoxemia.

While using the resuscitation bag/mask system, it was decided to hyperventilate the infant at a rate of 100/min with pressures of 28/4 mm Hg on 100% oxygen. This was done to rule out the presence of persistent pulmonary hypertension of the newborn (PPHN). The blood gases after 3 min of hyperventilation showed:

UAC Sample
pH   7.48
PaCO$_2$ 23 mm Hg
PaO$_2$ 95 mm Hg
Mode   Bag/mask ventilation
F$_I$O$_2$ 100%
P$_{INSP}$ 28 mm Hg
PEEP   4 mm Hg
Rate   100/min

☑ PaO$_2$ shows significant improvement (from 22 to 95 mm Hg) after 3 min of hyperventilation.

Based on the information obtained from the last blood gases, it was decided to continue hyperventilation using conventional ventilation. After 24 hours, the following results were obtained.

☑ Hyperventilation reduces the PaCO$_2$. In turn, it lowers the pulmonary vascular resistance and improves the pulmonary circulation and V/Q matching.

UAC Sample
pH   7.46
PaCO$_2$ 26 mm Hg
PaO$_2$ 89 mm Hg
Mode   A/C
PIP/PEEP   32/6 cm H$_2$O
Rate   100/min
T$_{INSP}$ 0.24 sec
F$_I$O$_2$ 98%

☑ Since the patient's condition is responsive to hyperventilation, pulmonary hypertension is likely the cause of hypoxemia. He is a candidate for trial of iNO therapy.

During this 24-hour period, unsuccessful attempts were made to decrease the oxygen requirement. Very little progress was seen in the patient as the pulmonary hypertension was not resolved using the hyperventilation strategy. Inhaled nitric oxide (iNO) therapy was started in hope of reversing the pulmonary hypertension.

The patient received 55 ppm (parts per million) of iNO, and the blood gases after 1 hour of iNO therapy showed:

✔ The PaO_2
 improved from
89 to 105 mm Hg at
a lower F_IO_2 (from
98% to 85%).

UAC Sample
pH   7.50
$PaCO_2$ 21 mm Hg
PaO_2 105 mm Hg
Mode   A/C
PIP/PEEP   32/6 cm H_2O
Rate   100/min
T_{INSP} 0.24 sec
F_IO_2 85%

The infant's F_IO_2 requirement continued to decrease over the next 48 hours. iNO therapy was discontinued and the F_IO_2 was weaned to 45%. Conventional ventilation continued at a rate of 55/min.

PATIENT MANAGEMENT

The pulmonary vascular resistance of the infant was increased due to severe hypoxemia and hypoxic vasoconstriction. Since hypoxemia could not be reversed with oxygen and ventilation, long-standing hypoxemia caused a persistent increase in PVR, thus the name persistent pulmonary hypertension of the newborn (PPHN).

Test to Rule out PPHN.   Persistent pulmonary hypertension of the newborn can be tested by hyperventilating the patient to an arterial pH of 7.5 and a $PaCO_2$ of between 20 and 25 mm Hg. The alkalotic condition reduces the pulmonary vascular resistance, thereby enhancing pulmonary perfusion and oxygen content. If PPHN is the cause of hypoxemia, the patient's oxygenation should show drastic improvement following hyperventilation.

Nitric Oxide to Treat PPHN.   Inhaled nitric acid therapy is done to lower pulmonary vascular resistance. The walls of the pulmonary arteries are lined with endothelial cells that release a substance known as endothelium-derived relaxing factor (EDRF, which has been identified as inhaled nitric acid). This substance is responsible for vasodilation in vascular smooth muscle. EDRF has been found to be an essential link in the transition from fetal to neonatal circulation. Because iNO dilates the pulmonary arteries, it decreases the pulmonary vascular resistance and its associated hypertension. Once the pulmonary vessels are dilated, this change should improve the patient's pulmonary circulation, V/Q ratio, and oxygenation status.

CASE 15: HOME CARE AND DISEASE MANAGEMENT

INTRODUCTION

F.W. was a 66-year-old moderately obese (weight 240 lbs) White female. She was brought to the emergency department by her husband and their 17-year-old daughter on a Saturday morning because they "couldn't keep her awake and her breathing sounded funny." Upon further questioning, the doctor was told by the patient's husband that she had no fever, but did have a productive cough with thick greenish sputum for the past 5 days. The patient had a history of COPD/asthma, cor pulmonale, hyponatremia, and hyperkalemia. She had no chest pain, except when coughing, but did have difficulty breathing when lying down (orthopnea). F.W.'s husband reported that she had no nausea and vomiting, and had not complained of pain other than when coughing.

Social history revealed that F.W. smoked one pack of cigarettes per day for 25 years, but quit 10 years ago. She did not drink alcohol. She lived with her spouse of 25 years and a 17-year-old daughter. Two other grown children from a previous marriage no longer lived at home.

✓ At the onset or worsening of dyspnea due to congestive heart failure or pulmonary congestion, breathing in an upright position reduces pulmonary congestion and work of breathing.

INDICATION

Physical assessment revealed an obese white female, lethargic, with central cyanosis and in respiratory distress. From the information provided by her husband, the physician determined that the patient had experienced paroxysmal nocturnal dyspnea in addition to orthopnea. She was placed on a monitor that revealed these vital signs: blood pressure of 160/80 mm Hg, heart rate of 128/min, respiratory rate of 28/min and labored, and SpO_2 of 85% on room air.

Further assessment showed 1 to 2+ pedal edema, jugular vein distension, bibasilar crackles and wheezes throughout.

Arterial blood gases on rom air revealed:

pH	7.26
$PaCO_2$	88 mm Hg
PaO_2	38 mm Hg
HCO_3^-	38 mEq/L
SaO_2	80%

Pertinent lab work results were as follows:

WBC: 7400 (*normal 3.2 to 9.8 × 10³*)
H&H: 16/49.3 (*normal for women: hemoglobin 12 to 16 g/100mL hematocrit 37 to 47%*)
Na^+: 119 (*normal 140 mEq/L*)

✓ Paroxysmal nocturnal dyspnea and orthopnea are signs of congestive heart failure.

✓ Blood gases show acute ventilatory failure superimposed on chronic ventilatory failure. Noninvasive positive pressure ventilation is indicated for this patient.

☑ IPAP provides mechanical ventilation and reduces the patient's work of breathing.

INITIAL SETTINGS

The patient was stabilized in the emergency department prior to transfer to the telemetry unit. For her severe hypercapnia and hypoxemia, she was placed on nasal bilevel PAP at 12/6 cm H_2O with 5 L/min of oxygen. IPAP of 12 cm H_2O was used to augment the patient's ventilatory effort. EPAP of 6 cm H_2O and 5 L/min of oxygen were used to maintain oxygenation and minimize auto-PEEP due to air trapping.

PATIENT MANAGEMENT

For the excessive fluid buildup due to cor pulmonale, 60 mg of Lasix were given via an intravenous line. Blood was drawn for lab workup. Chest radiograph and repeat ABG on bilevel PAP were done. Lab reports showed normal WBC, hemoglobin, and hematocrit, and low sodium, which could explain some of her confusion. Chest radiograph showed enlarged heart (cardiomegaly) with pulmonary vascular congestion and bilateral infiltrates especially on the left side. (See Figure 18-7.)

Repeat ABG 2 hours after initiation of bilevel PAP showed:

☑ IPAP of 12 cm H_2O is primarily responsible for the improvement of ventilation ($PaCO_2$ from 88 to 68 mmHg).

☑ EPAP of 6 cm H_2O and 5 L/min of oxygen is primarily responsible for the improvement of oxygenation (PaO_2 from 38 to 82 mmHg).

pH	7.34
$PaCO_2$	68 mm Hg
PaO_2	82 mm Hg
HCO_3^-	36 mEq/L
SaO_2	96%
Bilevel PAP	12/6 cm H_2O
F_1O_2	5 L/min

HOSPITAL COURSE

During the first 2 days of her hospital stay, F.W. was maintained on continuous nasal bilevel PAP at 12/6 cm H_2O with 2 L/min of oxygen. For the CHF and related conditions, she was treated with Lasix, Digoxin, and Cardizem. The pulmonologist ordered nebulizer treatments Q 4 hours with 2.5 mg albuterol and 0.5 mg ipratropium bromide in 3 cc of normal saline to relieve bronchospasm and promote secretion clearance. Prednisone (steroid) was ordered to decrease airway inflammation secondary to her asthma. Prophylactic antibiotics (Biaxin) were administered, used to address her probable pneumonia since sputum induction was unsuccessful.

Note: F.W.'s medical record retrieved shortly after admission indicated that PFTs had been done 1 year before and at that time her FEV_1 was 14% of predicted and her DLCO was 21%. Baseline room air blood gases were:

pH	7.37
$PaCO_2$	67 mm Hg
PaO_2	45 mm Hg
HCO_3^-	38 mEq/L

Figure 18-7 Chest radiograph shows cardiomegaly (1); pulmonary vascular congestion (2); bilateral infiltrates (3).

☑ CPAP alone increases the work of breathing. Patient requires some mechanical assistance via bilevel PAP (i.e., IPAP).

On the third day following admission, the pulmonologist attempted to wean F.W. from bilevel PAP. She was placed on CPAP at 7.5 cm H_2O and ABGs were drawn an hour later; the results were as follows:

pH	7.16
$PaCO_2$	91 mm Hg
PaO_2	66 mm Hg
HCO_3^-	31 mEq/L
SaO_2	90%

As a result of her deteriorating blood gas results and clinical condition, F.W. was placed back on bilevel PAP at 12/6 cm H_2O for 24 hours. Over the next several days, she was gradually weaned to 1 L/min nasal cannula during the day and bilevel PAP at night. The physician discussed several options with F.W. and her family, and it was decided that upon discharge from the hospital she would use nocturnal ventilation at home. Her total hospital stay was 11 days.

HOME CARE MANAGEMENT

Twenty-four hours prior to discharge from the hospital, the case manager contacted a local home medical equipment provided for respiratory services and a home care agency for nursing services. Among other health care professionals, this case was reviewed with the respiratory therapist. Due to the complexity of her pulmonary condition and special management requirements, the physician decided to directly communicate with the respiratory therapist from the medical equipment company.

Arterial blood gases on day of discharge were as follows:

pH	7.32
$PaCO_2$	60 mm Hg
PaO_2	62 mm Hg
HCO_3^-	30 mEq/L
SaO_2	93%
Bilevel PAP	12/6 cm H_2O
Oxygen	1 L/min via nasal cannula during the day and bilevel PAP therapy at 12/6 cm H_2O, F_IO_2 of 24% at night

ORDERS FOR HOME	EQUIPMENT
1. 1 L/min via nasal cannula continuously.	Oxygen concentrator
2. Portable oxygen	Conserving device with M-6 cylinders
3. Nebulizer treatments QID	Small air compressor
4. Nocturnal bilevel PAP 10/5 cm H_2O, 24%	NPPV with backup rate of 6/min
5. Keep head of bed elevated 30 degrees	Hospital bed
6. 1,200 calorie diet	
7. Ambulate as tolerated	
8. Incentive spirometry TID	Incentive spirometer (from hospital)

KEY MEDICATIONS

1. 2.5 mg albuterol and 0.5 mg atrovent in 3.0 mL of 0.9% NaCl QID and PRN for wheezing.
2. Lasix 20 mg po BID
3. Prednisone po tapering dose
4. Cardizem po

HOME CARE PLAN

The plan was devised by the physician and respiratory therapist. The patient was informed of the home care plan, as follows:

1. Maintain SpO_2 of 90% to 96%
2. Maintain tidal volume of 650 mL to 900 mL while on NPPV.
3. Use backup rate of 6/min to ensure adequate ventilation if patient were to become apneic.

4. Closely monitor patient for signs of CHF, hypercapnia, and exacerbation of asthma/COPD.
5. Notify physician of complications secondary to withdrawal or tapering of medications; specifically Prednisone and Lasix.
6. Increase exercise level as tolerated.
7. Improve diet and continue to lose weight. (F.W.'s height and weight: 5 ft 2 in and 235 lb)
8. Educate patient on disease and promote a healthier lifestyle (F.W. had already quit smoking 10 years ago).
9. Observe patient's attitude and family support and report to physician.

PATIENT MONITORING

F.W. required close monitoring for the first month. The same respiratory therapist visited her twice a week for the first 4 weeks and then once a week for the next 4 weeks. Routine monthly visits started in the third month.

Note: Nursing services were present in the home once a day for 2 weeks, and communication was established between the nurse (from a home care agency) and the respiratory therapist (from a DME company). During each visit, patient assessment was done and respiratory equipment was checked by the therapist.

Parameters monitored were as follows:

1. Tidal volume delivered via NPPV.
2. Vital signs (BP, HR, RR, SpO_2, weight, and breath sounds)
3. Bedside spirometry (PEFR, FVC, FEV_1) on initial visit, then every 6 months and prn.
4. Pedal edema (present or not)
5. Exercise tolerance—using vital signs and subjective response as indicators.
6. Saturation on room air—at rest and with exertion (walking with distance recorded)
7. Saturation on oxygen—at rest and with exertion (walking with distance recorded)
8. Sputum production—amount, color, and consistency.
9. Subjective response from patient and family members.
10. Patient compliance

Note: In order to have a successful outcome with home care, solid family support and proper emotional well-being of the patient are crucial. Motivation and positive attitude on the part of the patient are essential in order to achieve a positive outcome. Any signs of patient noncompliance, lack of family support, depression, lack of necessary resources, or other emotional problems should be promptly reported to the physician so that these issues may be addressed. If a home care nurse is also seeing the patient, then all information should be shared so that the patient may receive the best quality care.

PATIENT WEEKLY PROGRESS

Week 1. F.W. stayed in bed most of the time and got up only to go to the bathroom. Nocturnal bilevel ventilation was done at 10/5 cm H_2O with 1 L/min titrated through the nasal mask. Other parameters on the ventilator were: backup rate 6/min, expired tidal volume between 535 and 700 mL. Nebulizer treatments were done QID and incentive spirometry was done TID. Patient was able to achieve 800 to 1,000 mL on the incentive spirometry. Patient appeared to be compliant with her medications. Her weight was 235 lb with no signs of pedal edema. Vital signs were BP 150/84 mm Hg, RR 24/min, HR 82/min, resting SpO_2 91% on 1 L/min and 88% on room air.

Patient had a positive attitude and excellent family support. She was excited about getting better and used the nocturnal ventilator 6 to 8 hours every night. She claimed that she was still very tired and sore from her hospital stay.

Week 2. F.W. had improved a great deal. She was walking to the kitchen and watching television in the living room. She remained on 10/5 cm H_2O with 1 L/min O_2 at night and 1 L/min per nasal cannula continuously during the day. Vital signs were: BP 130/68 mm Hg, RR 16/min, HR 84/min, SpO_2 94% on 1 L/min resting and 89% to 90% on room air. Her weight was 218 lb. No pedal edema noted.

F.W. was in good spirits and compliant with regime.

Week 3. The expired tidal volume was 800 to 1000 mL on 10/5 cm H_2O. This indicated an improvement of pulmonary mechanics. She also was able to reach 1600 mL on her incentive spirometer TID. Her weight was down to 208 lb and she was ambulating more every week. No pedal edema noted.

Vital signs were BP 128/68 mmHg, RR 18/min, HR 70/min, SpO_2 97% on 1 L/min and 93% resting on room air. Ambulating SpO_2 was 88% on room air after walking just 25 ft, indicating that she continued to desaturate upon mild exertion.

Auscultation revealed bilateral expiratory wheezes. Small amounts of brownish sputum were noted. Bedside spirometry showed: PEFR 88 L/min, VC 1.69 L, FEV_1 0.709 L. F.W. continued to improve and remained positive about improving the quality of her life.

Week 4. One month out of the hospital and F.W. remained stable. At this time she was able to go grocery shopping and have her hair done. She used her portable M-6 cylinders with a conserving device while she was out. According to both the patient and her spouse, her sleep had increased to 8 to 10 hours per night and she no longer took naps during the day. A decision was made to decrease her nocturnal ventilator pressures to 8/5 due to the increasing expired volumes (1,100 mL). On bilevel PAP 8/5 cm H_2O, F.W. was more comfortable and had volumes of 650 to 850 mL.

Note: Tidal volumes were obtained with patient in supine position and were monitored for 20 min. This allowed the patient to relax in order to obtain more accurate readings).

Vitals and physical signs: BP 100/50 mmHg, RR 20/min, HR 78/min, weight 211 lb, SpO_2 94% on 1 L/min. No pedal edema was noted. After ambulating 60 steps: HR 100, RR28, SpO_2 86%. SpO_2 recovering within 3 min upon administration of 1 L/min O_2.

COMPLICATIONS

F.W. remained stable with no significant complications other than sinusitis for 6 months. During a routine visit almost 7 months after discharge, the therapist notified the physician with this assessment:

Vitals: BP 165/85 mm Hg, RR 22/min, HR 80/min, weight 224 lb., SpO_2 91% on 1 L/min, 1 to 2+ pedal edema.
Auscultation: inspiratory and expiratory wheezes bilaterally (audible); diminished in bases bilaterally.
Tidal volume on bilevel PAP of 8/5 cm H_2O = 500 to 600 mL.

Patient's husband reported that she was not sleeping well at night and with her legs "jittering" during the night. He also stated that F.W. was falling asleep during her meals and she frequently complained of headaches.

The respiratory therapist increased the nocturnal ventilator pressures to 10/5 cm H_2O (expired volume of 800 to 1000 mL) and notified the physician promptly. An appointment was made to see the physician on the following day. As a result of the office visit, the Lasix dosage was increased. She no longer experienced the signs and symptoms that were present prior to the visit, thus avoiding a possible hospital admission.

DISCUSSION

This case demonstrates one of the clinical indications for the use of nocturnal ventilation. F.W. was a COPD patient with hypercapnia and cor pulmonale. Is it also possible that F.W. suffered from a sleep disorder? Maybe; however, no sleep studies were ever done. F.W. qualified for nocturnal ventilation based on her $PaCO_2$ levels at the time of discharge from the hospital. Her pulmonary function studies indicated severe obstructive disease and poor diffusion capacity. Because of her obesity, F.W. also dealt with hypoventilation. The nocturnal ventilator assisted to overcome pressure placed on the diaphragm by her large abdomen, thereby increasing volumes when F.W. was in supine position.

Without nocturnal ventilation, home oxygen, bronchodilator therapies via nebulizer, and oral medications, F.W. would probably have had numerous physician visits and even hospital stays. In fact, she has avoided ER visits and hospital admissions for over 1 year. The home therapy allowed her greater independence and helped her "feel better"; therefore improving her quality of life. It is the responsibility of every home care provider to adequately assess patients, make sound clinical decisions, and report findings to the physician in a timely manner.

In this case the RCP quickly responded to signs and symptoms of hypercapnia and impending cardiac insufficiency. The pressure on the nocturnal ventilator was increased to improve minute ventilation and oxygenation and the physician was consulted to increase Lasix to eliminate pulmonary vascular congestion due to heart failure.

APPENDICES

APPENDIX 1: RESPIRATORY CARE CALCULATIONS

A   AIRWAY RESISTANCE: ESTIMATED (Raw)

EQUATION

$$Raw = \frac{(P_{max} - P_{st})}{Flow}$$

Raw : Airway resistance in cm H_2O/L/sec
P_{max} : Maximum inspiratory pressure in cm H_2O (peak airway pressure)
P_{st} : Static inspiratory pressure in cm H_2O (plateau airway pressure)
Flow : Flow rate in L/sec

NORMAL VALUE

0.6 to 2.4 cm H_2O/L/sec at flow rate of 0.5 L/sec (30 L/min).
If the patient is intubated, use serial measurements to establish trend.

EXAMPLE

Calculate the estimated airway resistance of a patient whose peak inspiratory pressure is 25 cm H_2O and whose plateau pressure is 10 cm H_2O. The ventilator flow rate is set at 60 L/min (1 L/sec).

$$Raw = \frac{(P_{max} - P_{st})}{Flow}$$

$$= \frac{(25 - 10)}{1}$$

$$= \frac{15}{1}$$

$$= 15 \text{ cm } H_2O/L/sec$$

B   ALVEOLAR–ARTERIAL OXYGEN TENSION GRADIENT: P(A-a)O$_2$

EQUATION

$$P(A\text{-}a)O_2 = P_AO_2 - PaO_2$$

$P(A\text{-}a)O_2$: Alveolar–arterial oxygen tension gradient in mm Hg
P_AO_2 : Alveolar oxygen tension in mm Hg
PaO_2 : Arterial oxygen tension in mm Hg

NORMAL VALUE

(1) On *room air*, the P(A-a)O_2 should be less than 4 mm Hg for every 10 years in age. For example, the P(A-a)O_2 should be less than 24 mm Hg for a 60-year-old patient.
(2) On *100% oxygen*, every 50 mm Hg difference in P(A-a)O_2 approximates 2% shunt.

EXAMPLE 1

Given : P_AO_2 = 100 mm Hg
$\qquad$ PaO_2 = 85 mm Hg
$\qquad$ F_IO_2 = 21%
$\quad$ Patient age = 40 years
Calculate P(A-a)O_2. Is it normal or abnormal for this patient?
$\qquad$ P(A-a)O_2 = P_AO_2 − PaO_2
$\qquad\qquad\quad$ = (100 − 85) mm Hg
$\qquad\qquad\quad$ = 15 mm Hg
P(A-a)O_2 of 15 mm Hg is normal for a 40-year-old patient.

P_AO_2 AT SELECTED F_IO_2

F_IO_2*	CALCULATED P_AO_2**
21%	100
25%	128
30%	164
35%	200
40%	235
45%	271
50%	307
55%	342
60%	388
65%	423
70%	459
75%	495
80%	530
85%	566
90%	602
95%	637
100%	673

*At F_IO_2 of 60% or higher, the factor 1.25 in the equation below is omitted.
**The calculated P_AO_2 is based on a PCO_2 of 40 mm Hg, saturated at 37°C, P_B of 760 mm Hg. P_AO_2 = (P_B − 47) × F_IO_2 − (PCO_2 × 1.25).

C   ANION GAP

EQUATION
Anion Gap $= Na^+ - (Cl^- + HCO_3^-)$

Na^+ : Serum sodium concentration in mEq/L
Cl^- : Serum chloride concentration in mEq/L
HCO_3^- : Serum bicarbonate concentration in mEq/L

NORMAL VALUE
10 to 14 mEq/L
15 to 20 mEq/L if potassium (K^+) is included in the equation

EXAMPLE
Given: $Na^+ = 140$ mEq/L
$Cl^- = 105$ mEq/L
$HCO_3^- = 22$ mEq/L
Calculate the anion gap.

$$\begin{aligned} \text{Anion gap} &= Na^+ - (Cl^- + HCO_3^-) \\ &= 140 - (105 + 22) \\ &= 140 - 127 \\ &= 13 \text{ mEq/L} \end{aligned}$$

D   ARTERIAL OXYGEN TENSION TO INSPIRED OXYGEN CONCENTRATION (PaO_2/F_IO_2) INDEX

EQUATION
Arterial Oxygen Tension to Inspired Oxygen Concentration Index = PaO_2/F_IO_2

PaO_2/F_IO_2 Index : Arterial oxygen tension to inspired oxygen concentration index
PaO_2 : Arterial oxygen tension in mm Hg
F_IO_2 : Inspired Oxygen Concentration

NORMAL VALUE
150 to 200 mm Hg or higher suggests a successful weaning outcome.
<150 mm Hg indicates presence of intrapulmonary shunt.

EXAMPLE
Given: $PaO_2 = 50$ mm Hg, $F_IO_2 = 40\%$ (0.4)
Is the calculated PaO_2/F_IO_2 index normal?

$$PaO_2/F_IO_2 \text{ Index} = \frac{50 \text{ mm Hg}}{0.4}$$

$$= 125 \text{ mm Hg}$$

The PaO_2/F_IO_2 index is below normal and it indicates presence of intrapulmonary shunt.

E   COMPLIANCE: DYNAMIC (C_{DYN})

EQUATION

$$C_{DYN} = \frac{\Delta V}{\Delta P}$$

C_{DYN} : Dynamic compliance in mL/cm H_2O
  ΔV : Corrected tidal volume in mL
  ΔP : Pressure change (Peak inspiratory pressure − PEEP) in cm H_2O

NORMAL VALUE

30 to 40 mL/cm H_2O
If the patient is intubated, use serial measurements to establish trend.

EXAMPLE

Given: $\Delta V = 500$ mL
Peak inspiratory pressure = 30 cm H_2O
PEEP = 10 cm H_2O
Calculate the dynamic compliance.

$$C_{DYN} = \frac{\Delta V}{\Delta P}$$

$$= \frac{500}{30 - 10}$$

$$= \frac{500}{20}$$

$$= 25 \text{ mL/cm } H_2O$$

F   COMPLIANCE: STATIC (C_{ST})

EQUATION

$$C_{ST} = \frac{\Delta V}{\Delta P}$$

C_{ST} : Static compliance in mL/cm H_2O
ΔV : Corrected tidal volume in mL
ΔP : Pressure change (plateau pressure − PEEP) in cm H_2O

NORMAL VALUE

40 to 60 mL/cm H_2O

If the patient is intubated, use serial measurements to establish trend.

EXAMPLE

Given: $\Delta V = 500$ mL

Plateau pressure = 20 cm H_2O

PEEP = 5 cm H_2O

Calculate the static compliance.

$$C_{ST} = \frac{\Delta V}{\Delta P}$$

$$= \frac{500}{20 - 5}$$

$$= \frac{500}{15}$$

$$= 33.3 \text{ or } 33 \text{ mL/cm } H_2O$$

G   CORRECTED TIDAL VOLUME (V_T)

EQUATION

Corrected V_T = Expired V_T − Tubing Volume

Expired V_T : Expired tidal volume in mL

Tubing volume : Volume "lost" in tubing during inspiratory phase

(Pressure change $\times$ 3 mL/cm H_2O)

EXAMPLE

Expired V_T = 650 mL

Peak inspiratory pressure = 25 cm H_2O

Positive end-expiratory pressure (PEEP) = 5 cm H_2O

Tubing compression factor = 3 mL/cm H_2O

Calculate the corrected tidal volume.

Because

Tubing volume = Pressure Change $\times$ 3 mL/cm H_2O

$\qquad\qquad = (25 - 5)$ cm $H_2O \times 3$ mL/cm H_2O

$\qquad\qquad = 20 \times 3$ mL

$\qquad\qquad = 60$ mL

then

Corrected V_T = Expired V_T − Tubing Volume

$\qquad\qquad = 650 - 60$

$\qquad\qquad = 590$ mL

H DEADSPACE TO TIDAL VOLUME RATIO (V_D/V_T)

EQUATION

$$\frac{V_D}{V_T} = \frac{(P_aCO_2 - P_{\bar{E}}CO_2)}{P_aCO_2}$$

V_D/V_T : Deadspace to tidal volume ratio in %
P_aCO_2 : Arterial carbon dioxide tension in mm Hg
$P_{\bar{E}}CO_2$: Mixed expired carbon dioxide tension in mm Hg

NORMAL VALUE
20% to 40% in patients breathing spontaneously
40% to 60% in patients receiving mechanical ventilation

EXAMPLE
Given: $P_aCO_2 = 40$ mm Hg
$\qquad\quad$ $P_{\bar{E}}CO_2 = 30$ mm Hg

Calculate the V_D/V_T ratio.

$$\frac{V_D}{V_T} = \frac{(P_aCO_2 - P_{\bar{E}}CO_2)}{P_aCO_2}$$

$$= \frac{40 - 30}{40}$$

$$= \frac{10}{40}$$

$$= 0.25 \text{ or } 25\%$$

I MEAN AIRWAY PRESSURE (mPaw)

EQUATION

$$mPaw = \left[\frac{RR \times I \text{ time}}{60}\right] \times (PIP - PEEP) + PEEP$$

mPaw : Mean airway pressure in cm H_2O
$\quad$ RR : Respiratory rate per minute
I time : Inspiratory time in sec
$\quad$ PIP : Peak inspiratory pressure in cm H_2O
PEEP : Positive end-expiratory pressure in cm H_2O

NORMAL VALUE
Below 30 cm H_2O (adults).

EXAMPLE 1
When PEEP is used.
Given: RR = 45/min
   I time = 0.5 sec
    PIP = 35 cm H_2O
    PEEP = 5 cm H_2O
Calculate the mean airway pressure.

$$mPaw = \left[\frac{RR \times I\ time}{60}\right] \times (PIP - PEEP) + PEEP$$

$$= \left[\frac{45 \times 0.5}{60}\right] \times (35 - 5) + 5$$

$$= \left[\frac{22.5}{60}\right] \times 30 + 5$$

$$= \{0.375\} \times 30 + 5$$

$$= 11.25 + 5$$

$$= 16.25\ or\ 16\ cm\ H_2O$$

J MINUTE VENTILATION: EXPIRED AND ALVEOLAR

EQUATION 1
$$\dot{V}_E = V_T \times RR$$

EQUATION 2
$$\dot{V}_A = (V_T - V_D) \times RR$$

$\dot{V}_E$: Expired minute ventilation in L/min
$\dot{V}_A$: Alveolar minute ventilation in L/min
V_T : Tidal volume in mL
V_D : Deadspace volume in mL
RR : Respiratory rate per minute

EXAMPLE
Given: V_T = 600 mL
   V_D = 150 mL
   RR = 12/min
Calculate the expired minute ventilation ($\dot{V}_E$) and the alveolar minute ventilation ($\dot{V}_A$).
$$\dot{V}_E = V_T \times RR$$

$$= 600 \times 12$$
$$= 7200 \text{ mL/min or } 7.2 \text{ L/min}$$
$$\dot{V}_A = (V_T - V_D) \times RR$$
$$= (600 - 150) \times 12$$
$$= 450 \times 12$$
$$= 5400 \text{ mL/min or } 5.4 \text{ L/min}$$

K OXYGEN INDEX (OI)

EQUATION

$$OI = \frac{(mPaw \times F_IO_2)}{PaO_2}$$

OI : Oxygen index
$mPaw$: Mean airway pressure
F_IO_2 : Inspired oxygen concentration in %
PaO_2 : Arterial oxygen tension in mm Hg

NORMAL VALUE

<30%
An oxygen index of 0.35 to 0.6 for 0.5 to 6 hours is inclusive for ECMO therapy.

EXAMPLE

Given : $mPaw = 20$ mm Hg, $F_IO_2 = 60\%$, $PaO_2 = 50$ mm Hg

$$OI = \left(\frac{mPaw \times F_IO_2}{PaO_2} \right)$$

$$= \left(\frac{20 \text{ mm Hg} \times 0.6}{50 \text{ mm Hg}} \right)$$

$$= \frac{12 \text{ mm Hg}}{50 \text{ mm Hg}}$$

$$= 0.24 \text{ or } 24\%$$

L SHUNT EQUATION (Q_{sp}/Q_T): CLASSIC PHYSIOLOGIC

EQUATION

$$\frac{Q_{sp}}{Q_T} = \frac{C_cO_2 - C_aO_2}{C_c{-}O_2 - C_{\bar{v}}O_2}$$

Q_{sp}/Q_T : Physiologic shunt to total perfusion ratio in %
  C_cO_2 : End-capillary oxygen content in vol%
  C_aO_2 : Arterial oxygen content in vol%
  $C_{\bar{v}}O_2$: Mixed venous oxygen content in vol%

NORMAL VALUE
Less than 10%

EXAMPLE
Given: C_cO_2 = 20.4 vol%
       C_aO_2 = 19.8 vol%
       $C_{\bar{v}}O_2$ = 13.4 vol%

$$Q_{sp}/Q_T = \frac{C_cO_2 - C_aO_2}{C_cO_2 - C_{\bar{v}}O_2}$$
$$= \frac{20.4 - 19.8}{20.4 - 13.4}$$
$$= \frac{0.6}{7}$$
$$= 0.086 \text{ or } 8.6\%$$

M SHUNT EQUATION (Q_{sp}/Q_T): ESTIMATED

EQUATION 1
For normal individuals:
$$\frac{Q_{sp}}{Q_T} = \frac{C_cO_2 - C_aO_2}{5 + (C_cO_2 - C_aO_2)}$$

EQUATION 2
For critically ill patients:
$$\frac{Q_{sp}}{Q_T} = \frac{C_cO_2 - C_aO_2}{3.5 + (C_cO_2 - C_aO_2)}$$

Q_{sp}/Q_T : Physiologic shunt to total perfusion ratio in %
  C_cO_2 : End-capillary oxygen content in vol%
  C_aO_2 : Arterial oxygen content in vol%

NORMAL VALUE
Less than 10%

EXAMPLE 1

Given : Normal patient

$C_cO_2 = 20.4$ vol%

$C_aO_2 = 19.8$ vol%

Use 5 vol% as the estimated $C(a - \bar{v})O_2$ and calculate Q_{sp}/Q_T.

$$\frac{Q_{sp}}{Q_T} = \frac{C_cO_2 - C_aO_2}{5 + (C_cO_2 - C_aO_2)}$$

$$= \frac{20.4 - 19.8}{5 + (20.4 - 19.8)}$$

$$= \frac{0.6}{5 + 0.6}$$

$$= \frac{0.6}{5.6}$$

$$= 0.107 \text{ or } 10.7\%$$

N VENTILATOR RATE NEEDED FOR A DESIRED PaCO$_2$

EQUATION 1

$$\text{New Rate} = \frac{\text{Rate} \times P_aCO_2}{\text{Desired } P_aCO_2}$$

EQUATION 2

$$\text{New Rate} = \frac{(\text{Rate} \times P_aCO_2) \times (V_T - V_D)}{\text{Desired } P_aCO_2 \times (\text{New } V_T - \text{New } V_D)}$$

New rate : Ventilator rate needed for a desired $PaCO_2$

Rate : Original ventilator rate per minute

$PaCO_2$: Original arterial carbon dioxide tension in mm Hg

Desired $PaCO_2$: Desired arterial carbon dioxide tension in mm Hg

V_T : Original tidal volume

V_D : Original deadspace volume

New V_T : New tidal volume

New V_D : New deadspace volume

NORMAL VALUE

Set rate to provide eucapnic (patient's normal) ventilation.

EXAMPLE 1

When tidal volume and deadspace volume remain unchanged. The P_aCO_2 of a patient is 55 mm Hg at a ventilator rate of 10/min. What should be the ventilator rate if a P_aCO_2 of 40 mm Hg is desired assuming the ventilator tidal volume and spontaneous ventilation are stable?

$$\text{New rate} = \frac{(\text{Rate} \times P_aCO_2)}{\text{Desired } P_aCO_2}$$

$$= \frac{(10 \times 55)}{40}$$

$$= \frac{550}{40}$$

$$= 13.75 \text{ or } 14/\text{min}$$

O   WEANING INDEX: RAPID SHALLOW BREATHING

EQUATION

$$\text{Rapid Shallow Breathing Index} = \frac{f}{V_T}$$

f : Spontaneous respiratory rate/min (without pressure support)
V_T : Spontaneous tidal volume (in liters)

NORMAL VALUE

<100 breaths/min/L is predictive of weaning success

EXAMPLE

Calculate the rapid shallow breathing index given the spontaneous respiratory rate and tidal volume are 14 breaths/min and 0.5 L (500 mL), respectively. Does this index indicate successful weaning outcome?

$$\text{Rapid Shallow Breathing Index} = \frac{f}{V_T}$$

$$= \frac{14}{0.5}$$

$$= 28 \text{ breaths/min/L}$$

Since the rapid breathing index is less than 100, it indicates a successful weaning outcome.

P   WEANING INDEX: SIMPLIFIED

EQUATION

$$\text{Simplified Weaning Index (SWI)} = \frac{f_{mv}\,(PIP - PEEP)}{MIP} \times \frac{PaCO_{2\,mv}}{40}$$

SWI : Simplified weaning index per minute
f_{mv} : Ventilator frequency
PIP : Peak inspiratory pressure
PEEP : Positive end-expiratory pressure
MIP : Maximal inspiratory pressure
$PaCO_{2\,mv}$: Arterial CO_2 tension while on ventilator

NORMAL VALUE
<9/min is predictive of weaning success
>11/min is predictive of weaning failure

EXAMPLE
Calculate the simplified weaning index given the following parameters and measurements. Does this index indicate a successful weaning outcome?

f_{mv} = 6/min, PIP = 40 cm H_2O, PEEP = 5 cm H_2O, MIP = 20 cm H_2O, $PaCO_{2\,mv}$ = 50 mm Hg.

$$SWI = \frac{f_{mv}\,(PIP - PEEP)}{MIP} \times \frac{PaCO_{2\,mv}}{40}$$

$$= \frac{6\,(40 - 5)}{20} \times \frac{50}{40}$$

$$= \frac{6\,(35)}{20} \times 1.25$$

$$= \frac{210}{20} \times 1.25$$

$$= 10.5 \times 1.25$$

$$= 13.1/min$$

Since the SWI is greater than 11/min, it is predictive of weaning failure.

APPENDIX 2: DUBOIS BODY SURFACE CHART

DIRECTIONS

To find the body surface of a patient, locate the height in inches (or centimeters) on Scale I and the weight in pounds (or kilograms) on Scale II and place a straight edge (ruler) between these two points which will intersect Scale III at the patient's surface area.

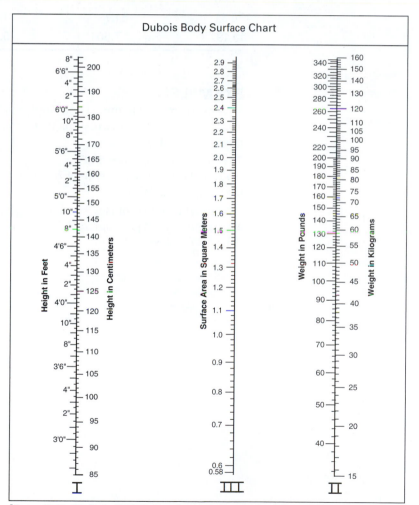

[From E. F. DuBois (1924). Basal metabolism in health and disease. Philadelphia: Lea & Febiger. Used with permission.]

APPENDIX 3:
PRESSURE CONVERSIONS

Pressure Conversions

cm H$_2$O	mm Hg	psig	kPa
1	0.735	0.0142	0.09806
1.36	1	0.0193	0.1333
70.31	51.7	1	6.895
10.197	7.501	0.145	1

EXAMPLES

To convert cm H$_2$O to mm Hg, multiply cm H$_2$O by 0.735. For example, a central venous pressure reading of 9 cm H$_2$O is about 6.6 mm Hg ($9 \times 0.735 = 6.615$).

To convert mm Hg to cm H$_2$O, multiply mm Hg by 1.36. For example, sea-level barometric pressure of 760 mm Hg is about 1034 cm H$_2$O ($760 \times 1.36 = 1,033.6$).

To convert psig to mm Hg, multiply psig by 51.7. For example, a piped-in oxygen gas source of 50 psig equals 2,585 mm Hg ($50 \times 51.7 = 2,585$).

APPENDIX 4:
FRENCH (Fr) AND MILLIMETER (mm) CONVERSIONS

French (Fr) and Millimeter (mm) Conversions	
French (Fr)	**Millimeter (mm)**
(4) mm + 2	1
1	$\dfrac{Fr - 2}{4}$

EXAMPLES

To convert millimeters to French, multiply millimeters by 4, then add 2. For example, an endotracheal tube with an internal diameter (*ID*) of 2.5 mm equals to 12 Fr {(4) 2.5 + 2 = 10 + 2 = 12}.

To convert French to millimeters, subtract 2 from French, then divide by 4. For example, a 30 Fr chest tube equals to 7 mm $\left(\dfrac{30 - 2}{4} = \dfrac{28}{4} = 7\right)$.

APPENDIX 5:
NORMAL ELECTROLYTE CONCENTRATIONS
IN PLASMA

Normal Electrolyte Concentrations in Plasma

Cations	Concentration (Range) mEq/L	Anions	Concentration (Range) mEq/L
Na^+	140 (138 to 142)	Cl^-	103 (101 to 105)
K^+	4 (3 to 5)	HCO_3^-	25 (23 to 27)
Ca^{++}	5 (4.5 to 5.5)	Protein	16 (14 to 18)
Mg^{++}	2 (1.5 to 2.5)	HPO_4^{--}, $H_2PO_4^-$	2 (1.5 to 2.5)
		SO_4^{--}	1 (0.8 to 1.2)
		Organic acids	4 (3.5 to 4.5)
Total	151	Total	151

APPENDIX 6:
OXYGEN TRANSPORT NORMAL RANGES

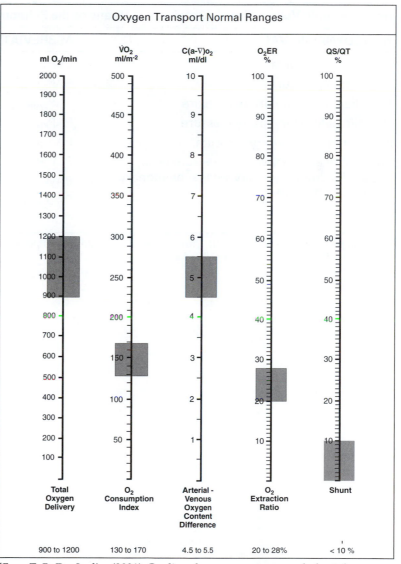

[From T. R. Des Jardins (2001). Cardiopulmonary anatomy and physiology (4th ed.). Clifton Park, New York: Thomson Delmar Learning. Used with permission.]

APPENDIX 7:
HEMODYNAMIC NORMAL RANGES

Hemodynamic Values Directly Obtained by Means of the Pulmonary Artery Catheter

HEMODYNAMIC VALUE	ABBREVIATION	NORMAL RANGE
Central venous pressure	CVP	1 to 7 mm Hg
Right atrial pressure	RAP	1 to 7 mm Hg
Systolic pulmonary artery pressure	$PAP_{systol \times 2}$	15 to 25 mm Hg
Dystolic pulmonary artery pressure	$PAP_{diastolic}$	6 to 12 mm Hg
Mean pulmonary artery pressure	$\overline{PA}$	15 mm Hg
Pulmonary capillary wedge pressure (also called pulmonary artery wedge; pulmonary artery occlusion)	PCWP PAW PAO	8 to 12 mm Hg
Cardiac output	CO	4 to 8 L/min

[Modified from T. R. Des Jardins (2001). Cardiopulmonary anatomy and physiology (4th ed.). Clifton Park, New York: Thomson Delmar Learning. Used with permission.]

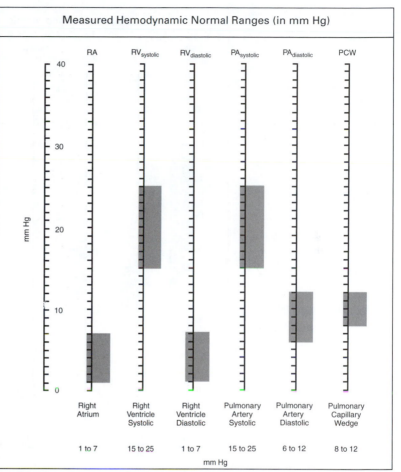

[Modified from T. R. Des Jardins (2001). Cardiopulmonary anatomy and physiology *(4th ed.). Clifton Park, New York: Thomson Delmar Learning. Used with permission.]*

Computed Hemodynamic Values

HEMODYNAMIC VARIABLE	ABBREVIATION	NORMAL RANGE
Stroke volume	SV	40 to 80 mL
Stroke volume index	SVI	33 to 47 L/beat/m^2
Cardiac index	CI	2.5 to 3.5 L/min/m^2
Right ventricular stroke work index	RVSWI	7 to 12 g·m/beat/m^2
Left ventricular stroke work index	LVSWI	40 to 60 g·m/beat/m^2
Pulmonary vascular resistance	PVR	50 to 150 dynes·sec/cm^5
Systemic vascular resistance	SVR	800 to 1500 dynes·sec/cm^5

[Modified from T. R. Des Jardins (1998). Cardiopulmonary anatomy and physiology—Essentials for respiratory care *(3rd ed.). Clifton Park, New York: Thomson Delmar Learning. Used with permission.]*

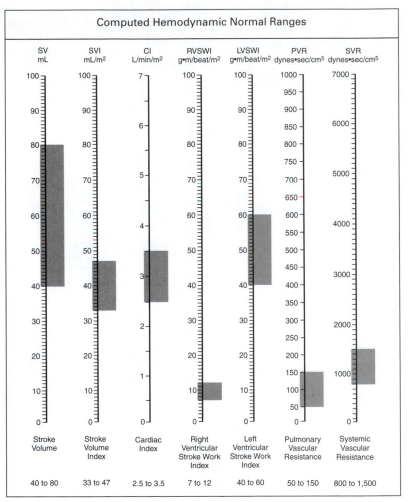

[*Modified from T. R. Des Jardins (2001).* Cardiopulmonary anatomy and physiology *(4th ed.). Clifton Park, New York: Thomson Delmar Learning. Used with permission.*]

APPENDIX 8:
GLASGOW COMA SCORE

Glasgow coma score (GCS)* ranges from 3 to 15 and is composed of three parameters: best eye response, best verbal response, and best motor response. The GCS is typically reported in its components such as E2V1M3 = GCS 6.

A GCS score of 13 to 14 correlates with a mild brain injury, 9 to 12 suggests a moderate injury, and 8 or less a severe brain injury.

BEST EYE RESPONSE (1 TO 4)
1. No eye opening
2. Eye opening to pain
3. Eye opening to verbal command
4. Eyes open spontaneously

BEST VERBAL RESPONSE (1 TO 5)
1. No verbal response
2. Incomprehensible sounds
3. Inappropriate words
4. Confused
5. Orientated

BEST MOTOR RESPONSE (1 TO 6)
1. No motor response
2. Extension to pain
3. Flexion to pain
4. Withdrawal from pain
5. Localizing pain
6. Obeys Commands

*Teasdale G., and Jennett B. (1974). *LANCET 2*, 81–83.

APPENDIX 9:

APACHE II SEVERITY OF DISEASE CLASSIFICATION SYSTEM*

PHYSIOLOGIC VARIABLE	HIGH ABNORMAL RANGE				0	LOW ABNORMAL RANGE				POINTS
	+4	+3	+2	+1	0	+1	+2	+3	+4	
Temperature—rectal (°C)	≥41°	39 to 40.9°		38.5 to 38.9°	36 to 38.4°	34 to 35.9°	32 to 33.9°	30 to 31.9°	≤29.9°	
Mean arterial pressure— mm Hg	≥160	130 to 159	110 to 129		70 to 109		50 to 69		≤49	
Heart rate (ventricular response)	≥180	140 to 179	110 to 139		70 to 109		55 to 69	40 to 54	≤39	
Respiratory rate (non-ventilated or ventilated)	≥50	35 to 49		25 to 34	12 to 24	10 to 11	6 to 9		≤5	
Oxygenation: A-aDO$_2$ or PaO$_2$ (mm Hg) a. FiO$_2$ ≥0.5 record A-aDO$_2$	≥500	350 to 499	200 to 349		<200					
b. FiO$_2$ <0.5 record PaO$_2$					PO$_2$>70	PO$_2$ 61 to 70		PO$_2$ 55 to 60	PO$_2$ <55	
Arterial pH (preferred)	≥7.7	7.6 to 7.69		7.5 to 7.59	7.33 to 7.49		7.25 to 7.32	7.15 to 7.24	<7.15	
Serum HCO$_3$ (venous mEq/l) (not preferred, but may use if no ABGs)	≥52	41 to 51.9		32 to 40.9	22 to 31.9		18 to 21.9	15 to 17.9	<15	
Serum sodium (mEq/l)	≥180	160 to 179	155 to 159	150 to 154	130 to 149		120 to 129	111 to 119	≤110	
Serum potassium (mEq/l)	≥7	6 to 6.9		5.5 to 5.9	3.5 to 5.4	3 to 3.4	2.5 to 2.9		<2.5	
Serum creatinine (mg/dl) Double point score for acute renal failure	≥3.5	2 to 3.4	1.5 to 1.9		0.6 to 1.4		<0.6			
Hematocrit (%)	≥60		50 to 59.9	46 to 49.9	30 to 45.9		20 to 29.9		<20	
White blood count (total/mm³) (in 1000s)	≥40		20 to 39.9	15 to 19.9	3 to 14.9		1 to 2.9		<1	
Glasgow coma score (GCS) Score =15 minus actual GCS										

A. Total Acute Physiology Score (sum of 12 above points)				
B. Age points (years)	$\leqslant$44 = 0;	45 to 54 = 2;	55 to 64 = 3;	65 to 74 = 5;	$\geqslant$75 = 6
C. Chronic Health Points (see below)				
Total APACHE II Score (add together the points from A+B+C)				

Chronic Health Points: If the patient has a history of severe organ system insufficiency or is immunocompromised as defined below, assign points as follows:

5 points for nonoperative or emergency postoperative patients

2 points for elective postoperative patients

Definitions: organ insufficiency or immunocompromised state must have been evident **prior** to this hospital admission and conform to the following criteria: **Liver**—biopsy proven cirrhosis and documented portal hypertension; episodes of past upper GI bleeding attributed to portal hypertension; or prior episodes of hepatic failure/encephalopathy/coma. **Cardiovascular**—New York Heart Association Class IV. **Respiratory**—Chronic restrictive, obstructive, or vascular disease resulting in severe exercise restriction (i.e., unable to climb stairs or perform household duties; or documented chronic hypoxia, hypercapnia, secondary polycythemia, severe pulmonary hypertension (>40 mm Hg), or respirator dependency. **Renal**—receiving chronic dialysis. **Immunocompromised**—the patient has received therapy that suppresses resistance to infection (e.g., immunosuppression, chemotherapy, radiation, long term or recent high dose steroids, or has a disease that is sufficiently advanced to suppress resistance to infection, e.g., leukemia, lymphoma, AIDS).

Interpretation of Score:

0 to 4 = ~4% death rate	10 to 14 = ~15% death rate	20 to 24 = ~40% death rate	30 to 34 = ~75% death rate
5 to 9 = ~8% death rate	15 to 19 = ~25% death rate	25 to 29 = ~55% death rate	Over 34 = ~85% death rate

*Adapted from *Crit Care Med* 1985; 13:818–829.

677

INDEX